Good Operations—
Bad Operations

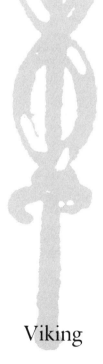

Good Operations—Bad Operations

THE PEOPLE'S MEDICAL SOCIETY'S GUIDE TO SURGERY

Charles B. Inlander and
The Staff of the People's Medical Society

Viking

VIKING
Published by the Penguin Group
Penguin Books USA Inc., 375 Hudson Street, New York, New York 10014, U.S.A.
Penguin Books Ltd, 27 Wrights Lane, London W8 5TZ, England
Penguin Books Australia Ltd, Ringwood, Victoria, Australia
Penguin Books Canada Ltd, 10 Alcorn Avenue, Toronto, Ontario, Canada M4V 3B2
Penguin Books (N.Z.) Ltd, 182–190 Wairau Road, Auckland 10, New Zealand

Penguin Books Ltd, Registered Offices: Harmondsworth, Middlesex, England

First published in 1993 by Viking Penguin, a division of Penguin Books USA Inc.

1 3 5 7 9 10 8 6 4 2

A NOTE TO THE READER
The ideas, procedures, and suggestions contained in this book are
not intended as a substitute for consulting with your physician.
All matters regarding your health require medical supervision.

Grateful acknowledgment is made for permission to reproduce five
anatomical charts. Copyright Rudiger Anatomie, Germany. U. S.
rights, Markham Anatomical, Stamford, CT.

LIBRARY OF CONGRESS CATALOGING IN PUBLICATION DATA
Inlander, Charles B.
Good operations—bad operations : the People's Medical Society's
guide to surgery / by Charles B. Inlander and the staff of the
People's Medical Society.
p.   cm.
Includes index.
ISBN 0-670-83778-4
1. Surgery—Popular works.   2. Consumer education.   I. People's
Medical Society (U.S.)   II. Title.
RD31.3.I55   1993
617'.9—dc20   92–50769

Printed in the United States of America
Set in Galliard
Designed by Beth Tondreau Design

Contents

Surgical Procedures

III.   ADDITIONAL RESOURCES

Acknowledgments

T his book could not have been written without the support and assistance of many individuals and organizations. The authors would like to acknowledge specifically the contributions made by the following:

Charles K. MacKay was principally responsible for locating, researching, and translating the thousands of studies found in medical journals on each of the more than 100 procedures examined in this book. Without his understanding of medical scientific research, coupled with his expertise in on-line data retrieval, this book would never have materialized.

Karla Morales, Vice President for Editorial Services and Communications at the People's Medical Society, served as the principal in-house editor and project supervisor. Her commitment to excellence and concern for detail assure the accuracy of the material found. She is an invaluable resource for the People's Medical Society.

Michael Donio, People's Medical Society Director of Projects, deserves our unending gratitude for the liaison work necessary for this project. His efforts in gathering data, locating statistics, compiling information, and working with other organizations were indispensable.

Special thanks to Mindy Werner, our editor at Viking.

Her insightful comments and questions, and her masterful editing, were essential ingredients in helping us create the final product. Her continuing enthusiasm and support over the entire length of the project kept weary workers at the grindstone.

Gail Ross, People's Medical Society board member and our literary agent, has been a vital part of our publishing endeavors since 1986. She was particularly instrumental in making this book a reality.

Carol Prevost, Operations Manager at Healthcare Knowledge Resources, Ann Arbor, Michigan, deserves our thanks for helping identify and compile the top 100 procedures performed in the nation's hospitals. Amazingly, almost no one has a good handle on these numbers.

Special acknowledgment to the following organizations, all of which provided us with special information and material: American Academy of Cosmetic Surgery; American Academy of Dermatology; American Academy of Facial Plastic and Reconstructive Surgery; American Academy of Neurological and Orthopedic

Surgeons; American College of Cardiology; American College of Foot Orthopedists; American College of Foot Surgeons; American College of Obstetricians and Gynecologists (with particular appreciation to Kate Ruddon); American Society for Laser Medicine and Surgery; and American Society of Colon and Rectal Surgeons.

The unsung heroes of any book are those who make the words appear on the pages. At Viking that is a crew of copy editors, designers, and production personnel who toil with few accolades. To them we express our unending appreciation.

And, finally, to the remaining staff of the People's Medical Society (Karen Kemmerer, Ellen Greene, Krishni Patrick, Linda Swank, Gayle Ebert, Miriam Flexer, and Julie Wendt) and the Society's Board of Directors (Lowell Levin, Lori Andrews, Pamela Maraldo, Tom Belford, John Alogna, Bonnie Prudden, Harrison Wellford, Alma Rose, and Irving Zola), we express our gratitude for tireless support.

Introduction

Having an operation is no longer an uncommon occurrence: more than fifty million Americans will be operated on this year. Not long ago, almost all operations were designed to cure or alleviate a problem or condition. Thirty years ago when people spoke of having an operation, they were usually talking about an appendectomy, a tonsillectomy, maybe even a hysterectomy.

Things are very different today. The now-familiar coronary bypass was unheard of in the early 1960s. Cesarean sections were performed in only 5% of births (today it's 23%). Many of the most frequently performed operations done today are diagnostic. In other words, they do not solve or alleviate a problem; instead, they are used to help caregivers determine what the problem is.

Most of us think of surgery as cutting someone open, removing or repairing an organ or body part, and sewing the person back up. In reality, surgery is any procedure that is invasive (that is, requires entering the body) and for which instruments are used. Indeed, with today's medical technology, our past idea of surgery has been altered dramatically. One hundred years ago the surgeon's tools were often just a hacksaw, scalpel, needle, and thread. Today surgeons use electronic monitors, lasers, and other space-age technology.

Fifteen years ago most surgery was performed in a hospital. Today more than 40% of all operations are performed on consumers as outpatients, either at a one-day surgical facility or at a physician's office.

The art of surgery has changed, too. Forty years ago a surgeon was a surgeon. Today surgery is a big business: there are numerous surgical specialties and subspecialties. For example, today not only are there surgeons who work exclusively on hands, but there are some who just operate on fingers.

When most of us hear the word *operation*, spoken by a doctor, our first reaction is fear. Am I going to die? Are there alternatives? What are the complications? Where's the bathroom?! The idea of anyone poking and probing inside of us is scary. Most of us know virtually nothing about what the doctor is proposing to do. Although the physician may explain why the operation is necessary, few other details are forthcoming. In fact, most doctors try to reassure a patient by saying such things as "don't worry; this is a very common procedure now" or "it will all be over in no time." Despite the possible truth of these statements, they are not the kind of factual information a person needs to make a decision about whether to have the operation.

In the past, consumers took the doctor's word, went home, packed a suitcase, and submitted without question—but not anymore. We have learned too much about the unknowns in medicine to accept outright a single physician's opinion. With the wide range of procedures available to accomplish the same goal, people are now seeking second opinions, not only about a diagnosis but about a course of treatment as well.

That is where *Good Operations—Bad Operations* comes in. Since its formation in 1983, the People's Medical Society has become America's largest nonprofit consumer health advocacy organization. Our organization was founded upon the concept of consumer empowerment. An empowered individual is one who knows the right questions to ask in order to find out the information he seeks. Consumers, by learning more about their medical conditions, the health care professionals who serve them, and the procedures performed upon them, can acquire the tools they need to get better care.

Over the years we have received tens of thousands of calls and letters from people asking about specific procedures. The information they seek is pretty much the same: How is the procedure performed? What are the death rates? What are the possible complications, and how often do they occur? What alternatives are there to having the procedure? What are the controversies (if any) surrounding the operation? We answered the questions to the extent that we could, using the medical literature as our source material.

We always asked people why they were calling or writing us. Why didn't they ask their physician or surgeon? Their answers were revealing. We heard time and again how their doctors either gave them scant information or did not respond to such requests at all. They wanted a resource that not only told them all they needed to know but documented where the information came from.

From the beginning, the staff and members of the Board of Directors of the People's Medical Society have met, talked, and debated with members of the medical profession on hundreds of occasions. When physicians are asked why they are not giving out the information

consumers need to be fully informed, the response is generally the same. Physicians argue that too much information will scare a person. They assume that the more complications a person discovers are possible—no matter how small each one may be—the more likely that person is to say no to a particular operation. We of the People's Medical Society think just the opposite.

Yet we have also learned that physicians are often slow to change. New procedures, which are sometimes more beneficial than older ones, are usually not quick to come into practice. On one level, this is a safeguard. On another, the delay may be detrimental to a consumer.

Keeping all this in mind, we believe the time is long overdue for consumers to have a single source to turn to when confronted with the prospect of having an operation. Our aim in creating this book is to answer the primary questions people have about specific procedures. We want to help people select the best surgeons or physicians for their particular needs. We also want people to know that almost every surgical procedure is associated with some degree of controversy.

This is how *Good Operations—Bad Operations* was born. There has never been a consumer guide quite like *this* one.

What makes this book unique is our assumption that you have the intelligence to understand what the risks and benefits of a particular operation are. We have done all we can to make the language understandable. When we use a term that is common in medical jargon, we attempt to translate it into everyday English—but we also do not insult your intelligence by using simple words that are not accurate or precise in their meaning. While we are committed to making sure you understand each word in this book, some anatomical or medical terms must stand on their own. Those words are either explained in the text itself or in the extensive glossary at the back of this book. These are words that your doctor might use when explaining the details of a procedure you are considering. You may have to use them to *get* precise information from your doctor before you can make an informed medical decision.

Like all professions, medicine has its own jargon and its own vocabulary, which is often rooted in Latin or Greek. Physicians speak to one another in this language because it is precise and unmistakable. More often than not, many of these strange-sounding words creep into a physician's conversation with you. While you should certainly insist on a translation, there are times when such terminology is the best description. Thus, the more medical terms you understand about your condition, the better off you will be not only in translating your doctor's conversation, but in asking questions as well.

Don't be afraid of "medicalese." Remember, there was a time just before medical school when your physician didn't understand a word of it either.

When we use statistics, we explain what they mean. We have not held back on passing along numbers or percentages. Knowing what the medical studies say about the risks associated with certain procedures is of critical importance when making a decision about surgery. Yet most doctors reveal very little, statistically, about these risks. In this book, we provide you with statistical information, directly from medical studies, about every operation covered. From mortality (death) rates to morbidity (complication) rates, we provide you with the full range of risks associated with a given operation.

Good Operations—Bad Operations is not designed to tell you whether you should have an operation. Its purpose is to empower you as a medical consumer, by giving you the tools to make the informed medical decisions—on your own and in partnership with your health care practitioner.

Charles B. Inlander
President
People's Medical Society

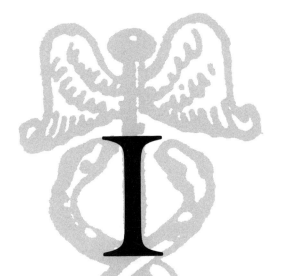

I

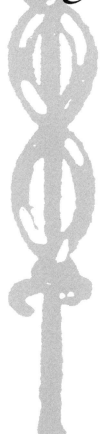

The Consumer's Guide
To Surgery

How to Use This Book

ood Operations—Bad Operations is divided into three parts. Part I is your guide to surgery. In it we discuss issues related to surgical operations and provide a guide to help you choose a surgeon. We also list specific types of specialists and describe what they do. A checklist is included, which you can use when considering surgery, to determine whether a particular operation is best for you.

Part II is a complete guide to the most frequently performed surgical procedures in the U.S. Each procedure is divided into the following subdivisions:

- Medical name of the procedure
- Translation for a layperson, if necessary, as well as a brief description of the procedure
- What condition does the procedure treat?
- What is the procedure? (A complete explanation)
- Who performs the procedure?
- Where is the procedure performed?
- What are the mortality (death) and morbidity (complication) rates?
- What are the other complications and possible side effects?
- Is this the most appropriate procedure for the condition?
- Are there alternatives to this procedure?
- What is controversial about the procedure?

This section provides you with facts and statistical information that will help you better understand the procedure itself and its appropriateness for you. We encourage you to use it in collaboration with your doctor. Remember that you and your doctor should form a partnership. As partners, you both bring knowledge, preferences, and skills to the alliance. Do not be afraid to use the material you have read in this book as the basis for discussion with or questions for your doctor.

There are likely to be references in this section with which your doctor is unfamiliar. That does not mean your doctor is not informed; rather it may mean that she is merely unfamiliar with a particular reference. Do not hesitate to discuss with your doctor anything you read in this section.

We also caution you not to make a decision based solely on what you learn in this section. The information we provide does not stand alone. We do not know your condition or your doctor. We do not know what other circumstances exist that would determine the appropriateness or inappropriateness of a given procedure. The information we pass along should be used as only part of your information and decision-making arsenal.

Part III has additional useful information. The extensive glossary explains medical terms that are used throughout the text. Also included in this section is a resource list to assist you further in your quest for information.

In the interest of readability, we have alternated use of male and female pronouns, except when a procedure is specific to one gender.

How to Choose a Surgeon

At some point in your life, you may need to choose a surgeon. Despite how intimidating the process may seem, it is not as difficult as you might think. The key to selecting the best surgeon for you is to be organized, patient, and persistent. You need to know as much as you possibly can about the person you select. In this section we give you the major points you need to consider while going through the process.

IT BEGINS WITH CREDENTIALS

Your search begins with learning a surgeon's credentials. Credentials are a combination of education, training, certification, experience, and reputation. Here is what you should know about each of those components:

Education

A surgeon's education begins with four years of undergraduate work at a college or university. Next come four years of medical school. That is usually followed by a general residency, which is hands-on training in a hospital or clinical setting under the supervision of experienced physicians. Then, if the doctor wants to specialize in surgery, a three- to four-year surgical residency usually follows.

In your search for a surgeon, education is an important consideration. While a degree from a top-notch medical school is not a guarantee of medical competence, it is a point to be noted. Medical schools are very selective, which means that often the best schools have the best academically prepared students. Yet academic preparation is only one part of a surgeon's training.

The residencies a surgeon has experienced are often more valuable than mere academic preparation in helping you to determine what skills a surgeon has acquired. If the surgeon went through a surgical residency at a very highly reputed facility with a large surgical volume, there is a likelihood that his training was more extensive than someone not having a similar experience.

Learning the educational background of someone who may be your surgeon is an important first step. Do not hesitate to ask where she was educated, where he had advanced training, and how recently and where he or she has gone for continuing education.

Surgical Training

As we noted, serious surgical training begins with the surgical residency, which is served in a hospital with an approved program and may last two to six years—depending upon the particular specialty. On average, however, a surgical residency lasts four years.

During the time of the surgical residency, the resident (who is already a licensed physician) attends classes and participates in surgery under the direction and supervision of a qualified surgeon. The instructors permit the resident to get the feel of the scalpel and other instruments used during the actual procedure.

The surgical residency is important for two reasons: It permits the orderly training of new surgeons, and it prepares them for their certification examinations.

In making your selection of a surgeon, a primary factor is completion of a surgical residency and passing of a surgical board examination that certifies the individual as qualified to perform such surgery. (See *Certification* below.) Although this process may seem routine, it is not.

Legally, there is no requirement that a physician enter and complete a surgical residency or pass a board certification examination in order to call herself a surgeon. Once the state medical licensing examination is passed, the physician can proclaim himself to be any specialist he desires. Although this practice is less common now than it was in the past, it still goes on. Thus, it is essential that you question your would-be surgeon thoroughly about her surgical training.

Certification

Certification is the next step in establishing surgical credentials. Upon completion of the surgical residency, the physician is considered "board eligible." This means that she may take an examination offered by one of the 10 medical specialty boards offering surgical certification programs. The 10 certifying boards for surgery are: American Board of Colon and Rectal Surgery; American Board of Neurological Surgery; American Board of

Obstetrics and Gynecology; American Board of Ophthalmology; American Board of Orthopedic Surgery; American Board of Otolaryngology; American Board of Plastic Surgery; American Board of Surgery; American Board of Thoracic Surgery; and American Board of Urology.

Being "board eligible" and "board certified" are two different things. To be declared "board certified," a surgeon must have taken and passed the examination. Being "board eligible" only means that a surgical residency has been completed. *Don't be fooled.* Some physicians who have either never taken the examination or have failed it are now listing themselves as "board eligible" in the Yellow Pages or in other advertisements. While it is true that they are "eligible," they are not certified.

One final note about "boards." The boards that certify practitioners are not government or third-party–regulating entities. Although individual states license doctors, states do not certify or license specialties. A medical board is a professional association of doctors who specialize in a certain type of practice. Each board develops its own education, credentials and/or examination requirements that must be met by any person who wants to be certified in that specialty. The problem is that boards are not uniform in their requirements. Some require reexamination in order to maintain certification. Others are less stringent.

On one level, boards are merely the foxes guarding the chicken coop, with fellow specialists being the judge and the jury—thereby raising a true conflict-of-interest issue. On another level, it is a step to help assure competence of surgeons.

As part of your "choosing a surgeon" plan, it is important to find out if your surgeon is board certified—and by what board. A surgeon may call himself board certified, but may be certified in a specialty outside of surgery. So ask the surgeon if she is certified in surgery, and ask which board did the certification. Contact the board and verify that the surgeon is currently certified, *and* ask for the requirements the surgeon had to meet to become certified and maintain that certification.

There are two other sources you can use to find out whether a surgeon you are considering is board certified. Any local library, even one of average size, should have a book entitled *The Directory of Medical Specialists 1989–1990,* 24th edition, 3 volumes (Chicago: Marquis Who's Who, Inc., 1988). Every certified doctor is listed in it.

The second source is the American Board of Medical Specialties, an umbrella organization of 23 different boards, which has a toll-free "800" number you can call to check on a doctor's certification status. The number is 800–776–CERT. *Be forewarned that not all board certified doctors are listed; doctors must pay a $300 annual fee to be listed in the service—and while over 400,000 physicians have a board certification, only 40,000 are listed in this "800" number service.*

Experience

Some experts believe that practical experience is the most important factor in selecting a surgeon, and there is no question that the more experience a surgeon has in doing what you need to have done, the better off you are.

Studies show that physicians who do a procedure more often than others tend to do it better—but that is not the only experience factor you need to consider. Also important is where the doctor has performed the surgery. A surgeon associated with a top-notch, high-volume hospital is often more experienced with a wider range of problems that may arise during a given procedure. This is important, because complications during surgery must be dealt with quickly and with confidence. A rookie with a scalpel may be less responsive to such an emergency and therefore lower your likelihood of a satisfactory outcome and recovery.

How do you measure experience? Is an older surgeon, with many years behind the mask, better than a fresh, young hotshot who has learned the absolutely latest techniques? It's a tough call, but it really depends upon your needs and preference. While an older surgeon may have been doing the same procedure well for many years, he may not be as up to date on or receptive to new techniques or alternative procedures. For example, a few surgeons continue to do the Halsted mastectomy on uninformed women, when the procedure has been rebuked and replaced by most other surgeons.

On the other hand, a young surgeon may have plenty of knowledge of the latest thinking on certain techniques, but may not have the kind of experience that comes with performing a given operation over and over on a high number of individuals.

This is where second opinions come into play. Too often, second opinions are sought for diagnostic purposes only. Yet second opinions should also be sought for treatment alternatives and surgical recommendations. It is not unusual for two different surgeons to propose two distinctly different types or modifications of surgery for the very same condition. So seeing just one surgeon and asking what she will do may give you only a limited perspective on what can be done, surgically, to resolve your problem.

It is also important to seek a second opinion about what surgeon to use. You may have been referred to a surgeon by another practitioner. It would be wise to ask another practitioner to also recommend several surgeons. If you know any nurses, be sure to ask them what they know about a particular surgeon. While this gets into the area of reputation (see below), it is also a way to seek information about the surgeon's experience from his peers.

Reputation

It all depends upon whom you ask. Certainly a surgeon would love to be well thought of by his or her colleagues. Too often, though, a physician's reputation may be based on factors that have less to do with medicine than with friendships or professional associations.

It is important to remember that medicine is a business, and a major part of the business is doctoring. For the most part, doctors get the majority of their business on referral from other practitioners. This is especially true of surgeons. So how does a nonsurgical physician determine where to refer a consumer? The referral ought to be made to the surgeon with the best record for the service needed. The doctor making the referral should know the record of the doctor to whom you are being referred. Unfortunately, that is not always the case. You may be referred because the two doctors are friends. They may play golf at the same country club. They may be coinvestors in a resort condominium. Who knows?

When your physician refers you to a surgeon, you should be ready with a series of questions. Ask why a particular surgeon is being recommended. Ask how many other patients from your doctor's practice have been referred to the surgeon and what the success rates of those surgeries were. Find out if your physician is associated in any business arrangement with the sur-geon. If there is such an association, it may cloud your doctor's objectivity.

It never hurts to get other, independent opinions of the surgeon. Ask nurses about the surgeon—they're the true frontline troops of medicine. In a given community, they have insider knowledge not easily found in other professionals. Ask the nurse, "Would you let this surgeon operate on you?" Then ask why or why not.

Find out which hospitals have granted the surgeon privileges. Check with the state medical licensing board for complaints filed or actions taken against the surgeon.

Throughout medicine, there is a well-documented "conspiracy of silence" that tends to keep the bad news about doctors and hospitals out of the public domain, while flooding the media with all of medicine's "miracles." Don't be misled. We cannot emphasize enough that you should get hard information from as many sources as possible about the reputation of your surgeon.

THERE'S MORE TO FIND OUT

Now that you know how to check out the surgeon's credentials, there are some other issues you need to weigh in selecting a surgeon.

Other than My Physician, Where Else Can I Get Names of Surgeons I Might Consider?

Putting together a list of potential surgeons is relatively easy. Aside from being referred by another physician, there are a number of other sources you can call upon.

The local medical society in most communities operates a referral service. While the service refers only physicians who are members, it is one way to get some names. Remember, these doctors are being referred because they pay dues to an organization, not because they have been judged competent by their peers. Hos-pitals often sponsor their own referral programs. In these instances, the doctors they refer you to have surgical privileges at the sponsoring hospital. Don't discount these sources, but remember that they do have built-in conflicts of interest.

In recent years, surgeons have begun to advertise on television and radio, and in newspapers and telephone books. While such advertisements are certainly no indication of competence, at least they provide you with names.

Don't forget to use your friends as a resource. No matter what operation you may need, there is a good chance that you have a friend, or a friend of a friend, who has had the same surgery. Ask who they used and whether they were satisfied with the results.

Should I Schedule an Interview with the Surgeon?

Absolutely! Recently it has become quite common for people to be scheduled for surgery by one specialist without ever meeting or talking with the surgeon. Don't let this happen to you. It is absolutely essential to sit down with several of the surgeons you are considering to go over their credentials, but also to have them explain in detail just what is going to happen. This interview appointment, as we call it, is probably the most important presurgical step you can take.

I Know I Need to Ask the Surgeon About His or Her Credentials, but What Other Things Should I Be Sure to Ask at the Interview?

Let's start with reviewing some of the questions you should automatically ask in this interview:

- *Are you board certified? What specialty are you certified in and what board certifies you?*
- *How often have you performed the procedure I require?* Remember, the more frequently a surgeon performs a particular procedure, the better the chances that it will be a success.
- *Are you in a group or solo practice?* If a doctor is in a group practice, you may be contracting with the group and not necessarily with the doctor to whom you are speaking. If you want "Dr. Bigshot," be sure to have the group guarantee it.
- *What are your fees?* Don't be afraid to ask this and have the doctor put it in writing. Today most people have to pay something out of pocket for surgery. If the procedure is elective, you may have to pay the whole bill. Have the doctor go over fees with you directly. Don't let him refer you to "my girl," who will handle it later. Don't forget that doctor's fees are negotiable. If you cannot afford the fee, or

you think it is too high, negotiate a price you can afford. You'll be surprised at how easy it is to get the price down.

- *What are the most common complications associated with this procedure?* Unfortunately, things can go wrong in surgery. Therefore, you want to be as well prepared as possible before you agree to go under the knife. If the doctor skirts the issue or says there are no complications, consider leaving. No surgery is without some possible complication. A good surgeon will go over the possibilities and give you the percentages that these complications occur. Ask any and all the questions necessary to get the answers you need to make a decision.
- *What is the nosocomial infection rate associated with this procedure?* Nosocomial infections are those acquired in the hospital. Nationally, the hospital-acquired infection rate is close to 10%, which means that approximately one out of every 10 people who are admitted to a hospital develop an infection they did not have when they arrived. As a surgical patient, with an open wound, you are a prime target for a number of nasty microbes.

More than half of all nosocomial infections are preventable if hospital personnel follow proper anti-infection procedures. Although it is unlikely that the hospital will release its overall figure, ask your surgeon to give you the infection rate she has experienced at that hospital for patients under her charge. If the number is in the mid-range of single digits, the hospital is probably doing a halfway decent job of controlling this national problem.

- *What are the success rates of the procedure?* The success rate means more than simply surviving—although this is important to find out too. Ask the surgeon what your chances are of 100% success, meaning regaining perfectly normal function. If less than 100%, and that is often the case, have the surgeon detail what you can expect your functional level to be after you have completely recovered from the surgery. This is an important consideration, because if the functional level is quite low, you may want to weigh it against the risk of surgery.

Does It Make Any Difference If My Surgeon Is an M.D. or a D.O.?

At one time the differences between a doctor of medicine (M.D.) and a doctor of osteopathy (D.O.) were significant. Today the differences are negligible. The same surgical techniques are used by both types of surgeons.

What Other Resources Are Available?

You should start with this book. Information about specific procedures is absolutely essential for you to be able to make an informed decision about your surgery and surgeon. Feel free to contact the other organizations we list throughout this book. Although many are professional organizations, they have agreed to serve you. Don't forget your public library; most have a good supply of medical and health-related books to help you in your decision-making.

Finally, don't forget the People's Medical Society. As America's largest consumer health advocacy organization, we publish a wealth of information to help you deal with the health care system and your medical needs.

Medical Specialists

If you're a candidate for surgery, chances are your personal physician has already sent you to see a specialist or two, so you may think you know what's happening. The more you ponder the situation, however, the more you realize that you're not quite sure who does what or where.

You already know that surgeons obviously do surgery, but did you know that a urologist may also perform surgical procedures? Or that other specialists may perform invasive diagnostic procedures (in which the skin is punctured, such as with a catheter, or in which a diagnostic tool such as an endoscope, an illuminated optical instrument, is put into a body opening)? To help you learn what these specialists do, we've compiled the following definitions:

ALLERGIST AND IMMUNOLOGIST: This specialist is qualified to diagnose and treat conditions of the skin (for example, acne, eczema, and hives), as well as diseases of the immune system, whether acquired or congenital. Some physicians in this specialty may receive additional training in diagnostic laboratory immunology, which is the use of laboratory procedures to analyze the functions of the immune system.

ANESTHESIOLOGIST: This specialist is concerned with the administration of local and general anesthetic agents and the monitoring of patients during surgery. Anesthesiologists are also involved in the management of pain and the care of critically ill patients.

CARDIOLOGIST: This specialist diagnoses and treats diseases of the heart and blood vessels.

CARDIOVASCULAR SURGEON (OR CARDIAC SURGEON): This specialist performs surgery on the heart and the associated vascular system, including open heart surgery and heart transplants.

COLON AND RECTAL SURGEON: This specialist diagnoses and treats diseases of the intestinal tract, colon, rectum, anus, and perianal area.

CRITICAL CARE SURGEON: This specialist cares for critically ill and postoperative patients, especially trauma victims, and works in intensive care units, burn units, and other similar settings.

DERMATOLOGIST: This specialist diagnoses and treats diseases affecting the skin, hair, and nails, using both medical and surgical procedures.

EMERGENCY MEDICINE SPECIALIST: This physician focuses on the immediate needs of patients in response to acute illness and injury in the hospital setting.

FAMILY/GENERAL PRACTITIONER: This physician is concerned with the total health care of the individual and the family. The scope of practice is not limited by age, sex, organ system, or disease.

GASTROENTEROLOGIST: This specialist diagnoses and treats diseases of the digestive system, the stomach, and the intestines.

GENERAL SURGEON: This specialist performs operations on various parts of the body, including the head and neck, breast, abdomen, hands, arms, legs, and feet.

GYNECOLOGIST (OR GYNECOLOGIC SURGEON): This specialist diagnoses and treats problems associated with the female reproductive system, using both medical and surgical methods.

HAND SURGEON: This specialist diagnoses and treats disorders of the hands, including the bones, muscles, and ligaments.

HEAD AND NECK SURGEON: This specialist deals with disorders of the head and neck, excluding the brain and eyes.

HEMATOLOGIST: This specialist diagnoses and treats diseases of the blood, spleen, and lymph glands. He or she may also perform special transfusions and bone marrow biopsies.

INTERNAL MEDICINE SPECIALIST (OR INTERNIST): This specialist is a general practitioner who diagnoses and treats both common and complex illnesses. Many internists complete additional training in subspecialties, such as endocrinology, infectious diseases, hematology, and pulmonary diseases.

INTERVENTIONAL CARDIOLOGIST (OR INVASIVE CARDIOLOGIST): This specialist is skilled in the use of instruments within the heart to diagnose and treat coronary diseases.

NEPHROLOGIST: This specialist deals with diseases that affect the kidneys.

NEUROSURGEON: This specialist deals with disorders of the central nervous system (brain and spinal cord) as well as the peripheral and autonomic nervous systems (the nerves that carry messages to the brain).

NUCLEAR RADIOLOGIST: This specialist injects radioactive substances into the body to diagnose or treat a condition.

OBSTETRICIAN: This specialist is concerned with the medical aspects of pregnancy, including prenatal care, labor, and delivery.

ONCOLOGIC SURGEON: This specialist is a board-certified general surgeon with a subspecialty in the removal of cancerous tumors from organs, bones, blood vessels, and connective tissue.

OPHTHALMOLOGIST: This specialist diagnoses and treats diseases of and injuries to the eyes. This includes removal of cataracts and reattachment of retinas, among other operations.

ORTHOPEDIC SURGEON: This specialist treats deformities of or damage to the musculoskeletal system. While primarily involved with the leg area, the practice also involves bones, muscles, and ligaments all over the body.

OTOLARYNGOLOGIST (OR EAR-NOSE-THROAT SPECIALIST [ENT]): This specialist diagnoses and treats disorders of the ears, nose, and throat.

PEDIATRIC SURGEON: This specialist is involved in the surgical treatment of premature and newborn infants, as well as children and adolescents.

PLASTIC AND RECONSTRUCTIVE SURGEON: This specialist restores and rebuilds body parts damaged or destroyed by accident or disease and also performs cosmetic procedures to improve appearance.

PULMONARY SURGEON: This specialist is a board-certified thoracic surgeon with a subspecialty in treating diseases and disorders of the lungs.

PULMONOLOGIST: This specialist is concerned with diseases of the lungs, including pneumonia, cancer, occupational diseases, bronchitis, emphysema, and other complex disorders.

RADIOLOGIST: This specialist is skilled in the application of radiant energy (basic x ray and computerized scanning), ultrasound, and magnetic fields in the diagnosis and treatment of disease.

SURGICAL ONCOLOGIST: See **Oncologic Surgeon.**

THORACIC SURGEON: This specialist concentrates on

the organs and related structures that lie within the chest cavity. Heart, lung, and circulatory system disorders fall within the scope of this physician.

THYROID SURGEON: See **General Surgeon.**

TRAUMA SURGEON: See **Critical Care Surgeon.**

UROLOGIST: This specialist diagnoses and treats disorders of the genitourinary system, including the kidneys, ureters, bladder, and urethra (as well as the prostate gland in men).

VASCULAR SURGEON, GENERAL: This specialist diagnoses and treats disorders of the blood vessels, especially those related to the heart, lungs, or brain.

VASCULAR SURGEON, PERIPHERAL: See **Vascular Surgeon, General.**

Surgical Settings

I n the not-too-distant past, choosing the proper setting for your surgery was no more complicated than checking into the nearest hospital. Your physician made most of the arrangements, and you showed up on the appointed day to be admitted; however, that is no longer the case.

Now you have options in surgical settings. Improvements in anesthesia and surgical techniques are primarily responsible for the new choices, especially in the area of outpatient surgery—that is, surgery that does not require an overnight stay in the hospital. Many surgical procedures that were once exclusively inpatient have been moved to the outpatient setting. We will say more about this later.

INPATIENT SETTINGS

Just what are your choices in selecting the surgical setting that is best for you? Your choices include hospitals, hospital outpatient departments, physicians' offices, and freestanding surgery centers. Hospitals can be further subdivided into: community, multispecialty center, osteopathic, specialty, teaching, and Veterans Administration.

Community hospitals vary in size from less than 100 beds up to 250 beds. They offer a fairly wide range of routine and more complicated surgical procedures, including appendectomies; cholecystectomies (gallbladder removal); tonsillectomies/adenoidectomies; repair of broken bones; hysterectomies; cesarean sections; dilation and curettage (D&C); and repair of hernias.

Because community hospitals tend to be small, they are not likely to provide all the services of a large, multispecialty teaching hospital. Also, they usually do not perform the new or more "exotic" surgeries you read about in the feature section of major newspapers.

That should not dissuade you from considering a community hospital for your operation. In fact, major studies comparing large, teaching hospitals with smaller community hospitals found that for the more routine surgeries (such as those noted above) the quality of community hospitals was equal to that of the multispecialty facility. Surveys of customer satisfaction showed that community hospitals often ranked higher because the atmosphere tended to be quieter and less frantic, and sometimes the personnel were more attentive.

More importantly, studies have also shown that the

size of a hospital is of little consequence when assessing a facility's quality. More important is the frequency with which a procedure is performed, the training of the primary and support staff, and the ability of the facility to respond to a major complication that might arise either while the operation was in progress or shortly thereafter.

Thus, the important information to find out about any hospital is:

- How many times in the last year have they done the procedure you are considering?
- What are the experience and training of the support staff (including anesthetists, assistant staff surgeons, and operating and recovery room nurses)?
- What services are available within the facility if something goes wrong during the operation?

Multispecialty hospitals—which may be affiliated with medical schools but are not medical schools per se—teaching hospitals, specialty hospitals, and Veterans Administration hospitals vary in size from 400 to 1,000 beds; in addition to basic medical and surgical services, they also offer specialized services such as: bone marrow transplants; burn care; coronary artery bypass surgery; coronary angioplasty; neonatal intensive care; and organ transplants.

Teaching hospitals, as the name implies, are in the business of educating the physicians of tomorrow. Such hospitals are affiliated with and staffed by medical schools, which are part of larger educational institutions such as colleges and universities.

Specialty hospitals are usually dedicated to one particular disease or condition and can be identified by their name: Memorial Sloan-Kettering Cancer Center; Miami Heart Institute; Shriners Children's Hospital; Massachusetts Eye and Ear Infirmary; and Wills Eye Hospital. Some specialty hospitals, such as the Mayo Clinic or the Cleveland Clinic, have slightly broader ranges of services. Specialty hospitals are usually staffed by "super"-specialists who are recognized as the leading experts in their fields. Very often patients sent to specialty hospitals are referred by doctors at community hospitals or transferred from other facilities.

Another category of hospital is the osteopathic hospital, which is designed to meet the needs of osteopathic physicians (D.O.s). In actuality, osteopathic hospitals differ little from allopathic hospitals (staffed with doctors of medicine, or M.D.s) and offer privileges to both D.O.s and M.D.s. As with their allopathic counterparts, osteopathic hospitals vary in size, from small community hospitals to major medical centers affiliated with osteopathic medical schools.

Veterans Administration (VA) hospitals are operated by the federal government especially for veterans—and not just veterans of foreign wars. Because of their mission, VA hospitals are large, with some facilities having up to 1000 beds. VA hospitals provide general medical and surgical services as well as specialty services. The VA also operates outpatient clinics across the country.

The ultimate question is which is the best setting for you. As noted earlier, the number of beds or size of the hospital is often of the least importance. What does matter is which facility does best the procedure that you need to have performed. Sometimes that facility may be the community hospital just around the corner; other times, it may be a world-famous medical center halfway across the country.

OUTPATIENT SETTINGS

Depending upon your particular community and what options are available there, you may choose among many settings for outpatient surgery:

- hospital outpatient department
- freestanding surgery center
- physician's office

Hospital outpatient departments may be found in the hospital, in a building adjacent to the hospital, or in a building some distance from the hospital. Although in the latter two locations the facility might appear to be independent, it is staffed and managed by the hospital.

Freestanding surgery centers (also called surgicenters) are not affiliated with hospitals but are independently owned, usually by a group of physicians. Freestanding surgery centers are generally less expensive than hospital-based surgery, whether inpatient or outpatient.

Physicians' offices are yet another setting for surgical procedures. Technology that led to the development of lasers, cryosurgery (freezing), and flexible scopes is responsible for expanding the range of procedures available to the office-based physician.

SURGICAL RISKS

Any time you agree to surgery, whether as an inpatient or an outpatient, you potentially put yourself at risk for:

- nosocomial infections (hospital-acquired)
- iatrogenic illnesses (doctor-caused)
- reactions to anesthesia

Nosocomial Infections

A nosocomial infection is one you acquire while you're hospitalized, and it's especially risky for surgical patients because microbes love an open wound. Studies indicate that between 5% and 10% of all patients develop a nosocomial infection, which is spread by hand contact and occurs as a result of direct contact between medical staff and patients. However, when hospitalized, you can protect yourself by doing the following:

- *Demand that all medical and nonmedical personnel wash their hands before touching you.*
- *Request a room change if your roommate develops a nosocomial infection.*
- *Request that shaving of body hair be done the morning of surgery, not the night before.* (It is just as important to find out whether shaving is absolutely necessary.) Some studies indicate a higher risk for infection when shaving occurs the night before surgery.
- *Make sure the nursing staff checks your catheter (a tube that drains a body cavity or the bladder) for proper drainage.* A clogged catheter is a prime breeding ground for germs.

Iatrogenic Illnesses

Iatrogenic illnesses are doctor-caused or doctor-produced in the sense that you didn't have the condition until the doctor did something to you, such as accidentally cutting into adjacent tissue with the scalpel or failing to remove a surgical sponge.

Medication errors are another example of iatrogenic illnesses. In some hospitals, the medication error rate can run as high as 11% of the time, while 2% to 3% is not uncommon even in the best of hospitals. In a 300-bed hospital, an error rate of 2% to 3% easily translates into 60 to 90 errors a day. Only constant vigilance by you or a family member or friend serving as your advocate can guard against potential medication errors.

Rule number one for preventing medication errors is never take any medication that hasn't been prescribed by your physician. You or a family member should ask your doctor to provide a list of all the medications that have been prescribed for you. Then when medications are brought to your bed, you can ask what the medicine is and compare it with the drugs on your list. Something as simple as knowing the color of your medication can help prevent a mix-up. If you've been taking a green pill every four hours, don't take the big orange pill that is brought to you. Thousands of consumers catch hospital medication errors each day using this color-matching technique. Being alert pays off.

Anesthesia Risks

Most consumers are surprised when they find out how relatively safe anesthesia is. As you read through this book, you will see that most studies have demonstrated that anesthesia *itself* is quite low on the list of what can go wrong during an operation.

Yet the fact remains that an estimated 10,000 Americans a year die from anesthesia-related mishaps and hundreds of thousands more are injured. These injuries can range from relatively mild but prolonged numbness, to conditions that handicap an individual for life.

The problem is human errors that are made in the administration of anesthesia. The medical literature is replete with reports of major goofs made by negligent anesthesiologists, nurse-anesthetists, and others who administer these highly toxic potions. Despite the safeguards most hospitals take to prevent these tragic mistakes from occurring, they still happen.

Anesthesia in the hospital setting is usually administered by a physician (anesthesiologist) who is board certified in anesthesiology, or by a certified nurse-anesthetist (who works under the supervision of an anesthesiologist). Both professionals are highly skilled with specialized training in the use and administration of anesthesia. Like every other medical professional, though, some are better than others. The important thing for you, as a consumer, to find out is:

- Who will be handling your anesthesia?
- What training and experience does that individual have?
- Has the person ever been sanctioned by the hospital or the state licensing agency?

You should never have an operation requiring anesthesia without first meeting directly with the person who will be administering it. Insist that such a meeting take place. At this meeting, ask any questions you may have about what will be used and what you should expect before, during, or after the surgery. Also, discuss any anxieties you may have about the anesthesia.

Aside from answering your questions about what will happen, the meeting should also make you more familiar to the person serving you. There is no question that someone who knows you personally is likely to be more attentive.

Anesthesia administration in the nonhospital setting requires even more caution. This is a relatively new area, which has bloomed as the ability to perform surgery in ambulatory settings has increased.

While personnel who administer anesthesia in nonhospital settings should be equally trained and as competent as inhospital personnel, this may not be the case. If the facility is physician-owned, the standards that the physician uses to hire personnel may not be as stringent as those of a hospital.

An additional problem is what type of backup the nonhospital setting has to handle emergencies that might occur as a result of the anesthesia. Do they have an ambulance available to move you to a hospital? Do they have written agreements with particular hospitals in case an emergency does arise? Are all staff members trained in CPR (cardiopulmonary resuscitation) and available to use it? Many are not!

The key here, just as in the hospital setting, is to question, question, question. Do not allow anesthesia to be administered to you in any outpatient setting unless you are absolutely comfortable with the competence of the practitioners involved and the emergency procedures in place.

While anesthesia itself is relatively safe, it is not 100% foolproof. Therefore, it is important for you to understand how anesthesia is administered and what can go wrong.

Ill effects of anesthesia can range from general discomfort to loss of life—a broad range to be sure but something you must be prepared to deal with. There are three basic types of anesthesia: local, regional, and general.

- Local anesthesia is used for procedures in which only a small portion of the body needs to be anesthetized for a short period of time (such as when your dentist uses novocaine before drilling).
- Regional anesthesia is used to numb a portion of the body for up to three hours. The four types of regional anesthesia are caudal, epidural, nerve block, and spinal. Each designation refers to the regions of the body affected by the anesthesia. A caudal block is anesthesia injected in the area below the lumbar vertebrae in the sacrum (the triangle-shaped bone between the hips). It deadens the area where it is injected. An epidural is delivered via a catheter to an area in the lower back between the lumbar vertebrae. It is a complete pain block for the abdominal region. A nerve block occurs when anesthesia is injected into an area where main nerves are located, such as the hand or foot. It differs from local anesthesia in that it "deadens" or numbs the area that the main nerve affects. Spinal anesthesia is that injected directly into the spinal fluid. It anesthetizes the region from the stomach to the toes (in other words, the lower part of your body).

  A major risk associated with regional anesthesia is lumbar (lower region of the spine) puncture if the needle is inserted incorrectly.
- General anesthesia is used to anesthetize the entire body for extended periods of time.

Some of the common side effects of regional and general anesthesia are: breathing difficulties, headaches, lightheadedness, nausea and vomiting, and pain. More serious complications of anesthesia can affect major organ systems and bring about heart attack, kidney failure, stroke, and death.

For specific information about anesthesia risks associated with the procedures we outline in Part II of this book, see "Understanding the Procedures" beginning on page 29.

Unnecessary Surgery: A National Problem

"There are regrettably some unconscionable pothunters who will operate on anybody that will hold still. Every hospital should eliminate that kind of man."

Sadly, that advice, written in 1922 by William D. Haggard, M.D., in a famous editorial entitled "The Unnecessary Operation," has gone unheeded.

More than 30 million people in the U.S. will enter a hospital this year for an operation. Some will stay just one night; most will stay at least five days. Another 10 million will be admitted to a hospital for at least one night for an invasive diagnostic test. A significant percentage will stay longer.

Ten million more citizens will be operated on in ambulatory care facilities. Unless a life-threatening complication arises, in these settings the patient arrives in the morning and is home by evening.

Joining the above-mentioned 50 million, countless others will have minor, or sometimes not so minor, operations performed in a doctor's office. There are no accurate counts of these in-office procedures.

Thus, more than 20% of the U.S. population will have an operation this year. Next year, the percentage will creep higher, and projections indicate that the increase in surgery will continue indefinitely. As new procedures are developed and as Americans age, surgical and other invasive treatments will become almost the norm. Given this trend, it may not be long before half the people in the U.S. have at least one operation each year!

The increase in the number of surgeries cannot au-tomatically be equated with Americans being better off medically. In fact, the medical literature—those writings physicians and researchers exchange among themselves—suggests that far too many operations are performed unnecessarily, inappropriately, or without taking into consideration factors that may affect the outcome.

Dr. Haggard issued his warning more than 70 years ago, at a time when surgery was just beginning to come into its own. It was written in an era when most unnecessary surgery was performed out of ignorance on the part of the physician. History shows that it was only a generation or two before Dr. Haggard's time that more people died than survived as a result of a doctor operating on them. By 1922 doctors were beginning to feel a bit "heady" about their ability to solve theretofore unsolvable medical problems with a scalpel.

Dr. Haggard observed that many doctors were performing operations without knowing whether there was a benefit from the procedure. He was concerned that little scientific research had been done to look at the effectiveness, complications, or even efficacy of given procedures. He was especially concerned about certain doctors who exercised their egos or contemplated their pocketbooks, rather than their knowledge and common decency, in deciding whether to operate.

Unfortunately, Dr. Haggard's warnings went unheeded. Not only has the number of unnecessary surgeries grown, but the record is clear that hospitals, because of their unique economic reliance on doctors, especially surgeons, have done little to rid their staffs of these "pothunters."

Today the number of unnecessary operations is estimated to range between six million and 10 million annually. On the high end, that represents 20% of the operations performed in the United States. Some experts suggest that both the numbers of unnecessary operations and the percentages are significantly higher than 20%. Further, unnecessary surgery is not confined to certain regions of the country or types of operations. It is rampant in every community. It also occurs in every operation on the list of most frequently performed procedures.

For example, 23% of all children will be born this year by cesarean section. It is estimated that at least half of those cesarean births will be unnecessary. Yet the American medical community has done little to remedy this obvious problem. By comparison, in England, where the cesarean-section rate has just reached 11%, the medical community itself has reacted in outrage. They claim the rate should be half that, or 5.5%. Their claim is probably valid when one considers that in 1970 the American cesarean-section rate was a mere 5%.

It cannot be argued that we have better birth outcomes as a result of this 400% cesarean-section increase. Since 1970 the United States has continued to lose ground in the infant mortality ratings when compared

with other industrialized countries. Today we stand near the bottom in those rankings.

Medically there is no reason for women who have had a previous cesarean to necessarily have another one (the "once a cesarean, always a cesarean" myth). The American College of Obstetricians and Gynecologists has issued very strong guidelines to all its members, and these guidelines should have eliminated 70% of the repeat cesareans. They have not.

Cesareans are not the only high-volume, often unnecessary operations. The National Center for Health Statistics reported that of the annual 750,000 hysterectomies performed, 22% were unnecessary and "in only 10% of the cases were the indications for a hysterectomy so clear-cut that all doctors would agree to perform the operation."

In its own study, the prestigious Rand Corporation found that 30% of all coronary bypass operations performed each year are medically unnecessary.

Even the 1.5 million circumcisions performed each year have come under fire as medically unnecessary. Side effects, including excessive bleeding and infection, occur in one out of 500 circumcised infants. These figures and other facts have led both the American Academy of Pediatrics and the American College of Obstetricians and Gynecologists to declare the procedure unnecessary.

Given the findings of extensive medical research, it is accurate to conclude that a significant percentage of most surgical or invasive diagnostic procedures performed are done unnecessarily.

Unnecessary operations also may lead to death. The overall mortality rate for all major surgery in the United States is 1.33%. By multiplying 6.5 million unnecessary surgeries by the overall surgical mortality rate, 86,450 unnecessary deaths can be accounted for.

Necessity of an operation is not the only problem. Nor is it the only factor that a person must take into consideration when surgery is presented as an answer to a medical problem.

There is also the matter of risk. Most people go under the knife without being fully informed of the hazards involved. The information they have is scant and not documented, and very rarely includes alternatives to what is being proposed.

Data are also often skewed to the positive aspects of the proposed procedure. For example, most procedures have very low mortality statistics on a percentage basis. If a patient asks the survival rate of a proposed operation, the surgeon will often state the figure as a percentage. Thus a person having a bone marrow biopsy will be told that 92% survive. Yet an 8% mortality rate translates into 8,850 deaths out of 110,653 bone marrow biopsies performed each year. The mortality rate for that procedure is six times higher than the average for all major surgeries. So while the percentage is correct, in this case the actual number is more enlightening. When compared with the overall surgical mortality rate, a more meaningful basis for comparison can be made.

Other risks are often ignored or quickly glossed over. For example, 10% of all people who enter a hospital will acquire a nosocomial infection. The risks of these hospital-caused infections vary from hospital to hospital and from procedure to procedure, but few surgeons ever divulge such information to their patients. It is also alarming that some studies suggest that physicians may not even know the infection rates of the procedure or the hospital.

Complications other than infection are not usually mentioned either. Many people, for example, are not informed that a likelihood of a certain complication may exist with a given operation. Nor are they informed of possible long-term side effects that accompany many operations.

Doctors also fail to advise patients of medical controversies surrounding particular operations. For example, one of the most frequently performed controversial procedures is the insertion of tubes in children's ears to help prevent ear infection. This procedure has long been the topic of heated medical debate; there is no consensus either in the literature or among physicians that it is worthwhile. Yet most parents who have approved the operation for their child report that they were not advised of the controversy.

Even as classic an operation as the tonsillectomy is under serious reconsideration for appropriateness. Yet again, most families are unaware of this very important medical debate.

As surgeons become better trained and more proficient, the number of elective procedures increases. These procedures are neither emergencies nor medical imperatives. They range from the frivolous, such as "vanity" plastic surgery, to the fine-line necessary, such as "prophylactic" hysterectomy. Despite the many risks elective procedures pose, however, more are performed each year.

To illustrate the risk potential of elective surgery, consider the situation that unfolded in Los Angeles County during the first 35 days of 1976. At that time, physicians staged a work slowdown and performed nothing but emergency surgeries. The newspapers, responding to the physicians' public relations machine, ran alarmist stories implying that the public health was in severe jeopardy. The fact is the public health was affected, but only for the better. Researchers M. I. Roemer and J. L. Schwartz reported in the December 1979 issue of *Social Science and Medicine* that "the withholding of elective surgery . . . was associated with a significant reduction in the county's overall mortality experience, compared with the previous five years." They found that the number of deaths decreased as the number of slowdown days increased. It is not surprising that, as soon as the slowdown ended, there was a "substantial jump in the mortality rate."

The Los Angeles experience is not an isolated occurrence. In 1973, when doctors went on strike in Israel and elective surgery was stopped, the country's death rate plummeted 50%, while a 52-day doctors' work stoppage in Brazil in 1976 led to a 35% decline in the mortality rate.

How can so many operations be performed each year unnecessarily? Why do so many Americans agree to go under the knife when the facts clearly point to such a high volume of useless, not to mention dangerous, procedures? Why do so many doctors, knowing both the risks and the lack of medical need, perform so many overly dangerous and unnecessary operations? Finally, what can be done to correct the situation?

The answers have a great deal to do with the state of medical consumerism and the "business" of medicine in the United States. Consumers know virtually nothing about the operations they agree to have performed on them. While most doctors will describe the procedure briefly, the majority disclose little information about appropriateness, side effects, or complications.

Furthermore, medicine still retains its status as the last bastion of nonconsumerism in the U.S. For the most part, consumers have little information about the record of their doctors or hospitals. Any information about the competence of either is more likely to be generated by a public relations office than by a medical record room.

Until this book, a consumer could find virtually no understandable information about a given invasive diagnostic or therapeutic procedure. Unless you turned to a medical textbook, information was unavailable about how a particular operation was performed. Even if consumers were able to cut through the Greek and Latin in medical texts, they would find that most do not contain updated information related to the experience gained by the tens of thousands of surgeons who perform the procedure in question.

Furthermore, until now there has been no one single source of information that outlines the medical necessity, the procedure itself, the risks and complications, or the medical controversies surrounding a particular operation available for consumers.

Since doctors began doing invasive procedures, the patient has been coaxed and prodded to trust the physician. As consumers, we have become passive, accepting what physicians tell us, based upon our faith in the person rather than upon the facts.

However, in recent years as consumers have begun to do research in the medical literature, they have learned that quite often physicians are not aware of what the scientific community has published on routinely performed tests and procedures. In fact, there is a growing body of literature suggesting that a significant segment of doctors do not know the mortality risks, much less the morbidity (complication) risks of procedures they perform regularly.

It is in the prestigious medical journals, often published by medical specialty societies, that important information about the successes and problems associated with particular operations can be found. The major studies on outcome, complications, and necessity of medical procedures are regularly published in these journals, yet many go unread by those who should be reading them.

Because of this, the consumer is in a medical abyss. What the doctor may be telling the consumer may not be the whole truth. While the physician may not be lying outright, the complete picture is often not revealed. Even if a consumer seeks an independent second opinion, most patients are still not fully informed.

The inadequacy of consumer information is only one of the reasons that unnecessary and inappropriate operations are performed. Another is a pure dollar-and-cents matter. Performing operations is big business. Surgeons' earnings rank among the highest of all medical specialists. Surgeons generate hundreds of billions of dollars for both themselves and the hospitals with which they have affiliations. A high-volume surgeon is to a hospital what a high-volume real estate agent is to the agency—money in the bank.

Like it or not, medical practitioners are in competition with one another. So are hospitals. Their bottom line is to make money, whether it is for reasons of compassion or greed. In both the inpatient and outpatient settings the competition is fierce. These days it is not unusual to see roadside billboards advertising a particular doctor, hospital, or outpatient setting specializing in a particular procedure such as lens implants or knee surgery. It's a modern-day "medicine show" being operated through the electronic and print media, instead of the back of a wagon.

Surgery rates have a lot to do with this race to the bottom line. New techniques and the aging of the U.S. population are not the only reasons for the annual increase in the number of surgeries. Astonishingly, the largest contributing factor, according to some recent studies, has been and continues to be nonmedical. These studies demonstrate that surgery rates increase in direct proportion to the increase in the number of surgeons available. It's a matter of making the pie bigger so that everyone continues to get the same size share.

For example, from 1971 to 1977 the number of operations increased 34%, while the population increased only 6%. During that same period, the supply of surgeons increased at a rate seven times that of the general population.

Even more revealing is the fact that in 1977, with 100,000 surgeons available, there were 20 million operations. Five years later the number of operations had risen to 34 million. During that interval the number of surgeons had increased by 15,000, or 15%, while the general population had grown by only 4%.

The increase in the number of surgeons continues unabated, as does the number of settings in which surgery is performed.

Only 12 years ago 95% of all surgery was performed in the hospital. Today, only 65% is in the hospital. Now 35% is done on an outpatient basis, and the number of ambulatory care facilities is growing at about the same rate as McDonald's is opening new restaurants.

As of 1988 there were 964 freestanding surgery centers in America. That was an 11.4% increase over 1987. In 1991 there were more than 1,320 facilities open. This growth trend is projected to last throughout the decade.

As of 1988, besides these freestanding facilities, more than 5,000 American hospitals had ambulatory surgery departments. That is close to 90% of all hospitals.

It is interesting that outpatient surgeries at the freestanding centers doubled between 1988 and 1991. They also increased in the hospital ambulatory centers *and* at inpatient hospitals. In other words, in every setting more people are having surgery performed each year.

What is going on here? There is no question that modern medicine has done much for most of us. There is no doubt that surgery and invasive diagnostic tests can, more often than not, lead to a better life.

There are still two sides to the coin. As consumers, we also become victims of a medical system driven too much by business and greed, one that often pays less attention to the consumer's medical need and more attention to the financial bottom lines of the physician and hospital. The fact that the federal government had to issue warnings to hospitals about "dumping" Medicare beneficiaries from their hospital beds before they had fully recovered is merely one sign of this clash between greed and compassion.

More than ever before, consumers must rely heavily on themselves and on independent sources to make truly informed medical decisions.

We no longer can rely solely on the information our doctor passes along. When we must decide whether to undergo a particular operation we cannot base the decision on blind faith in our practitioner. We have learned that not every operation is applicable to every patient. Even people presenting the same symptoms often do not require the same procedure to control, cure, or deal with them.

Medicine is now the biggest business in the U.S. It consumes almost 14% of the gross national product. In this light, consumers must remember the "buyer beware" maxim when it comes to surgery. Today there are more "pothunters" than ever lurking behind white coats. Only informed and empowered consumers can make sure that they do not become victims.

Surgeon/Surgery Checklist

Many factors must be considered when surgery is being contemplated. Do I really need it? Are there alternatives? Is my surgeon the best one for my condition? Does the procedure have to be performed in a hospital? Which is the best hospital for my needs?

Most of us begin oozing a cold, clammy sweat when a physician mentions the word *surgery*. We are frightened. We think of wills, insurance policies, our family. We recall all the horror stories we have read in the newspaper about surgery gone wrong.

Often our fear of surgery changes our normal behavior. At a time when we should be asking a lot of questions, we withdraw. Many people lapse into a temporary depression which, although not serious over the long term, is significant enough that we forget about important things we should be doing.

Every person confronting surgery should have lengthy discussions with the physician who recommended surgery and with the surgeon being considered.

Note that we say "surgeon being considered." In most cases it is wise to consult more than one surgeon. That's because different surgeons may approach your problem in different ways. Studies show that the level of medical misdiagnosis is significant. At least 25% of all second opinions do not agree with the first opinion diagnostically.

The percentage is often higher when it comes to what to do about your problem. That's because medicine is more of an art than a science. In fact, a study by the United States Congress's Office of Technology Assessment found that only about 20% of all medical procedures have been proven effective by thorough clinical trials. That means that what to do is often as much an educated guess as it is a scientific conclusion.

You should not say no to surgery simply because there are differences of opinion about what should be done. You must take the bull by the horns and get as much information as you can possibly get in order to make an informed decision about if, when, where, and by whom you should have the procedure performed.

We have assembled a checklist for you to use as a guide. At a minimum, we recommend that you ask your physician and the surgeon all of the questions on the list. If you are too shy, afraid, or unable to do it because of your condition, bring a family member or friend with you. Inform the doctor(s) that you have brought your advocate along to help you better understand what is being contemplated and to help you make decisions. If your physician balks at speaking in front of another person, consider changing doctors. Remember, you have the legal right to have anyone you choose with you at any doctor's appointment.

Not every question you should ask is on the list. You probably have other issues that need to be addressed. The questions on the checklist are some of the more important ones you should consider asking. They are the types of questions that require more than cursory answers. As a result, when they are answered you will have a wealth of information to help you make your important medical decisions.

USING THE SURGEON/SURGERY CHECKLIST

The surgery checklist is quite simple to use. Each of the questions is designed to provide you with information to help you decide whether to have a particular surgical procedure and/or whether the surgeon you are contemplating is the best one for the job.

Part one of the checklist is designed to help you learn about the competence of the surgeon you are considering. There are no right or wrong answers to these questions. Rather, they are designed to help you sort out the experience and training of one doctor versus another.

For example, it is important to ask the doctor if she is board certified in the specialty under which you are being treated. Although board certification does not ensure better results, it does give a measurable indication that the doctor has sought advanced and continuing education in his field.

Part one also discusses insurance acceptance and fees. These matters should *always* be discussed directly with the doctor. Do not let the practitioner direct you to an office manager or receptionist to discuss costs. You are doing business with the doctor, not with an office assistant.

Part two of the checklist is specifically related to the procedure being contemplated. The questions are self-explanatory, but you should go over them in your own mind before you discuss each one with your doctor. Think about how you feel about each question. For example, the issue of pain is an important one. Do you have a high or low threshold of pain? Knowing where your needs or beliefs are on these questions will help you to evaluate the answers your doctor provides.

Remember, there are many more questions you might ask based on your individual situation. So take this list and add your own questions to it. By being aggressive in your questioning before you pick a surgeon or approve an operation, you will help ensure that there will be no surprises after the surgery has been performed.

Your Surgeon/Surgery Checklist

GENERAL INFORMATION

Is this surgeon an M.D. or D.O.? _____

Is this surgeon board certified in his/her specialty? _____

Is this surgeon board certified in another specialty? _____

If yes, which one? _____

Is this surgeon in solo or group practice? _____

If group practice, have you been assured that the surgeon you select will perform your surgery? _____

Does this surgeon have privileges at the hospital of your choice? _____

Has the surgeon fully discussed his/her fees for the procedure and discussed other costs that might be associated with the operation? _____

Does this surgeon publish a list of his/her fees? _____

Does this surgeon's fee include postoperative follow-up care? _____

Will your insurance coverage be accepted as payment in full? _____

If not, is a flexible payment plan offered? _____

Has this surgeon been highly recommended by others? _____

PROCEDURE-SPECIFIC INFORMATION

What type of procedure are you recommending for my condition?

_____

Is this the most appropriate procedure for my condition? _____

Will this procedure be painful? _____If yes, how can the pain be decreased? _____

Is this procedure dangerous? _____If yes, in what ways? _____

How often have you performed this procedure in the last year? _____How often have you performed it on someone in my age bracket? _____

What is the national mortality (death) rate associated with this procedure? _____

What are the most common complications associated with this procedure? _____

_____

_____

_____

What is the average recovery time following this procedure? _____

What, if any, alternatives are there to the procedure you recommend? If there are any, what might I expect as possible and probable results should I elect to choose one? _____

_____

_____

_____

What can I expect if I choose not to have any procedure performed? _____

_____

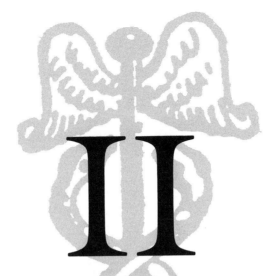

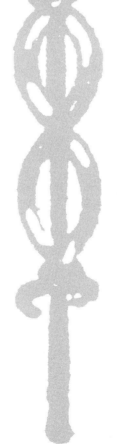

II

*Understanding the
Procedures*

Introduction

In this section we review 100 of the most commonly performed operations in the U.S. Some are diagnostic in nature, used to determine a disease or problem not otherwise diagnosable. The others are surgical treatments, used to solve or alleviate a medical problem. And some, like balloon angioplasty, are used both diagnostically and therapeutically.

The 100 procedures reviewed were selected in two ways. The majority are those procedures most frequently performed in U.S. hospitals, either on an inpatient or an outpatient basis. Others, like lens implantation and circumcision, are not necessarily performed in hospitals, but are still major procedures in terms of volume and/or the controversial issues surrounding various aspects of the procedure. (It is because they are often not performed in hospitals that these two common operations are not given a number rank here.) This represents a major trend now occurring in American medicine: the shift from hospital-based surgery to outpatient surgery. Because of improved practice techniques and advanced technology, operations like the lens implant are done in a matter of minutes, with little risk to the patient, and therefore do not require overnight or prolonged hospitalization.

Determining the 100 most frequently performed procedures is not as easy as you might think. Doctors and hospitals are not required to report each operation they perform to some central data bank. Even the federal government does not track a full 100 of the most common procedures. Thus, we had to do a great deal of research to find out just what were the most often performed operations.

But find them we did. Our data come from two sources. The major one was Healthcare Knowledge Resources of Ann Arbor, Michigan, which produces such a list by keeping a data base of 16% of all hospital discharges in the U.S. Healthcare Knowledge Resources, then extrapolates those figures to find the national number. Our other source of information was the federal government, which does gather and publish selected data concerning procedures. By putting these two sources together, we were able to come up with the 100 procedures covered in this section.

It is also important to have a perspective of the actual volume for each procedure in a given year. For example, cesarean sections, which top the list, were performed 962,622 times in 1989. There were 267,868 appendectomies (the eighth most frequently performed procedure), and 149,444 ureteral catheterizations (number 100 on our list). But these numbers may be less than the actual number performed for certain procedures.

The fact is that the number of operations done outside the hospital setting is virtually impossible to track. Individual insurance companies may have statistics for their policy holders, but these numbers cannot be extrapolated with any authority because of the uneven distribution of ambulatory surgical settings in various parts of the country.

Some procedures may be performed more frequently than some of those we have listed. Many are cosmetic in nature, such as the vast majority of the breast implants that were performed in the United States in the 1980s. We arbitrarily left those procedures out because we believe there is an adequate number of books covering them and because the medical literature on them is scant at best. We also believe that such surgeries are truly elective and may even fall into the category of "boutique" medicine.

We should also say a word about "elective" surgery. There are actually two different types of elective surgery. One falls into the category described above—not necessary for any medical reason, but possibly useful for other, mainly psychological, reasons. Such procedures might include nose jobs, tummy tucks, or breast enlargements.

The second type of elective surgery is not absolutely necessary at the moment, but might dramatically improve a patient's health or prospects for longevity, or delay the progress of a degenerating condition. For example, a coronary bypass operation, under nonemergency circumstances, would be classified as elective. Most hysterectomies are classified as elective. "Elective" does not mean frivolous or unnecessary. It merely suggests that the individual consumer has an option.

Finally, we make no mention in the discussion of the individual procedures about how long each operation takes, what the recovery time might be, or what type of follow-up therapy could be recommended. This is because there are no hard and fast rules about these issues. The minutes or hours it may take to perform a particular operation are of little significance. The important issue is whether the procedure is performed competently and with excellent results. The same is true for recovery time. Some people take longer to heal than others. The time is of little significance if the outcome is ultimately good. And follow-up therapy depends upon so many factors that a general guide like this one could not begin to predict the range of programs that may be necessary. But each of these issues is important, and they should be discussed in advance with the practitioners involved.

Using This Section

UNDERSTANDING THE TERMINOLOGY

We have attempted to present the information in a logical, easy-to-read way, using language that you will understand. Despite these efforts, there are many words with which you will not be familiar. We address this problem by providing a complete glossary at the end of the book. In the text, words that appear in the glossary are highlighted in bold print on first mention. If you are unfamiliar with a term, turn to the glossary for a definition.

It is important not to be intimidated by the language of medicine. We have made every effort to "translate" medical jargon into normal English; however, it was not possible or appropriate in all situations. In addition, it is likely that your doctor will be using many of the terms found in both the text and the glossary. The playing field becomes more level when you are familiar with many of those terms.

ABOUT THE SOURCES

The information provided about each of the following procedures comes completely from medical journals and studies reported in the medical literature. For each procedure, all the major facts and figures are documented with appropriate endnotes. The exact source is then listed in the back of the book.

We have reviewed all the information we could find on each one of the operations listed. This was a massive undertaking that involved computer on-line searching and review, scrutiny of medical journals and references, and any other bona fide data source we could find.

Medical studies are often quite complicated. It is often difficult, even for the most skilled researcher, to know exactly how significant any one study may be. For example, a recent Canadian study on mammography reported that women under the age of 50 who had routine mammography were *more* likely to develop breast cancer than women in the same age range who had not had routine mammograms. Some highly esteemed researchers from around the world began criticizing the results of the findings based only on the news reports. Their criticism was based on the fact that all previous studies of a similar nature had shown opposite results. Even after the results were scrutinized more closely, expert opinions varied about the validity of the findings.

For the consumer using this book, the contradiction

highlighted in this example raises several important questions: Should your decision about whether to have a procedure performed be based on one or even a few studies? Is there some way to judge the validity of one study over another?

Very rarely is the result of a single medical study, in and of itself, enough for you to use as the basis for a medical decision. Unless the results of a study can be replicated (achieved by other independent researchers using the same protocols), the validity of the findings must always be suspect. This does not mean that the findings were wrong. It merely means unless it can happen again somewhere else, using similar study subjects and comparable conditions, the results will always be under question. Thus, the answer to the first question is a clear "no." One study should not be the basis for making any medical decision.

What do you do when there is more than one study? How do you evaluate the validity of one over another? There is no short answer to these questions. While studies can be compared, the hard part is knowing how to do it. In this section of the book we refer you to more than 1,000 studies. To some extent we have done much of the comparison work for you. We used strict criteria to research each of the procedures. We made sure that the studies we cite are from legitimate medical journals. We looked to see that the journals had established standards for accepting studies that they published. We also looked closely to see if the studies referenced earlier studies. This is important because medical research is a building process wherein one step usually leads to another. That is why studies from many years ago are cited with newer ones. We also made sure that the studies were done in the context of the procedure being discussed or were directly related to something that might occur during the discussed procedure.

For example, many of the procedures discussed in this section require the use of general anesthesia. That meant that we had to do separate research on the safety and risks of general anesthesia and note the findings in the context of each procedure.

When we found controversies in the medical literature, meaning contradictions between two or more studies, we searched even further. What we attempted to do was find the widest range of studies in order to establish a consensus on the subject among the medical experts. In all cases we present the full range of information to you along with the source it came from so that you may seek out the primary source yourself, should you so desire.

Because the quality of studies varies, we have elected to list as many as possible for each particular reference. As a result, you may see a tremendously wide variation in outcome or complication data for a given procedure. This also means that you will find a certain level of detail not ordinarily available in other reviews of procedures you have come across. For example, when discussing complications that may be associated with a particular procedure, we often cite studies that have noted specific problems for certain segments of the population who might be candidates for the operation, such as persons above the age of 80 or individuals having other underlying conditions. Sometimes those studies involved only a small number of subjects, but the information they contained was not contradicted by other studies, and their importance was apparently substantial enough that they were accepted for publication by a medical journal. Based upon that, we decided that the information was useful for a consumer to have. Also, we believe it is essential that consumers know and understand how inexact medical data often may be.

It is also essential to note that many foreign sources are referenced in this book. Too often, U.S. studies and medical literature reviews have ignored studies published abroad. In our effort to find the widest possible range of information, we reviewed both foreign and domestic studies. In so doing, we believe we are providing a more complete picture of a given topic. American medicine is just now recognizing the high quality often found in foreign studies and in care provided in other countries. While the United States is undoubtedly the world leader in medicine, many other countries use techniques and procedures that surpass ours in outcomes.

Finally, it is important for you to understand why we went to as many sources as we did to bring this information to you. The reason is simple: There is no other single book or document available for *any* of the procedures we discuss that has all the information you need to make a sound medical decision. That includes medical textbooks. The fact is that even your doctor must go to literally hundreds and even thousands of sources of information to keep abreast of what is happening in her own field. In fact, you might want to share what you read with your practitioners.

So do not be overwhelmed by the numerous sources and lengthy section of endnotes. They are presented for your use when and if you need them.

LOOKING UP A PROCEDURE

The procedures in this section are broken up into two groups: diagnostic procedures and surgical treatments. The diagnostic procedures appear first, followed by the surgical treatments, and in each group, the procedures are listed in alphabetical order.

Beginning Your Review

Look up the name of the procedure you want to review. Procedures are listed by their general medical title as well as the common lay title for the procedure, if there is one.

The Good Operations—Bad Operations Quick Rating Guide

Next to the title on the first page of each procedure is the *Good Operations—Bad Operations Quick Rating Guide*. It consists of three categories and an area where brief explanations are found, if necessary.

The first category listed is **MORTALITY.** Mortality refers to the percentage of people who die during or as a result of the procedure being discussed. In the box under **MORTALITY** will be either a " + " or a " − ."

The overall mortality rate for all operations in this country is 1.33%. That means that 1.3 people out of every 100 die during or as a result of an operation. If the overall mortality rate of a procedure is lower than or equal to 1.33%, the box will have a " + ." The plus signifies that the chances of dying from the procedure are less than the national norm for all operations. A " − " in the box means there are more deaths associated with that particular procedure than the national norm for all procedures.

The second box is labeled **MORBIDITY.** Morbidity consists of the complications associated with a particular procedure. Unfortunately, there are no national norms or standards to determine what is acceptable and unacceptable morbidity. However, we have used the same " + " and " − " system to note procedures with low rates of significant complications versus those with high rates. Thus, if you find a " + " in the **MORBIDITY** box you will know that the research reports relatively low complication rates. A " − " means frequent and/or significant complications are reported in the literature.

The third box is labeled **CONTROVERSY.** In this box you will find either a white or dark circle. If the circle is white, there are few, if any, controversial issues associated with the procedure. If the circle is dark, significant and/or numerous controversies surround the operation.

Description and Discussion of Procedures

Under the title (and lay title, if there is one) is a brief description of what the procedure is intended to accomplish.

After the above description, each procedure is discussed with respect to the following questions:

What Condition Does the Procedure Treat?
What Is the Procedure?
Who Performs the Procedure?
Where Is the Procedure Performed?
What Are the Mortality (Death) and Morbidity (Complication) Rates?
What Are the Other Complications and Possible Side Effects?
Is This the Most Appropriate Procedure for the Condition?
Are There Alternatives to This Procedure?
What Is Controversial About the Procedure?

Here is what you will find in each section.

WHAT CONDITION DOES THE PROCEDURE TREAT?

Obviously, every procedure is designed to treat at least one specific condition. However, you may be surprised to learn that some operations are performed for both diagnostic and therapeutic reasons. In fact, a given operation may be performed for a variety of underlying reasons.

In this section, we explain all the conditions for which the particular procedure may be used. We explain the details of the condition(s) so that you are familiar with the reasons a particular operation is done. We also note interesting and important facts you probably did not know about your condition or why certain procedures are employed to correct it.

WHAT IS THE PROCEDURE?

In this section we describe in detail how the procedure is performed. Here you will find many terms with which you are not familiar. When the word is in **boldface type,** it is defined in the glossary.

WHO PERFORMS THE PROCEDURE?

You might expect that every operation in this book is performed by a surgeon, but that is not the case. In this section, we explain who frequently performs each procedure. Some procedures must be performed by very highly trained specialists; others can be done by a family practitioner.

WHERE IS THE PROCEDURE PERFORMED?

In the not-too-distant past, every operation was performed in the hospital. That is no longer the case. Since 1980, several thousand procedures that once required you to be hospitalized have been approved by Medicare and other third-party payers to be done on an outpatient basis. This has dramatically changed the process of surgery.

Many of the procedures found in this book can be done in either an inpatient or outpatient setting. The choice of which route to take may not always be in your control. Much of the decision is based on coverage under Medicare or your insurance carrier. Both Medicare and private insurers have become very strict regarding where they will pay for a procedure to be performed. If there is an option between inpatient and outpatient surgery, your insurer will most likely inform you that the company will only pay the equivalent of what it would cost as an outpatient procedure, even if you choose to have it done as an inpatient.

In this section, we explain where the procedure can be performed. We also note what situations might warrant having the procedure done in the hospital versus as an outpatient.

WHAT ARE THE MORTALITY (DEATH) AND MORBIDITY (COMPLICATION) RATES?

There is probably no word that evokes more fear than *surgery*. The first fearful thought most people have after hearing the word is "Am I going to die?"

Modern medicine has come a long way since the turn of the century, when surgical death rates made dying from an operation as likely as surviving one. Today, only slightly more than one out of 100 persons (1.33%, to be exact) dies as a direct result of all surgery performed. The percentage of people who die during or as a direct result of an operation is termed the mortality rate. For the procedures covered in this book the mortality rate is 1.33%. The same percentage rates between all operations and the ones we review reflects the fact that the operations found in this book are generally the most frequently performed and perhaps the most invasive.

Yet overall mortality rates are of little significance to those of us who must deal with our own operations. Of importance to you is what the mortality rate is for the procedure you are contemplating and what factors increase or decrease those percentages.

For each procedure, we discuss the mortality rate and the factors that affect it. We also discuss the morbidity rate—but more on that later. For now, let's concentrate on how to assess your chances of surviving a surgical procedure.

The mortality rates associated with the procedure are calculated on the total number of procedures performed. For example, closed reduction and internal fixation of fracture of the femur (surgical repair of a broken leg; see page 133) has a mortality rate of 3.7% based on 28,000 procedures studied. It translates into 1,036 deaths resulting from the procedure, or one death out of every 27 procedures. The important point to consider is the percentage of deaths, rather than the actual numbers. The percentage gives you a much better perspective on what your survival chances are. Thus, in this case your chance of surviving the operation is 96.3%.

As you will find as you review each operation, certain factors may raise the overall mortality rate. Depending upon the procedure, age may be a factor. In other instances, other medical conditions that you might have may lower your chances of survival.

Therefore, it is important not only to read this part carefully, but also to assess (and discuss with your doctor) your overall condition as compared with the points noted in the discussion.

Mortality is not the only hazard facing consumers considering surgery. There is also the prospect of complications. These are conditions that develop as a result of the procedure; some of them may be life-threatening. The rate at which these complicating factors occur is called the morbidity rate. It, too, is expressed as a percentage.

Although there are standard definitions of what a "complication" is, there are no standards for what is major, minor, or deserving of consideration. Thus, a very meticulous study of one set of practitioners that looks at every event that extends the hospital stay or increases the cost of care could report a very high complication rate, while a sloppy study that counts only events that ultimately led to a bad outcome could report a very low one.

We have carefully reviewed the methodologies and data, or the equivalent sections of the studies reviewed, in an attempt to assure quality information. Because there are no true common research standards with respect to morbidity, however, such a review must also be accompanied with a note of caution.

Because of this, we have chosen to provide a very wide range of studies to show the significant variations that can occur. They are not meant to scare you, but rather to inform you and to help you use the data as a basis to discuss these matters with your doctor.

As you look at many of the discussions of mortality and morbidity found in this section, you will find that there are wide variations in outcomes between two or more studies of the same procedure. How can this be? Do medical journals publish bad studies? Isn't medicine a science, and aren't scientific measurement standards pretty exact?

Let's answer the last question first. As previously stated, the practice of medicine is more of an art than a science. This explains why a second opinion often does not confirm a first one. It also explains how one surgeon's results may be much different from a colleague's. In answer to the second question, quality medical journals do not publish bad studies, if they can avoid it. However, with rare exceptions, studies reflect only the experience of a few doctors in a single group or single hospital. Because of varying conditions, such as the severity of the patient's illness, the training and competence of the doctors, and the support and experience of other, back-up hospital personnel, surgical outcomes can be significantly diverse.

It is well understood among medical researchers that wide variations in surgical outcomes and complications associated with specific surgical procedures are fairly routine. Work conducted by Dartmouth Medical School professor Jack Wennberg, M.D., and studies conducted by the Pennsylvania Council on Health Care Cost Containment (both have done extensive studies on variations in mortality and morbidity rates) indicate that there is a difference of at least two standard deviations between any two doctors in the same hospital. In other words, if the mean (average) mortality rate for a particular procedure per doctor is 5% and the standard deviation is 5%, this would allow for a mortality rate range of zero to 15%.

CALCULATING YOUR RISK

With all that said, how do you translate the numbers and percentages you will find in each of the operations covered in this section? In other words, how do you calculate your risk of death or complications?

It is important that you understand the combined risks of mortality and morbidity. Keep in mind that as the percentage increases so does your risk. Obviously, your risk is lower as the percentage decreases. As noted earlier, the overall mortality rate for all surgical procedures is calculated to be 1.33%. That means that one death occurs for every 75 surgical procedures. Nationally, there are some 30 million surgical procedures performed in hospitals each year, resulting in 400,000 deaths.

Of course, you must keep in mind that some procedures have very low mortality rates, whereas others are much higher than the national average.

The mortality rate for the diagnostic procedures listed in this book is 1.12%. This means that one death is expected to occur for every 89 procedures performed. The mortality rate for the nondiagnostic procedures covered in the book is 1.38% (one death expected for every 72 procedures performed). Thus, the combined rate is 1.33, or exactly the national average.

The following table will help you translate the mortality and morbidity percentages associated with procedures described in the book.

PERCENTAGE	YOUR RISK
100%	1 OUT OF 1
50%	1 OUT OF 2
25%	1 OUT OF 4
10%	1 OUT OF 10
5%	1 OUT OF 20
4%	1 OUT OF 25
3%	1 OUT OF 33
2%	1 OUT OF 50
1%	1 OUT OF 100
.75%	1 OUT OF 133
.60%	1 OUT OF 166
.50%	1 OUT OF 200
.40%	1 OUT OF 250
.25%	1 OUT OF 400
.20%	1 OUT OF 500
.15%	1 OUT OF 666
.10%	1 OUT OF 1,000

To calculate a risk from a percentage not shown:

1. Put the percentage in decimal form (always move the decimal point two places to the left). For example, 1.33% becomes .0133.

2. Next, divide the decimal into the number 1. In the case described, it would be 1 divided by .0133. Your answer will be expressed as a whole number. In this case, the answer is 75.

Two final notes to help you better use this section: In many of the procedures we note a risk related to the use of general anesthesia. Because the risk is the same regardless of the procedure, we have noted when the risk applies and referred you to the "anesthesia risk" entry in the glossary.

Finally, be sure to keep risks in perspective. Many people who die as a result of surgery may have been so ill that their likelihood of surviving was minimal to begin with. The same applies to complications.

Remember that your condition and situation are unique; the material found in this part of the procedure description should be used only as a guide.

WHAT ARE THE OTHER COMPLICATIONS AND POSSIBLE SIDE EFFECTS?

In this section, complications and other possible side effects not necessarily associated with the complications covered in the above section may be noted. Often these are observations noted in the studies that could not be directly attributed to the operation itself, but which may occur. For example, in several procedures involving joint replacements it has been observed that the surgical glue used to adhere elements of the device to existing bone in the body may begin to disintegrate after a certain number of years.

Thus, this section addresses issues that are important, but not normally presented to you when an operation is being discussed with a practitioner.

IS THIS THE MOST APPROPRIATE PROCEDURE FOR THE CONDITION?

If there is one question every consumer should ask a practitioner who suggests an operation, this is it. The advances in medical knowledge and technology have made many conditions treatable in a variety of ways.

For example, gallbladders can be removed at least three different surgical ways. In addition, you will also find that there is now medication available that can satisfactorily relieve some patients' symptoms without surgery.

In this section, we discuss if and what options are available for a given procedure. Use this as a guide in discussions with your doctor.

ARE THERE ALTERNATIVES TO THIS PROCEDURE?

Similar to the above, this section differs in several ways. Whereas the section above discusses the appropriateness of the specific operation for certain conditions, this section goes into greater detail about available alternatives.

We believe that it is very important for you to know as much as possible about the range of alternative treatments for your condition. This is especially useful if the procedure under discussion might put you in a high-risk category for mortality or morbidity.

WHAT IS CONTROVERSIAL ABOUT THE PROCEDURE?

Most doctors will not discuss controversies surrounding a particular procedure. For example, cesarean section is rife with controversies among medical professionals. With national cesarean section rates at about 23%, many medical and nonmedical experts believe it is at least double what it should be.

Such issues are important for you to know.

In this section we discuss the significant controversies associated with the procedure. You will find the range of controversies quite surprising.

If you are contemplating an operation around which there is controversy, it is important that you discuss these issues with your doctor. You might also want to do more research on the subject; many sources are listed in the endnotes. You might also consider getting a second opinion. Although most doctors are aware of the controversies associated with procedures they perform, they have usually developed their own viewpoint or practice pattern, which may not be what other experts have concluded is the right way to go. Thus, an independent second opinion is an important tool for helping you make your decision.

DON'T BE INTIMIDATED

Now you are ready to use this section of the book. Do not be intimidated by what you read. You are quite capable of understanding everything covered under each procedure. If you have further questions (which you should), talk to your doctor about them.

Use the material we included in the first section of the book to help you in deciding what is best for you.

We especially encourage you to use the Surgeon/Surgery Checklist found on page 24.

We have called this book *Good Operations—Bad Operations* because what may be a good operation for you may be a bad operation for someone else. By utilizing the information you find in these pages, you will be reducing the likelihood of undergoing a bad operation.

Diagnostic Procedures

Arterial Catheterization (47)

MORTALITY	MORBIDITY	CONTROVERSY
+	+	o

Placement of a **catheter** in an artery to measure intra-arterial pressures, administer chemotherapy drugs, or remove **emboli** blocking an artery

❓ WHAT CONDITION DOES THE PROCEDURE TREAT?

Arterial catheterization is carried out for a variety of purposes: to measure intraarterial pressures to assess heart and lung function; to administer chemotherapy drugs locally to organs so that they will be delivered in concentrated forms and perhaps not be as toxic to other organs;[1-4] and to remove clots.

❓ WHAT IS THE PROCEDURE?

Depending upon the complexity of the procedure and whether or not placement of the catheter can be done with a **trochar** or requires an incision, the patient is given a local or short-acting general anesthetic by vein. For complex surgery requiring an incision, such as a liver operation, an inhaled general anesthetic is used.

Generally, an artery that passes fairly close to the skin surface, or a vein that leads to the heart, is punctured with a trochar or opened with a scalpel while the patient is under local anesthesia, after the skin is washed with soap and antiseptic and shaved if necessary. The catheter is threaded into the artery or vein. For example, a **Swan-Ganz catheter**, which measures vessel pressure, is threaded into the **subclavian vein**. It is poked through the **septum** between the right and left sides of the heart,

and a balloon on its tip is inflated. The inflated balloon carries the catheter out into the **pulmonary artery** with the flow of blood. Further inflation of the balloon, once it is in the pulmonary artery, blocks the artery and permits measurements of the force with which the **left ventricle** is contracting. The catheter also allows measurement of several other things, including the amounts of oxygen and carbon dioxide in the freshly oxygenated blood being sent out into the body by the heart.

If repeated pressure measurements or chemotherapy treatments are needed, the catheter is left in place and may be held to the skin with a few loops of **suture** material. If repeated measurements or treatments are not needed, the catheter is removed.

When a **Fogarty catheter** (another specialized catheter) is being used to remove a clot, ideally the clot should first be located on a special type of x ray of the arteries called an angiogram, which is made by injecting **radiopaque** dye into an artery, thus allowing the artery to be seen on film. Knowledge of the normal anatomy and the ability to visualize the location of an artery not usually seen on film allow the surgeon to determine the location of the clot. If the clot cannot be located and the patient's situation is desperate, the doctor may go on an arterial "fishing expedition" based on symptoms that indicate where the clot may be.

In either case, guided by the angiography films or a best clinical guess, the catheter is threaded through the artery until the clot is reached. The catheter is advanced either past or through the clot to just beyond it, and the balloon at the tip of the catheter is inflated. The catheter is slowly withdrawn, dragging the clot along with it. The amount of force the surgeon needs to exert depends upon how strongly the clot is adhered to the arterial wall. The force required may be enough to damage the artery.

? WHO PERFORMS THE PROCEDURE?

Depending upon the purpose of the treatment, the catheter can be inserted by a cardiologist, emergency medicine specialist, general surgeon, oncologist, surgical oncologist, pulmonary surgeon, pulmonary medicine specialist, vascular surgeon, or radiologist. Simple placement of a catheter that does not need to traverse the heart to get to the necessary artery is within the competence of any physician. Placement of a catheter that must go through the heart is best left to a cardiovascular surgeon, vascular surgeon, or pulmonary medicine specialist. Removal of clots with a Fogarty catheter is best done by a vascular surgeon or radiologist.

? WHERE IS THE PROCEDURE PERFORMED?

Because of ancillary equipment needed for many treatments, arterial catheterization is usually done in the inpatient or outpatient departments of a hospital. Placement of a catheter into an artery for chemotherapy can be done in a hospital, an outpatient surgery center, or doctor's office.

? WHAT ARE THE MORTALITY (DEATH) AND MORBIDITY (COMPLICATION) RATES?

Use of a Swan-Ganz catheter was associated with a higher complication rate in elderly patients undergoing aorta surgery in a small (72 patients) 1989 study.[5] Although this type of catheter has a higher rate of complications and mortality, it is the only one that produces the information doctors want.

Simple arterial catheterization itself carries no risk of death and essentially no complications. The mortality and morbidity that are seen are associated with the treatment the catheter is used for, not with the catheter itself. For example, when a Fogarty catheter is used to remove

a clot, the amount of force that the surgeon has to use is determined by the extent to which the artery is blocked, how big the clot is relative to the inside of the artery, how long the artery has been blocked, and how adherent the clot is to the arterial wall. If it is firmly stuck, the surgeon may have to exert enough force to tear the inner lining of the artery in order to remove the clot. Such complications generally heal without incident; others can lead to almost immediate **re-occlusion** of the vessel, and some can tear the artery completely, requiring an emergency operation for vessel repair. Similarly, chemotherapeutic drugs can have a toxic effect on the walls of an artery and lead to vessel **necrosis.**

Mortality and morbidity rates for regional or single-organ chemotherapy delivered through an arterial catheter vary depending upon the organ and the chemotherapeutic drugs used. Most of the morbidity arises from the chemotherapeutic agents, not from the catheter itself. For liver cancer that has spread from the colon, the operative mortality is zero, the operative morbidity rate is 10%, and the rate of treatment-associated complications consists of gastrointestinal tract inflammation or erosion in 48% of patients and noninfectious hepatitis in 65%.[6] Mispositioning of the catheter can be expected in up to 3.4% of all chemotherapy cases, a situation not always detectable on a standard x ray.[7]

A 1988 study of women with ovarian cancer found minor complications (for example, infection at the site of the catheter) in 13.6% of patients and major complications (for example, intestinal **perforation, peritonitis**, fever, hemorrhage, catheter obstruction, and pain) in 17%; an operation for removal of the catheters was required in 11.9% (70% of those who had major complications).[8]

When a Fogarty catheter was used to remove a clot in one large study, the **perioperative mortality** rate was 20% and the rate of complications leading to amputation were zero for upper limbs and 13% for lower limbs.[9] In another series of late **embolectomies** over a period of 22 years, the mortality rate was 15.55% and the rate of complications leading to amputation was 17.8%. The rate of limb salvage for the later cases in the series was 91.6%, with an 8.4% rate of limb loss.[10]

? WHAT ARE THE OTHER COMPLICATIONS AND POSSIBLE SIDE EFFECTS?

Perforation of the pulmonary artery can occur during the placement or removal of a Swan-Ganz catheter,[11] and has a high mortality rate.[12] Damage sufficient to require another replacement of the mitral valve, situated in the left side of the heart, occurred in one patient with an artificial mitral valve.[13] It is also possible for the catheter to get tangled in the sutures used for a heart repair.[14]

Totally implantable catheters, which leave nothing outside the body, are still experimental. The idea behind them is that drugs can be delivered continuously through the catheter from a reservoir (a bladder attached to the catheter, filled with medication, and implanted) without tying the patient to an IV stand. As the person breathes, bends, or otherwise moves, the bladder is squeezed, forcing the medication out. The lack of anything outside the body would encourage patient acceptance of long-term intravenous or intraarterial therapy. The reservoir in most systems is filled by an ordinary hypodermic needle when needed, and is made of plastic, somewhat like a gum eraser, that reseals itself as the needle is withdrawn. Unfortunately, some devices have shown a major complication rate as high as 40%.[15]

Healing around the puncture wound through which the typical catheter enters tends to create a "funnel" that can channel bacteria into the body. Thus, infection can occur at the site of any catheter. The use of a cuffed catheter, which has an inflatable cuff around the end that holds it in place, can prevent this to some extent, by creating a better seal of the insertion point. So can careful attention to sterility in implanting and changing

the catheters.[16] **Thrombosis** may occur in up to 28% of patients but may reach clinical significance—that is, have discernible signs—in only 6%.[17]

When chemotherapy drugs are given for brain cancer, with a catheter implanted in the **carotid artery**, there can be damage to one or both eyes if the drug is not administered with the catheter tip above the intersection of the carotid artery and the supraophthalmic artery, which is located above and over the eye. Safe use of this therapy is simply a matter of proper dilutions of medication and positioning technique on the doctor's part.[18, 19] Even under ideal conditions, however, minor complications can be expected in about 20% of patients having carotid artery chemotherapy.[20]

When the brachial artery of the arm is used, complications can occur in about 23% of patients, but few complications result in any permanent damage.[21] Studies of the use of arterial catheters in gynecologic cancers have also found complication rates in the 20% range.[22] In cases of cancer of the tongue, a malposition of the catheter can occur in up to 71% of cases.[23] However, careful technique by the doctor makes it possible to have complication rates as low as zero to 2%.[24–26]

? IS THIS THE MOST APPROPRIATE PROCEDURE FOR THE CONDITION?

Pulmonary artery catheterization with a Swan-Ganz catheter for monitoring does not seem to be any more effective than central venous pressure monitoring in patients undergoing heart surgery, and the placement of the central venous line is technically simpler.[27, 28] (In this procedure, the catheter is introduced through the vein in the inside crook of the arm and threaded on through to the **superior vena cava**. Attached to the end of the catheter is an instrument for measuring the force of blood flow.) One study estimates that only 2% of postoperative complications in elderly patients would be prevented by the use of a Swan-Ganz catheter.[29]

Swan-Ganz catheterization has been shown to be more effective than clinical judgment alone in diagnosing the cause of shock and pulmonary **edema**, but the usefulness is limited in the case of shock because no effective therapy may be available to reverse the problem.[30] However, in selected high-risk patients, pulmonary artery catheterization has been associated with higher survival, although there was no difference between pulmonary artery catheterization and central venous catheterization for patients who were not at high risk.[31] Pulmonary artery monitoring was also associated with higher survival in a group of patients having aorta surgery when compared with unmonitored control patients.[32] For patients at low risk, pulmonary artery monitoring made no difference in outcome.[33]

In summary, except for patients who are at high surgical risk or patients who present difficult diagnostic problems in a critical care unit, the Swan-Ganz catheter is associated with higher risk and has no appreciable benefit. Most of the information needed can be derived in other ways. This conclusion is not an atypical finding for many of the most recent high-tech innovations in medicine—they turn out to be lifesaving for a subgroup of patients but useless or even harmful for the majority. The key research task is defining the exact subgroups that will benefit.

Clearly, regional or single-organ chemotherapy is less toxic to the entire body than whole-body chemotherapy, especially if the drug is rapidly metabolized in the organ for which it is intended. So the administration of chemotherapy (and other potentially irritating solutions such as complex nutrients for patients who are receiving total feeding via the circulatory system—a process called **hyperalimentation**) via the arterial catheter route is preferable for cases in which the position of the cancer and the patient's anatomy make it possible. There are normal variations in anatomy, for example in the arteries of the liver, that may make it impossible to treat the entire organ without extensive arterial surgery.

Removal of blood clots by a Fogarty catheter, if possible, is obviously preferable to an open operation, which involves making a large incision.

❓ ARE THERE ALTERNATIVES TO THIS PROCEDURE?

Measurement of pressures using a central venous pressure line seems as effective as Swan-Ganz catheterization for many purposes.

Whole-body chemotherapy and open surgery for removal of clots are alternatives. There is no alternative for introduction of **contrast media** for diagnostic purposes.

❓ WHAT IS CONTROVERSIAL ABOUT THE PROCEDURE?

Except for Swan-Ganz catheterization, there is little controversy about any of these procedures, except for the lack of controlled trials of regional versus whole-body chemotherapy for some cancers. There is little reason to suspect, however, that regional therapy would be any less effective than **systemic** therapy, except for cancers that have spread beyond their original site.

Aspiration and Curettage, Postdelivery (82)

MORTALITY	MORBIDITY	CONTROVERSY
+	+	o

Use of a suction **catheter** to remove all of, or samples of, the womb lining for diagnostic or therapeutic purposes following the birth of a baby

? WHAT CONDITION DOES THE PROCEDURE TREAT?

Aspiration and curettage (usually abbreviated A&C) is a diagnostic and occasionally therapeutic procedure that is performed following birth if there are indications of incomplete expulsion of the placenta; otherwise, it may be performed anywhere from a few days to a few weeks postdelivery, depending upon the symptoms (such as a foul-smelling discharge or pain in the abdominal region). This procedure differs from dilation and curettage (D&C), postdelivery (see p. 140). With A&C there is usually no need to **dilate** the mouth of the womb, the **cervix**, in order to insert the suction device (called a **cannula**), because it is flexible—unlike the rigid instrument (a **curette**) that is used in a D&C—and can easily pass through the cervix. A&C is not necessarily or generally used to detect cancer; however, if the material sucked out is sent to the pathology lab and cancer is detected, then the procedure did detect cancer—but it was not the primary reason for performing it.

? WHAT IS THE PROCEDURE?

The woman is usually only sedated and not anesthetized, except for those few instances in which even the flexible instrument causes pain. (In those cases, general anesthesia is used and the standard D&C is performed.) With the patient placed on the classic gynecological exam table, the doctor inserts a **speculum** into the vagina and locks it to hold the vagina as wide open as possible. She then inserts the suction cannula and moves it along the top and sides of the womb. The material removed is examined by a pathologist to determine if any disease is present. If it is and if the disease is limited to the **endometrium**, and if the suction has been thorough enough, diagnosis and therapy have been accomplished in one step.

? WHO PERFORMS THE PROCEDURE?

This procedure is done by an obstetrician-gynecologist or by a general or family practitioner with appropriate training.

? WHERE IS THE PROCEDURE PERFORMED?

This can be done on an inpatient or outpatient basis in a hospital, although the trend is to do it as an outpatient procedure. It can also be performed in an ambulatory surgery center or in a well-equipped doctor's office. As with all surgery, the most important requirement in any case is that the patient be observed long enough to make sure that the sedative or anesthetic used has worn off completely, and that there is no excessive blood loss before she is sent home.

? WHAT ARE THE MORTALITY (DEATH) AND MORBIDITY (COMPLICATION) RATES?

The mortality and complication rates for this procedure are essentially zero.

? WHAT ARE THE OTHER COMPLICATIONS AND POSSIBLE SIDE EFFECTS?

The chief complication of this procedure is failure to stop postdelivery hemorrhage, which in some studies has been shown to be 89%.[1]

Studies of self-reported stress and stress-related chemicals in the bloodstream suggest that there is much more patient stress in a D&C done under local anesthesia, compared with general anesthesia.[2, 3] This may be true of the A&C as well, although the issue appears not to have been studied.

? IS THIS THE MOST APPROPRIATE PROCEDURE FOR THE CONDITION?

Clearly, this procedure is less invasive and less traumatic than a dilation and curettage, and there is no reason not to try it before D&C postdelivery—unless there are clear reasons for the use of the rigid curette. For instance, the rigid instrument must be used when a large mass of tissue cannot be sucked out.

Another reason for preferring the A&C to the D&C is that most complications appear to be associated with the dilation phase of the procedure rather than the curettage phase. In one study, 98.8% of patients did not require any dilation when a Vabra suction curette (a variation on the A&C that uses a particular type of curette) was used. When one considers situations other than postpartum bleeding, curettage by suction is as effective as the D&C at removing tissue and has a lower complication rate.[4] The accuracy of diagnosis with Vabra curettage of the cervix has been found to be twice as high as the traditional D&C in one study.[5] Another study found that the tissue removed was adequate for pathological examination in 98.8% of the cases.[6] Others have reported zero mortality and zero morbidity using the Vabra device.[7]

In many patients, the Vabra procedure can be used without anesthetic, eliminating the small but real risk of anesthetic complications.[8] A single dose of a **nonsteroidal anti-inflammatory drug** given one hour before operation reduced cramps and backache significantly after Vabra curettage, but did not reduce the pain felt during the procedure itself.[9] In a 1990 Dutch study, Vabra curettage was found to be as reliable as three other methods (conventional D&C, cone biopsy of the cervix—a surgical procedure in which a cone-shaped piece of tissue is cut out of the center of the cervix for diagnostic purposes—and hysterectomy) in detecting invasive cancer, which has spread beyond the tissue layer in which it started.[10] Vabra curettage is not generally used to detect cancer; however, if the tissue sucked out

is sent to pathology and cancer is detected, then the procedure produces results as good as the more conventional procedures usually employed to detect cancer.

A newer device, the endometrial pipelle, is a variation on the Vabra device that produces less pain for the patient.[11] Regardless of the alternative method used, if after repeated attempts the doctor cannot get the suction device into the uterus—because the cervix is too narrow and cannot be dilated under mild sedation or local anesthesia—a conventional D&C should be done under general anesthesia, to ensure the correct diagnosis.[12]

? ARE THERE ALTERNATIVES TO THIS PROCEDURE?

Yes. Besides the D&C postdelivery, another alternative is **hysteroscopy**—the introduction of a small fiber-optic telescope into the womb through a minimally dilated cervix. Sometimes the cervix even will open sufficiently from the application of **prostaglandin** gel, making a dilation unnecessary. Because this procedure gives the doctor a magnified view of any abnormal tissue through the scope, she can sample suspicious areas directly, rather than removing the entire lining of the womb. Hysteroscopy can be done in a doctor's office with a local anesthetic.[13] A comparison of hysteroscopy and the D&C indicated that the D&C provided more information than the hysteroscopy in only 3.26% of the women studied.[14]

? WHAT IS CONTROVERSIAL ABOUT THE PROCEDURE?

The most controversial thing about the procedure is whether there are any compelling reasons not to do it. Recent articles strongly suggest that the hysteroscope or the suction curette be used, and that the classic D&C should be reserved only for patients whose cervixes cannot be dilated enough to use either of the two instruments.

Bone Marrow Biopsy (30)

MORTALITY	MORBIDITY	CONTROVERSY
–	+	o

- The **MORTALITY** figure for this procedure is 7.7%, which is much too high. This figure reflects the fact that serious underlying diseases, most often cancer, lead to the need for bone marrow biopsy.

Removal of marrow from the central channel of a bone for study to assist in the treatment of various serious diseases

? WHAT CONDITION DOES THE PROCEDURE TREAT?

This is a diagnostic procedure that is used to determine what kind of treatment a patient should receive. Diseases for which it can be used in planning treatment include the leukemias (blood cancers), **aplastic anemia,**[1] and several immune system and metabolic diseases.[2]

? WHAT IS THE PROCEDURE?

The site selected—usually the breastbone or front tip of the hipbone, where it is most prominent under the skin at the front of the abdomen—is washed with soap and antiseptic and draped. Depending upon the surgeon's preferences and the patient's tolerance, the patient is given either a local anesthetic plus a sedative, or a short-acting general anesthetic. A combination needle and drill is used to puncture the skin and penetrate into the bone until the central canal, which holds the marrow, is reached. A large needle and syringe is used to suck up a bit of marrow. When enough has been collected, the needle is withdrawn and the entry wound is closed with a bandage.

? WHO PERFORMS THE PROCEDURE?

This procedure is within the competence of any physician, but is usually done by a **hematologist**, immune system diseases specialist (also known as an allergist or **immunologist**), or **oncologist**.

? WHERE IS THE PROCEDURE PERFORMED?

Because of the severity of the conditions that lead to the need for a bone marrow biopsy, this procedure is usually done in a hospital, but it can be done in an outpatient surgery facility or in a well-equipped doctor's office.

? WHAT ARE THE MORTALITY (DEATH) AND MORBIDITY (COMPLICATION) RATES?

Data drawn from the Commission on Professional and Hospital Activities (CPHA), which include a large sample of U.S. hospitals, show a mortality rate of 7.7% for patients who undergo this procedure.[3] This very high figure reflects the fact that serious underlying diseases, most often cancer, lead to the need for the bone marrow biopsy in the first place. Aplastic anemia, for example, has a 38% mortality rate when treated without bone marrow transplant,[4] and the mortality rate for some leukemias is 50% within two years of diagnosis.[5]

A multiyear study of more than 1,000 patients found zero mortality and minor complications in 0.2% of patients. Failure to obtain adequate specimens that were apparent to the surgeon at the time of operation occurred in 1.6% of the cases, and later discovery by the laboratory that a specimen was unsuitable occurred in 5% of the cases, meaning that 6.6% of procedures had to be repeated.[6]

? WHAT ARE THE OTHER COMPLICATIONS AND POSSIBLE SIDE EFFECTS?

Although infections are not a direct risk of bone marrow biopsy (as opposed to the conditions and treatments for which bone marrow biopsy is a diagnostic step), they can be devastating in patients who have had bone marrow transplants. Frequent use of antibiotics and failure to maintain the patients in laminar flow rooms are both associated with increased infections in these patients.[7] (Laminar flow rooms are those in which the air flow is controlled to prevent the entry of airborne bacteria.) The patient's immune system recovers within about a year if the transplant is successful.[8]

As with any procedure in which anesthesia is used, death from reaction to the anesthetic drugs, error on the part of the anesthetist, or machine failure is a remote possibility. (See Glossary, p. 309)

? IS THIS THE MOST APPROPRIATE PROCEDURE FOR THE CONDITION?

The real question is not the appropriateness of bone marrow biopsy but of the treatments that are based on the results of this diagnostic procedure. Bone marrow transplantation, for example, is being done with increasing frequency, despite very high mortality and morbidity rates from graft-versus-host disease—a condition in which the transplanted marrow attacks the recipient—and from the drugs given to suppress this harmful attack.

? ARE THERE ALTERNATIVES TO THIS PROCEDURE?

If a specimen of bone marrow is actually needed, no.

? WHAT IS CONTROVERSIAL ABOUT THE PROCEDURE?

Because a rare childhood disease of the blood known as transient erythroblastopenia—a type of acquired anemia—can mimic leukemia, it is important to rule out this anemia disease before proceeding to do a bone marrow biopsy on a child.[9] Bone marrow studies are not needed prior to the treatment of transient erythroblastopenia.

Combined Right and Left Cardiac Catheterization (17)

MORTALITY	MORBIDITY	CONTROVERSY
+	+	o

X ray of the arteries and chambers of the heart using a **contrast medium** injected via a **catheter** threaded into the heart through an artery in the arm or leg.

? WHAT CONDITION DOES THE PROCEDURE TREAT?

This is a diagnostic procedure that is performed prior to any surgical treatment for coronary artery disease, specifically to help determine the kind of treatment needed. A virtually identical set of equipment and techniques is used for percutaneous transluminal coronary angioplasty (PTCA) (see p. 194), laser angioplasty, and similar procedures to remove blockages in coronary arteries, but this exact procedure is used only for diagnosis. The principal problem that it helps to diagnose is narrowing of the coronary arteries that is caused by **plaque** formation. (Although not the same as coronary **angiography**, this procedure is part of the family of procedures called angiography, which is the general term for an x ray of a vessel or organ through the use of a contrast medium.)

This procedure treats what is now the leading cause of death in the United States and in much of the developed world—coronary artery disease associated with plaque formation. The arteries feeding blood to the heart are relatively few in number and fairly small—about the size of a pencil lead on its inside channel. Disease begins when these arteries become increasingly clogged with deposits called plaques. Plaques are a complex mass of cells that form the lining of the arterial wall, cholesterol crystals, and assorted other organic substances. The process of plaque formation apparently needs a slight injury to the wall of the artery to start, but once it has started, it not only narrows the artery but in some way enhances the tendency of blood near it to clot.[1, 2] The walls of the arteries are composed in part of smooth muscle cells. Arteries can expand, relax, and go into spasm; points of repeated spasm seem to encourage plaque formation.[3]

If the clot, or combination of clot and spasm, is large enough to block the artery completely, a person can have a heart attack; if the clot is not large enough to do that but still interferes with the flow of blood, then a person may experience **angina**—a crushing, squeezing chest pain that results from the heart muscle not receiving enough oxygen.

Both heart attacks and repeated episodes of angina pose problems because they deprive the heart of blood for a sufficient period of time to damage the heart muscle, called the **myocardium**. The damaged muscle tends to be replaced by scar tissue as it heals. The scar tissue impedes the normal contraction of the heart's pumping chambers, sometimes to the point that the **ejection fraction**—the amount of blood pumped out into the body by the **left ventricle**—is cut by half or more.

If the attack leads to serious disruption of the heartbeat or if the heart stops pumping completely, the brain is also deprived of blood, and therefore of oxygen. The heart and the brain are both exquisitely sensitive to oxygen deprivation; it now appears that the heart is far more sensitive to oxygen deprivation than previously thought—more sensitive, in fact, than the brain. If the deprivation of oxygen goes on long enough, a portion of the heart muscle dies. Depending upon how large the dead portion is, the result can range from almost undetectable to immediately fatal. Evolution has not prepared us well for having heart attacks; there is even more damage to the cells of the heart wall when blood flow is restored and a complex series of chemical events ensues, causing a great deal of internal damage to the recovering cells. Much current research is aimed at finding drugs that will block the destructive reactions.

Not all of the mechanisms by which this disease progresses are fully understood, but it is quite clear that higher blood cholesterol levels (even those in the "normal" range),[4] being overweight,[5] smoking,[6] stress,[7–12] and not getting enough aerobic exercise (which is exercise that causes heavy breathing and high use of oxygen, and in which the muscles tend to burn fats in the blood, as well as sugar, for fuel)[13] all contribute to it.

Some mechanisms of coronary artery blockage and disease are known. Cholesterol, of course, is a major constituent of plaques. Although cholesterol is an essential constituent of cell walls and the basis for several hormones that are critical for life, we did not evolve to take in large quantities in our diet. The liver, which makes about 75% of our total cholesterol, keeps pumping it out even if the dietary supply is ample. Inadequate aerobic exercise results in ratios of cholesterol-transporting lipoproteins in the blood that favor deposition of cholesterol in plaques rather than carrying it out of plaques to the liver for processing.

Another risk factor is smoking, which loads the blood with carbon dioxide, lowers the oxygen reserve available to heart cells, lowers the level of vitamins that may have some protective effect against plaque formation, and contributes to arterial spasm. The list of known factors grows with each month's collection of medical journals.

❓ WHAT IS THE PROCEDURE?

The surgeon selects the artery (either the **femoral artery** in the thigh or the **brachial artery** in the arm). The patient is then given a local anesthetic. Depending upon the size of the catheter to be used, the size of the patient's arteries, and the difficulty of getting to them, either a **trochar** is used to punch a hole through the leg or arm into the artery, or a small incision is made down to the level of the artery. Depending upon the tests planned, either the catheter or a guide wire is run up the femoral artery into the **ascending aorta**, and turned downward at the arch of the **aorta** (just above the heart, where it turns downward to enter the left ventricle). The catheter or guide wire is threaded through the aortic valve (the valve between the start of the aorta and the heart) into the left ventricle of the heart, which is the main pumping chamber. If a guide wire is used, the catheter is threaded over it once the guide wire is where the surgeon wants it to be.

When the catheter is in the proper position, a contrast medium is injected. The contrast medium is usually a solution of an iodine compound. Images of the left ventricle and the coronary arteries running from the aorta are captured. The catheter is then rotated, and the tip is pushed through the **septum** between the left and **right ventricles**. This is necessary in order to study the pulmonary circulation, which consists of deoxygenated blood pumped into the arteries of the lungs by the right ventricle. It is also possible to enter the right ventricle from the aorta, as described in the next paragraph, but the approach through the aorta is more direct. If the heart is entered on the right side, the puncture runs from right to left, rather than the usual left-to-right course.

If because of disease or mechanical replacement the catheter cannot be inserted into the aortic valve, it can be inserted into the right side of the heart and then pushed through the wall between the right and left ventricles, or through the septum between the **right**

atrium and the left ventricle. Serious complications occurred in 3% of cases using these techniques in one study; 95% of the procedures produced the needed diagnostic information.[14]

With the catheter in place, the **radiopaque** solution is injected into the coronary arteries and the left ventricle, and the flow is photographed with a specialized x-ray camera. The films are reviewed to determine the presence and extent of various problems with the heart's arteries, valves, chambers, and the connections between the chambers (the septa). The catheter is then pushed through the septum between the ventricles, and imaging is repeated for the **pulmonary** circulation. If images are needed of the two upper chambers of the heart, which receive the blood from the body, the catheter is pushed through the floors of those chambers and more photographs are made. After all imaging is complete, the catheter is withdrawn.

❓ WHO PERFORMS THE PROCEDURE?

This procedure is performed by a cardiac surgeon, a radiologist, or an interventional cardiologist.

❓ WHERE IS THE PROCEDURE PERFORMED?

This type of catheterization is controversial. As with many other procedures, it has been found that the mortality and morbidity rates fall as the number of catheterizations a hospital does goes up.[15] In one study, the combined incidence of death, heart attack, and **cerebral embolism** in institutions performing fewer than 100 procedures per year was five times higher than the rate in institutions performing 400 or more.[16] While some studies have concluded that outpatient catheterization is safe for the great majority of patients,[17–19] maximum safety is attained if the outpatient procedure is done in or near a hospital that does a large volume of cardiac surgery. Since up to one-third of deaths can occur suddenly in patients who show no evidence of problems after the procedure,[20] a period of careful observation after catheterization is essential.

? WHAT ARE THE MORTALITY (DEATH) AND MORBIDITY (COMPLICATION) RATES?

Mortality rates reported for left heart catheterization, depending upon the particular study's findings, range from zero[21] to 0.089%[22]; 0.875% to 0.1%[23]; 0.14%[24] to 0.16%[25] to 0.19%[26] to 0.2%[27] to 0.24%[28] to 0.875%, with peaks of 1.8% (for children with cardiac disorders) to 5% (for newborn infants).[29] In a 1987 report, doctors could confidently state that the risk was 0.3% for death and 0.2% for major complications.[30] Because cardiac catheterization is being conducted on older and sicker patients even as its perceived risk declines, these mortality and complication rates are unlikely to be reduced further.[31]

In infants younger than one year, mortality rates of zero to 0.3% and complication rates ranging from 1.5% to 12% were observed.[32] Mortality rates of 1% have been observed in infants in the first month of life.[33]

Judging from studies in which a central venous injection of contrast medium—the dye is injected directly into the veins without using a catheter—was used for **digital subtraction angiography** and no arterial catheter was used, complications attributable to the contrast medium itself occur in about 4.2%, with **renal** failure in 0.2% of patients and **thrombosis** of the vein used for the injection in 0.8%.[34] Other studies have shown that sensitivity to the contrast medium, which can produce very mild to fatal reactions, exists in about 0.4% to 3.1% of patients.[35, 36]

According to a 1991 meta-analysis (a study which used combined data) for all studies published since 1980, the death rate for all procedures that use contrast media is 0.9 per 100,000 (0.0009%). The 95% confidence interval (the range within which the results of 95% of all studies using randomly selected patients would be expected to fall) is 0.0003% to 0.0026%.

The risk of severe reactions was 157 per 100,000 (0.157%) for high-**osmolality** contrast media and 126 per 100,000 (0.126%) for low-osmolality media. No reduction in deaths was found when low-osmolality contrast media were used, although studies universally report better patient comfort with low-osmolality media. The authors of the study note that 80% of severe reactions can be avoided by using low-osmolality contrast media.[37]

A 1978 study found a complication rate of 18%, but no mortality, following left heart catheterization.[38] A 1989 British study found a mortality rate of 0.2%, and complication rates of 0.7% for heart attack during or shortly after the procedure; 0.2% for major vascular complications (such as blood clots in the leg or a stroke); 1.1% for chest pain; 0.67% for minor vascular complications (such as a slight tearing of the aorta or double vision); 0.56% for bleeding at the catheter entrance site; 0.44% for **arrhythmia**; 0.33% for pulmonary **edema**; and 0.22% for reaction to the contrast medium.[39] Another 1989 study found an overall complication rate of 6.9% and a major complication rate of 2.6%.[40] A 1979 study found a risk of 0.13% for heart attack and 0.6% for stroke during catheterization.[41]

Complications from outpatient catheterization severe enough to require hospital admission occurred in 3.9% of patients in a 1989 study; 5.9% were admitted for urgent coronary artery bypass surgery or other procedures after the discovery of major artery blockages.[42]

Use of a pressure-drip flushing technique considerably lessened **thromboembolic** complications and reduced mortality to 0.16% and complications to 1.2% in one study.[43] This technique involves putting a saline solution into the catheter before it is withdrawn from the patient; the thought here is that such a flushing will reduce the formation of blood clots around the top of the catheter as it is being withdrawn.

A 1990 British study found the major complication of **circulatory collapse** in 0.24% of patients having left heart catheterization, with a survival rate of 77% for those who had emergency coronary artery bypass surgery[44] (see p. 88). A Canadian study of cardiac catheterizations for the period 1978–1984 found a mortality rate of 0.1% and a major complication rate of 1.5%.[45]

The use of **heparin** reduced the mortality rate for all catheterizations to 0.04% from 0.2% in the same study. The difference, which appears large, was barely statistically significant—meaning it had little effect on the overall outcome rate of this procedure.[46]

A study that examined mixed cases of heart and brain angiography found that 95% of patients had some side effects. These resolved within one hour in 86.25% of the patients, within one week in 7.5%, and lasted longer than one week in 6.25%; the rate of neurological complications (such as bleeding in the brain) was 6.4%.[47]

Death from **embolism** by pieces of atherosclerotic plaques that are torn off during catheterization has been reported.[48, 49]

Perforation of the aorta and the right atrium during cardiac catheterization has also been reported.[50]

? WHAT ARE THE OTHER COMPLICATIONS AND POSSIBLE SIDE EFFECTS?

Hemopericardium, **ventricular fibrillation**, and **transient vagal reactions** have been noted in patients undergoing left heart catheterization.[51]

The contrast medium used for observation makes a great difference in the patient's comfort and the incidence of side effects. Reactions to contrast medium range from flushing, nausea, vomiting, pain in the leg and chest during and after the procedure, to fatal anaphylactic shock, which is a severe allergic reaction to the medium.[52] If a severe reaction occurs, the morbidity

rate following unsuccessful treatment can be as high as 33%.[53]

Newer contrast agents cause significantly fewer problems than older ones.[54] The degree of pain experienced is apparently related to the **osmolality**.[55] Solutions with less than twice the osmolality of blood seemed to produce no objectively detectable pain sensation.[56] Whether or not the contrast medium is **ionic** may be related to the degree of pain experienced.[57] Severe reactions requiring treatment occurred in 16% of patients given Renografin-60 but only 2% of patients given Hexabrix, a newer medium, in a 1988 study.[58] Injections of Iopamidol, one of the new media, produced the same sensation of heat as the older agent, but no pain in most patients in a small study.[59] Use of Iopamidol has been shown to reduce the incidence of ventricular fibrillation, **hypotension**, and heart rhythm disturbances to a statistically significant degree.[60]

A **thrombus** in the main vein of the liver can cause Budd-Chiari syndrome, which results in great enlargement of the liver, extensive development of new vessels within it, uncontrollable accumulation of fluid in the abdomen (**ascites**), and hypertension in the portal veins and arteries. It is also called Chiari's disease or syndrome, Rokitansky's disease, or Budd's syndrome.[61]

Cardiac arrest, puncture of the heart, and damage to the heart muscle without puncture have also been reported during angiography, occurring at the rates of 1.04% and 0.44%, and have been reported for patients undergoing pulmonary angiography, which is similar to left heart catheterization in technique.[62]

Damage to the artery used to insert the catheter can also occur, and may be associated with loss of a limb if the repair is not adequate. Vascular damage can also lead to embolism in the brain, lungs, or other organs.[63]

Extravasation of contrast medium can occur; this problem is associated, in part, with the use of straight catheters rather than curled "pigtail" catheters.[64] If the medium leaks out of the catheter and gets into the tissue, it can cause reactions in the brain and lungs, or wherever else it went; therefore, it must be gotten out of the system or body cavity in which it accumulated.

The medical literature reported one case of septic shock due to **septicemia** that arose from contaminated contrast medium.[65]

A "complication" of coronary catheterization can be failure to recognize that the patient's problems or chest pain may have a source other than the heart. In a 1990 British study, a majority of patients with chest pain indistinguishable from angina who had normal coronary angiograms and normal left ventricular wall motion turned out to have various treatable esophageal problems. The authors of the study recommend that heart specialists investigate possible esophageal problems in patients who have anginal chest pain and no demonstrable heart abnormalities.[66]

? IS THIS THE MOST APPROPRIATE PROCEDURE FOR THE CONDITION?

Because of the cost and risk involved, most authorities agree that cardiac catheterization should be used only in cases where information about the exact physical location and degree of artery or valve damage is needed to make important diagnostic or therapeutic decisions. If this information is not needed, a combination of blood tests, electrocardiography (EKG), exercise stress tests, **echocardiography**, and **radioisotope studies** can diagnose coronary artery disease.[67]

A 1979 study concluded that "left main coronary artery disease cannot be reliably predicted in patients with unstable **angina pectoris** before coronary arteriography" because of the low correlation between items in the patient's history, results of noninvasive tests, and the actual finding of **stenosis**.[68]

? ARE THERE ALTERNATIVES TO THIS PROCEDURE?

At present, if the information needed is the exact location and degree of arterial narrowing, there is no alternative to this procedure.

? WHAT IS CONTROVERSIAL ABOUT THE PROCEDURE?

This procedure is far less controversial than it used to be, basically because the mortality and morbidity rates have been reduced appreciably over those found when the procedure was invented around 1960. The current controversy concerns the proper role for medical and surgical therapy for heart disease, which is still very much in flux as techniques are developed and information accumulates. No clinical trial comparing coronary artery bypass surgery with percutaneous transluminal coronary angioplasty and medical (nonsurgical) therapy has even been done. A better-informed decision process for determining which patients should be considered for surgery and which should have medical treatment would probably lead to a reduction in the number of catheterizations.

Contrast Aortogram (90)

MORTALITY	MORBIDITY	CONTROVERSY
+	+	o

X ray of the **aorta** with a **contrast medium** inserted into an artery

❓ WHAT CONDITION DOES THE PROCEDURE TREAT?

This is a diagnostic procedure that is used before and after surgery on the aorta to plan operations and evaluate outcomes and to assess the extent of damage to the aorta due to trauma. Surgery of the aorta is required for birth defects and for bulges in the artery walls, called **aneurysms**, which can develop in adults. Aneurysms are a problem because they may rupture, sometimes causing fatal blood loss or, in the case of a cerebral aneurysm, severe damage to the brain's structure.

❓ WHAT IS THE PROCEDURE?

With the patient sedated, the surgeon or radiologist administers a local anesthetic and makes a small cut or skin puncture at a site selected to give easy access to the portion of the aorta that she wishes to study. The various sites where the dye may be introduced are: the **femoral artery** in the leg, the **brachial artery** on the inside of the elbow, arteries and veins in the armpit, or arteries of the lower back; the cut or puncture will be in one of these areas. A sterile **catheter** is threaded up to the beginning of the portion of the aorta to be studied. Dye is injected in high volume (usually about two ounces for a 150-pound person) and still or moving pictures are taken using an image-intensifying x-ray screen.

When the study is finished, the catheter is withdrawn. The entry site is sutured if necessary. Otherwise, a bandage is applied and the patient is observed for any problems while the sedative wears off.

❓ WHO PERFORMS THE PROCEDURE?

This procedure is done by a radiologist, vascular surgeon, or an invasive cardiologist.

❓ WHERE IS THE PROCEDURE PERFORMED?

This procedure can be performed in an inpatient or outpatient department of a hospital, in an outpatient clinic, or in a well-equipped doctor's office. The possibility of a fatal late reaction to the contrast medium makes it necessary for the patient to be observed for a few hours after the procedure.

❓ WHAT ARE THE MORTALITY (DEATH) AND MORBIDITY (COMPLICATION) RATES?

Very few deaths are reported for aortography.[1] The rate of complications is probably lower than for some other exams that use contrast media because in this procedure the medium is diluted by the large volume of blood flowing through the aorta. Complications reported in the literature include **microembolization** and reaction to the contrast medium, which can happen in any procedure using contrast media.

For a discussion of the death rates for procedures that use contrast media, see "Combined Right and Left Cardiac Catheterization," p. 50.

A study from the Mayo Clinic on **urography** found a death rate of 1 in 75,000 (0.0013%), about the same as for penicillin injections.[2] In this study, all patients who died were age 50 or older. A 1987 British study found that the experience of the physician doing the procedure accounted for more morbidity than the type of contrast used, with better results coming from more experienced physicians.

❓ WHAT ARE THE OTHER COMPLICATIONS AND POSSIBLE SIDE EFFECTS?

Temporary paralysis of the bladder and rectal **sphincters** as a result of microembolization following aortic surgery has been reported; this is a theoretical possibility following aortography.[3] (In this context, the word *theoretical* means that any one of a long list of possible complications could happen at any given time with any given patient, but seldom does.) Reactions, other than severe allergic reactions to the dye, vary greatly from patient to patient but have occurred in as many as 68% of patients in studies in which high-**osmolality** contrast media were used. Reactions included headache (34%) and vomiting (31%). The incidence of some, but not all, such nonsevere reactions can be greatly reduced by using low-osmolality or nonionic contrast media.[4] (An ionic medium is one that separates into positively charged and negatively charged molecular fragments, or ions, when it is dissolved; a nonionic one does not.)

? IS THIS THE MOST APPROPRIATE PROCEDURE FOR THE CONDITION?

In cases in which nonemergency surgery on the aorta is required, some surgeons may feel confident enough about results of studies other than aortograms to operate without them, particularly if the problem with the aorta is glaringly obvious and the test results determine exactly the location of the damage relative to other body structures (heart, ribs, etc.). Other surgeons may insist on an aortogram. Because knowing exactly where to cut limits the scope of the operation and, therefore, operative mortality and morbidity to some extent, this is the most appropriate procedure if other studies do not locate the damage precisely enough for the surgeon to operate confidently. That judgment is largely up to the surgeon.

? ARE THERE ALTERNATIVES TO THIS PROCEDURE?

A number of diagnostic procedures, many of them noninvasive, can do much of the work of aortograms, but at present this is the only one that provides the surgeon with a clear visual image of the exact location and extent of damage to the aorta. But even aortograms can be misleading. The most obvious signs of damage are leakage of the contrast medium from the aorta and detection of a flap of the lining of the aorta floating free within the central channel of the vessel. When contrast material is detected on x rays, it means there is a hole in the aorta; similarly, the detection of a flap, which is really a piece of the aorta, signifies that the aorta is deteriorating. Unfortunately, the flow of blood within the aorta can push these flaps against the artery wall where they would not be detected by x rays, because they are no longer floating free within the artery. A flap may also be pushed against a hole in the aorta, thus sealing off the flow of contrast material and preventing detection of the problem. Ideally, x rays should be taken both with the heart fully contracted and fully expanded, and with the patient in several positions. Cine-aortography, which uses movies rather than still pictures, can overcome some of the limitations of still films.

In cases of trauma, ordinary chest x rays may show indications of damage to the aorta; **CT scans** may show many cases of aortic aneurysms. Some problems with the aorta can be found by **echocardiography**, an **ultrasound** examination of the heart.[5, 6] It is generally agreed that the decision to operate, in nonemergency cases, should be made on the basis of aortograms.[7] The word on future diagnostics is that **MRI scans** will be able to replace some percentage of aortograms.[8, 9]

? WHAT IS CONTROVERSIAL ABOUT THE PROCEDURE?

The conditions under which an aortogram should be done following blunt (nonpenetrating) injury to the chest are debated among doctors. About 4.9% of trauma patients have damage to the aorta that is detectable on an aortogram. Several studies have identified findings on ordinary chest x rays that predict the discovery of damage to the aorta at surgery, making it possible to more carefully select patients who need aortograms.[10-12]

Also, if it is possible, there is good reason to delay surgery: mortality for emergency surgery for aortic rupture is much higher than for patients with nonemergency operations—35% versus zero in one series.[13]

The general tendency is for newer, noninvasive procedures to replace older, invasive ones. We can expect that many aortograms will be replaced by MRI in the future, as the technology and software used to produce the images improve. However, such procedures may still require some type of contrast medium to fully define damage to the aorta.

Contrast Cerebral Arteriogram (49)

MORTALITY	MORBIDITY	CONTROVERSY
+	+	o

X ray of one or more arteries of the head with a **contrast medium** injected into the arteries

? WHAT CONDITION DOES THE PROCEDURE TREAT?

This is a diagnostic procedure intended to help determine what treatment to give. Conditions for which it might be used include stroke, threatened stroke, **transient ischemic attacks**, **atherosclerosis** of the cerebral (related to the brain) arteries, and the diagnosis of various causes of dementia and senility. It can also be used to locate the blood supply of benign and malignant tumors of the brain prior to brain surgery.

? WHAT IS THE PROCEDURE?

The patient is taken to the x-ray suite, and a **catheter** is inserted into an artery lying close to the skin surface and associated with the area of the brain to be studied. The contrast medium is injected while x-ray studies are taken.

? WHO PERFORMS THE PROCEDURE?

This procedure is performed by a radiologist.

? WHERE IS THE PROCEDURE PERFORMED?

This procedure can be done in any x-ray facility (hospital, outpatient surgery facility, or radiology suite) that has facilities to observe the patient for reaction to the contrast medium for a while following the procedure.

? WHAT ARE THE MORTALITY (DEATH) AND MORBIDITY (COMPLICATION) RATES?

Severe, life-threatening complications due to reaction to the contrast media used occur in 0.01 to 0.1% of patients who have this procedure.[1]

For discussion of the death rates for procedures that use contrast media, see "Combined Right and Left Cardiac Catheterization," p. 50.

? WHAT ARE THE OTHER COMPLICATIONS AND POSSIBLE SIDE EFFECTS?

Tissue death in the spinal cord of the neck is a complication following this procedure, and arises from both brief loss of oxygenated blood to the cord and leakage of the dye into the spinal canal.[2]

About one cancer is produced per 16,000 to 60,000 procedures performed, depending on where on the body the procedure is done and the radiation dose.[3]

? IS THIS THE MOST APPROPRIATE PROCEDURE FOR THE CONDITION?

The risk associated with this procedure is low, but since there are alternative, less invasive techniques available, it should be reserved for after a diagnosis has been established by other means and before surgery.

? ARE THERE ALTERNATIVES TO THIS PROCEDURE?

CT scans made with dilute contrast media (meaning, at less than full strength) can substitute for arteriograms in many instances.[4, 5] **Digital subtraction angiography**, which permits the use of less concentrated contrast media, can also be used.[6]

There are two other alternatives: phonoangiography, which uses sound waves in the arteries of the eyes; and oculoplethysmographic studies, which use timing of transmission of pressure waves in the arteries of the eyes. These are noninvasive and can provide most of the information that the cerebral arteriogram does, but are slightly less precise in giving the exact location of **lesions.** Both may possibly fail to detect the actual severity of lesions. The key point, in clinical decision-making, is that lesions can appear severe on arteriograms but no major circulatory problems may be revealed with these

two alternative tests, which measure the actual dynamics of blood flow rather than "how bad it looks on the film" (meaning that the imaging tests—x ray or arteriogram—show what appear to be major lesions but the actual blood flow measurements are normal). The availability of actual blood measurements makes possible a policy of "watchful waiting" until definite problems appear.[7, 8] Surgeons, of course, prefer to know exactly where to operate, so at least one arteriogram will nearly always precede surgery.

? WHAT IS CONTROVERSIAL ABOUT THE PROCEDURE?

This procedure itself is not controversial, but many of the procedures which it leads to are. For example, about 44% of patients show marked improvement between arteriograms, indicating that the obstruction that was causing the symptoms may be transient in nature—for example, a blood clot that the body succeeds in dissolving. The author of one study suggests that cerebral artery surgery (in this case, the internal-external cerebral artery bypass) be delayed at least six weeks and preceded by another study unless symptoms require immediate treatment.[9]

Contrast Phlebogram of the Leg (44)

MORTALITY	MORBIDITY	CONTROVERSY
+	+	o

X ray of one or more veins of the leg using a **contrast medium** injected into a vein

? WHAT CONDITION DOES THE PROCEDURE TREAT?

This is a diagnostic procedure intended to locate vein damage due to injury—either **stenosis**, **aneurysm**, or **thrombosis**—and other conditions affecting the veins of the leg. Poor blood circulation in the lower limbs can lead to a number of problems, including **gangrene** and the need to amputate a foot or part of the leg. Amputations of part of the leg may lead to operative mortality as high as 15% (see "Above-the-Knee Amputation," p. 101, and "Below-the-Knee Amputation," p. 114). Problems with the veins of the leg can be caused by such factors as diabetes, smoking, and injury.

Veins contain one-way valves that allow the blood to flow only toward the heart. Blockage of the vein at any site by a blood clot leads to changes in the wall of the vein. These changes can cause scarring and permanently block all or part of the blood flow, even after the clot dissolves or breaks loose and moves elsewhere into circulation. If the clot lodges in or at a valve in a vein (which is common because of the way the valve lies across the inside of the vein), changes in the valve tissue can lead to destruction of the valve. This leaves a length of vein with uncontrolled blood flow, which can create circulatory problems affecting the whole leg.[1] Examples of such problems are varicose veins, swelling of the leg, and pooling of blood in the leg.

? WHAT IS THE PROCEDURE?

Usually, the patient is given only a local anesthetic, and perhaps valium as a mild sedative. However, if the surgeon has reason to suspect that a vein must be removed, then and only then would she give the patient a general anesthetic.

For veins that are right on the surface of the leg, the contrast medium is simply injected through a needle inserted into the vein. Other veins can be reached with a deeper needle puncture and insertion of a small **cath-eter**. And some others may need to be reached through a small incision, but the surgery needed to reach the vein is minor in all cases.

When the contrast medium is injected into the vein, x rays are taken. Depending upon the length of the vein to be examined, what is found, and the need for measurements of narrowing, further injections of contrast medium may be needed.

? WHO PERFORMS THE PROCEDURE?

This procedure is performed by a radiologist or vascular surgeon.

? WHERE IS THE PROCEDURE PERFORMED?

This procedure can be done on an inpatient or outpatient basis in a hospital, in an outpatient surgery or diagnostic center, or in a doctor's office, if it is well equipped. Equipment to deal with cardiac arrest and breathing problems should be available, because some reactions to contrast media can be fatal.

? WHAT ARE THE MORTALITY (DEATH) AND MORBIDITY (COMPLICATION) RATES?

No mortality from this specific examination has been reported in the abstracts maintained by the National Library of Medicine since 1976. The complication rate was as high as 50% in a study that used sophisticated diagnostic techniques to find clots in the vein after the procedure was performed and when **ionic contrast media** were used.[2]

For discussion of death rates for procedures that use contrast media, see "Combined Right and Left Cardiac Catheterization," p. 50.

? WHAT ARE THE OTHER COMPLICATIONS AND POSSIBLE SIDE EFFECTS?

Destruction of the skin at the site of the injection resulting from retention of the contrast medium, and the development of blisters that took months to heal have been reported.[3] When used for a vein in which a clot is already present, the procedure may make the problem worse; it may even lead to the formation of new clots. These two problems combined occur in about 5% of cases.[4]

? IS THIS THE MOST APPROPRIATE PROCEDURE FOR THE CONDITION?

Because this is a diagnostic procedure, its appropriateness depends upon the therapy that is planned. If only medical therapy is planned, the doctor does not need to know exactly where a lesion is, she only needs to know that constriction or blockage of the veins is present and needs to be treated. That information, together with a good indication of the site of the problem, can be obtained with **ultrasound**. A procedure called plethysmography, which measures volume changes in a limb, can indicate that there is a problem with a vein, but can give only a very rough indication of where it is.[5]

On the other hand, if surgery is planned, the surgeon needs to know which portions of the vein need to be operated on, and at present, only a phlebogram can give this information, since methods other than the phlebogram are only 85% to 95% accurate and tend to miss problems with smaller and deeper vessels.[6] There is a possibility in the future that with improved computer software for image generation, **MRI scans** can be used to detect some vein problems.

? ARE THERE ALTERNATIVES TO THIS PROCEDURE?

See "Is this the most appropriate procedure for this condition?"

? WHAT IS CONTROVERSIAL ABOUT THE PROCEDURE?

The biggest controversy concerns the use of contrast media; ionic versus nonionic, and low-**osmolality** versus high-osmolality. The traditional contrast medium causes a variety of reactions in many people; the newer (nonionic, low-osmolality) media cause much less discomfort and provoke fewer reactions. These newer agents are more expensive than the older ones, however, and so there is a tendency not to use them, especially for patients on Medicare or Medicaid who are thought to be "underpaying" their way. Because 80% of severe reactions can be avoided with the newer (nonionic, low-osmolality) media, patients should request that newer media be used, in spite of their higher cost.

Cystoscopy (18)

MORTALITY	MORBIDITY	CONTROVERSY
+	+	o

Examination of the inside of the bladder through a scope inserted through the **urethra**

? WHAT CONDITION DOES THE PROCEDURE TREAT?

Strictly speaking, this is a diagnostic procedure designed to determine what is wrong and how it should be treated, but very often diagnosis and treatment are combined if the needed treatment can be done with the **cystoscope**—a bladder-viewing fiber-optic scope. (See

Glossary for more information on scopes.) Conditions that cystoscopy is used to diagnose and/or treat include benign and malignant tumors of the bladder; benign prostatic hypertrophy (an enlarged prostate); bladder stones, kidney stones, and ureteral stones; bladder infections; stress incontinence of urine; and dribbling of urine following urination.

? WHAT IS THE PROCEDURE?

In this procedure, which is performed on both men and women, the patient is asked to urinate. The amount of urine voided is measured. The patient is then given a spinal anesthetic or an injectable general anesthetic and is placed on a table with stirrups much like that used for a gynecological exam. The scope is lubricated and inserted through the penis (in men) and through the vagina (in women). The residual urine in the bladder is sucked out and measured. This measurement is added to the first measurement to give a number indicator of total bladder capacity. (The relationship of bladder capacity to what remains after urinating tells the urologist how well the bladder is functioning. If, for instance, the bladder holds 20 cc and there are 5 cc remaining, the bladder is functioning at 75%.) Then the bladder is inflated with saline or other solutions and visually examined with the scope. If a condition that can be treated through the scope is found, **catheters**, **Randall stone forceps**, **cautery probes**, and biopsy knives can be passed through the scope to do the needed work.

? WHO PERFORMS THE PROCEDURE?

This procedure is performed by a urologist.

? WHERE IS THE PROCEDURE PERFORMED?

The procedure is done in a hospital (on either an inpatient or outpatient basis), in an outpatient surgery center, or in a well-equipped doctor's office.

? WHAT ARE THE MORTALITY (DEATH) AND MORBIDITY (COMPLICATION) RATES?

The mortality rate for diagnostic cystoscopy is zero.

Injury to the urethra is described as "extremely common."[1] Possible injuries are tearing and bruising of the urethra; these usually occur as a result of rough handling. A complication limited to men is a condition in which **fibrosis** and scarring following injury cause the penis to bend and become impossible to straighten. This may require reconstructive surgery.[2] **Iatrogenic** (doctor-caused) injuries to the penis, including narrowing of the urethra, are increasing, but can be prevented by special care on the part of the doctor.[3]

? WHAT ARE THE OTHER COMPLICATIONS AND POSSIBLE SIDE EFFECTS?

Failure to adequately sterilize all parts of the cystoscope and the instruments used through it has been associated with repeated outbreaks of infection.[4]

Reflux of urine out of the bladder and back into the kidneys can occur in up to 20.6% of patients who have had cystoscopic treatment of bladder tumors.[5] Even carefully sterilized catheters can still carry bacterial toxins that can cause fever, even when all bacteria have been killed.[6]

Explosions inside the bladder can occur when electrosurgery probes break down water into hydrogen and oxygen, an explosive combination that can be ignited by the heated probe. Careful evacuation of all gas from the bladder as it is formed can prevent this complication, which is rare.[7] Although not usually fatal, this complication may cause severe damage to abdominal organs.

? IS THIS THE MOST APPROPRIATE PROCEDURE FOR THE CONDITION?

Because cystoscopy is used for a wide variety of conditions, the answer depends upon the condition. There is little, if any, need for cystoscopy simply to measure residual urine or as a first step in evaluating stress incontinence. All of the other alternatives to cystoscopy are more invasive and are probably not preferable to cystoscopy, but it is becoming quite clear that this procedure is not as innocuous as it was once claimed to be.

? ARE THERE ALTERNATIVES TO THIS PROCEDURE?

Monthly testing of urine for cancer cells has been shown to be an effective substitute for repeated cystoscopies to check for recurrence in treated cancer patients.[8]

? WHAT IS CONTROVERSIAL ABOUT THE PROCEDURE?

Little is controversial except the mounting evidence that doctors have a cavalier attitude towards the procedure; that they perform it unnecessarily with little regard for possible complications; and that they handle these delicate tissues too roughly.[9] More attention should be paid to avoiding complications, even though they are relatively rare.

Diagnostic Laparoscopy (56)

MORTALITY	MORBIDITY	CONTROVERSY
+	−	o

- Minor **COMPLICATIONS** can be as high as 5.1% to 9.4%. Major complications run as high as 1.8% to 2.3%, and include: **hematomas** in the abdominal wall; bleeding that irritates the **peritoneum**; and **respiratory depression** (slow breathing).

Examination of the organs within the abdominal cavity via a small lighted telescope inserted through an incision in or just below the navel

? WHAT CONDITION DOES THE PROCEDURE TREAT?

This is a diagnostic procedure that can also be used to guide a variety of treatments and surgical procedures within the abdominal cavity. Here we discuss the two main diagnostic uses for laparoscopy: (1) the diagnosis of conditions that can be identified by visual inspection of the organs and surrounding structures; and (2) the retrieval of biopsy specimens that cannot be obtained by inserting a biopsy needle through the skin. If, for example, the results from a needle biopsy of the liver are unclear, a better and larger sample can be taken with the laparoscope.[1] Laparoscopy is also valuable in determining the cause of infertility in women.[2, 3] Certain infertility procedures such as **gamete intra-fallopian transfer** (**GIFT**) can be performed at the same time the diagnostic study is done, if the diagnosis indicates that GIFT might work. In this way, two separate operations are avoided.[4] The same approach can also be used for other infertility treatments.[5]

In cases of suspected appendicitis, laparoscopy can provide a definitive diagnosis. This enables the patient to avoid the removal of a normal appendix, which can occur up to 25% of the time.[6]

In cases of undescended testicles in males, laparoscopy

is superior to ultrasound in locating the undescended testicle within the abdominal cavity.[7] (An undescended testicle occurs when the testicle fails to move out of the abdominal cavity, where it is formed in the fetus, and into the scrotum before birth.)

? WHAT IS THE PROCEDURE?

First the patient is placed under general anesthesia, combined light general and local anesthesia, or local anesthesia.[8] Then the region around the navel and any other incision sites that are needed are shaved if necessary, scrubbed with soap and antiseptic, and draped with sterile sheets, exposing only the points where the scope will be inserted. A small incision is made in the navel, or just below it. Bleeding vessels are cauterized with an **electrocautery device**. Any other incisions needed for access by biopsy forceps or other instruments are made, and bleeding is controlled. The laparoscope is inserted through the navel incision and the abdominal cavity is inflated with carbon dioxide, to separate the organs. The surgeon looks through the scope (or at a TV monitor connected to a TV camera in the scope)[9] and takes biopsy samples of tissue.

If any surgical treatment is needed and the surgeon can easily perform it with the operative set-up, it may be done at this time. Videotapes of the TV signal or still photographs may be taken. When the examination and tissue sampling are complete, the abdomen is deflated and the scopes and other instruments are withdrawn. Bandages are applied to the incisions. The patient is taken to the recovery room and then to her room.

If **adhesions** (see "Peritoneal Adhesiolysis," p. 197) are present, a **culdoscopy** can establish a safe point for insertion of the laparoscope.[10] Culdoscopy is an examination of the union between the vagina and uterus at the top of the vagina, which offers a route into the abdomen.

? WHO PERFORMS THE PROCEDURE?

This procedure can be done by a general surgeon, a gastroenterologist, a gynecologic surgeon, or a family physician or general practitioner who has special training in laparoscopy.

? WHERE IS THE PROCEDURE PERFORMED?

This procedure can be performed in the inpatient or outpatient departments of a hospital, an outpatient surgery center, or a well-equipped doctor's office.

? WHAT ARE THE MORTALITY (DEATH) AND MORBIDITY (COMPLICATION) RATES?

The mortality rate from laparoscopies that involve only visual inspection of the abdomen is essentially zero. A mortality rate of 0.09% is reported for uncontrollable bleeding following liver biopsy; another study reports 0.01%.[11]

Minor complications can be as high as 5.1% to 9.4% and major complications may run as high as 1.8% to 2.3%. Major complications include **hematomas** in the abdominal wall, bleeding irritating the **peritoneum**, and **respiratory depression**. Diagnosis is not achieved in 18% of cases, primarily because of adhesions that block the scope.[12, 13] Mortality and major complication rates of zero have also been reported.[14]

In some cases, suppressed breathing may be due to changes in **blood electrolytes** that are found with the use of carbon dioxide (CO_2) but not with nitrous oxide (N_2O).[15]

Medical studies can involve surveys of records that are not made with later studies in mind (called **retrospective studies**) or can involve formal reporting protocols established before the study begins (called **prospective studies**). There is universal agreement that prospective studies are more accurate than retrospective studies. A prospective study of laparoscopy complications found that the minor and major complication rates and mortality reported in the literature (1.07%, 0.3%, 0.03%, respectively) were about seven times too low and that more realistic rates were 5.1%, 2.3%, and 0.49%, respectively. Of course, it is entirely possible that those studies reporting zero mortality and essentially zero major complications did in fact have such records;[6] the question is how typical these studies are.[17]

? WHAT ARE THE OTHER COMPLICATIONS AND POSSIBLE SIDE EFFECTS?

Herniation of the small intestine through the navel incision has been reported.[18]

Necrotizing fasciitis, which is potentially lethal, has been reported in patients with compromised immune systems (resulting from radiation therapy, cancer, AIDS, etc.).[19]

In use of the laparoscope for treatment of infertility, the ovaries may be inaccessible up to 7.4% of the time.[20]

As with any procedure in which anesthesia is used, death from reaction to the anesthetic drugs, error on the part of the anesthetist, or machine failure is a remote possibility. (See Glossary, p. 309)

? IS THIS THE MOST APPROPRIATE PROCEDURE FOR THE CONDITION?

Virtually all **endoscopic** procedures, including laparoscopy, have genuine appeal for doctors—even aside from the higher fees that endoscopy, as a form of surgery, commands—because few diseases of the abdominal cavity have an unmistakable appearance on x ray or **CT scan**. The assessment of diagnostic x rays, even when read by highly experienced radiologists, always has an element of inspired guesswork about it. With endoscopy of any form, the doctor can look right at the diseased organ and even take videotapes and still pictures for later study. When emergency diagnoses of abdominal conditions are made by other means (for instance, x ray, colonoscopy, or palpation), follow-up with laparoscopy revealed diagnostic errors (and made possible a correct diagnosis) in up to 40% of those emergency diagnoses,[21] and in close to 60% of diagnoses of pelvic pain.[22] So its appeal should be apparent.

? ARE THERE ALTERNATIVES TO THIS PROCEDURE?

Yes. X-ray studies, **CT scans**, **MRI scans**, and open examination of the abdomen involving a small incision (called a **laparotomy**) are all alternatives. Laparoscopy is more accurate than most less invasive methods and much less invasive than laparotomy.

? WHAT IS CONTROVERSIAL ABOUT THE PROCEDURE?

Laparoscopy appears to be subject to periodic fads in that its use has waxed and waned. Considering the relative inaccuracy of other methods compared with laparoscopy, it may be underutilized because of a misplaced faith in the accuracy of less invasive methods.

Dilation and Curettage (43)·

MORTALITY	MORBIDITY	CONTROVERSY
+	+	o

• For further information, see "Dilation and Curettage, Postdelivery," p. 140, and "Aspiration and Curettage, Postdelivery," p. 46.

Widening of the mouth of the womb and removal of samples of the womb lining for diagnostic purposes

? WHAT CONDITION DOES THE PROCEDURE TREAT?

Dilation and curettage (D&C) is a diagnostic and occasionally therapeutic procedure that is used for a wide variety of conditions, including abnormal bleeding; postmenopausal bleeding; suspected leiomyoma (a benign tumor, most commonly of the uterus) with bleeding; follow-up for adenomatous hyperplasia (overgrowth of the uterine lining); bleeding from an intrauterine contraceptive device (IUD); incomplete miscarriage; infertility with bleeding; abnormal **hysterosalpingogram**; and abnormal endometrial cells on Papanicolaou ("Pap") smear. Before abortions were legal where they now are, D&Cs were performed for the same result. After the delivery of a baby, a D&C is done if there are indications that the womb did not empty completely at birth.[1] This last use is regarded as the most important role of the D&C.[2]

? WHAT IS THE PROCEDURE?

The standard D&C may be done in a hospital on an inpatient or outpatient basis. The growing trend is to do it as an outpatient procedure. The woman is under general anesthesia and her feet are placed in stirrups on a classic gynecological exam table. The doctor inserts a **speculum** into the vagina and locks it to hold the vagina as wide open as possible. She then begins passing metal dilators through the **cervix** until it is wide enough to insert a **curette**, then scrapes off the top and sides of the womb. The material removed by the curette is examined by a pathologist to determine if any disease is present. If there is disease, if it is limited to the **endometrium**, and if the scraping has been thorough enough, diagnosis and therapy have been accomplished in one step.

The chief problem with the procedure is that the doctor is "flying blind" and may puncture the uterus with the curette while missing a cancerous **lesion** a fraction of an inch away. Puncture of the uterus occurs in about 0.08% of the cases. Studies of **false-negative** and **false-positive diagnoses** made on the basis of tissue samples taken via D&C suggest that it is not a highly accurate procedure.

? WHO PERFORMS THE PROCEDURE?

This procedure is done by an obstetrician-gynecologist or by a general or family practitioner with special training.

? WHERE IS THE PROCEDURE PERFORMED?

This can be done as an inpatient or outpatient procedure in a hospital, in an ambulatory surgery center, or in a well-equipped doctor's office. It is most important that the woman be observed a while before discharge from the hospital, until health care personnel are sure that the anesthetic or sedative used has worn off completely, and that there is no excessive blood loss. Prudence seems to require that the great majority of D&Cs in which a general anesthetic is used be done in or near a hospital in case of anesthetic problems.

? WHAT ARE THE MORTALITY (DEATH) AND MORBIDITY (COMPLICATION) RATES?

The mortality rate for this procedure in community hospitals in the United States in 1989 was zero. Incidences of zero mortality, 0.08% for uterine punctures, and 2.8% for complications other than uterine puncture for second-trimester abortions performed by D&C have been reported.[3] Rates of complications of 1.7% have also been reported.[4]

? WHAT ARE THE OTHER COMPLICATIONS AND POSSIBLE SIDE EFFECTS?

D&Cs are not very impressive as diagnostic tools; false-negative rates of 15% and above have been reported.[5]

Forced **dilation** of the cervix may cause **cervical incompetence** during subsequent pregnancies.[6, 7]

Although relatively rare, infection serious enough to cause septic arthritis and require surgical drainage of abscesses has occurred following D&Cs.[8]

As with any procedure in which anesthesia is used, death from reaction to the anesthetic drugs, error on the part of the anesthetist, or machine failure is a remote possibility. (See Glossary, p. 309)

Studies of self-reported stress and measurements of chemicals in the bloodstream released when the body is under stress suggest that there is much more stress on the woman with a D&C done under local anesthesia, compared with general anesthesia.[9, 10]

? IS THIS THE MOST APPROPRIATE PROCEDURE FOR THE CONDITION?

The answer seems to be clearly "No." The procedure has a questionable **diagnostic yield** at best, and causes pain to the woman and unnecessary trauma to the female genitalia. It can clearly be replaced, in the vast majority of cases, by procedures that are cheaper, give the doctor better information, and do not carry risks associated with general anesthesia.

Consider how much information a D&C provides in regard to cancer. In one 10-year review of diagnostic D&Cs, the detection or diagnosis of uterine cancer did not significantly increase until after the age of 50. The incidence of premalignant tissue changes rose smoothly from 4% in a group of adolescents to 16% in the 45 to 49 year age group and then declined again, until age 70, when it started to rise once more. The authors of the study conclude that the D&C should be replaced

by another procedure with less complexity and better diagnostic yield for abnormal uterine bleeding.[11]

Most complications appear to be associated with the dilation of the cervix rather than with the curettage. In one study, 98.8% of women did not require any dilation when a Vabra suction curettage was used (which performs the curettage portion of the procedure by suction rather than scraping). Apparently, this stage of the procedure—dilation—could just about be eliminated if the Vabra device were used (see more under alternatives, below).

? ARE THERE ALTERNATIVES TO THIS PROCEDURE?

Yes. **Hysteroscopy** is the introduction of a small fiber-optic telescope into the womb through a minimally dilated (to about the diameter of a pencil) cervix. Sometimes the cervix will open sufficiently from the application of **prostaglandin** gel (a drug with many effects, in this case to widen or dilate), making a dilation unnecessary. Since the doctor has a magnified view of any abnormal tissue through the scope, she can sample suspicious areas directly, rather than removing the entire **endometrium**, which if removed properly will regrow. A further advantage is that hysteroscopy can be done in a doctor's office with a local anesthetic.[12] A comparison of hysteroscopy and the D&C indicated that the D&C provided more information than the hysteroscopy in only 3.26% of the women studied.[13]

Curettage by suction (with the Vabra curettage) is as effective as D&C at removing tissue and has a lower complication rate.[14] The accuracy of diagnosis with Vabra curettage of the cervix has been found to be twice as high as the traditional D&C in one study.[15] Another study found that the tissue removed was adequate for pathological examination in 98.8% of the cases.[16] Others have reported zero mortality and zero morbidity using the Vabra device.[17]

In many women, the Vabra procedure can be used

without anesthetic, eliminating the small but real risk of anesthetic complications.[18] A single dose of a **nonsteroidal anti-inflammatory drug** given one hour before the operation reduced cramps and backache significantly after Vabra curettage, but did not reduce the pain felt during the procedure itself.[19] In a 1990 Dutch study, Vabra curettage was found to be as reliable as three other methods (conventional D&C, cone biopsy of the cervix, and hysterectomy) in detecting invasive cancer (cancer is called "invasive" if it has spread beyond the tissue layer in which it started).[20]

A newer device, the Endometrial Pipelle (see "Aspiration and Curettage, Postdelivery," p. 46), is a variation on the Vabra device that produces less pain for the woman.[21] Regardless of the alternative method used, if the doctor cannot get the suction device into the uterus because the cervix is too narrow and cannot be dilated under local anesthesia, correct diagnosis requires that a D&C be done under general anesthesia.[22]

? WHAT IS CONTROVERSIAL ABOUT THE PROCEDURE?

The most controversial thing about the procedure is whether it should be done at all for diagnosis. Recent articles strongly suggest that the hysteroscope or the suction curette be used, with the classical D&C reserved only for those women whose cervixes cannot be dilated enough to use these instruments. Of course, some D&Cs would be required after diagnosis, but the diagnostic use of this procedure would virtually disappear if this advice were followed.

Endoscopic Biopsy of the Bronchus (38)

MORTALITY	MORBIDITY	CONTROVERSY
+	+	o

Examination of the inside of the **bronchial tree** of the lungs through a fiber-optic scope and the removal of tissue specimens for analysis

? WHAT CONDITION DOES THE PROCEDURE TREAT?

This is a diagnostic procedure that helps to determine what is wrong with the patient and what treatment to give. The **endoscope** can also be used to treat diseases of the bronchial tree and retrieve foreign objects that have been inhaled.

? WHAT IS THE PROCEDURE?

The patient is given sedatives and a short-acting general anesthetic. The endoscope is lubricated and inserted through the mouth and into the **trachea**, and the **bronchi** are examined visually. If a **lesion** is found, a sample is taken with a small biopsy forceps that is passed through a channel of the endoscope. The scope is withdrawn and the patient is taken to the recovery room.

? WHO PERFORMS THE PROCEDURE?

This procedure is performed by a pulmonologist, thoracic surgeon, general surgeon, or otolaryngologist (ear, nose, and throat specialist).

? WHERE IS THE PROCEDURE PERFORMED?

The procedure is done either on an inpatient or outpatient basis in a hospital, in an outpatient surgery facility, or in a well-equipped doctor's office.

? WHAT ARE THE MORTALITY (DEATH) AND MORBIDITY (COMPLICATION) RATES?

A 1991 study shows zero mortality and complication rates of 1.8% for coughing up of more than 100 ml (about three ounces) of blood; 8.9% for chest pain; and 1.2% for **pneumothorax**.[1]

? WHAT ARE THE OTHER COMPLICATIONS AND POSSIBLE SIDE EFFECTS?

There are essentially no other complications from endoscopic biopsy.

As with any procedure in which anesthesia is used, death from reaction to the anesthetic drugs, error on the part of the anesthetist, or machine failure is a remote possibility. (See Glossary, p. 309)

? IS THIS THE MOST APPROPRIATE PROCEDURE FOR THE CONDITION?

Yes, in the sense that it is less invasive than most other alternatives.

? ARE THERE ALTERNATIVES TO THIS PROCEDURE?

X rays and **CT** and **MRI scans** can reveal the presence of a lesion in the lungs, but a biopsy is usually required before it can be determined whether the lesion is benign or malignant. Endoscopic biopsy is much less invasive than **thoracotomy**, which involves opening the chest cavity and cutting into the bronchi to obtain the tissue samples.

? WHAT IS CONTROVERSIAL ABOUT THE PROCEDURE?

There are some controversies concerning the safety of laser use in the lung, but these concern the use of the endoscope for treatment, not for diagnosis.

Endoscopic Large Bowel Examination (32)

MORTALITY	MORBIDITY	CONTROVERSY
+	+	o

Examination of the large bowel (colon) via a **colonoscope** or **sigmoidoscope**

? WHAT CONDITION DOES THE PROCEDURE TREAT?

This is a diagnostic procedure that can be used to check for benign or malignant tumors of the colon, **volvulus** of the sigmoid colon, bowel obstruction due to **adhesions**,[1] inflammatory bowel disease (**Crohn's Disease** and ulcerative colitis[2]), foreign objects in the colon,[3] pseudomembranous colitis—which is inflammation arising from the use of antibiotics in some patients[4, 5]—bowel **ischemia** following intestinal surgery,[6] emergency diagnosis of postoperative bowel complications,[7] and numerous other conditions. When the scope is used with a balloon dilator or similar device, the technique can be used to treat **strictures** of the rectum and colon.[8, 9]

The sigmoidoscope can be used for examinations of

the first two feet of the large intestine; the longer colonoscope has to be used for examinations in the colon higher than two feet from the rectum. The colonoscope and the sigmoidoscope also can be used to remove **polyps** from the lining of the intestine. (See "Endoscopic Colon Polypectomy," p. 141.) The exact reason for their growth is unknown but may be related to irritants in digested food and to a lack of fiber in the diet.

The probability of malignancy increases dramatically in patients with eight or more polyps, reaching 100% in patients with 50 or more polyps. In a study of patients with eight or more colonic polyps, 11.6% were found to have benign stomach polyps, which may become malignant and should be removed. The reverse has also been found to be true—polyps in the stomach can be a clue that there are polyps in the colon.[10] After endoscopic removal of polyps, further colon surgery (to treat **lesions** that cannot be removed with the colonoscope) is needed in about 40% of patients with eight or more polyps.[11]

Physicians now generally agree that endoscopic examination is the most accurate diagnostic technique for most colon conditions,[12] in large part because the procedure allows the doctor to look directly at lesions that may not show up on x rays and **CT scans**.

? WHAT IS
THE PROCEDURE?

The day before the exam, medical staff usually give the patient an enema or one of the preparations (such as GoLytely) that cleanse the colon by inducing painless watery diarrhea. The patient is told not to eat or drink anything until after the procedure. Depending upon the surgeon's preferences and practices, the patient may be lightly or heavily sedated, or given a sufficient dose of sedative to induce sleep. The colon has little sensation above the internal anal **sphincter** (one of two sphincters

that control defecation), but it is sensitive to **dilation** and pulling along its length, which are felt as cramps.

The patient is laid on her left side with the knees drawn up in the classic fetal position. The lubricated colonoscope is inserted through the rectum and is snaked up through the colon to the **ileocecal valve**. The surgeon or gastroenterologist "drives" the scope around the twists and turns of the intestine by manipulating controls on the eyepiece (or handle, if a TV monitor is used).[13] She then carefully and slowly withdraws the scope, looking for polyps and other lesions of the colon along the way. Biopsies can be taken and tumors removed as the scope is slowly withdrawn.

The patient is taken to a recovery area, and when she has clearly recovered from the sedation and shows no signs of bleeding, she is discharged. Patients who have been given sedation are asked to have someone else drive them home, because their reflexes may be slowed even if they feel fully recovered from the sedation.

? WHO PERFORMS
THE PROCEDURE?

This procedure is done by colon-rectal surgeons, gastroenterologists, or family physicians, all of whom should have had special training in the use of the colonoscope.

? WHERE IS THE
PROCEDURE PERFORMED?

This surgery can be performed on an inpatient or outpatient basis in a hospital, in an outpatient surgery facility, or in a well-equipped doctor's office. A study of almost 600 outpatient cases revealed no mortality and a complication rate no higher than that for inpatient procedures.[14]

? WHAT ARE THE MORTALITY (DEATH) AND MORBIDITY (COMPLICATION) RATES?

Now that most surgeons and gastroenterologists performing this procedure are past their "learning curve," mortality rates of zero are regularly reported.[15–17] A study of 5,000 patients reported a complication rate of 1.1% and a mortality rate of 0.06%–three deaths in 5,000 cases.[18] A larger study (36,000 cases) reported a 0.02% mortality rate and a complication rate of 0.148% for diagnostic procedures.[19] Some community hospital studies report zero mortality and zero complications.[20]

Members of the American Society of Colon and Rectal Surgeons reported a complication rate of 0.4% in a mail survey.[21] In a similar study, the American Society of Gastrointestinal Endoscopists reported a complication rate of 0.34% for diagnostic colonoscopies.[22] A case of perforation of the colon leading to rectal **abscess** has been reported.[23] A 1986 study reports a complication rate of 1.2% for colonoscopic polyp removal, with bleeding and intestinal burns from the heated wire loop used to remove polyps the most common.[24] In a Czech study of patients over the age of 65 who underwent colonoscopic polyp removal, a mortality rate of 1.2% and total complication rate of 4.7% were reported.[25] The primary complications are **perforation** of the colon (0.34% of patients), excessive bleeding requiring transfusion (0.23% of patients), and physician judgment that a tumor has not been completely removed when in fact it has, thereby leading to an unnecessary bowel operation (0.46% of patients).[26]

In cases of **toxic megacolon**, perforation can occur in up to 2% of patients.[27] Other studies quote complication rates in the range of zero to 1%.[28, 29] Inability to remove the polyp for one reason or another occurs in about 2.33% of patients.[30] In cases where complications occur, surgery to repair them is required in about 7% of the cases (0.07% of all cases.)[31] An individual physician who is literally just starting the practice of colonoscopies may have a very high complication rate, but this high rate usually drops dramatically with experience. Failure to detect flat lesions that do not extend far above the surface of the intestine is a further problem, but the extent to which this occurs is unknown.[32, 33]

? WHAT ARE THE OTHER COMPLICATIONS AND POSSIBLE SIDE EFFECTS?

Despite the diagnostic power of the scope, up to 25% of polyps less than 5 mm (one-fifth of an inch or less) in size can be missed on colonoscopic exams. Among the many reasons for repeated exams is that the percent of polyps missed on exam increases as their size decreases; only 5% of polyps larger than 5 mm in diameter are missed by a single endoscopic exam.[34] **Septicemia** occurs in about 2% to 4% of patients undergoing colonoscopy, but all the cases in the study cited were subclinical, which means they had no symptoms requiring treatment. However, it would be useful for doctors to keep in mind that septicemia can arise from a colonoscopy.[35]

A potential complication arising from the procedure is that endoscopic bowel surgery leaves signs, such as abrasions and oozing of blood, in the intestine that persist for a short time after surgery and may appear on a **barium enema** study and lead to false diagnosis of other diseases.[36]

The doctor has the choice of using cold or hot biopsy forceps when taking biopsy samples through the biopsy channel of the scope. The hot forceps simultaneously cut and stop the bleeding of tissue at the same time and, therefore, theoretically should lower the rate of bleeding complications because of the cauterizing effect. However, if the hot biopsy forceps are not used with care, the rate of complications can increase.[37]

? IS THIS THE MOST APPROPRIATE PROCEDURE FOR THE CONDITION?

If polyps are discovered in the colon, they can be removed with a colonoscope or sigmoidoscope. The operation can be considered curative if the polyps show certain characteristics on pathological exam. In this case, the risk of cancer after colonoscopic removal is less than the risk of death with an open bowel procedure.[38] It would seem that colonoscopy is the more appropriate procedure for polyps that meet the pathological criteria. If the cancer has spread along the surface of the bowel rather than having grown on a stalk, or if the cancer is not completely removed, an open procedure (necessitating an incision) is required.[39]

? ARE THERE ALTERNATIVES TO THIS PROCEDURE?

The surgeon may elect to remove polyps in the lower part of the colon with a fiber-optic sigmoidoscope, a shorter version of the colonoscope that can reach only about 60 centimeters (about two feet) into the colon. This is much more comfortable for the patient and can be used with no sedation at all, but may lead to missing tumors that are higher than two feet into the colon.[40] About 21% of tumors are located beyond the reach of the sigmoidoscope.[41]

Double-contrast barium enema can also be used to examine the large bowel. It is, however, almost as uncomfortable as a colonoscopy or sigmoidoscopy, can lead to **barium impaction** if the patient does not drink enough liquids after the exam, and can miss up to 50% of cancer.[42]

? WHAT IS CONTROVERSIAL ABOUT THE PROCEDURE?

Worldwide medical opinion now overwhelmingly supports endoscopic removal as the first choice for treatment.[43] A five-year survival rate of 100% has been reported following endoscopic polyp removal in patients who had malignant polyps that were judged to be completely removed through the scope and whose cancer cells were well-differentiated on pathological examination.[44] (Differentiation is a measure of the extent to which a cancer resembles a normal body cell in the location where the cancer was found. Cells with little differentiation are the most malignant.)

The remaining controversy concerns what to do when the polyps show poorly differentiated cells or there is evidence (found on microscopic pathological examination of the stump of the polyp) that cancer has spread into the bowel wall.[45] Use of a laser through an endoscope (as opposed to the heated wire snare that is normally used to remove polyps) can destroy cancer cells that have spread into the bowel wall; this would suggest universal use of the laser, rather than the wire snare, just to be safe, but it is also more expensive and requires more training for the physician.

The laser cannot, however, follow cancer cells that have spread into the blood or lymph channels. All authorities recommend surgical removal of the portion of the colon containing cancer that may have spread beyond the bowel wall and into the surrounding structures of the abdomen. This requires an open procedure and cannot be done with an endoscope. Many authorities also recommend follow-up chemotherapy to take care of any cancer cells that may have spread to other sites in the body.[46]

A Mayo clinic study found that most patients with **cancer in situ** can be treated with endoscopic polypectomy (removal of polyps through an endoscope) but should be carefully monitored to make sure that the cancer does not spread.[47, 48] Other studies recommend the same.[49] A 1989 10-year follow-up study suggests that cancer will occur or recur in at least 1.51% of patients who have had polyps removed endoscopically. Males, those who had multiple polyps removed at the first procedure, and those who have had recurrence of polyps, are at higher risk.[50]

Another study found malignancy in 4.1% of patients after varying periods (anywhere from one to 11 years) following initial removal of polyps.[51] Patients who have malignancy that has spread beyond the original site and is not definitely completely removed should have an open procedure called a bowel resection, in which the portion of the colon containing the cancer is removed.[52]

Microscopic examination of the specimens removed is absolutely essential for correct diagnosis and correct follow-up treatment. One study shows up to a 32% **false-positive diagnosis** rate and a 16% **false-negative diagnosis** rate.[53]

Endoscopic Lung Biopsy (59)

MORTALITY	MORBIDITY	CONTROVERSY
+	+	o

Examination of the lungs with a flexible fiber-optic endoscope and removal of tissue samples for pathological examination

? WHAT CONDITION DOES THE PROCEDURE TREAT?

This is a diagnostic procedure in which a small piece of lung tissue is removed and examined by microscope to determine what disease is present and to decide on a course of treatment.

The **diagnostic yield** for endoscopic lung biopsy is superior to x rays.[1, 2] Yields of up to 98% have been reported.[3]

? WHAT IS THE PROCEDURE?

Because this procedure involves inserting a tube that takes up virtually all the space in the **trachea** and creates a choking sensation even if air delivery to the lungs is adequate, it is often done under general anesthesia.[4–7] A special, small-diameter scope has been used with success in awake patients.[8]

The scope is a flexible tube carrying fiber-optic cables, air and water channels, and a channel through which biopsy forceps can be passed. After the tube is in one of the two main **bronchi,** experienced operators can maneuver the tube into the next two smaller divisions of the bronchial tree, the lobar and segmental bronchi, which carry air to and from the two main divisions of each lung and the segments within them. If the operator finds a **lesion** or a suspicious mass, a biopsy may be taken using the cutting instrument in the bronchoscope. The specimen is then sent to pathology.

? WHO PERFORMS THE PROCEDURE?

Fiber-optic bronchoscopy should be done only by a thoracic surgeon or pulmonologist with special training in the use of the bronchoscope. If a general anesthetic is to be used, the anesthesiologist should have experience or certification in anesthesia for bronchoscopic procedures.

? WHERE IS THE PROCEDURE PERFORMED?

The surgery can be done on an inpatient or outpatient basis in a hospital, in an outpatient or ambulatory surgery clinic, or in a well-equipped doctor's office. If general anesthesia (other than intravenous sedatives that put the patient to sleep without major respiratory suppression) is to be used, it should be done in a hospital.

? WHAT ARE THE MORTALITY (DEATH) AND MORBIDITY (COMPLICATION) RATES?

This is a relatively new procedure. Most of the mortality associated with it seems to be related to **intraoperative** disasters that, once understood as possibilities, can be avoided with due care. Therapeutic procedures seem to be more dangerous than purely diagnostic ones. The mortality rate for diagnostic procedures can be as low as zero, with complications occurring in 10.5% of cases. If bleeding, which is an expected consequence of taking a biopsy sample, is excluded, the complication rate is 1.9%.[9]

In the one large study (48,000 procedures) of purely diagnostic bronchoscopies that we could locate, there were 12 procedure-associated deaths, resulting in a mortality rate of 0.025%. Two deaths and 41 serious complications were attributed to the anesthesia, not to the bronchoscopy, giving an anesthesia death rate of 0.004%. Two deaths resulted from massive hemorrhage after a lesion was biopsied. There were 10 cardiac arrests, for a cardiac arrest rate of 0.021%. Also reported were four cases of brushes, used for obtaining tissue-surface samples, breaking off inside the patient. And all deaths occurred in patients who had preexisting heart disease, severe pneumonia, chronic lung disease, or cancer.[10]

A small series of pediatric patients reported a mortality rate of zero and a complication rate of 11%.[11]

Pneumothorax can occur in up to 4% of cases. Generally, though, only 1% of these patients will need to have a chest tube inserted to remove the air and reexpand the lung.[12]

Many complications in patients with airway disease of one sort or another arise from failure to deliver enough air to the lungs through the scope or damage from a rigid bronchoscope used during part of the procedure. Monitoring of the concentration of oxygen in the arterial blood can avoid many of these, as can other techniques,[13–15] such as blood pressure measurement and pulse oximetry, in which a probe is attached to a finger and leads run to a device that "reads" the oxygen concentration in percentages.

In cardiac transplant patients, minor bleeding after biopsy occurs about 10% of the time.[16]

? WHAT ARE THE OTHER COMPLICATIONS AND POSSIBLE SIDE EFFECTS?

The "complication" of a **false-positive** culture report can occur when the brush used to swab the bronchi to obtain samples for culture is uncovered. When this happens, the brush may pick up any other organism in the endoscope, or may come in contact with tissue that isn't being biopsied. The use of a covered-brush technique essentially eliminates the problem of false-positive cultures.[17] The covered brush is encased in a shield that prevents it from coming into contact with other tissue; the brush is pushed from its shield at the site of the biopsy and then retracted and brought out through the endoscope.

As with any procedure in which anesthesia is used, death from reaction to the anesthetic drugs, error on the part of the anesthetist, or machine failure is a remote possibility. (See Glossary, p. 309)

? IS THIS THE MOST APPROPRIATE PROCEDURE FOR THE CONDITION?

The diagnostic yield is so superior to x rays and the trauma to the patient so much reduced that this procedure is widely becoming regarded as the appropriate procedure for any diagnoses that cannot be made with a chest x ray, **CT scan**, or **MRI scan**.

? ARE THERE ALTERNATIVES TO THIS PROCEDURE?

Yes. If a biopsy is needed, it can be obtained through an open lung biopsy, in which an incision is made in the chest to obtain a specimen. This procedure can have zero mortality and a minor complication rate of about 13%.[18] In patients who had immune system problems associated with bone marrow transplant therapy, an intraoperative mortality rate of zero and a postoperative minor complication rate of 21% have been reported for the open lung biopsy. Postoperative mortality at 30 days, however, was 45%.[19]

A rigid bronchoscope can be used as an alternative to the flexible endoscope typically used for the procedure. The bronchoscope is regarded by some surgeons as a superior instrument for controlling bleeding and maintaining good air flow. It must be used with the patient under general anesthesia.[20]

? WHAT IS CONTROVERSIAL ABOUT THE PROCEDURE?

There are essentially no controversies about this procedure, although the search continues for a combination of sedation and suppression of the gag reflex that will eliminate the need for general anesthesia.

Esophagogastroduodenoscopy with Closed Biopsy (14)

MORTALITY	MORBIDITY	CONTROVERSY
+	+	o

Examination of the **esophagus,** stomach, and **duodenum** with a flexible fiber-optic scope, and removal of small pieces of tissue for examination

? WHAT CONDITION DOES THE PROCEDURE TREAT?

This procedure is primarily diagnostic. However, it can be used to treat, for example, gallstones in the **common bile duct**, common bile duct **sphincter** problems, upper-gastrointestinal bleeding, bleeding ulcers, bleeding from distended veins in the esophagus. Because the endoscope used has channels for instruments such as biopsy forceps, **electrocautery loops**, and lasers, diagnosis and treatment can often be combined. The various treatments done with this instrument have their own names; here, we discuss only diagnostic techniques, although everything said here also applies to the therapeutic procedures.

"Closed biopsy" refers to the removal of a tissue sample with a forceps that pinches off the specimen; no incision is necessary.

? WHAT IS THE PROCEDURE?

Replacement of the rigid instruments previously used for examinations of this type with much smaller and more flexible scopes is a relatively recent phenomenon. (For more details, see Glossary, p. 309.) The scope diameters range from 8.5 to 11.5 mm, or about one-third to one-half inch in diameter. The smaller scopes are better tolerated, especially by children.[1]

In this procedure, the patient's throat is sprayed with a local anesthetic to suppress the gag reflex. The patient is given one or more sedative and antispasmodic drugs, either by intramuscular or intravenous injection. Usually, one of the prominent veins on the back of the hand is used for intravenous injections.

A mouthpiece with a hole in the middle for the scope is inserted between the teeth. The scope is lubricated with a water-soluble jelly and inserted through the bite block down the throat and into the esophagus, stomach, and duodenum. Generally, biopsy specimens are taken, the organs examined through the magnifying eyepiece, and photos are taken through the eyepiece as the instrument is slowly withdrawn; some machines allow connection of the eyepiece to a TV camera, so the physician and patient can watch together on a TV screen.

Even without sedation, there is very little sensation as the scope is advanced and moved. If the local anesthetic does not completely suppress the gag reflex or nausea, this can be done with additional doses of intravenous drugs.[2]

? WHO PERFORMS THE PROCEDURE?

This procedure is done by gastroenterologists, some internal medicine specialists (internists), some general practitioners, some family physicians,[3] and some general surgeons. The use of an endoscope in the esophagus, which is relatively straight from top to bottom, is less dangerous than the use of a similar scope in the twists and turns of the large and small intestines. It is essential that the doctor have been expertly trained and proctored in its use. It is also essential that the doctor have performed a large number of whatever surgical (as opposed to diagnostic) procedure you need to undergo.

? WHERE IS THE PROCEDURE PERFORMED?

This procedure can be done in a doctor's office, an outpatient surgery center, or in the inpatient or outpatient departments of any hospital.

? WHAT ARE THE MORTALITY (DEATH) AND MORBIDITY (COMPLICATION) RATES?

Rarely, cardiac arrest has been associated with this procedure. And one study shows that one-fifth to one-third of patients with cardiac problems will have **transient electrocardiographic changes** while the scope is being inserted.[4, 5] This apparently results from stimulation of nerves in the region of the heart due to the pressure of the scope, and is a complication that can be adequately controlled by drugs in most patients.[6]

? WHAT ARE THE OTHER COMPLICATIONS AND POSSIBLE SIDE EFFECTS?

Most reported complications from diagnostic use of EGDS relate to the heart, and include **ventricular fibrillation** and chest pain. Stimulation of nerves in the chest cavity, as well as emotional stress, may account for some of these symptoms. Indeed, there is some evidence that the cardiac symptoms are triggered by patients' fear (in some cases subconscious) that the tube used for EGDS will impede their ability to breathe. In these cases, better patient preparation—a clear explanation of what will go on and what it may feel like—would probably be beneficial.[7]

One possible chain of events that would explain cardiac complications is this: Many people have never noticed that it is possible to breathe while simultaneously eating or drinking. Few have adequate knowledge of anatomy, and the complete separation of the food tube (**esophagus**) and the windpipe below the level of the mouth is not clear to them. Therefore, it is reasonable for some people to believe, if only on a subconscious level, that they will not be able to breathe with a rather wide tube down their throats—a perception that can induce emotional stress. This stress, in turn, alters the reactivity of blood components, a situation that can lead to cardiac **ischemia** and a possible heart attack, even in the absence of stimulation of the nerves near the heart.[8]

Brief and passing—impermanent—swelling of the upper part of the throat is another complication reported in some patients.[9]

Tearing of the esophageal lining and puncture of the esophagus are possible complications but are quite rare. They are most likely to occur when the tissue has been weakened by cancer or chemical injury.

? IS THIS THE MOST APPROPRIATE PROCEDURE FOR THE CONDITION?

EGDS with closed biopsy has certainly advanced our ability to study and diagnose upper-gastrointestinal-tract disease. An Italian study found that endoscopy was superior to history-taking in that patient histories did not accurately predict which patients would have real **lesions** found by the scope and which would not.[10] Some upper-intestinal parasites, such as *Giardia lamblia,* the most common intestinal parasite in the U.S., apparently are not detectable by the scope and biopsy, thus making scoping worthless as a tool for the diagnosis of these conditions.[11]

The procedure is also said to have "revolutionized" the treatment of patients with stones in the common bile duct and problems with the gallbladder valve, called the sphincter of Oddi.[12] (See "Total Cholecystectomy," p. 248, for more information.)

On the other hand, there are situations in which controlled trials have shown no benefit to early diagnosis of a lesion with EGDS. One study estimates around 1.2% to be the maximum reduction on mortality that could be attributed to earlier diagnosis with this procedure. A controlled trial of more than 5,000 patients would be required to detect an effect that small, and the studies that have been done have involved far fewer patients.[13] The failure to achieve better results may also be attributable to the absence of effective therapies for some upper-gastrointestinal-tract diseases after they are diagnosed.

? ARE THERE ALTERNATIVES TO THIS PROCEDURE?

Basically, the only alternatives are x rays, **CT scans,** and **MRI scans.**

What excites doctors about EGDS is that they are finally in a "What you see is what you get" position with respect to upper-gastrointestinal diseases. X rays and CT and MRI scans all give pictures that are two-dimensional and black-and-white. The radiologist and the treating physician have to associate what they see on the films with their mental pictures of the anatomy involved. Although CT and MRI scans can give a 360-degree view of the areas scanned, finding a lesion depends upon a radiologist looking at the right slice and seeing the lesion. Flat films, such as x-ray plates, are even less efficient because variations in tissue density and transparency to x rays are generally best seen when the lesion is perpendicular to the beam. Because lesions can be anywhere in an organ and usually only a few flat films are taken, the chances of missing a small lesion located at an angle to the x-ray beam are high.

Identifying what the lesion is calls for further guesswork. Many diseases have a highly characteristic appearance on x-ray and scan films; others do not. Radiologists, like all doctors, learn by doing, so part of their education consists of missing lesions and finding out the consequences later. In contrast, the gastroenterologist or other physician performing EGDS has an idea of what she is looking for, and has only to match her mental picture with what is visible in the eyepiece. Many lesions that are hard to detect on x-ray or scan films are easy to see with the scope-aided eye.

For the patient, the big plus for use of EGDS is avoidance of the radiation exposure inherent in x rays and the attendant small but real risk of cancer.

Continuous monitoring of the **pH**—the acidity or

alkalinity—of the esophagus was found superior to endoscopy for detecting early **gastroesophageal reflux**. This procedure should be used if symptoms persist and nothing can be found with the endoscope.[14]

? WHAT IS CONTROVERSIAL ABOUT THE PROCEDURE?

As a diagnostic tool, the procedure is not controversial; most of the controversies concern its use as an instrument for therapy. As users of EGDS gain experience, it will no doubt become clear that some are much better at visual detection of lesions than others, but this will likely promote discussion of how the technique of detecting lesions with the scope can be improved.

Exploratory Laparotomy (58)

MORTALITY	MORBIDITY	CONTROVERSY
—	—	●

- Reported **MORTALITY** rates range from 2.58% to 16% for trauma patients at first laparotomy, to 40% for trauma patients at repeat laparotomy, to 86% at repeat laparotomy for patients over age 65.

- **RUPTURE** of the abdominal wound occurs in only 0.6% of all patients, but the mortality rate in such cases is 34%. A rare but life-threatening complication is an infectious condition known as **necrotizing fasciitis**.

- One of the major controversies surrounding this procedure is the very high **MORTALITY** rate. Another area of controversy is appropriateness of the procedure, unless all other nonsurgical options have been tried.

Opening the abdomen to explore the contents when other diagnostic methods have failed or are not applicable

? WHAT CONDITION DOES THE PROCEDURE TREAT?

An exploratory laparotomy is a diagnostic procedure to determine what disease the patient has and what treatment to give. Many times the procedure does reveal that something is amiss and the surgeon is able to correct the condition through the laparotomy incision. This section refers to exploratory laparotomy as a diagnostic procedure only and does not include whatever treatments may be done as a result.

Exploratory laparotomy may be done in cases of **Hodgkin's disease**,[1] unexplained abdominal pain, **lymphogranulomatosis**,[2] gunshot and stab wounds to the abdomen, blunt (or nonpenetrating) trauma to the abdomen—such as injuries from auto accidents or punches and kicks—and any condition in which a diagnosis of an abdominal condition cannot be made by other means.

? WHAT IS THE PROCEDURE?

The patient is given a general or spinal anesthetic. The abdomen is shaved and scrubbed with soap and antiseptic. A small incision is made over the suspected site of a problem if it can be localized; otherwise, the surgeon makes any one of the wide abdominal incisions that she prefers. Bleeding vessels are **ligated** or **cauterized**. The contents of the abdomen are explored, and if a condition is found that can be treated as part of the same procedure, this is usually done. When treatment has been completed or it is determined that no treatment can be given because the condition is inoperable or the diagnosis is still uncertain, the abdomen is closed layer by layer. The surgeon may close all layers at once if she prefers to, or if the patient's condition makes it necessary to conclude the operation as quickly as possible. These conditions may include a weak heart, lung collapse, or excessive bleeding, especially when caused by abdominal trauma.

? WHO PERFORMS THE PROCEDURE?

This procedure is usually done by general surgeons. Increasingly, exploratory laparotomies for trauma are done by trauma surgeons, and those for cancer are done by surgical oncologists.

? WHERE IS THE PROCEDURE PERFORMED?

This surgery is always performed in a hospital, on an inpatient basis.

? WHAT ARE THE MORTALITY (DEATH) AND MORBIDITY (COMPLICATION) RATES?

Reported mortality rates range from 2.58%[3] to 16% for trauma patients at first laparotomy, to 40% for trauma patients at repeat laparotomy, to 86% at repeat laparotomy for patients over age 65.

The medical literature clearly indicates that initial and repeat laparotomies are very different entities.[4] Second laparotomies that are attempts to find a focus of infection in patients with **intraabdominal sepsis** and that are not directed by positive clinical findings—second laparotomies that are "fishing expeditions"—have a 93% mortality rate.[5]

Exploratory laparotomy for gunshot wounds of the abdomen has a 2.7% mortality rate if major arteries or veins were not injured, and a 39.2% mortality rate if major vascular structures were injured. An incidental finding was that the heroic effort of emergency resuscitative **thoracotomy** was successful in only 10% of the patients on whom it was attempted. The most common postoperative complication was **abscess** formation, which occurred in 3% of patients. The seriousness of the condition of patients with vascular injuries is perhaps best indicated by the fact that 50% of them required more than 18 units of blood.[6]

Mortality from exploratory laparoscopy rises with age, primarily because of the increased susceptibility of the elderly to infection and their inability to recover from the surgery as well as younger patients do.[7] Mortality for second laparotomies in patients over age 65 is 86%, versus 21% for those under age 65. For patients who had signs of organ failure prior to their second laparotomy, the mean survival following the procedure was four days for patients both over and under 65 years of age.[8]

Repeat exploratory laparotomy to determine the stage of disease and the response to treatment has very low mortality in patients with Hodgkin's disease. Even so, a special analysis indicates that in hospitals with a 1% mortality rate for laparotomies on patients with Hodgkin's, the operation is too risky for one in seven patients—and in institutions with a 3% mortality, too risky for one in three.[9] This means that it is unwise to perform even the safer variations in most hospitals.

Exploratory laparotomy for lymphogranulomatosis has essentially a zero mortality rate and a 13.2% complication rate.[10]

Emergency first laparotomy for cancer patients receiving chemotherapy and **corticosteroids** who develop intestinal **perforations** has a mortality rate of 53% and a major complication rate of 50%.[11]

? WHAT ARE THE OTHER COMPLICATIONS AND POSSIBLE SIDE EFFECTS?

Misdiagnosis can be a devastating "complication." A study of 36 patients who were referred for exploratory laparotomy for undiagnosable liver disease revealed that 100% of them had been misdiagnosed and that the correct diagnosis could have been made from information recorded in the history and physical in 31 of them, and from additional laboratory testing in the other five. The 36 patients had a 31% mortality rate and a 61% complication rate.[12]

Rupture of the abdominal wound occurs in 0.6% of all laparotomies and has a mortality rate of 34%.[13] Necrotizing fasciitis is a rare but devastating infectious complication that may require reconstruction of the entire abdominal wall if the patient is to live.[14]

As with any procedure in which anesthesia is used, death from reaction to the anesthetic drugs, error on the part of the anesthetist, or machine failure is a remote possibility. (See Glossary, p. 309)

? IS THIS THE MOST APPROPRIATE PROCEDURE FOR THE CONDITION?

Clearly, performing an exploratory laparotomy for the purpose of determining the extent of spread of Hodgkin's disease is valid; the same is true for lymphogranulomatosis, despite the high complication rate associated with it, because most laparotomies result in some change in treatment.[15] And obviously, bullets lodged in the abdomen should be found and removed.

In other situations, the exploratory laparotomy has an air of desperation after other attempts at making a diagnosis have failed. The most important thing for the patient (or his advocate) to do is repeatedly question the doctor to determine: (1) Have all possible nonsurgical tests been done to determine whether the patient is genuinely sick, and to diagnose the problem? (2) Have all possible diagnoses been considered? Why did the doctor rule out those she is not exploring further? (3) Has she considered using an artificial intelligence (AI) diagnosis program such as NTERNIST to suggest further diagnoses and their appropriate tests? (4) If the hospital does not make AI available to its doctors, why not? Only if all other alternatives have been explored should exploratory laparotomy be considered in nonemergency situations.

? ARE THERE ALTERNATIVES TO THIS PROCEDURE?

Alternatives to laparotomy vary with the range of suspected diagnoses, but reasonable alternatives in nonemergency situations are: "watchful waiting"; treatment of suspected intraabdominal infections with broad-spectrum antibiotics while waiting for culture results; **ultrasound**; **CT** and **MRI scans**; review of the history and physical and lab tests, or retaking of all of them, by a specialist in diagnosis; and second and third opinions prior to surgery.

? WHAT IS CONTROVERSIAL ABOUT THE PROCEDURE?

The major controversies surrounding the procedure concern its very high mortality rate in many circumstances.

In one study of critically ill patients, instead of surgery, a computer-generated mathematical model was used to predict intraabdominal infection. The model was found to be slightly more accurate than exploratory laparotomy.[16] The mathematical model is a decision-support program that runs on a computer and provides diagnoses based on input of test and other results. Doctors, however, are quite fearful of "empirical" therapy —that is, treatment given on the basis of signs and symptoms without a definite diagnosis—and of the few cases of missed diagnosis that could result from use of the model. This fear comes despite the fact that laparotomy exposes patients to a higher error rate at greater risk.

Assuredly, the doctors' thinking results in part from a valid tenet of the field of medicine: Make sure the treatment fits the disease. This requires knowing what the disease is, which in turn requires a definite diagnosis. Also, at least some of their reasoning has to do with their fear of malpractice suits. This situation appears to be yet another area in which "defensive medicine" defends the doctor at the possible cost of the life of the patient.

Fetal Electrocardiogram (61)

MORTALITY	MORBIDITY	CONTROVERSY
+	+	o

LAY TITLE: Fetal EKG

Monitoring of the health status of a fetal heart before and during birth using electrodes attached to the scalp

? WHAT CONDITION DOES THE PROCEDURE TREAT?

This procedure is just one of an increasing number of ways to monitor a fetus during labor. To best understand the entire concept and practice of fetal monitoring, read this section in conjunction with "Fetal Monitoring," p. 83.

? WHAT IS THE PROCEDURE?

An electrocardiogram, or EKG, is a tracing of the expansion and contraction of the heart as it pumps blood through the body. In an adult, it is obtained by taping several electrical contacts to the patient's chest and back. For a baby during delivery, it is obtained with the internal monitor; a **catheter** is threaded through the vagina and an electrode placed on the baby's presenting part (usually the scalp) by means of metal clips or screws.[1] It is also possible to monitor the combined fetal heart rate and force of uterine contractions by a noninvasive procedure called cardiotocography: A belt is placed around the mother's abdomen and the electronic contacts are connected to a monitor. As the uterus contracts, the force and time interval are recorded on graph paper. By monitoring both the fetal heartbeat and the mother's uterine contractions, the doctor has more information about the condition of the baby and mother during labor and delivery.

? WHO PERFORMS THE PROCEDURE?

This procedure can be performed by obstetricians, family and general practitioners who deliver babies, obstetrical nurses, and anesthesiologists.

? WHERE IS THE PROCEDURE PERFORMED?

Because of the small but real risk of fetal injury in **invasive procedures** and the small but real risk of triggering labor that cannot be controlled, invasive monitoring should be performed in or near a facility that is equipped for cesarean-section deliveries and neonatal intensive care.

? WHAT ARE THE MORTALITY (DEATH) AND MORBIDITY (COMPLICATION) RATES?

There is no death associated with this procedure. There is only occasional damage to the infant's scalp. Controversies have to do with its possible negative effect on the birth experience, and with the way that it influences clinical decision-making. Some obstetricians recommend it for high-risk births only.[2]

❓ WHAT ARE THE OTHER COMPLICATIONS AND POSSIBLE SIDE EFFECTS?

The chief complications of all methods are unnecessarily hastened labor and delivery, or delivery by cesarean section. Slow fetal heartbeat—a problem that disappears after birth—may be misinterpreted as fetal distress and can lead to unnecessary surgery.[3–5]

The basic problem with electronic fetal monitoring (EFM) is that the relation of changes in heart rate and rhythm to the actual health of the fetus at a given moment is simply not well understood. Obviously, if the fetal heart stops, a tragedy is underway and should be averted if possible, but beyond that, the meaning of various changes—particularly those that occur just long enough to induce panic in the obstetrician and then revert to normal—is not well understood. Many responses that are believed to indicate fetal distress and result in cesarean sections may be within the range of normal, albeit unusual, fetal responses to the stress of labor.

It is known, for example, that the pressure of the walls of the cervix and uterus on the baby's chest helps expel fluid from the baby's lungs. This may help the infant to avoid inhalation of meconium (which consists of fetal intestinal discharge—mucus, bile, and lining cells of the colon) and may help prepare the baby to breathe. It would be surprising if there were not heart rate and rhythm changes in response to such stresses, and the range of heartbeat responses to the process of labor may be very wide.[6] Because EFM has been in use for only about two decades and the response to any significant change has been panic and a cesarean, we simply do not know exactly which changes indicate real distress and which do not. Given that 90% of even high-risk pregnancies have good outcomes, the gains from fetal monitoring would not be large in any case: The number of fetuses in distress at birth is actually much smaller than the number that experience transient cardiac and other changes that alarm the obstetrician.[7]

One approach to improving the usefulness of fetal heart rate and rhythm data involves a computerized filtering system that is still under development. The system employs techniques that were used to reduce noise on telephone lines as far back as 1959; these were among the first computerlike applications to use electronic circuits, called neural networks, that were "grown" in response to data, very much like the connections among neurons in the human brain.[8] Devices using such techniques could "learn" the range of normal variation in the fetal heart responses, improving their "judgment" and advice to the obstetrician with each birth. Such techniques are not in general use, however.

The American College of Obstetricians and Gynecologists (ACOG), partly in an effort to bring some reason to the field and partly to lay a foundation for defending obstetricians against malpractice suits, has declared that continuous fetal monitoring and "intermittent auscultation"—medicalese for "listening every so often" by stethoscope[9]—are equivalent and equally acceptable methods. Furthermore, the college recommends that the choice be left to the informed consent of the patient![10]

❓ IS THIS THE MOST APPROPRIATE PROCEDURE FOR THE CONDITION?

Although the outcome of fetal monitoring of various types is spectacular in individual cases, on the whole it probably contributes to unnecessary treatment and surgery, and by inducing hasty action may cause more morbidity than it avoids. The development of effective artificially intelligent monitoring programs could change this, but for now, it is probably better (assuming a normal, healthy pregnancy) for the physician to listen occasionally through the stethoscope, as ACOG has suggested.

? ARE THERE ALTERNATIVES TO THIS PROCEDURE?

Yes—monitoring by stethoscope.

? WHAT IS CONTROVERSIAL ABOUT THE PROCEDURE?

Everything. There is little agreement on what a normal fetal heart rate tracing is and what variations within labor can be considered within the normal range. There is also disagreement among doctors interpreting the same heart tracing.[11] Given that there is at least as much variation among fetuses as there is among adult human beings; that labor is a time of stress for both mother and infant; and that the infant is receiving the mother's stress-related hormone output through the umbilical cord until the cord is cut, it would be reasonable to expect that "normal" fetal EKGs vary widely and that some tracings indicative of problems in an adult would be part of the normal variation present during birth. The extent to which allowances should be made for this is unknown. It has been shown repeatedly that supposedly quiet hospitals are in fact very noisy places. Because there are strong fetal responses to certain sounds, some of the variation that is seen may be an **artifact** of noise in the delivery suite.[12]

Fetal Monitoring (29)

MORTALITY	MORBIDITY	CONTROVERSY
+	+	o

Monitoring of the health status of a fetus using one or more instruments, some of which are electronic

? WHAT CONDITION DOES THE PROCEDURE TREAT?

This procedure—and its rank in the most frequently performed procedures—grows out of the "catch-all" coding developed jointly by the medical profession and the insurance industry, and encompasses monitoring of the fetus not covered under more specific codes or titles such as "Fetal Electrocardiogram" (see p. 81). All of the methods discussed under this topic represent attempts to monitor the health status of the fetus during pregnancy and delivery. Except for very high-risk pregnancies, monitoring is done for extended periods only during delivery.

The simplest fetal monitoring technique consists of the physician placing a stethoscope against the mother's stomach and listening for the fetal heartbeat. From there, the monitoring techniques get more sophisticated.

? WHAT IS THE PROCEDURE?

Exactly what is done depends upon the type of monitoring needed and apparatus used. The continuous measurement of the fetal heart rate is considered the "gold standard" of monitoring; it can be taken along with an electrocardiogram via wires screwed into the baby's scalp through the widening cervix.[1] Existing technology now makes it possible to monitor even the fetal blood circulation velocity and the velocity of blood circulation in the placenta, although this method remains experimental;[2, 3] to monitor the combined fetal heart rate and force of uterine contractions, in a procedure called cardiotocography;[4] to monitor maternal hormones that may have an effect on fetal brain development;[5] to obtain images of the fetus by using ultrasound and to examine the fetus's heart by echocardiography;[6] to monitor fetal development and treat various problems in the fetus prenatally;[7] to give transfusions in the womb to the fetus;[8] to monitor amniotic fluid and thereby assess fetal kidney function;[9] to check brain function through observation of fetal movement by ultrasound;[10] and to check fetal and uterine response to the mother's release of oxytocin, which causes the uterus to contract.[11]

Two well-known prenatal tests monitor the health of the fetus: **Amniocentesis,** performed between weeks 15 and 16 of pregnancy, involves the sampling and examination of fetal cells floating in amniotic fluid. In this procedure, a needle is inserted through the woman's abdomen and into the uterus, and a small amount of the fluid surrounding the baby is removed. The test is most often used to detect Down syndrome, but it can also detect other chromosome abnormalities, some structural defects, and inherited metabolic disorders. In **chorionic villus sampling**, or CVS (done between weeks 8 and 12), a thin tube is passed into the vagina and through the **cervix**, and a very small sample of tissue is taken from the chorionic villi, finger-shaped projections of the fetal sac that later will develop into the placenta. From this sample, chromosome abnormalities, such as Down syndrome, can be detected.

? WHO PERFORMS THE PROCEDURE?

All of these monitoring procedures are performed by obstetricians, by family and general practitioners who deliver babies, and by obstetrical nurses and **midwives,** in states that permit midwives to practice.

? WHERE IS THE PROCEDURE PERFORMED?

Because of the small but real risks of causing fetal injury in **invasive procedures** and of triggering labor that cannot be controlled, invasive monitoring should be performed in or near a facility that is equipped for cesarean-section deliveries and that has a neonatal intensive care unit. Noninvasive tests can be performed

safely anywhere, and many are done in obstetricians' offices and freestanding birthing centers.

? WHAT ARE THE MORTALITY (DEATH) AND MORBIDITY (COMPLICATION) RATES?

The only monitoring procedures that involve a significant risk of complications, up to and including loss of the infant, are chorionic villi sampling and amniocentesis. Both procedures can be done with or without **ultrasound** guidance of the needle. It has been shown that ultrasound guidance of the needle reduces complications substantially in amniocentesis.[12] In rare instances, amniocentesis can be fatal to the mother, usually if amniotic fluid embolism (leakage of the amniotic fluid into the mother's circulatory system) occurs.[13]

? WHAT ARE THE OTHER COMPLICATIONS AND POSSIBLE SIDE EFFECTS?

See "Fetal Electrocardiogram," p. 81.

? IS THIS THE MOST APPROPRIATE PROCEDURE FOR THE CONDITION?

See "Fetal Electrocardiogram," p. 81.

? ARE THERE ALTERNATIVES TO THIS PROCEDURE?

Yes—monitoring by stethoscope.

? WHAT IS CONTROVERSIAL ABOUT THE PROCEDURE?

The debate over electronic fetal monitoring (EFM)—with an instrument that measures uterine contractions and fetal heart rate during labor—is contentious. EFM was first used by American obstetricians in the early 1970s, on the assumption that the monitoring device would alert the doctor to problems that deprive the infant of oxygen. Reserved for high-risk pregnancies in its early application, EFM by the beginning of the 1980s had become routine practice in most hospitals even though no scientific evidence of its safety and efficacy existed. Today EFM is a widespread practice; approximately three-quarters of births are electronically monitored. Critics of the technology maintain that it often incorrectly indicates that a fetus is in distress, thereby leading to unnecessary cesarean sections. Proponents contend that EFM saves lives.

Fiber-Optic Bronchoscopy (66)

MORTALITY	MORBIDITY	CONTROVERSY
+	+	o

Examination of the bronchial tubes with a flexible fiber-optic endoscope, which may also be used for treatment

? WHAT CONDITION DOES THE PROCEDURE TREAT?

This is a diagnostic and therapeutic procedure that can be used to take biopsies and remove small **lesions** of the **bronchi** using lasers. (The term *fiber-optic bronchoscopy* alone means the diagnostic procedure only. We discuss treatment using the bronchoscope because most complications are treatment-associated, but deaths have been associated with purely diagnostic procedures.) Experienced operators can maneuver the tube into the next two smaller divisions of the bronchial tree, the lobar and segmental bronchi, which carry air to and from the two main divisions of each lung (the lobes) and the segments within them. Inhaled foreign objects, even an open safety pin, can be safely removed with a fiber-optic bronchoscope.[1] (For more information on fiber-optic scopes, see Glossary, p. 309.)

Indications, which are valid reasons for doing the procedure, are still being developed, but the procedure has proven useful in cases of inhaled foreign bodies; hoarseness; recurrent pneumonia; abnormal chest x-ray findings; evaluation of the airway in patients with a **tracheostomy**; chronic cough; inability to remove an **endotracheal tube**; airway injury; and coughing of blood.[2] Fiber-optic bronchoscopy is also done for evaluation of respiratory infections in transplant patients and patients with immune system problems;[3, 4] examination of malignant and nonmalignant tumors of the **trachea** and bronchi;[5, 6] examination of the bronchial tree during reconstructive surgery;[7] diagnosis of twisting of a lung in the chest cavity;[8] sealing of holes in the bronchi after removal of a lung;[9] diagnosis of lung fluid accumulation in transplant patients;[10] diagnosis of diseases of the **pleura**;[11] location of the source of bleeding in lung and bronchial hemorrhage;[12] and insertion of a **stent** to hold a bronchus open.[13] Multiple other uses are reported as well.

The **diagnostic yield** is superior to x rays.[14, 15] Yields of up to 98% have been reported.[16]

? WHAT IS THE PROCEDURE?

The bronchi are two tubes composed of fibrous, elastic rings that run off the trachea, or windpipe. The bronchi divide in two, with one running to each lung, just above the top of the heart.

Because this procedure involves inserting a tube that takes up virtually all the space in the trachea and creates a choking sensation even if air delivery to the lungs is adequate, it is often done under general anesthesia.[17–20] A special, small-diameter scope has been used with success in awake patients.[21] Laser surgery through the bronchoscope has been successfully done with sedation and local anesthetic applied to the airway.[22]

? WHO PERFORMS THE PROCEDURE?

Fiber-optic bronchoscopy, whether diagnostic or therapeutic, should be done only by a thoracic surgeon or pulmonologist with special training in the use of the bronchoscope. This is especially important for laser surgery. And if a general anesthetic is to be used, the anesthesiologist should have experience or certification in anesthesia for bronchoscopic procedures.

? WHERE IS THE PROCEDURE PERFORMED?

Technically, the surgery can be done in the inpatient or outpatient departments of a hospital, an outpatient or ambulatory surgery clinic, or a well-equipped doctor's office. Aside from intravenous sedatives that put the patient to sleep without major respiratory suppression, if general anesthesia is to be used, the procedure should be done in the hospital.

? WHAT ARE THE MORTALITY (DEATH) AND MORBIDITY (COMPLICATION) RATES?

This is a relatively new procedure, and most of the mortality associated with it seems to be related to **intraoperative** disasters that, once understood as possibilities, can be avoided with due care. Therapeutic fiber-optic bronchoscopy seems to be more dangerous than one done purely for diagnostic reasons. The mortality rate for diagnostic procedures is 0.004%, and the mortality rate for laser operations in cancer patients can be as high as 10.1%. (See below.) The risk of death has a lot to do with the seriousness of the preexisting illness. There is a report in the medical literature of a nonfatal explosion of oxygen and polyvinyl chloride gas in a patient's trachea during laser bronchoscopy;[23] a more serious instance of gas explosion could well be fatal.

A case of **air embolism** during a laser bronchoscopic procedure has been reported.[24] One surgical team, writing in the journal *Chest,* stresses that the laser is a potentially dangerous device. These doctors have developed a formal safety protocol for bronchoscopic laser surgery and report a mortality rate of zero during laser procedures and a postoperative mortality rate of 0.4%.[25]

In the one large study (48,000 procedures) of purely diagnostic bronchoscopies, there were 12 procedure-associated deaths, resulting in a mortality rate of 0.025%. In this same study, two deaths and 41 serious complications were attributed to the anesthesia, not the bronchoscopy, for an anesthesia death rate of 0.004%. Two deaths were caused by massive hemorrhage after a lesion was biopsied. There were ten cardiac arrests, for a cardiac arrest rate of 0.021%. Four cases of brushes breaking off inside the patient were reported. All of the deaths were in patients who had preexisting heart disease, severe pneumonia, chronic lung disease, or cancer.[26]

One study of 117 pediatric patients who underwent bronchoscopy reported a mortality rate of zero and a complication rate of 11%.[27]

In larger studies, mortality seems to be heavily related to the underlying condition that prompts the bronchoscopy. For laser bronchoscopy treatment of obstructions of the trachea and bronchi in patients with noncancerous and cancerous tumors, the mortality rate was zero for the patients with benign disease. Of the patients with cancer, 10.1% of the patients died immediately following the procedure, and another 8.5% died within five days.[28] Another study with cancer patients and laser bronchoscopy had a mortality rate of 10%.[29]

In pediatric patients, a minor complication rate of 2% and a major complication rate of zero have been reported.[30]

A rate of zero complications requiring treatment has been reported for a group of AIDS patients.[31]

Pneumothorax can occur in up to 4% of cases. Generally, only 1% will need to have a chest tube inserted to remove the air and re-expand the lung.[32]

Many complications in patients with airway disease of one sort or another arise from failure to deliver enough air to the lungs through the scope or damage from a rigid bronchoscope used during part of the procedure. Monitoring of the concentration of oxygen in the arterial blood can avoid many of these, as can other techniques[33–35]—such as pulse oximetry, in which a probe is attached to a finger and leads run to a device that "reads" the oxygen concentration in percentages.

Minor bleeding after biopsy occurs in about 10% of transplant patients.[36]

? WHAT ARE THE OTHER COMPLICATIONS AND POSSIBLE SIDE EFFECTS?

As we mentioned earlier, an explosion of gases in the mouth, trachea, and bronchial tree has been reported with the use of a laser bronchoscope and a polyvinyl chloride tracheostomy tube. The patient received first- and second-degree burns of the tongue and otherwise was unharmed. This complication can be avoided by using a mixture of helium and oxygen together with the anesthetic gas.[37] Rare but more serious are fires within the patient's chest during laser procedures.[38] Chest fires have also occurred with use of **electrocautery** through the bronchoscope. In the report of this complication, the patient was not injured.[39]

A false-positive result in a culture report can occur when an uncovered bronchoscope brush is used to swab the bronchi to obtain samples for culture. A covered-brush technique essentially eliminates the problem of false-positive cultures.[40] The covered brush is encased in a shield that prevents it from coming into contact with other tissue; the brush is pushed from its shield at the site of the biopsy and is then retracted and brought out through the bronchoscope.

As with any procedure in which anesthesia is used, death from reaction to the anesthetic drugs, error on the part of the anesthetist, or machine failure is a remote possibility. (See Glossary, p. 309)

? IS THIS THE MOST APPROPRIATE PROCEDURE FOR THE CONDITION?

The diagnostic yield is so superior to x rays and the trauma to the patient so much reduced that fiber-optic bronchoscopy is coming to be widely regarded as the appropriate procedure for any diagnoses that cannot be made with a chest x ray, **CT scan**, or **MRI scan**.

? ARE THERE ALTERNATIVES TO THIS PROCEDURE?

Yes. If a biopsy is needed, it can be obtained through an open lung biopsy, in which an incision is made in the chest to obtain a specimen. This procedure can have zero mortality and a minor complication rate of about 13%.[41] In patients who had immune system problems associated with bone marrow transplant therapy, an intraoperative mortality rate of zero and a postoperative minor complication rate of 21% has been reported for the open lung biopsy. Postoperative mortality at 30 days, however, was 45%.[42]

A rigid bronchoscope can also be used. This is regarded by some surgeons as a superior instrument for controlling the laser, controlling hemorrhage, and maintaining good air flow. It requires general anesthesia.[43]

? WHAT IS CONTROVERSIAL
ABOUT THE PROCEDURE?

The controversies surrounding this procedure include the necessity for the use of general anesthesia and the relative safety of laser surgery done through the rigid bronchoscope versus the fiber-optic scope. Some of the complications that have been observed indicate that laser surgery is being done by some surgeons with dangerously little knowledge of laser physics and laser safety. Formal, well-monitored certification programs for both physicians and facilities should be required if lasers are to be used.

Left Cardiac Catheterization (4)

MORTALITY	MORBIDITY	CONTROVERSY
+	+	o

X ray of the arteries and chambers of the heart using a **contrast medium** injected via a **catheter** threaded into the heart through an arm or leg artery

The only difference between "Left Cardiac Catheterization" and "Combined Right and Left Cardiac Catheterization" concerns whether the catheter is pushed through the **septum** of the heart to allow visualization of both of the lower chambers. In left cardiac catheterization, it is not; in the combined procedure, it is. This difference is discussed below. Everything else is identical. See "Combined Right and Left Cardiac Catheterization," p. 50, for details.

? WHAT IS
THE PROCEDURE?

The surgeon selects the artery (either the **femoral artery** in the thigh or the **brachial artery** in the arm). A local anesthetic is given and, depending upon the size of the catheter to be used, the size of the patient's arteries, and the difficulty of getting to them, either a **trochar** is used to punch a hole through the leg or arm into the artery, or a small incision is made down to the level of the artery. Depending upon the tests planned, either the catheter or a guide wire is run up the femoral artery into the **ascending aorta**, and turned downward at the arch of the **aorta** (just above the heart, where it turns downward to enter the left ventricle). The catheter or guide wire is threaded through the aortic valve (the valve between the start of the aorta and the heart) into the left ventricle of the heart, which is the main pumping chamber. If a guide wire is used, the catheter is threaded over it once the guide wire is where the surgeon wants it to be.

When the catheter is in the proper position, a contrast medium is injected, to make the arteries of the heart visible on the x rays taken during the procedure.

If disease or mechanical replacement of the aortic valve make entry through it impossible, an alternative route can be used to reach the left chamber of the heart. In this instance, the catheter can be inserted into the right side of the heart and the catheter pushed through the wall between the right and left ventricles or through the wall between the right atrium and the left ventricle. Serious complications occurred in 3% of cases using these techniques in one study, and 95% of the procedures produced the needed diagnostic information.[1]

With the catheter in place, the **radiopaque** solution is injected into the coronary arteries and the left ventricle, and the flow is photographed with **fluoroscopy** and the use of a fluoroscopic x-ray camera. The films are reviewed to determine the presence and extent of various problems with the heart's arteries, valves, chambers, and the connections between the chambers.

Myelogram with Contrast Enhancement (26)

MORTALITY	MORBIDITY	CONTROVERSY
+	−	●

- The major **COMPLICATION** from myelogram is headache, reported in at least 30% to 67% of patients. Another reported problem is allergic reactions to the **contrast medium** used for the procedure.

- The major **CONTROVERSY** concerns whether a myelogram should be used when magnetic resonance imaging is available, which is noninvasive in nature. The other controversy surrounds the type of contrast medium used for the procedure.

LAY TITLE: Myelogram

X ray of the spinal column with **contrast medium** inserted into the spinal canal via a spinal tap

? WHAT CONDITION DOES THE PROCEDURE TREAT?

This procedure is not a treatment, but a diagnostic test used prior to treatment if the physician suspects a bulging **disk,** a herniated or ruptured disk in the back or neck, a narrowing of the spinal canal, called spinal stenosis, or another condition affecting the soft tissues of the spinal column.

Your understanding of what follows may be helped by a bit of information about anatomy. The spine consists of a series of separate bones, called **vertebrae,** each of which has a hole in the center that the spinal cord passes through. Each also has other holes and recesses through which nerves pass in and out to the cord, and blood vessels enter and leave to ensure that the spinal bones have nourishment. Nowhere in the body does bone grind directly on bone; in fact, the loss of the smooth, lubricating covering of the joints is part of degenerative arthritis, which is painful at best and agonizing at worst.

The spine needs special protection, and the joints between the vertebrae need to have their range of motion restricted so that the cord is not stretched, torn, or broken. Each pair of vertebrae is held together by a tough fibrous donut, called an intervertebral disk, which has a jellylike center. These structures, which normally protect the cord, can be a source of pain, muscle weakness, odd sensations called dysthesia, or loss of sensation called anesthesia, and ultimately a source of paralysis if the fibrous capsule bulges, creating pressure on the spine or a nerve root. The same symptoms can occur, usually more severely, if the disk ruptures and the jellylike substance in the center comes into contact with the cord or nerve roots, or both. **Spinal stenosis** can have many of the same symptoms.

Obviously, being able to see what is going on is an advantage to the doctor who is planning treatment. A standard x ray of the spinal column is not overly revealing, unless the damage is on the outside of the disk, and in a position perpendicular to the x-ray beam. The vertebral bones block visualization of bulges or tears on the inside of the disk. The use of a contrast medium in the spinal canal, and of x rays powerful enough to penetrate rather than just outline the vertebrae, allows disk damage and spinal stenosis to be seen.

The idea of having something put into the spinal canal should rightfully strike terror in the hearts of the bravest, if they are at all anatomically informed. Surely sticking a needle into the spinal cord does not help the situation.

Nature provides an out. There is space between the membrane covering the spinal cord and the cord itself, into which a needle can be inserted without damaging the cord. Anywhere on the back below the atlas, which is the first cervical vertebra (the cervical vertebrae are the portion of the spine that makes up the neck bones) that connects the spine to the skull, a skilled pair of hands can slip a needle into the spinal canal and remove spinal fluid for analysis, or inject contrast media, anesthetics, or narcotics. The procedure in each case is called a spinal tap. It is easiest to do this in the lower back, where the rearward bony projections of the vertebrae, called processes, are basically parallel to the ground. In the upper back, they slant downward, but it is still possible to insert a needle with proper care.

? WHAT IS THE PROCEDURE?

For a contrast myelogram, the patient is placed on her side in the "knee-to-chest," or "fetal," position, which extends the spine maximally. The radiologist feels the vertebrae to locate the region between the end of the cord and the tailbone, and anesthetizes with novocaine or a similar drug the place where the spinal needle will be inserted. Then a spinal needle, consisting of a solid, pointed stylet inside a hollow needle about five inches long, is inserted into the canal, passing between two of the vertebrae that don't have a full-fledged disk connecting them. If everything is going well, the sensation is not so much pain as strong pressure, rather like someone bearing down hard with a thumb. Severe pain, such as any "electric shock" sensation in the legs, should be loudly articulated by the patient and is a sign for the radiologist to stop.

The radiologist withdraws the stylet when she thinks that she has the needle in the canal. If clear spinal fluid flows out, all is well. Blood is an indication that, either the needle is in an artery or vein rather than the canal, or there is blood in the spinal fluid. Pus indicates a spinal canal or brain infection, and the procedure should be stopped. Assuming that clear fluid is found, the radiologist withdraws a volume equal to the amount of contrast medium to be inserted, the needle is withdrawn or replaced with a **cannula,** and the patient is asked to lie on her back. The table (and patient) are then tilted head-down so that the contrast medium can run to the area of suspected disk damage or spinal stenosis. (Although this is a somewhat uncomfortable position, it is how the procedure is done because gravity helps the contrast medium to infiltrate the spinal column.) Then x rays are taken.

? WHO PERFORMS THE PROCEDURE?

The procedure is usually done by a radiologist. If she is unable to perform the spinal tap portion of it for some reason, an anesthesiologist or anesthetist can do it.

? WHERE IS THE PROCEDURE PERFORMED?

This procedure is usually done as an inpatient procedure. Theoretically, it can be performed wherever proper equipment is available, whether in a hospital, an x-ray laboratory, outpatient clinic, or freestanding clinic. For the person hospitalized with a back condition, the myelogram is of course done as an inpatient procedure.

Some authorities maintain that this should always be done as an inpatient procedure so that patients can be carefully monitored for signs of reaction to the contrast agent. The same kind of monitoring can be done in a short-stay unit. A study of the incidence of complications found that myelograms can be performed safely on an outpatient basis.[1] Actually, the complication rates are lower for outpatient procedures, primarily because the patients selected for outpatient myelograms generally have fewer risk factors—they're younger and in better general health.

? WHAT ARE THE MORTALITY (DEATH) AND MORBIDITY (COMPLICATION) RATES?

The overall mortality associated with this procedure is 0.5%.[2] The vast majority of these deaths are attributable to allergic reactions to the contrast medium. Some result from malignant hyperthermia—an uncontrollable fever—or from the effects of seizures; both are complications of reactions to the contrast medium. There are indications that the use of preoperative medications such as Valium, Dilantin, and Prednisone can reduce mortality and morbidity, but there is not enough evidence to make their use routine for those people who have not shown past sensitivity reactions to contrast media. The first administration of a contrast medium to a patient is always somewhat of an experiment.

For discussion of the death rates for procedures that use contrast media, see "Combined Right and Left Cardiac Catheterization," p. 50.

Whether done as an inpatient or outpatient procedure, myelograms are associated with complications. These are usually not severe and consist primarily of a spinal headache—mild in the 67% of the patients who have such headaches and moderate to severe in 15% to 24%, depending upon the volume of contrast medium used. The complication rates for inpatients and outpatients are 37% and 40%, respectively.[3]

The use of air as a contrast medium, a practice that, happily, has been almost abolished in favor of better contrast media, **CT scans**, and **MRI scans**, has been associated with fatalities and severe complications, particularly if high air volumes (much like putting too much air into a tire and causing it to explode) and high pressures (air pushed forcefully into the spinal column) were used.[4]

? WHAT ARE THE OTHER COMPLICATIONS AND POSSIBLE SIDE EFFECTS?

Thirty percent to 67%[5] of people who have a myelogram have at least some spinal headache.[6] The severity of headache pain varies from barely noticeable to agonizing, depending upon how much fluid was withdrawn, how much contrast medium was inserted, what premedication was used, and how long the needle or cannula was in the canal. The exact cause of spinal headache is uncertain, but it appears to be related to pressure changes and changes in the **osmolality** (the concentration of dissolved solids) of the spinal and cerebral fluid,[7] as a result of the loss of fluid from the canal. Spinal headache is minimized by replacing the spinal fluid removed with another fluid, volume for volume, as closely as possible. The great majority of patients who have a spinal tap will have at least some spinal headache; it will not be severe for most.

Hyperextension, or extreme stretching, of the cervical spine has been reported as a result of the radiologist's trying to clear a space for insertion of the needle between the cervical vertebrae. Injection of contrast medium into the spinal cord has also been reported, and the author of a paper reviewing such complications notes that **fluoroscopic** (a "real-time," moving x ray on a display screen) guidance of the needle should be done to ensure that the spinal cord is not injected.[8]

The choice of contrast medium can make a difference in the quality of the images obtained, the amount of pain the patient feels, and the incidence of allergic or sensitivity reactions to the contrast medium.[9] The side effects associated with older, **ionic**, high-osmolality contrast media are legion. These side effects include **electroencephalographic (EEG) changes**, seizures, auditory and visual hallucinations, and assorted other neurological problems. Iohexol, a new agent, produces few such complications. With iohexol, 44% of patients in one study had some reaction to the medium, but only one reaction (2.32%) was considered severe.[10] A study comparing iohexol with metrizamide, an older and popular agent, showed a lower rate of adverse reactions for iohexol.[11]

Another study of older contrast media in myelography found that 3% of 400 patients had some neurotoxic reaction (one or more signs of poisoning of the nervous system). In one person, the injection produced spasms of the leg muscles so severe that the **femur** was broken at the neck (just below the "ball" of the ball-and-socket hip joint). Another patient developed paranoid psychosis, which resolved after four days.[12] In yet another study, iohexol reduced the incidence of headache, nausea, vomiting, and neurologic reactions. No psychiatric problems were observed.[13]

Uncommon complications, 12 cases of **lesions** of the cauda equina, the so-called horse's tail that contains the roots of the spinal nerves below the first lumbar (low-back) vertebra, after myelography were reported in the literature as of 1977. All of the patients in a later study recovered from this uncommon complication without permanent disability.[14]

Instances of death, convulsive segmental myoclonus (a seizure limited to the portions of the body innervated by the nerve roots flowing from just a few of the vertebrae), and **hypotension** have been associated with an even older contrast medium called Dimer-X.[15]

As with any procedure in which anesthesia is used, death from reaction to the anesthetic drugs, error on the part of the anesthetist, or machine failure are remote possibilities. (See Glossary, p. 309)

? IS THIS THE MOST APPROPRIATE PROCEDURE FOR THE CONDITION?

Executed by a good radiologist, a contrast myelogram identifies the location of the damaged disk about 90.2% of the time.[16] As medical tests for specific diseases go, this is highly accurate.

From another perspective, however, detection of disk problems by a myelogram depends on the size of the bulge or tear and its relationship to the x-ray beam. Imagine, for a moment, a small dent in the side of a tin can. As one rotates the can, the dent will be most obvious when one is looking down into the can, and least obvious (in fact, invisible) when one is looking at the opposite side of the can. The "top-down" view—looking down through the spinal column—is not available with standard x rays such as myelograms, which have to be taken from one side or another of the spinal column. So detection of a disk problem depends upon the relationship between the x-ray beam and the lesion. If

the lesion is 180 degrees away from the beam, it may show up poorly or not at all. Detection is best when the lesion is perpendicular to the beam. Therefore, it is possible to miss lesions in unusual positions around the disk.

This is one of many reasons that other alternatives should be considered. One of these alternatives is diskography—an x ray taken with injection of the contrast medium directly into the spinal canal at the level of the suspected disk lesion. About two-thirds of the cases of failure of **chemonucleolysis**—a procedure that dissolves disk fragments with chemicals—are related to failure to locate and inject a large disk fragment. Diskography is capable of locating such fragments and indicating whether further attempts at chemonucelolysis, a **percutaneous diskectomy**—the removal of disk fragments through a very small skin incision using a long needle—or an open procedure (which involves an incision) is indicated.[17]

? ARE THERE ALTERNATIVES TO THIS PROCEDURE?

The presence of a disk problem in the lumbar spine can be diagnosed with a high degree of accuracy from the history and physical examination alone. Confirming information can be obtained from electromyography (explained below), from CT scans, from MRI scans, and from myelograms. The first three of these have the advantage of being far less invasive than the myelogram.

Electromyography, in which information about the speed and strength of signals carried in the nerves is obtained, uses very fine needles placed into the muscles to obtain a tracing of electrical activity in them, and is relatively painless. Both CT scans and MRI can be performed with or without contrast media. Both the CT scan and the MRI scan have the advantage of being able to "look down" into the spinal canal as well as looking "across it," which is all the myelogram can do. In both CT and MRI, the patient is completely surrounded by a ring of sensors through which the patient is moved. The sensors pick up x rays in the CT scan and radio waves in the MRI. The information obtained is fed to a computer, which can construct two-dimensional "slices" and three-dimensional images, as seen from almost any angle. Both provide potentially much more information than the myelogram; MRI, in particular, has been found to be highly specific and accurate in recent studies.[18]

? WHAT IS CONTROVERSIAL ABOUT THE PROCEDURE?

Myelograms have been around for a long time, and there is little controversy associated with them except in two areas: the type of contrast medium used and the use of a myelogram at all instead of an MRI. The traditional contrast medium causes a variety of reactions in many people; the newer ("nonionic") media cause much less discomfort and provoke fewer reactions. These newer agents are more expensive than the older ones, however, and there is a tendency not to use them, especially with patients on Medicare or Medicaid who are thought to be "underpaying" their way.

Similarly, the MRI is noninvasive and as effective as the myelogram, but is more expensive. Whereas many urban areas already have an oversupply of MRI machines, other areas may not have access to one within a radius of several hundred miles. Obtaining an MRI may be difficult or impossible, leaving the myelogram as the only alternative. It is reasonable to assume, however, that the MRI will eventually replace the myelogram entirely.

Percutaneous Liver Biopsy (76)

MORTALITY	MORBIDITY	CONTROVERSY
+	+	o

LAY TITLE: Needle biopsy of the liver

Obtaining a piece of liver tissue with a needle placed through the skin and into the liver

? WHAT CONDITION DOES THE PROCEDURE TREAT?

Not used as a treatment but to help determine what to treat, if anything, this procedure is used for diagnosis of liver diseases. Liver disease does not always present clinical signs until a late stage of development; however, a biopsy can show the condition of the liver before signs of illness develop. Experimental performance of liver biopsies during operations for gallbladder disease disclosed previously unsuspected liver disease in 11% of patients[1] in the study, a finding that led the authors of the study to recommend that liver biopsies be done routinely as a part of gallbladder operations.

? WHAT IS THE PROCEDURE?

The skin over the liver is scrubbed with soap and antiseptic, and the patient is draped so that only the biopsy site is exposed. A local anesthetic is given. Then a relatively large-bore, or wide, needle is placed through the skin into the liver, and the specimen is loosened by suction on the syringe to which the needle is attached. The needle is withdrawn and the specimen is examined. If the specimen is adequate in size, the procedure is over. If not, the surgeon has the choice of making as many additional punctures as the patient will tolerate.

? WHO PERFORMS THE PROCEDURE?

This procedure is within the competence of any physician trained in the technique of needle biopsies, but is usually done by a general surgeon or gastroenterologist.

? WHERE IS THE PROCEDURE PERFORMED?

This procedure is usually done within the hospital—in the outpatient or short-procedure unit—because of the possible complication of bleeding; however, it can also be done in an outpatient surgery center or a well-equipped doctor's office.

? WHAT ARE THE MORTALITY (DEATH) AND MORBIDITY (COMPLICATION) RATES?

Liver biopsy is fatal only in extremely rare instances, when bleeding cannot be controlled or infection develops.[2] Reported complications include pain after the procedure in 1.9% to 5.9% of patients; a need to repeat the biopsy immediately in 6.4%; and major complication rates ranging from 0.2% to 1.9%, depending upon the technique used. The lower complication rates result from using ultrasound visualization to guide the needle; the higher ones occur when the doctor is "flying blind."[3]

Reports of pain—from "none" to "severe"—during the procedure vary greatly from patient to patient. If pain is a major concern, it is reasonable to ask the doctor to use a sedative in addition to the local anesthetic.

? WHAT ARE THE OTHER COMPLICATIONS AND POSSIBLE SIDE EFFECTS?

There are no other common complications.

? IS THIS THE MOST APPROPRIATE PROCEDURE FOR THE CONDITION?

If liver cancer is suspected, the answer is yes, because cancer cannot be differentiated from benign tumors in most x rays or similar techniques, such as **CT scans** and **MRI scans**. If cancer is not suspected, noninvasive techniques such as x rays, **ultrasound** studies, and blood studies may yield enough information to make the diagnosis. If the results are equivocal and the patient is still having problems, a biopsy should be done.

? ARE THERE ALTERNATIVES TO THIS PROCEDURE?

Liver biopsies can be done through a **laparoscope**, and can also be done when the abdomen is open for surgery. For other alternatives, see the paragraph above.

? WHAT IS CONTROVERSIAL ABOUT THE PROCEDURE?

Indications for this procedure are still evolving; as we come to understand more diseases and how they are reflected in the liver, the use of liver biopsy as a diagnostic tool is likely to increase. Use of some means of visualizing the course of the needle (via ultrasound or **fluoroscopy**, for example) appears to reduce complications, but also increases the cost of the procedure.

Spinal Canal Exploration (39)

MORTALITY	MORBIDITY	CONTROVERSY
–	–	●

- A **MORTALITY** rate of up to 14% has been reported for this procedure. The implication of anesthesia mortality must also be considered.

- Permanent **NERVE DAMAGE** of various degrees of severity has been reported to affect 1.3% to 14% of all patients.

- The major **CONTROVERSY** is whether this procedure is appropriate when less invasive procedures have not yet been tried.

Surgical exploration of the **spinal canal**

? WHAT CONDITION DOES THE PROCEDURE TREAT?

This procedure is carried out for diagnosis and treatment of **spinal stenosis**; removal of fatty tumors of the canal that can result from high-dosage steroid treatment;[1] removal of other types of tumors;[2] **congenital** malformations of the spinal column;[3] spinal damage caused by trauma (such as fractures associated with vehicular accidents);[4] infections of the spinal canal;[5] and diagnosis of soft-tissue problems in the spinal canal that cannot be definitively diagnosed with x rays or **MRI** scans.[6]

? WHAT IS THE PROCEDURE?

With the patient under general anesthesia, the back is shaved if necessary, washed with soap and antiseptic, dried, and draped with a sterile sheet that exposes only the area to be operated on. The skin, **fascia**, and muscles are opened. Bleeding vessels are **ligated** or **cauterized** with an **electrocautery device**. The **spinous processes**, which are the backward-pointing extensions of the bones of the spine, are broken off, and the **vertebrae** carefully opened at the point where the problem is

thought to lie. Any further surgery carried out at this time, such as removal of a tumor or rerouting of an abnormally positioned blood vessel, is based on the disease found.

When the exploration and any treatment have been completed, the vertebrae are reassembled; bones from the spinous processes may be used as **grafts** to fuse the vertebrae. The muscles, fascia, and skin are closed in layers. Depending upon the treatment given, a body cast may be applied. The patient is taken to the recovery room and then to her room.

? WHO PERFORMS THE PROCEDURE?

Like all neurosurgery, this procedure has the potential to go drastically wrong, and should be performed only by a board-certified and experienced neurosurgeon, preferably one who does at least 100 open-back procedures a year.

? WHERE IS THE PROCEDURE PERFORMED?

This is major surgery which should be performed only on an inpatient basis in a hospital.

? WHAT ARE THE MORTALITY (DEATH) AND MORBIDITY (COMPLICATION) RATES?

Most studies of patients having this procedure were small, so mortality and morbidity figures may be exaggerated. Mortality rates of up to 14% have been reported, the immediate cause of death being tuberculosis infection of the spine. Spinal canal exploration can be expected to cause permanent nerve damage of various degrees of severity, depending upon the study, in about 1.36% to 14% of patients.[7, 8]

? WHAT ARE THE OTHER COMPLICATIONS AND POSSIBLE SIDE EFFECTS?

As with any procedure in which anesthesia is used, death from reaction to the anesthetic drugs, error on the part of the anesthetist, or machine failure is a remote possibility. (See Glossary, p. 309)

? IS THIS THE MOST APPROPRIATE PROCEDURE FOR THE CONDITION?

Yes, if noninvasive diagnostic and therapeutic measures, such as CT and MRI scans or use of **anti-inflammatory medications**, fail.

? ARE THERE ALTERNATIVES TO THIS PROCEDURE?

If noninvasive diagnostic and therapeutic measures fail (see above), there is no alternative. For problems that prove to be disk-related, percutaneous disk excision or chymopapain injection—a procedure called chemonucleolysis in which disk fragments are dissolved with a protein-dissolving enzyme to dissolve the disk would be possible, but if spinal canal exploration is done, it is highly probable that the disk problem was not detected. (See "Intervertebral Disk Excision," p. 160.)

When the surgeon opens the spine to do an exploration and finds other problems—such as a ruptured (bulging) disk, fused vertebrae, or bone spur—the problem will be treated while the patient is under anesthesia for the spinal canal exploration. Similarly, if there are mechanical problems (a fractured vertebrae or ruptured disk, for example) with the spinal canal, it is unlikely that they could be repaired without spinal canal exploration.

? WHAT IS CONTROVERSIAL ABOUT THE PROCEDURE?

Clearly, all less invasive diagnostic studies should be carried out first. These include myelography (see "Myelogram with Contrast Enhancement," p. 89) and venography (in this case, x rays of the veins of the spinal column)[9], as well as CT scans.[10] In large measure because of the variety and rarity of some of the conditions treated by this procedure, a 1991 article states that "no consensus exists" about the indications for each operative approach.[11]

Another article suggests that, for spinal cord cancer, surgery be restricted to those cases in which radiation and chemotherapy have failed.[12]

Surgical Procedures

Abdominal Aorta Resection and Replacement (64)

MORTALITY	MORBIDITY	CONTROVERSY
–	–	●

- **MORTALITY** rates of 2% to 5% have been reported for this procedure when performed on an elective basis. When performed on an emergency basis, mortality rates climbed as high as 50%, according to one study.
- **OBSTRUCTION** of the ureters and paralysis of the lower body are two major complications associated with this procedure.
- The major **CONTROVERSY** has to do with the type of materials that are used to construct the graft.

Replacement of the abdominal portion of the **aorta** with a flexible **graft**

❓ WHAT CONDITION DOES THE PROCEDURE TREAT?

This procedure is used to treat the following: traumatic injury to the aorta that cannot be repaired by simple suturing; rupture of the aorta; and **aneurysms.**

❓ WHAT IS THE PROCEDURE?

Because the aorta is a long vessel and runs from above the heart to the upper groin, many different surgical approaches are possible. The surgeon selects the one that will give her the best access to the portion of the aorta that needs to be replaced. Depending upon the exact site, the incision can be made in the upper or lower abdomen or the middle or lower back.

The patient is given a general anesthetic. The skin is shaved and scrubbed with soap and antiseptic, then draped so that only the site of the incision is exposed. The skin, fat, **fascia**, and muscle are cut and the incision site is spread open with retractors. Bleeding vessels are **ligated** or **cauterized**. When the aorta is reached and the damaged portion is well exposed, the surgeon may elect to construct a temporary bypass around the damaged portion, but the aorta is usually clamped above and below the site to be replaced.

If a bypass is not constructed, speed is essential to avoid damage to the portions of the body that lose their blood supply when the aorta is clamped. This is one of the few remaining surgical procedures for which speed is essential, which is why we recommend that a board-certified vascular surgeon do the surgery. If a board-certified surgeon is not available and the doctor cannot state her average clamp time for aortic procedures, the patient should insist on the construction of a temporary bypass before the aorta is clamped.

With the damaged section clamped off or bypassed, the surgeon cuts between the two clamps and removes the section, leaving cuffs to which the graft will be attached. The graft, or **prosthesis**, is inserted and sewn or clamped into place. As soon as the graft is in place, the aorta is unclamped and the suture lines (or points of connection if a sutureless graft is used) are checked for leaks. Any leaks that are found are repaired. The body wall is closed in layers and the incision is bandaged. The patient is taken to the recovery room and then to her room.

❓ WHO PERFORMS THE PROCEDURE?

As discussed, this procedure should be performed only by a board-certified vascular surgeon, although it may be necessary to have a general surgeon or a trauma surgeon perform it in an emergency. Many trauma surgeons have the requisite skills; nevertheless, it is best to use a board-certified vascular surgeon except in cases of emergency when one is not available.

? WHERE IS THE PROCEDURE PERFORMED?

This is major surgery that is always performed in a hospital.

? WHAT ARE THE MORTALITY (DEATH) AND MORBIDITY (COMPLICATION) RATES?

Mortality rates as low as 2% to 5% are reported regularly, but there is considerable variation in the results depending upon the age of the patient, the seriousness of the condition, whether the operation is elective or emergency, and what technique is used.[1] Complication rates as low as zero have been reported.[2]

About one-third of patients whose grafts were examined by **ultrasonography** on several occasions following surgery showed incipient major or minor problems, suggesting a complication rate of about 33%.[3]

A 1989 study of the use of a sutureless, ringed prosthesis for the aorta showed that the stage of the operation during which blood supply to the lower body was cut off lasted only 17 minutes and was associated with a mortality rate of 6% (death from heart attacks) and a zero complication rate. A 1990 study of the same device showed a mortality rate of 8%, with a restricted flow time of only nine minutes. The authors of this study recommend that surgeons use sutureless, ringed grafts, because they can be inserted quickly. In contrast, the careful and minute suturing required for the sutured grafts consumes most of the surgeon's time. As mentioned earlier, speed is essential because surgery on the aorta requires cutting off the blood supply to the lower body, which can result in kidney or nerve damage.[4, 5]

As with many other operations, the mortality rate is vastly higher for emergency than for elective procedures. An Israeli study showed a 4.6% mortality rate for elective replacements and a 45.2% mortality rate in emergency operations.[6] A German study found 50% mortality for emergency operations.[7]

Replacement of an infected aortic replacement graft has an operative mortality rate of 10% and an additional mortality of 15% within the first year. The 85% of patients who survive the first year have no further problems. The traditional operation for infected aortic grafts requires complete removal of the graft and a bypass operation to establish an alternate flow channel for the arterial blood, rather than graft replacement. This operation results in a high rate of loss of one or both legs as a result of restricted circulation to the lower body during excessively long operations. The direct replacement operation described above resulted in no leg loss in one study.[8, 9]

Use of a rigid, sutureless graft—made of Dacron woven over metal, either titanium or Vitallium—has an early postoperative mortality rate of 11.25% and a late mortality rate (within an average follow-up of about two years) of 6%. About 40% of patients will require some further suturing of the aorta when this device is used.[10]

? WHAT ARE THE OTHER COMPLICATIONS AND POSSIBLE SIDE EFFECTS?

About 7.3% of patients will require replacement of a tube graft within an average follow-up period of about 4½ years.[11]

Obstruction of the **ureter** or ureters where a Dacron tube graft crosses it is a possible but uncommon complication. Whether a patient is at risk for it depends upon the patient's anatomy and the positioning of the graft. Only about 3.1% of patients who are at risk for this complication will actually develop it. Whether the Dacron graft is passed over or under the ureter seems to make no difference.[12]

While misdiagnosis is not, strictly speaking, a complication, the discovery of an aneurysm of the thoracic aorta, which is the part in the chest above the **diaphragm**, strongly points to the possibility of abdominal aortic disease, and patients who have a thoracic aorta problem should have full aorta studies to make sure that there are no problems in the abdomen.[13, 14]

Paralysis of the lower body can occur if the blood supply to the spine is destroyed, but this can be avoided by proper surgical technique.[15] Some surgeons construct a temporary blood supply to the kidneys and use electronic monitoring of electrical activity in the spine to avoid complications; others rely on speed of operation to avoid them.[16] Although the complicated procedure of constructing a temporary blood supply seems logical, this increases operating time, which exposes the patient to greater risk.

As with any procedure in which anesthesia is used, death from reaction to the anesthetic drugs, error on the part of the anesthetist, or machine failure is a remote possibility. (See Glossary, p. 309)

? IS THIS THE MOST APPROPRIATE PROCEDURE FOR THE CONDITION?

Again, the answer depends upon the condition. Most problems with the aorta are mechanical problems that have no nonsurgical treatment, so the question quickly becomes not whether to have surgery but what surgery to have and which surgeon to use. The mortality rate in emergency operations is so high that "watchful waiting" has no real role here except in patients who are so old or so sick that there is a real chance they will die as a result of some other condition before the aortic problem becomes serious.

? ARE THERE ALTERNATIVES TO THIS PROCEDURE?

No—the question is which aortic replacement procedure to have, not whether to have it.

? WHAT IS CONTROVERSIAL ABOUT THE PROCEDURE?

The ultrasonography study cited above supports the general dissatisfaction with current graft materials that has been reported in the literature. A great deal of animal research is ongoing to find better replacement materials, and is inconclusive so far.

Above-the-Knee Amputation (85)

MORTALITY	MORBIDITY	CONTROVERSY
–	–	●

- The national **MORTALITY** rate following amputation for trauma is 2.3%, while another study reported an operative mortality of 15%.
- **CONTRIBUTING FACTORS** to death were **sepsis** (54% of cases); heart disease (16%); and stroke (11%).
- The **CONTROVERSY** centers on the best way to construct the flap of skin that covers the stump, and also concerns the experience of the surgeons who perform this procedure.

Amputation of the leg at a point above the knee

? WHAT CONDITION DOES THE PROCEDURE TREAT?

This procedure is performed for several reasons, most of which in one way or another involve problems with the blood supply to the knee and the lower leg. These **indications** include severe **ischemia** of the lower leg that does not respond to medical (nonsurgical) therapy or more conservative surgery; uncontrollable pain in the limb when it is at rest; infection in the lower leg that cannot be controlled by antibiotics and is causing **systemic** problems (for example, **gangrene** or an infection causing **septicemia**); failure of attempts to reconstruct veins and arteries[1] or remove clots that are blocking veins and arteries; traumatic total dislocation of the knee that leads to irreparable damage to blood vessels;[2] gunshot, shotgun, or stab wounds, and **blunt trauma**; and bone and soft-tissue cancers. It may also be required in severe cases of Buerger's disease (caused by recurrent attacks of inflammation of the arteries and sometimes the veins), Raynaud's phenomenon (a circulatory disorder that affects fingers and sometimes toes, and occurs when the small arteries that supply fingers and toes with blood become extra sensitive to cold and suddenly contract, reducing the flow of blood to the affected area), and frostbite. Above-the-knee amputation may also result following injury, because of failure to treat damage to the **popliteal artery**. The limb is at risk if popliteal artery damage is not repaired within three to six hours.[3]

Risk factors that may lead to vascular damage requiring above-the-knee amputation include diabetes, smoking, high blood pressure, and coronary artery disease (a clue that arterial blockages may occur elsewhere in the body).[4]

WHAT IS THE PROCEDURE?

Like most amputation procedures, this one goes far back in history, and has become only slightly less crude with the passage of time. The patient is given a general anesthetic. The leg to be amputated is shaved and washed with soap and antiseptic, and draped so that only the knee is exposed.

If the condition of the knee and the upper part of the lower leg allows for it, the surgeon makes several incisions in the flesh of the lower leg to provide padding for the stump, and ensures that each of the resulting flaps has a good blood supply from the upper leg. All soft tissue attachments to the lower leg are severed. Vessels that bleed are **ligated** or **cauterized** one by one. The **femur** is cut through with a bone saw. The bone is filed smooth and bone wax is applied to the exposed bone stop bleeding if necessary. The tissue flaps are folded over the stump to provide as much padding as possible. The blood supply is checked at each stage to make sure that the tissue will not be deprived of blood.

The skin is sutured over the stump to provide as good a cosmetic result as possible. Once the stump has been formed and lightly bandaged, a mold for a custom **prosthesis** (in this case, an artificial leg) may be taken, or the surgeon may attempt to fit an off-the-shelf prosthesis. The stump is then cleaned, dressed with topical antibiotics, and bandaged, and the patient is taken to the recovery room.

What follows is a long and often frustrating period of physical therapy and learning to walk with an artificial leg.

WHO PERFORMS THE PROCEDURE?

This procedure is performed by a general or orthopedic surgeon.

WHERE IS THE PROCEDURE PERFORMED?

This is major surgery that must be performed in the hospital on an inpatient basis.

WHAT ARE THE MORTALITY (DEATH) AND MORBIDITY (COMPLICATION) RATES?

As with some other procedures discussed in this book, many of the conditions that require the surgery can in themselves be fatal. The mortality rate following amputation for trauma is about 2.3%.[5] Another series of patients without trauma were found to have an operative mortality rate of 15% and two-year postoperative mortality of an additional 26%. Causes of death were sepsis in 54%, heart disease in 16%, and stroke in 11%. All of the patients in this series required above-the-knee amputation for various systemic diseases, such as diabetes, that cause vascular problems.[6]

Burn patients who have above-the-knee amputations

of both legs as a result of concomitant trauma—albeit a rare occurrence—have a mortality rate of 33%.[7]

Mortality is higher after failed **thromboembolectomy** and for infection that cannot be controlled with antibiotics.[8]

An artificial blood vessel **graft** may be used to repair traumatically damaged vessels as part of an amputation procedure or may be used to increase blood flow in an attempt to avoid amputations. In either case, it can be a source of blood clots that block nearby arteries and veins.[9] A 1976 study using a mathematical model predicted greater success using vein transplants from other parts of the body rather than artificial materials.[10] Current materials—for example, polytetrafluoroethylene and Dacron—have a better record, but 45% of patients still experience blood vessel blockage four years after the operation.[11, 12]

A study in the late 1980s of World War II veterans who had above-the-knee amputations during the war found that 5.8% of them had abdominal aortic **aneurysms**, a condition marked by ballooning of the **aorta**, which can rupture with fatal results, compared with 1.1% of veterans with two good legs. The change in blood flow that accompanies above-the-knee amputation appears to alter the circulatory pattern in a way that causes aneurysms in some people.[13]

Measures of the energy expenditure required to walk with a prosthesis for an above-the-knee amputation indicate that it is much more difficult than walking with a below-the-knee prosthesis or with two good legs. This is one reason for a surgeon to try to save the knee if at all possible. A high level of physical fitness is required to use an above-the-knee prosthesis successfully.[14]

Well-engineered, newer artificial legs can reduce the energy demand required for walking by about 50% with improvements in gait and walking speed.[15, 16] An artificial leg has been developed that is better for jogging than the usual artificial leg, designed primarily for walking. However, it is regarded as needing improvement.[17] Designing the ideal artificial limb continues to present problems because there are many variables to consider, such as the normal gait of the person; the amount of pressure put on the socket as the person shifts weight; and the general condition of the stump relative to blood flow and health of the tissue. Attempts have been made to write computer programs that take these variables into account, so that artificial limbs may be better designed; however, preliminary studies have shown that the use of such computer-aided design and manufacturing techniques did not result in an artificial limb that was notably superior to those produced using conventional manufacturing methods.[18, 19]

Problems have also arisen with "robotized" artificial limbs that use computers and an elaborate system of motors to create the walking motion. Researchers have discovered the difficulty of creating an artificial limb that responds to twitching of the thigh muscle or contraction of the buttocks and produces a normal gait. They also discovered that going from one mode (straight level walking) to another (going up an incline) can produce problems for the computer system. Further research is needed to determine how best to match patient and computer system.[20]

As with virtually all surgery of the lower body, **pulmonary embolism** is a possibility.[21]

The risk of amputation for patients who have an infected knee prosthesis is about 4%.[22, 23]

Seventy-two percent of patients have "phantom limb" pain, in which pain is felt in the missing part of the limb, or stump pain.[24]

? WHAT ARE THE OTHER COMPLICATIONS AND POSSIBLE SIDE EFFECTS?

Unrecognized damage to vessels has been reported. This may lead to further surgery.[25]

A poorly fitted prosthesis can result in a noncancerous skin condition resembling Kaposi's sarcoma.[26]

As with any procedure in which anesthesia is used, death from reaction to the anesthetic drugs, error on the part of the anesthetist, or machine failure is a remote possibility. (See Glossary, p. 309)

? IS THIS THE MOST APPROPRIATE PROCEDURE FOR THE CONDITION?

Yes, if all tissue below the knee is genuinely devitalized. The medical literature suggests that a through-the-knee amputation or a below-the-knee amputation be used if at all possible for recovery-related reasons detailed earlier.

? ARE THERE ALTERNATIVES TO THIS PROCEDURE?

Amputation through the knee, in which the knee is taken apart and the femur is not cut, is technically simpler than above-the-knee amputation and can be performed more rapidly, but still carries a mortality rate of 20%.[27] Rehabilitation is satisfactory in 62% of the patients with a through-the-knee amputation, in contrast to rates of 33% to 44% for patients with two types of above-the-knee amputations.[28] This experience has been repeated in other studies.[29]

Results are even better with below-the-knee amputation, but it is not a real alternative because above-the-knee amputation is not even considered if a below-the-knee amputation is possible.

Amputation can be avoided entirely in the case of vascular problems if the blood supply to the limb can be guaranteed. As far as preventing amputation is concerned, results in patients with **intermittent claudication** who have artificial vein or artery replacement are no better than results in patients with untreated disease. Yet patients with intermittent claudication who have the artificial vein/artery replacement/grafts have less painand disability.[30] Other studies have found more optimistic results.[31] Mortality within 30 days of an operation for artificial artery grafts is 3%; the rate of complications, excluding graft failure or amputation resulting from graft failure, is 5%.[32]

? WHAT IS CONTROVERSIAL ABOUT THE PROCEDURE?

There is some controversy about the best technique for constructing the flaps to cover the stump. Some surgeons preserve the soleus muscle—a broad, flat muscle that lies under the large muscle of the calf on the back of the leg—believing that it is needed for an adequate blood supply to the stump; others remove it during the amputation.[33]

One possible cause of the high mortality and morbidity associated with this procedure is that each surgeon who does above-the-knee amputations does very few, because there are few to be done, relative to other types of surgery. As a result, this procedure is a sort of "amateur hour" for virtually every surgeon who does it, no matter how good her general surgical skills are. Development of specialty referral centers for amputation might reduce the high morbidity and mortality currently seen, but there is little prospect of their development, in part because those who need amputations tend to belong to lower socioeconomic strata, lacking medical insurance and continuous medical care. There is also little knowledge of how to use anticlotting drugs and long-term regimens of antibiotics to reduce postoperative problems such as clotting and infection, which account for much of the postoperative mortality.[34]

Aortocoronary Bypass (10/40/51/55)

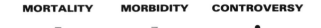

MORTALITY	MORBIDITY	CONTROVERSY
–	–	●

- The national **MORTALITY** rate for this procedure is between 1% and 3%; however, while exceeding the national surgical mortality rate of 1.33%, it is an improvement over the early years of bypass surgery.

- Major **MORBIDITY** factors include failure of the breastbone to heal and infection of the sac that surrounds the heart; this was reported in 35% of cases. Another risk of this procedure is stroke, the rate of which rose from .57% to 2.4% in cases studied from 1979 to 1983.

- The major **CONTROVERSY** is whether this procedure should be used before more conservative procedures are tried, such as balloon angioplasty (see p. 194) (PTCA, or percutaneous transluminal coronary angioplasty) or medical management.

LAY TITLE: Coronary Artery Bypass Graft (CABG, pronounced "cabbage")

Replacement of blocked coronary arteries with transplanted veins or arteries

This procedure is essentially the same, regardless of the number of arteries bypassed; therefore, we have combined into one discussion the following (with their rank in the top 100 surgeries in brackets):

Aortocoronary Bypass—2 coronary arteries [51]
Aortocoronary Bypass—3 coronary arteries [40]
Aortocoronary Bypass—4 or more coronary arteries [55]
Aortocoronary Bypass—2-, 3-, and 4-vessel procedures [10]

❔ WHAT CONDITION DOES THE PROCEDURE TREAT?

This procedure treats what is now the leading cause of death in the United States and much of the developed world—coronary artery disease. For further discussion of coronary artery disease, see "Combined Right and Left Cardiac Catheterization," p. 50.

❔ WHAT IS THE PROCEDURE?

A coronary bypass is one of the more heroic surgical procedures done today. It takes anywhere from two to four hours to perform, depending upon the patient and any difficulties encountered along the way. The procedure is essentially the same regardless of the number of arteries to be bypassed. There is general agreement that, if at all possible, one-vessel problems should be treated with percutaneous transluminal coronary angioplasty (called balloon angioplasty, or PTCA), in which a balloon is inserted into an artery and inflated to crush the plaque (see p. 194). Bypass is used for two, three, or more **occluded** arteries that cannot be successfully treated with balloon angioplasty.

When necessary, the chest is shaved the night or morning before surgery. General anesthetics are given both by vein and by inhalation, through a tube placed into the **trachea** after intravenous anesthetics have put the patient to sleep. While the general anesthesia is being started and stabilized ("induced"), the patient's chest is scrubbed with soap and antiseptic, as is the place on the leg from which veins will be extracted, if the surgeon plans to use leg veins for the **grafts**. (The internal mammary artery of the chest can also be used; if it is, no surgery is done on the legs because the "spare parts" are located in the chest and can be reached through the same incision used to reach the heart.) After the chest is dried, the patient is draped so that only the area to be operated on is exposed.

An incision about 12 to 18 inches long is made down the center of the chest. As soon as the integrity of the chest wall is lost—in other words, when the chest is opened by the surgeon—the lungs, which depend on a partial vacuum in the chest to expand, can no longer work, and breathing is done for the patient by the anesthetist's machines. (As mentioned above, a tube is placed in the windpipe and breathing is then controlled by the anesthesiologist until the patient is out of surgery and breathing on her own.) The **sternum**, or breastbone, is cut with a bone saw, and the two halves of the rib cage are pulled back far enough to allow the surgeon to reach the heart. Once the heart is stopped, incisions are made in major arteries and veins to allow the circulation to be taken over by the heart-lung machine. **Cannulas** running to the heart-lung machine are inserted, and the heart is stopped with a mild electric shock or drugs.

The heart must be stopped because the surgeon will be doing delicate stitchery on some rather small veins that are attached to the heart, which leaps and bounds in the chest, especially when the tissues around it are pulled back (**retracted**). While the heart is stopped, adequate blood flow is maintained by the heart-lung machine, which oxygenates and pumps the blood and also controls its temperature.

The leg vein grafts, if used, are usually taken by the surgical assisting team while the cardiac surgeon and her assistants are opening the chest. The occluded arteries and their blocked portions are identified, using x rays that were taken during an earlier procedure called a cardiac catheterization (see "Combined Right and Left Cardiac Catheterization," p. 50). Using the veins taken from the leg or sections of the internal mammary artery, each of the blockages is bypassed. No attempt is made to remove the wholly or partially blocked arteries, merely to establish circulation around them. When the grafts are complete, dye is injected. The grafts are then checked with a special x ray for the heart and its vessels (called an **angiogram**) to make sure that blood is flowing freely.

If there are no leaks or additional blockages and all appears well, the heart is restarted with an electric shock (and with drugs, if needed), and the patient is removed from the heart-lung machine. The sternum is sutured with metal wires, and the other layers are closed indi-vidually with nonmetallic sutures. The skin is closed with sutures, staples, or clips, depending upon the surgeon's preference. The patient is usually taken to the cardiac intensive care unit after a stay in the recovery room, or directly to the intensive care unit if the hospital is set up that way. Because breathing with a recently split sternum is painful, many patients are kept on a respirator for several hours until it is clear that they can breathe on their own. As soon as independent breathing is assured, the tube in the windpipe is removed. The patient is taken to the cardiac intensive care unit. When intensive care is no longer needed, usually after one to two days, the patient is moved to a cardiac unit with a less intensive level of care—the names of these units differ from hospital to hospital, but are often referred to as advanced cardiac care units. After three to five days, the patient usually no longer needs constant monitoring, and is taken to a general surgical unit. This process of tailoring the care to the patient's progress in recovery is called "staging" or "step-down care."

WHO PERFORMS THE PROCEDURE?

The procedure is performed by a cardiovascular surgeon, who is usually assisted by at least one other cardiovascular or vascular surgeon. The surgeon should be board certified, and ideally should perform at least one bypass procedure a week, and operate in a hospital that does at least 200 per year. This seems to be the minimum level needed to obtain acceptable morbidity and mortality rates, according to American College of Cardiology guidelines.

? WHERE IS THE PROCEDURE PERFORMED?

This surgery always requires an inpatient hospital stay; only hospitals, and usually only the larger ones, have all the personnel and equipment needed to perform the surgery and monitor patients afterwards.

? WHAT ARE THE MORTALITY (DEATH) AND MORBIDITY (COMPLICATION) RATES?

Mortality for this procedure has fallen steadily since its conception, and recent (1990–1991) literature notes that overall operative mortality of 0% to 3% can be achieved with current techniques.[1] Based on a review of some 400 articles from the National Library of Medicine data base, this rate of 1% to 3% reflects the results seen with carefully selected patients in the best centers. Five-year survival following surgery, even in patients over age 65, can be as high as 96.9%.[2] As with all surgeries, mortality rises with age, with the number and severity of coexisting diseases, and with the presence of any medical problems that are likely to cause problems with anesthesia. One 1990 study of emergency bypasses found 14.5% **operative mortality** and 35.9% **major morbidity** (for example, the breastbone does not show signs of healing or there is infection of the sac that surrounds the heart). Operative mortality was 4% for those taken directly to the operating room from the cardiac catheterization suite and 22.4% for those who had to be taken to the operating room from a general ward or the intensive care unit.[3] Results in other series range between these two extremes. Mortality increased with the number of vessels replaced.

Major complications include problems with sternal (breastbone) wounds, which occurred in 1.1% of patients in a study covering the period from 1985 to 1987. Of those who had sternal wound problems, 14.1% died of multiorgan failure; the presence of bacteria in cultures of the sternal wound was an indication of a stormy course, even if the patient lived.[4] Other problems include cardiac complications, which can be expected in about 18% of patients both over and under age 70; patients over age 70 can expect noncardiac complications to occur in 31% of cases.[5] One study comparing patients under and over age 70 found **perioperative** heart attacks in 4.1% and 7.9% of patients, respectively; a need for prolonged respiratory support in 3.1% and 7.9%; and major neurologic complications in 1.1% and 4%.[6] (Examples of major neurologic complications include stroke resulting from fat clots in the brain and brain damage caused by lack of oxygen.)

? WHAT ARE THE OTHER COMPLICATIONS AND POSSIBLE SIDE EFFECTS?

In addition to the usual surgical risks, depression following cardiac surgery is somewhat more severe than that following other surgeries, and about 16% to 31% of those operated on display mild to severe psychiatric symptoms.[7–12] Very extensive pre- and postsurgical testing in one study indicated that about 11% of patients will fail to recover fully from the effects of cardiac surgery on the nervous system.[13] Postoperative depression, especially in the elderly,[14] is a persistent finding; however, it seems to respond well to standard pharmacological treatment for depression.

The cause of cognitive impairments following cardiac surgery is unknown; one theory is that patients suffer "microstrokes" from clots released from the walls of arteries and veins while the cardiac bypass machine is in use. The machine reverses the usual direction of blood flow, and this may create turbulence that releases tiny **emboli** from the vessel walls.[15] Other theories point to alternating sensory deprivation and sensory overload in the cardiac intensive care unit, and the patient's having to face the extreme seriousness of her medical situation and the possibility of death. Most patients recover fully, but the full impact of mental health problems following CABG is unknown.

Stroke during or immediately following the operations has been rising, from about 0.57% to 2.4% over the five-year period 1979 to 1983, largely as a result of the increasing age of patients being operated on.[16] A later study (1988) showed a risk of 2.9% for patients who had a prior history of stroke and had general anesthesia for any surgery.[17] In yet another study, for patients with diagnosis of severe **carotid artery** narrowing, the risk of stroke was 9.2%, versus 1.9% for those without severe narrowing.[18] Other studies have found stroke rates in the 2.4% range as well, and have found that probability of stroke correlates very highly with increasing age of those having CABG.[19]

Several risk factors, none of them significantly avoidable or modifiable by either patient or physician, have been identified.[20] **Carotid bruits** raise the risk to 2.9% for having a stroke during or immediately after the surgery, a risk not dramatically greater than the overall stroke risk of 2.4% found in several studies. Depending upon the size of the clot, the region of the brain affected, and the speed and competence of poststroke therapy, the consequences of perioperative stroke can range from trivial to devastating.

? IS THIS THE MOST APPROPRIATE PROCEDURE FOR THE CONDITION?

Because this procedure has been in use for only about 20 years, because medical therapy in general has improved greatly, and because balloon angioplasty (PTCA) and its related treatments are still under development, this question is hard to answer. Studies have revealed a variety of subgroups of patients who react differently to nonsurgical treatment (such as blood pressure medication, calcium and **beta blockers**, diet, and exercise), CABG, and PTCA. These studies have also

been criticized as not representing the "typical" heart patient.[21]

Based on current knowledge, if one is already in the situation of having to face a CABG, it is the most appropriate procedure if one has blockage in the left main coronary artery and impaired function of the **left ventricle**. In a comparison of results with "worst-case" patients, the three-year survival rate was 82% for those treated with CABG and 34% for those treated medically.[22] For patients with three-vessel disease and mild angina, six-year survival was 43% better in the surgically treated group than in the medically treated group. A 10-year follow-up study showed that the quality of life (objectively and subjectively measured) of the medically treated patients and the surgically treated patients slowly converged. This reflects both a decline in the functioning of the bypass grafts—the tendency to clog—in the surgically treated patients and the slow improvement of those who were treated without surgery.[23]

If one is not in one of the subgroups that have been identified as having probably better survival with CABG, the decision should turn on quality of life as perceived by the patient. Some patients have all subjective symptoms (such as chest pain, shortness of breath, and lack of energy) resolved by medical treatment or PTCA. If further relief from symptoms is not needed, CABG is a foolish risk. However, if one is in one of the subgroups for which surgery doubles the survival rate achieved with medical treatment, not having CABG would seem to be foolish.

Of course, the real issue here is that a randomized, controlled trial comparing medical treatment, CABG, and PTCA has never been conducted.[24] Without this scientific "gold standard" to work from, one must resort to a newly developed technique called **meta-analysis**. A mathematical model that has been developed suggests that PTCA is a reasonable choice except in patients with three-vessel disease who have no other diseases that make surgery unusually risky. This latter group of patients should have bypass surgery. For single-vessel and even accessible multivessel disease, PTCA appears to offer equally good short-term results.

Appropriate diet and exercise can slow the progress of **atherosclerosis** or prevent it entirely, and there is recent evidence that a rigidly vegetarian, low-fat diet can reverse it.[25–30] There are new drugs that block cholesterol production, speed up the liver's removal of cholesterol from the bloodstream, or both.[31–33]

Neither PTCA nor CABG alone can prevent reblockage of the arteries operated on; significant dietary and exercise changes must be made.[34] The best choice is clearly an active program of prevention. In short, CABG is the appropriate choice only if medical and less radical surgical management do not produce an acceptable work performance and quality of life.

? ARE THERE ALTERNATIVES TO THIS PROCEDURE?

As mentioned above, prevention, medical management, and less radical surgery are all alternatives to this procedure. A number of new techniques, including laser angioplasty, in which plaques are burned away, and a "roto-rooter" that destroys them mechanically, are in research and development stages. All of them, however, carry risks, costs, and discomfort that would be entirely avoidable if people would care for their cardiac health.

? WHAT IS CONTROVERSIAL ABOUT THE PROCEDURE?

The most controversial aspect of CABG is the extent of its use. If, in the early days of CABG, we knew what we now know from controlled trials, the total use of CABG would never have approached current levels. Controlled trials, conducted after the procedure was already widespread, identified several subgroups of patients who quite clearly did far better with surgical than with medical treatment—for example, those with three-vessel disease and a left ventricular **ejection fraction**

between 35% and 49%.[35] At 10-year follow-up in one of the largest studies conducted, there was no statistically significant difference between survival with medical treatment or survival with surgical treatment except for those with an ejection fraction below 50% and either three-vessel disease or a blockage of greater than 70% in the proximal left anterior descending coronary artery,[36] which is the artery on the left side of the heart that runs down past the **aorta** and is closest to the breastbone.

It is quite clear, for example, that it is safe to defer surgery for patients who are medically treated until they find symptoms intolerable, unless they are in one of the subgroups for which bypass surgery has definitely been shown to improve survival. Many people will never experience intolerable symptoms, so if medicine were the primary treatment, the use of CABG could be reduced significantly.[37]

Instead, the use has increased continuously. This has been attributed to the fact that the procedure is a "cash cow" both for the doctors who perform it and for the hospitals where it is done. Many critics have stated that if physician payment for the procedure were minimal, its use would drop dramatically. One critic of the procedure is Thomas Preston, M.D., who was an electrical engineer before entering medicine and has a keen appreciation for the mythology of the profession. He wrote a book, *Coronary Artery Surgery: A Critical Review* (New York: Raven Press, 1977), which should be required reading for potential bypass patients. Although it was published in 1977, its critique of the theoretical and methodological assumptions underlying bypass surgery remains valid.

Appendectomy (8)

MORTALITY	MORBIDITY	CONTROVERSY
+	+	o

Removal of the appendix through a small incision

? WHAT CONDITION DOES THE PROCEDURE TREAT?

The appendix is a small tube of tissue about three inches long. It dangles from the start of the large intestine, or **colon**, on the right side of the body, just below the point where the small intestine joins the large intestine. The appendix has no known function at present, but is thought to have been involved in protecting the intestines against infection in our dim and distant past.

At present, far from being a protection against infection, it is a major source of internal infections. Although the contents of the small intestine are generally sterile, the lower intestines teem with bacteria; in fact, much of feces is bacteria. Some bacteria in the intestines produce useful vitamins, but in the main, they are "free riders"—they get nutrients from the food we eat, but don't do anything that benefits us in return. The bacteria generally stay in the colon, below the **ileocecal valve** which, when healthy, ensures that food being digested passes only from the almost-sterile small intestine into the bacteria-laden colon, and not the reverse. If the ileocecal valve malfunctions, bacteria can colonize the small intestine, with results that range from undetectable to serious, depending upon the number and type of bacteria present.

Because the appendix lies below the ileocecal valve, it lies in the bacteria-laden colon. When anything—a seed, a nut, a swallowed tooth, a tumor, an undigested pill, a bit of fibrous scar tissue—blocks the appendix, it

cannot clear its bacterial contents. In turn, the rapid multiplication of bacteria produces an **abscess**, which causes inflammation of the appendix. The result is appendicitis. About one person in 500 gets appendicitis each year.

Rarely—about 5% of the time—the pressure within the appendix clears the obstruction and allows the abscess to drain into the colon. In such cases the person will have had appendicitis without ever knowing it. Repeated bouts of infection and healing, in fact, can form the scar tissue, which in turn can produce the blockage that leads to a bout of appendicitis the person cannot avoid noticing.

An attack of appendicitis usually begins with pain in the region of the upper stomach or around the navel and includes an episode or two of vomiting. Within a few hours, the pain shifts to the lower right quadrant of the abdomen (the region below and to the right of the navel). The pain is made worse by walking or coughing. Within a few more hours, fever, constipation or diarrhea, and a feeling of weakness begin, and the pain becomes more localized. Often the patient can put her finger right on the most tender spot, which will prove to be right over the inflamed appendix. If the patient has wisely decided to see a doctor by this time, the doctor will find that pressing on the sore spot and suddenly releasing it causes a sharp increase in the pain and spasm of the abdominal muscles. A classic sign, this is called rebound tenderness.

There are usually no specific x-ray findings unless a **radiopaque** obstruction (something blocking the intestine that shows up on x rays) is the cause of the blockage. A **barium enema** rules out appendicitis if the appendix is seen to be filling (which means the appendix is not blocked). If no filling is seen, the x-ray finding strongly suggests appendicitis. The symptoms can vary if the appendix is not in the most common anatomical position, which is directly under the connection between the large and small intestines, and to the left of and slightly below the tip of the hipbone. Various odd locations of the appendix can lead the doctor to suspect diseases other than appendicitis.

"Watchful waiting" to further refine the diagnosis is generally safe during the first eight hours, a period in which the appendix rarely **perforates** (ruptures or bursts). After this interval, the appendix is prone to rupture at any time.[1] (When this happens, the contents of the swollen appendix are released into the abdomen and possibly spread infection there.) Patients with appendicitis-related surgical acute abdomen—symptoms indicating that something major is wrong with the intestines—require immediate surgery. A 1989 French study found a 4% mortality rate among such patients, who were operated on within 12 hours of the onset of pain. And those operated on 24 hours or more after the onset of pain had a mortality rate of 23%.[2] Studies of other abdominal conditions that can lead to **peritonitis** have found out again and again that early operation lowers the mortality rate.[3–5]

? WHAT IS THE PROCEDURE?

Even in emergency cases, patients are prepared for the procedure by administration of antibiotics to reduce the infection as much as possible and limit tissue damage in the abdomen, and by administration of intravenous fluids. (Anything by mouth, other than an antibiotic pill or two, is usually forbidden before procedures in the abdomen.) The patient is given a general or spinal anesthetic. The abdomen is washed with soap and antiseptic and draped so that only the area where the incision will be made is exposed.

An appendectomy can be performed in a variety of ways. The method used depends upon factors including the training and preferences of the surgeon; how inflamed the appendix is; whether it is in the classic anatomical position; and whether or not the **peritoneum**

in the area of the appendix looks clear, or cloudy and bloody. These variations are of little importance to the patient, because the broad outlines and the end result are the same. The surgeon makes an incision in the lower right abdomen that is no larger than she thinks will be necessary to perform the operation. If the appendix is in the classic position, she just reaches in through the incision, and grabs the end of the large intestine nearest the appendix (the **cecum**) with a gauze pad, bringing it outside the body. If the appendix is located elsewhere, enough of the ligaments holding the colon are cut to allow it to be brought outside the body.

The appendix is cut away from the membrane that holds it against the cecum and the end of the small intestine. A "purse-string" suture, so-called because it resembles the closure string of a sack-type purse, is placed through the cecum in a wide ring around the base of the appendix. The base of the appendix is tied off with a **suture**, and the appendix is placed on a pad of sterile gauze, clamped off (to avoid spreading the infection), and cut at the base. At this point in the procedure, some surgeons prefer to use an **electrocautery** device to make sure the base of the appendix is sealed. The stump of the appendix is pushed into the large intestine, and the purse-string suture is pulled tight, sealing the wound left by removal of the appendix. Depending upon conditions in the abdomen, the surgeon closes some or all of the layers of tissue with sutures, and may or may not insert soft rubber drainage tubes. If the abdomen is badly infected, only the peritoneum is sutured shut, and the other layers (fat, muscle, and skin) are closed when the infection subsides.

? WHO PERFORMS THE PROCEDURE?

The procedure is usually done by general surgeons. In remote or medically underserved areas where the older tradition of "physician and surgeon" still survives out of necessity, general and family practitioners perform appendectomies.

? WHERE IS THE PROCEDURE PERFORMED?

Appendectomies are rarely performed outside of hospitals because of the generally risky nature of "open" abdominal operations involving larger incisions. Other procedures performed through a **laparoscope**, after which the incision can be closed with a Band-Aid, or an **endoscope** can be done in outpatient settings.

Following an appendectomy, there is also the need to monitor the patient for postoperative bleeding or infection for a few days, and this requires a hospital setting. In the future, some appendectomies may be performed as short-stay procedures, but this is not the practice now.

? WHAT ARE THE MORTALITY (DEATH) AND MORBIDITY (COMPLICATION) RATES?

The mortality rate for appendectomy in community hospitals in the U.S. in 1988 was 0.1%.[6] Even in Soviet hospitals, which have well-documented problems with quality of care, the mortality rate from appendicitis can be as low as 0.14%[7] For patients with heart problems, the mortality rate one month after an appendectomy can be as high as 9%.[8] In cases complicated by patient self-treatment with strong laxatives, which can contribute to rupture, the mortality rate can be as high as 12.2%.[9] Age above 58 was found to increase mortality in a 10-year study of appendectomies.[10]

In California in 1984, mortality rates for persons over age 60 with unperforated, or unruptured, appendixes was 0.7%, and was 2.4% for those over age 60 with perforations. The proportion of cases with perforations increased from 22% to 75% as ages increased from 20 to 80.[11] The higher mortality rate among the elderly has been attributed, in part, to physician error. Symptoms of appendicitis in the elderly tend to be milder than those in younger patients, leading to delays in operating.[12]

The major cause of death is peritonitis, resulting in part from delayed operation.[13] Ninety-five percent of appendicitis cases that are not surgically treated or rapidly stabilized with antibiotics progress to rupture, and rupture causes peritonitis. Peritonitis can rapidly progress to **toxemia** and then to toxic shock, which can be fatal. Antibiotic treatment can be lifesaving, but cure almost always requires removal of the source of the infection—in this case, the inflamed appendix. Mortality from peritonitis ranges from 10%[14] to 43.75%,[15] depending on the organisms causing the infection and other medical conditions. If peritonitis is complicated by hospital-acquired pneumonia, the mortality rate is 75%.[16] Mortality rates as high as 92.2% have been reported for generalized peritonitis in the entire abdominal cavity.[17]

Because of the clear association between delay and death, and the variable nature of the symptoms of appendicitis, doctors believe that to be prudent—and avoid malpractice suits, we might add—they should operate when there is a high probability that appendicitis is present, even if the diagnosis is not certain. This leads to a negative operation rate, which is the rate at which normal appendixes are removed by appendectomy. The negative operation rate is 15% to 20% for emergency appendectomies at most hospitals, a figure most medical experts consider acceptable. Unfortunately, the complication rate associated with negative operations for appendicitis is about 15%. Some researchers suggest that computer-aided diagnosis could reduce the incidence of negative operations for appendicitis.[18] Even without computer assistance, the diagnostic error rate can be as low as 6% for nonemergency but "urgent" operations.[19] (Generally, doctors define an emergency procedure as one that is done in response to a medical situation that arises suddenly and unexpectedly, and requires quick judgment and prompt action. An urgent procedure is one that calls for immediate attention.)

Early in the course of appendicitis when the decision to operate has to be made, laboratory data (blood and urine studies, primarily) tend not to vary greatly from normal. Eight test values have been identified that differ between patients with and without appendicitis. However, each of the tests and an index composed of all eight of them had low sensitivity—in other words, could not be used to differentiate between who was sick and who wasn't—and low specificity, which meant the test values were not good indicators of which sick people had appendicitis and which didn't.[20]

In most cases the cause of death in patients who die after appendectomy is peritonitis (60.9%), followed by **thromboembolism** of the pulmonary artery (7.8%), intestinal **fistulas** (2.6%), and bleeding (1.7%).[21] A 1983 French study of complicated cases—in which other medical problems were superimposed on appendicitis and which altered the patient's symptoms or course for the worse—found a mortality rate of 24.5%, with peritonitis again the leader.[22] If re-operation is required for a complication following an appendectomy, the mortality rate can be as high as 6.6%.[23]

A Soviet study, relevant because Soviet hospitals can produce mortality results comparable to those of American hospitals, found that physician error accounted for 65% of the deaths.[24]

Up to 29% of the appendixes removed turn out not to be infected or inflamed. The removal of the undamaged appendix certainly imposes a minor risk on the patient, but may be advantageous in that a person without an appendix cannot get appendicitis in the future. Operations in patients who do not have appendicitis can also lead to proper diagnosis and therapy for the condition that is causing the abdominal pain.[25] Some doctors advocate removal of the appendix whenever abdominal surgery is performed that puts the appendix within easy reach.[26, 27]

Postoperative infection rates can be as high as 6% for patients who do not have appendicitis and 19.3% for those who do.[28] A single dose of the antibiotic metronidazole (Flagyl) before surgery was found to reduce the rate of complications by 89% in a group of French children.[29]

? WHAT ARE THE OTHER COMPLICATIONS AND POSSIBLE SIDE EFFECTS?

As with any procedure in which anesthesia is used, death from reaction to the anesthetic drugs, error on the part of the anesthetist, or machine failure is a remote possibility. (See Glossary, p. 309)

? IS THIS THE MOST APPROPRIATE PROCEDURE FOR THE CONDITION?

Given the tendency of the appendix to rupture, yes.

? ARE THERE ALTERNATIVES TO THIS PROCEDURE?

In rare instances where a walled-off abscess has formed around an inflamed appendix and the patient's age and condition make surgery risky, the surgeon may elect to use intensive antibiotic treatment followed by drainage of the abscess with a long needle and a **catheter** inserted under a local anesthetic with x-ray or **ultrasound** guidance. In all other cases, an appendectomy is performed.

? WHAT IS CONTROVERSIAL ABOUT THE PROCEDURE?

Controversy continues with respect to the high negative operation rate (operations in which a normal appendix is found), the wisdom of doing "incidental" appendectomies during other abdominal surgery, and the many means of improving diagnosis. None of these controversies is particularly heated.

Below-the-Knee Amputation (87)

MORTALITY	MORBIDITY	CONTROVERSY
–	–	●

- **MORTALITY** rates around 14% are the expected norm and are about 10 times higher than the national average for all surgical procedures.

- Deep **VENOUS CLOTTING** is a problem in 40% to 70% of cases in which anticlotting treatment is not started. Pulmonary embolisms are reported in 2% to 10% of the cases, and injury to the vessels in the region of the knee is also a risk.

- The **CONTROVERSY** centers on the best way to construct the flap of skin that covers the stump, and on the experience of the surgeons who perform this procedure.

Removal of the lower leg below the knee joint

? WHAT CONDITION DOES THE PROCEDURE TREAT?

Below-the-knee amputation is performed for **ischemia** that cannot be corrected surgically; for failed attempts at repair of veins and arteries below the knee and failed attempts at removal of clots; for life-threatening infections that cannot be controlled with antibiotics[1]; and for traumatic damage to the lower leg (e.g., auto accident injuries and gunshot wounds) that is too severe to repair surgically.[2] Below-the-knee amputation may also result following injury, because of failure to treat damage to the **popliteal artery** in a timely manner. The limb is at risk if popliteal artery damage is not repaired within three to six hours.[3] In up to 90% of injuries it is possible to avoid amputation with vessel repairs.[4]

Generally, learning to walk with a below-the-knee amputation is far easier than learning to walk with an above-the-knee amputation, so surgeons attempt to preserve the knee if at all possible.[5, 6] Diabetes and smoking are risk factors that may make the healing process more

difficult or impossible, or lead to the need for amputation in the first place. Both can cause ischemia and damage to blood vessels.[7, 8]

? WHAT IS THE PROCEDURE?

Like most amputation procedures, this one goes well back in history, and has become only slightly less crude with the passage of time. With the patient under general anesthesia, the area to be operated on is shaved, scrubbed with soap and antiseptic, and draped so that only the area of incision is exposed. The surgeon makes incisions in the skin, fat, **fascia**, and muscles that will allow her to form a covering for the stump.[9] Bleeding vessels are **ligated** as they are encountered. When the tissue flaps are prepared and the bone is exposed, it is sawn through and filed smooth; bone wax is used to stop bleeding if needed. The stump is constructed from surrounding flaps of tissue, and the muscle, fascia, and skin are closed in layers, with careful attention paid to preserving a good blood supply to the stump. The patient is taken to the recovery room and then to her own room.

A course of physical therapy and practice in learning to use a **prosthesis** (in this case, an artificial lower leg) follow. Some types of prostheses can be fitted within five days of surgery.[10] The surgeon may elect to use a plaster cast and pylon arrangement, which is a metal rod that extends from the bottom of the cast to an artificial foot, to aid in early return to walking.[11] About a year is required to reach maximum improvement in walking and general functioning.[12] If the stump proves to be too short for effective walking, a Soviet-developed limb-stretching technique called an Ilizarov extension can be used to lengthen it.[13]

? WHO PERFORMS THE PROCEDURE?

This procedure should be performed by a board-certified orthopedic surgeon, preferably one who does a large number of such operations each year.

? WHERE IS THE PROCEDURE PERFORMED?

This is major surgery that should be performed in the inpatient department of a hospital. Careful monitoring for postoperative **thrombosis** and infection is required. The rehabilitation phase can probably best be done in a rehabilitation hospital on either an inpatient or outpatient basis.

? WHAT ARE THE MORTALITY (DEATH) AND MORBIDITY (COMPLICATION) RATES?

The mortality rate for two different techniques of constructing stumps was 11% and 17% for the two methods in a 1991 controlled trial. Not statistically significant, the difference suggests that mortality rates around 14% are to be expected.[14] About 5% of cases have complications serious enough to require above-the-knee amputation.[15] In patients over age 80, problems with healing of the stump flaps can be expected in about 10% of cases.[16] Seventy-two percent of patients have "phantom limb" pain, in which pain is felt in the missing part of the limb, or stump pain.[17]

Complication rates recently cited for joint replacement surgery are broadly applicable to most lower limb surgery: 40% to 70% risk of deep venous thrombosis without anticlotting treatment; 2% to 16% risk of non-fatal **pulmonary embolism**; and 1.8% to 3.4% risk of fatal pulmonary embolism.[18] Various courses of treatment with anticlotting drugs can reduce these risks appreciably.

? WHAT ARE THE OTHER COMPLICATIONS AND POSSIBLE SIDE EFFECTS?

Injury to the vessels in the region of the knee can occur, and can be serious but unrecognized at the time of operation. When the injury is discovered, vessel repair operations are possible.[19]

As with any procedure in which anesthesia is used, death from reaction to the anesthetic drugs, error on the part of the anesthetist, or machine failure is a remote possibility. (See Glossary, p. 309)

? IS THIS THE MOST APPROPRIATE PROCEDURE FOR THE CONDITION?

Any amputation should be a last-resort measure. Procedures to deal with circulatory problems should be tried first, unless the patient's condition makes failure virtually certain; the physician has a number of computer-aided-decision tools to use here. (These are computer programs that analyze the variables associated with each patient, such as height, weight, age, sex, blood flow in the vessel, and length of vessel. Once this profile is generated, it is compared with a data base of other patients, and a probable success rate can be determined.) The presence of gangrene and certain other infections can be life-threatening and should be treated by speedy amputation if more conservative measures, such as just cutting away the infected tissue and administering intravenous antibiotics, fail.

? ARE THERE ALTERNATIVES TO THIS PROCEDURE?

Attempts at vein or artery grafts to bypass blockages are usually tried before amputation; if successful, they make amputation unnecessary.[20] The mortality rate for Dacron-graft artery replacements—artificial arteries made of woven Dacron, a synthetic fiber—is 0.5%, with about 8% of patients requiring amputation during a 10-year follow-up period.[21] There is no alternative to amputation in some cases of life-threatening infection—gangrene, for example. If further surgery is needed, through-the-knee amputations, which preserve the bottom part of the **femur,** are a good alternative to above-the-knee amputations.[22] Conventional balloon angioplasty (see "Percutaneous Transluminal Coronary Angioplasty," p. 194), in which a balloon is inflated in a narrowed artery to open it up, has a mortality rate of 3% and a complication rate of 10%. Ninety-five percent of balloon angioplasty patients have initial success, but 40% require re-operation within three to 15 months.[23] Laser-assisted balloon angioplasty (opening up of a constricted artery with laser beams and balloon inflation) produced clinical success in 71% of patients in a small trial and is a reasonable alternative to try before amputation; however, it remains to be seen how well it will work for large groups of patients and to what extent it can help avoid amputation.[24]

? WHAT IS CONTROVERSIAL ABOUT THE PROCEDURE?

There is some controversy about the best technique for constructing the flaps to cover the stump. Some surgeons preserve the soleus muscle—a broad, flat muscle that lies under the large muscle of the calf on the back of the leg—believing that it is needed for an adequate blood supply to the stump; others remove it during the amputation.[25]

It has been argued that most surgeons do too few amputations to be really proficient at them. As a result, this procedure is a sort of "amateur hour" for virtually every surgeon who does it, not matter how good her general surgical skills are. Development of specialty referral centers for amputation might reduce the high morbidity and mortality rates that are now seen. There is little prospect of their development, however, in part because those who need amputations tend to belong to lower socioeconomic strata, lacking medical insurance and continuous medical care. There is also little knowledge of how to use medical treatment—for example, anticlotting drugs and long-term regimens of antibiotics—to reduce postoperative problems such as clotting and infection that cause much of the postoperative mortality.[26]

Bilateral Salpingo-Oophorectomy or Salpingo-Ovariectomy (91)

MORTALITY	MORBIDITY	CONTROVERSY
+	+	●

- The major **CONTROVERSY** centers on the appropriateness of removing the ovaries and tubes unless medically indicated. The recommendations are that more conservative methods be tried before both ovaries and tubes are removed.

Removal of the ovaries and the **fallopian tubes**; "female castration"

? WHAT CONDITION DOES THE PROCEDURE TREAT?

This procedure is done primarily to treat cancer of the ovaries; cancer of the fallopian tubes;[1, 2] cancers of the uterus that have a tendency to spread to and recur in the tubes and ovaries;[3] hormone-dependent breast cancer (affected by the level of hormones, estrogen or progestogen, in the blood);[4–7] and infections of the ovaries that do not respond to antibiotics. (The latter is usually done in conjunction with a hysterectomy.) It is worth noting that current recommendations call for preservation of the ovaries in younger women even when the uterus is removed; if the problem being treated is limited to the uterus, the ovaries should not be removed.[8]

? WHAT IS THE PROCEDURE?

Ovaries and tubes can be removed either via a **laparoscope** or with an open procedure, which involves cutting into the abdomen. In either case, the patient is given a general anesthetic. If the open procedure is used, the abdomen is shaved and scrubbed with soap and antiseptic, and an incision is made in the lower abdomen. The tubes and ovaries are located and removed. To avoid the **ovarian remnant syndrome**, the surgeon should be careful to remove all of the ovaries. Once all the ovaries are out, the abdomen is closed in layers. The patient is taken to the recovery room and then to her room.

If this procedure is to be done with a laparoscope, the patient is prepared in exactly the same way as in the open procedure. A small incision is made in or just below the navel. Bleeding vessels are **cauterized** with an **electrocautery device**. The laparoscope is inserted through the navel incision, and the abdominal cavity is inflated with carbon dioxide to separate the organs. This also gives the surgeon the necessary room to maneuver the laparoscope and carry out the procedure. A **trochar** is then positioned over the ovary and tube to be removed, and the abdomen is punctured.

The surgeon looks through the scope (or at a TV monitor connected to a TV camera in the scope) and locates the ovaries and tubes. Using the channels in the scope, the surgeon is able to pass small surgical instruments to where they are needed, and the ovaries and tubes are removed. Then the abdomen is deflated and the scope and instruments removed. The incisions are bandaged and the patient is taken to the recovery room and then to her room.

? WHO PERFORMS THE PROCEDURE?

This procedure is performed by a general surgeon or a gynecologist.

? WHERE IS THE PROCEDURE PERFORMED?

If the open procedure is done, it is performed in a hospital. The laparoscopic procedure can be done on an inpatient or outpatient basis in the hospital or in an outpatient surgery facility.

? WHAT ARE THE MORTALITY (DEATH) AND MORBIDITY (COMPLICATION) RATES?

Mortality is essentially zero, with most deaths relating to anesthesia rather than to the procedure itself. As with any procedure in which anesthesia is used, death from reaction to the anesthetic drugs, error on the part of the anesthetist, or machine failure is a remote possibility. (See Glossary, p. 309)

There is little morbidity immediately following the procedure; of chief concern are the later side effects of loss of the ovarian hormones, such as reduction in bone mass which results in osteoporosis.

? WHAT ARE THE OTHER COMPLICATIONS AND POSSIBLE SIDE EFFECTS?

The chief side effects of removal of both ovaries in premenopausal women include all those assigned to menopause—flushing, hot flashes, increased risk of cardiovascular disease,[9] and depression. Medical treatment of premenopausal women who have had both ovaries removed is controversial, but opinion seems to be increasingly leaning towards using estrogen supplements to counteract the above-mentioned side effects.[10]

Failure to remove the ovaries completely can commonly lead to the ovarian remnant syndrome, which is difficult to treat,[11] and occasionally leads to blockage of the **ureters**.[12]

? IS THIS THE MOST APPROPRIATE PROCEDURE FOR THE CONDITION?

Except in cases of cancer of the ovaries, the best answer is probably "we don't know." Tamoxifen (brand name Nolvadex) can be used to suppress the growth of breast cancers that are responsive to estrogen in the minority of patients who have hormone-dependent breast cancers; therefore, there is no reason to do this procedure for breast cancer alone. A few other cancers (primarily varieties of endometrial, or uterine, cancer) have shown a high statistical probability of spreading to the ovaries; their removal to prevent later cancer is recommended.

Beyond these cases, there seems to be no compelling reason to remove the ovaries other than because of infections that cannot be eradicated with antibiotics, or injury so severe that repair is impossible. A study of 1,000 women who had hysterectomies—some with and some without removal of the ovaries—showed that the rate of undiagnosed cancer present in the removed ovaries was zero. This lends support to the idea of leaving the ovaries in place if they appear normal during a hysterectomy.[13]

Although the logic of the aforementioned studies would suggest that leaving a normal ovary in when the other one is removed is safe, this is not the current practice of surgeons.

Studies of postmenopausal women show that the loss of estrogen that accompanies shutting down of the ovaries can lead to bone loss and osteoporosis. This can be prevented if estrogen supplements are started within three years of the last menstrual period.[14] The same protection from bone loss can be obtained if estrogens are started after surgery. At least one form of vitamin D, when used with a diet containing adequate calcium, has reversed bone loss in female rats whose ovaries had been removed.[15]

? ARE THERE ALTERNATIVES TO THIS PROCEDURE?

Except in cases of ovarian cancer or hormone-responsive breast cancer that cannot be treated with tamoxifen, infections that do not respond to antibiotics, or severe injury, there seem to be few reasons to remove the ovaries.

If the ovaries are removed, calcitonin and diphosphates can be prescribed for women who do not wish to take estrogen. Calcitonin is a hormone that increases the intake of calcium and phosphates by bone, resulting in preservation and reconstruction of bone.

? WHAT IS CONTROVERSIAL ABOUT THE PROCEDURE?

Because of the tendency of bowel cancer in women to spread to the ovaries, some doctors recommend removal of the ovaries in postmenopausal women who have cancer of the large intestine. The recommendation is considered controversial.[16]

Surgery should be a "last-resort" treatment for severe premenstrual syndrome after drug treatments have failed.[17, 18] There are no statistics on how often this procedure is done for this particular purpose; however, it is important to note that in all but a very few cases premenstrual syndrome is treatable by medication, either by hormones or psychoactive drugs, or a combination of both.

A completely open question is whether removal of one or both tubes and ovaries should be done for conditions that do not require suppression of hormone production by the ovaries.[19] Leaving a normal ovary in the body has the theoretical advantage of promoting a normal hormonal cycle even if supplemental estrogen is used.

Regarding hormone replacement therapy, there are two areas of concern, one scientific and one ideological. Some doctors are concerned that the use of replacement estrogens will increase the incidence of breast cancer, but studies so far have not proven this theory to be true. Current research strongly suggests, however, that the benefits of hormone replacement therapy—a reduction in bone loss (and thus the risk of osteoporosis) and heart disease (a major and currently growing problem in women) more than outweighs any risk of breast cancer that might be associated with this treatment. This academic opinion is slowly filtering down to the practicing obstetrician-gynecologists and family and general practitioners.

Bilateral Tubal Destruction (98)

MORTALITY	MORBIDITY	CONTROVERSY
+	+	o

Destruction of the **fallopian tubes** to avoid pregnancy

? WHAT CONDITION DOES THE PROCEDURE TREAT?

Strictly speaking, this procedure does not treat anything, unless there is a need to avoid pregnancy for health reasons. Its purpose is sterilization.

? WHAT IS THE PROCEDURE?

The literature regarding tubal destruction is mingled with that covering tubal **clipping**, clamping, and **ligation**, all of which are methods used for permanent or reversible sterilization. Methods that do not destroy the tubes, such as ligation or clipping, are associated with a small rate of failure resulting in unwanted pregnancies. For that reason, some doctors prefer to remove a section of the tube and plug the remaining ends when it is quite clear that the patient does not want a reversible procedure. Nonreversible methods used include cutting the tubes with surgical scissors or using an **electrocautery device** to clog and seal the ends, and plugging the tubes.

All procedures can be done with a **laparoscope**, in an **open procedure** called a mini-**laparotomy**, which involves a very small incision, and via an open procedure called a **laparotomy**, which entails a larger incision. The mini-laparotomy can be done with an incision through the abdomen or through the top of the vagina, where it attaches to the **cervix**.

Regardless of the approach, the opening stages of the procedure are identical. The patient's abdomen is shaved and washed with soap and antiseptic. A sterile drape is placed over the patient, covering everything except the small area where the incision will be made.

General anesthesia or local anesthesia plus sedation is used.[1] For laparoscopic cases, local anesthesia can be used.[2] In the laparoscopic procedure, a small incision is made in or just below the navel, and the laparoscope is inserted. The abdomen is inflated with air or carbon dioxide to separate the organs and enable the surgeon to avoid damaging the **peritoneum**. Depending upon the surgeon's preferred technique, another small incision may be made through which other instruments will be passed.

In the mini-laparotomy or the laparotomy, with either the abdominal or the transvaginal approach, an incision is made that allows access to the fallopian tubes.

From this point on, the two procedures are identical regardless of the route taken into the abdomen. The surgeon takes care to distinguish the fallopian tubes from the **ureters** and the veins and arteries that supply the pelvic area. When identified, the tubes are cut. Depending upon the surgeon's preferred technique, most or part of the tubes may be removed. Some surgeons cut both tubes and fold the ends back, sewing them to the remaining stumps. Others cut and plug the tubes. Regardless of the approach, when the procedure is finished the surgeon closes the entry incision with sutures or bandages, and the patient is taken to the recovery room and then to her room.

? WHO PERFORMS THE PROCEDURE?

This procedure can be performed by a general surgeon or an obstetrician-gynecologist. As usual, if a board-certified specialist is available, she is likely to give better results than a surgeon who is not certified.

? WHERE IS THE PROCEDURE PERFORMED?

Open procedures are usually performed in the inpatient department of a hospital. The laparoscopic procedure can be performed in a hospital, an outpatient surgery clinic, or a well-equipped doctor's office. If a general anesthetic (as opposed to sedation) is to be used, the procedure should be performed in a hospital.

? WHAT ARE THE MORTALITY (DEATH) AND MORBIDITY (COMPLICATION) RATES?

There is virtually no mortality from this procedure. A Centers for Disease Control and Prevention study reported 29 deaths from tubal procedures of all types in the U.S. from 1977 to 1981. Thirty-eight percent were attributable to complications of general anesthesia, 10% were caused by heart attacks, and the other 52% resulted from other causes. The procedure has undoubtedly become safer since 1981.[3] A 1982 study estimates a mortality rate of 0.004% from the procedure itself and 0.008% for deaths due to all causes in women having the procedure.[4] Other studies estimate a rate between 0.001% and 0.009%.[5] A 1986 review of mortality rates worldwide found that even developing countries have rates of well under 0.5%.[6] The risk is less than that of a single pregnancy or taking birth control pills for one year.[7]

The Centers for Disease Control and Prevention estimate that complications associated with tubal surgery occur in 1.7% of cases and are five times more common for procedures done under general anesthesia.[8] Indeed, other studies have implicated general anesthesia, rather than the procedure itself, as the chief cause of complications.[9] In a German study of sterilization by laparoscope, **intraoperative** complications were found in 8.4% of cases.[10]

Even after a laparoscopic tubal sterilization, an open procedure—a laparotomy—is necessary in more than 1% of women to manage complications or complete the sterilization.[11] The risk of pregnancy within 24 months of the procedure is about 1% for procedures in which the tubes are clipped and not destroyed; the rate following tubal destructions is probably somewhat lower.[12] Injuries to the abdominal organs during surgery have been found in up to 1.045% of cases when the laparoscopic technique is used.[13] A very large 1989 German study showed a complication rate of 1.97% with the laparoscopic technique.[14]

A 1991 study indicates that about 6% of women having this procedure will develop pelvic inflammatory disease (PID), a potentially serious infection.[15]

Infections other than PID occur in 0.4% of cases in which the open technique is used.[16]

? WHAT ARE THE OTHER COMPLICATIONS AND POSSIBLE SIDE EFFECTS?

In 1978 to 1979, two deaths were associated with the use of unipolar electrical coagulators, devices that are used to stop bleeding.[17] **Ectopic pregnancy**, a pregnancy outside the uterus that can cause severe abdominal pain and vaginal bleeding, can occur after tubal destruction.[18] A rare but clearly life-threatening complication is cardiovascular collapse during tubal procedures done by laparoscope. This condition may be caused by an **embolism** of the carbon dioxide used to inflate the abdomen during the procedure.[19] One death resulting from carbon dioxide embolism has been reported.[20]

Spasm of the tubes may make it impossible to insert plugs into the tubes to seal the ends.[21]

One case of a fatal explosion in a patient's abdomen, apparently caused by leakage of anesthetic gas while an electrocautery device was being used, has been reported.[22]

As with any procedure in which anesthesia is used, death from reaction to the anesthetic drugs, error on the part of the anesthetist, or machine failure is a remote possibility. (See Glossary, p. 309)

? IS THIS THE MOST APPROPRIATE PROCEDURE FOR THE CONDITION?

This is probably the most appropriate procedure if both partners in the relationship no longer desire children. Male sterilization is technically much simpler and much less expensive than female sterilization and has a zero mortality rate. No fewer than 14 women die from sterilization procedures each year.[23]

Theoretically, pregnancy cannot occur at all if the tubes are destroyed; however, use of a clip, as opposed to destruction of the tubes, has been associated with pregnancy rates as high as 8.6%.[24] Other studies have shown pregnancy rates of 1% or less for clip use.[25, 26]

? ARE THERE ALTERNATIVES TO THIS PROCEDURE?

Use of a contraceptive drug is one alternative, but it appears that the associated risk of pregnancy and other complications may be higher than the health risk associated with this procedure. The exact risk depends upon the woman's age, her health status when the contraceptive drug is started, the drug used, and her overall health-related habits (nutrition, exercise, and smoking, for example). Contraceptive devices (IUD, diaphragm, condom, and spermicidal foam or jelly) can be used, but their failure rates are significantly higher.

? WHAT IS CONTROVERSIAL ABOUT THE PROCEDURE?

There is very little controversy over this procedure, but it appears that the ideal tubal clip has not yet been developed.

Bilateral Tubal Division (78)

MORTALITY	MORBIDITY	CONTROVERSY
+	+	o

LAY TITLE: Having your tubes tied

Division (cutting) of the **fallopian tubes** for sterility

In every issue but appropriateness of the procedure, this particular procedure is identical to "Bilateral Tubal Destruction," p. 119.

? IS THIS THE MOST APPROPRIATE PROCEDURE FOR THE CONDITION?

This is probably not the most appropriate procedure if both partners are certain they no longer desire children, but if there is some chance of their changing their minds and desiring children, then the procedure is appropriate. Male sterilization is technically much simpler and cheaper than female sterilization and has a zero mortality rate. On the other hand, no fewer than 14 women die from sterilization procedures each year.[1] Theoretically, pregnancy cannot occur at all if the tubes are destroyed; however, use of a clip, as opposed to destruction of the tubes, has been associated with pregnancy rates as high as 8.6%.[2] Other studies have shown pregnancy rates of 1% or less for clip use; the wide variation may be attributable to differences in techniques used by the surgeons, or to mechanical differences between clips.[3, 4]

Research repeatedly indicates that the risk from tubal sterilization is less than that of normal delivery.

Cataract Removal with Intraocular Lens Implant (not ranked)·

MORTALITY	MORBIDITY	CONTROVERSY
+	+	o

• As explained in the introduction to Part II, this procedure is not given a rank among the 100 most common operations because it is usually not performed in a hospital.

LAY TITLE: Cataract surgery

Surgical removal of a hard opacity of the lens of the eye and implanting an intraocular plastic lens

Before we begin, it is helpful to review the anatomy of the eye, the organ of sight. There are five main components to the eye: the cornea (the transparent outer surface); the iris (the color portion); the pupil (controls the amount of light entering the eye); the lens (which focuses the image or light on the retina); and the retina (which converts the light images to electrical impulses and sends them to the brain via the optic nerve). The white portion of the eye is called the vitreous humor. The aqueous humor is the fluid in front of the lens.

Eye movement is essentially controlled by three pairs of muscles: the superior and inferior rectus, the muscles on the top and bottom of the eye; the lateral and medial rectus, the muscles on the right and left sides of the eye; and the superior and inferior oblique, the muscles that surround the top and bottom of the eyes.

The earliest recorded cataract surgery occurred in India 3,000 years ago.[1]

At one time, cataract surgery required general anesthesia and a hospital stay of at least five days. Most patients had to wear dark glasses because the glare from sunlight was too strong for the unprotected eye. Today cataract surgery is safely performed on an outpatient basis with a local anesthetic. The development of the implantable lens has greatly improved visual acuity and all but eliminated the need for thick glasses and contact lenses, which many elderly cataract patients found difficult to handle.

? WHAT CONDITION DOES THE PROCEDURE TREAT?

A cataract is formed when the transparent material that makes up the eye's natural lens becomes clouded and blocks or distorts the light entering the eye.[2] This cloudiness has been likened to viewing the world through Vaseline-coated glasses or attempting to see through a waterfall—everything becomes distorted and difficult to see. In fact, the word *cataract* means waterfall in Greek.

For most people, lens deterioration begins in their 20s, when the lens takes on a slight discoloration. Through the aging process, the lens continues to change until the amount of light entering the eyes and striking the retina is reduced. In fact, it's a natural part of the aging process and most people over the age of 60 have some evidence of cataract formation.[3]

Cataracts interfere with vision by distorting the light as it passes through the lens. Most people aren't aware that they are developing a cataract because the process generally occurs over a long period of time. The first indication that something might not be right is when people report seeing lights that appear to "shatter" like a star or they see lights with "halos." This is especially true of automobile headlights. It is also difficult for people with cataracts to differentiate colors, because blues and reds tend to be filtered out (removed) and what's left very often appears much like an old sepia-toned photograph.

Cataracts may develop as a result of injury (such as a physical blow to the eyes or exposure of the eyes to chemicals); disease (such as diabetes); use of certain medications (such as steroids); and the effects of infrared rays, microwaves, and x rays.[4] Loss of the ozone layer is another possible contributor to the increase in the incidence of cataracts; however, this supposition requires further study.

? WHAT IS THE PROCEDURE?

With the patient in the surgical suite and properly draped for surgery, the surgeon administers the local anesthetic. One injection is made in the eyelid to prevent blinking. A second injection is made in the muscles of the eye in order to immobilize the eyeball.[5] This is very important because of the delicate nature of the surgery involved.

Once the local anesthetic takes effect and makes the eyelid and muscles numb, the surgeon selects a thin wire retainer and places it over the eye to hold the eyelid open. This is done for two reasons: to give the surgeon a good view of the eyeball and to keep the operative field clear. A very powerful ophthalmic microscope—an instrument that magnifies small objects and is used for microsurgery—is placed over the eye to be operated on.

Viewing the eye through the microscope, the surgeon makes a small incision around the edge of the cornea to gain access to the lens. The lens is contained within a transparent sack called the capsular bag. The surgeon cuts through the front portion of the lens and removes the cataract; the back portion of the transparent lens capsule is left in place, to support the intraocular lens.[6, 7] Before the 1980s, the entire lens was removed using **cryosurgery**; however, this is no longer the preferred procedure.

Another procedural variation called phacoemulsification uses high-frequency sound waves to liquefy the cataract and the remaining portion of the lens. The remnants of the cataract and the lens are sucked out by a vacuum device much like a small vacuum cleaner. This process also preserves the lens capsule and helps to support the plastic lens implant.[8] Preservation of part of the lens capsule is essential if the intraocular lens is to remain in place.

After the cataract is removed, using either of the techniques described here, the surgeon carefully places the plastic lens in the space that was occupied by the natural lens. The lens implant is held in place by two springlike fibers. (This concept may be clear if you try to visualize a contact lens with two question-mark–like features extending from the top and bottom.) *Sutures* are used to close the incision and the procedure is completed.

The procedure takes about 30 to 40 minutes to perform. Cataract surgery reportedly improves vision in 90% to 95% of all cases, but this does not mean that vision returns to 20/20. If there are other underlying visual problems such as **glaucoma** or **macular degeneration**, then additional treatment is required.[9] One study reported that a visual acuity of 20/50 or better was achieved by 31% of patients the day after surgery. After three months, 89% of the patients demonstrated a visual acuity of 20/50 or better.[10]

? WHO PERFORMS THE PROCEDURE?

A board-certified ophthalmologist is best qualified to perform this procedure.

? WHERE IS THE PROCEDURE PERFORMED?

Improvements in cataract removal techniques make it possible to perform this procedure on an outpatient basis or in a well-equipped doctor's office. In some parts of the country, ophthalmologists operate clinics that specialize in cataract removal and lens implant procedures. Cataract removal is also performed in hospitals on patients who have complicating health problems that would not make them good candidates for outpatient surgery.

? WHAT ARE THE MORTALITY (DEATH) AND MORBIDITY (COMPLICATION) RATES?

A review of recent medical literature from the field of ophthalmology failed to reveal a single death from cataract surgery.

In about 3.7% to 10.8% of cases, the back portion of the lens capsule thickens or becomes hazy, obstructing vision.[11] A YAG (yttrium-aluminum-garnet) laser is used to remove the thickened capsule or remove the cloudy areas. This same study also recommended removal of the cell lining of the lens capsule to prevent the formation of any opacity.

One study reported that, during administration of the local anesthesia, the wall of the eyeball was punctured resulting in a tear in the retina; however, the damage was repaired the next day using heat to seal the tear.[12]

Postoperative infection has been recognized as contributing to chronic inflammation of the eye following a lens implant. When the infection is nonresponsive to antibiotic treatment, it may be necessary to intervene surgically.[13] Late-onset infection associated with intraocular lens implant has also been reported to occur in patients having cataract surgery.[14]

? WHAT ARE THE OTHER COMPLICATIONS AND POSSIBLE SIDE EFFECTS?

Some additional complications of cataract surgery are **astigmatism** and dislocation of the lens implant. According to one study, the degree of astigmatism was dependent upon the size of both the incision (either 4 mm or 6.5 mm) and the intraocular lens implant (6.5 mm or 6 mm). It was also shown that the technique of wound closure (type of sutures used) influenced the degree of astigmatism. Measurement of visual acuity at one day, one week, one month, and three months confirmed that patients with the smaller incision had less astigmatism than those patients who received the conventional 6.5 mm incision.[15]

Dislocation of the intraocular lens is a serious problem associated with lens implant techniques.[16] Studies show that preservation of the intact capsular bag, which holds the natural lens, is essential to assure proper placement of the intraocular lens and keep it from moving around in the white of the eye.[17, 18]

? IS THIS THE MOST APPROPRIATE PROCEDURE FOR THE CONDITION?

Yes. There is no medical treatment for cataracts that will restore the natural lens to its clear state. Because the goal is to improve vision by removing the cataract, this procedure is appropriate.

? ARE THERE ALTERNATIVES TO THIS PROCEDURE?

Technically speaking, a person with cataracts could use specially designed glasses or contact lenses to improve vision. However, these are rather dated methods for improving vision, and they do nothing to rid the lens of the cataract. When surgery absolutely cannot be done—for example, in people with extremely poor health—these may be the only alternatives.

? WHAT IS CONTROVERSIAL ABOUT THIS PROCEDURE?

There is nothing controversial about cataract surgery itself, because a cataract cannot be cleared up with medication. Refinements in surgical techniques and local anesthesia enable this procedure to be performed very safely on an outpatient basis.

When the intraocular lens was first introduced, there was some controversy associated with it. The design of these early lenses caused patients to develop serious complications (such as infections and corneal problems) that resulted in the need for further corrective surgery. These problems were resolved when newer and safer implantable lenses were developed and brought into the market.

Cervical Cesarean Section (1)

MORTALITY	MORBIDITY	CONTROVERSY
+	+	•

• The major **CONTROVERSY** of this procedure is the appropriateness of its continued use. The increased use of fetal monitoring devices is often cited as contributing factor to the increased number of cesarean births.

LAY TITLE: C-Section

Removal of infant from the womb through an incision in the lower abdomen

WHAT CONDITION DOES THE PROCEDURE TREAT?

This procedure is used when, in the opinion of the attending physician or midwife, labor will not progress to a satisfactory vaginal delivery, the infant is in the wrong position, the placenta is in the wrong position, the infant is in severe distress, or continued labor will be harmful to the mother, the infant, or both.

WHAT IS THE PROCEDURE?

The area where the incision will be made (just above the beginning of the pubic hair) is shaved, and the woman's abdomen is washed with an antiseptic solution and surgically draped. A spinal or general anesthetic is used. The skin and the underlying fat and muscle layers are cut horizontally across the front of the abdomen. An incision is made in the wall of the uterus and, with

all the layers of tissue **retracted**, the infant and the placenta are removed. The incision is closed in layers.

WHO PERFORMS THE PROCEDURE?

This procedure is usually done by an obstetrician or obstetrician-gynecologist.

WHERE IS THE PROCEDURE PERFORMED?

This procedure is usually performed in a hospital, with the woman as an inpatient.

WHAT ARE THE MORTALITY (DEATH) AND MORBIDITY (COMPLICATION) RATES?

The mortality rate is less than 0.1%. Even so, depending upon the study quoted, the mortality rate is between three and 11.5 times higher than for vaginal deliveries.[1]

Morbidity of one sort or another seems to be fairly common. One study quotes rates for postoperative anemia and **endometritis** of 29% and 22%, respectively.[2] Another quotes infection rates of 5% to 85% depending upon the study.[3] Mortality is higher with general than with regional anesthesia, even though the latter involves a spinal tap, which itself carries a degree of risk.[4]

WHAT ARE THE OTHER COMPLICATIONS AND POSSIBLE SIDE EFFECTS?

Complications and side effects other than infection appear to be relatively rare. These include anesthesia-related problems: hemorrhage, which occurs in about 1% of the cases; **embolism**; and introduction of endometrial tissue into the operative scar, which causes the same problems as endometrial tissue inside the abdomen if **endometriosis** is present.

As with any procedure in which anesthesia is used, death from reaction to the anesthetic drugs, error on the part of the anesthetist, or machine failure is a remote possibility. (See Glossary, p. 309)

? IS THIS THE MOST APPROPRIATE PROCEDURE FOR THE CONDITION?

Today one of four pregnant women in the U.S. will give birth by cesarean section—a rate higher than any other country in the world, according to the National Center for Health Statistics. Cesarean section rates have become so high that many consumer and medical groups have expressed concern. A case in point is New York State, where laws have been passed requiring hospitals to reveal their cesarean-section rates. This type of surveillance and consumerism was unheard of until recently. Cesareans have become so safe—even with high postoperative infection rates—and fetal monitoring so technologically, if not clinically, sophisticated, that there is a strong tendency to perform a cesarean at the first sign of difficulty. Doctors' sometimes inaccurate perceptions about malpractice add further pressure, but the time may be coming when public and consumer pressure and lawsuits against doctors for performing an unnecessary cesarean section may exert pressure in the other direction.

Some members of the medical community now suggest that at most 15% of all births should be cesareans, and only 9% of first births should be done by cesarean section.[5] Quite a few studies have shown that almost any conscious effort to review all alternatives before proceeding to a cesarean reduces the rate dramatically. Since 1974, infant deaths resulting from the trials of normal delivery rather than cesarean section in cases of breech presentation (in which the baby's head is up,

rather than down, in the womb) have resulted in a 0.2% fetal death rate and a 0.4% neurological damage rate.[6]

? ARE THERE ALTERNATIVES TO THIS PROCEDURE?

The only alternative to a cesarean section is a normal or assisted (forceps or vacuum extraction) vaginal delivery. For further information, see "Low-Forceps Delivery with Episiotomy," p. 177, and "Vacuum Extraction Delivery with Episiotomy," p. 285.

? WHAT IS CONTROVERSIAL ABOUT THE PROCEDURE?

The most controversial aspect of cesarean sections is their rate of use, which seems to be highly influenced by wholly nonmedical factors. This has often been noted, and a study published in the *Journal of the American Medical Association* on January 2, 1991, and worth quoting here, shows that matters have not improved, at least in California:

In 1986, 45,425 hospital births to women with previous cesarean sections took place in California. Of these births, 89.1% were by repeat cesarean section, while 10.9% were by VBAC [vaginal birth after cesarean]. . . . While the clinical and demographic characteristics of patients had a considerable impact on repeat cesarean section use, this study suggests a prominent role for nonclinical factors. Hospital ownership, hospital teaching level, payment source, and obstetric volume each had a substantial independent influence on repeat cesarean use. . . . An influence of direct or indirect financial incentives on clinical decisions is one explanation consistent with this study's findings. . . . The sizable nonclinical variations in VBAC rates . . . question the clinical appropriateness of current practice patterns.[7]

A portion of the rise in cesarean sections is attributable to the growing use of fetal heart rate monitoring (see "Fetal Monitoring," p. 83), in which electrodes inserted through the opened cervix or a sensor placed on the mother's abdomen are used to check the baby's heart. Sometimes even minute changes detected in such monitoring lead doctors to assume that the fetus is in distress, so they perform a cesarean. In a recent study, the correlation of the heartbeat patterns with blood chemistries indicated that a large proportion of the heart patterns thought to indicate fetal asphyxiation are, in fact, part of the normal variation in heart rate during delivery.[8] The study suggests the need for either wider use of fetal blood sampling and heart rate monitoring, or better research into the meaning of fetal heart rhythms.

When the vertical incision through a large portion of the uterus was in vogue, the medical doctrine "once a cesarean, always a cesarean" had some merit, because that incision greatly increased the chance of uterine rupture in subsequent deliveries. The danger is far less with the low cervical incision in use today, and trials of vaginal delivery after cesareans have shown good results.[9–15] The current guidelines of the American College of Obstetricians and Gynecologists encourage a trial of normal labor after a previous cesarean. Even one of the key indications for cesarean—breech delivery—seems to proceed to a good outcome with vaginal delivery in a majority of cases.[16] Whether cesarean sections reduce risks to the infant enough to justify the risk to the mother, and in what situations, are the key questions.

Circumcision (not ranked)

MORTALITY	MORBIDITY	CONTROVERSY
+	+	

- The major **CONTROVERSY** is whether it is necessary to remove the foreskin. Technically, circumcision treats no medical conditions; however, there is some evidence that circumcisions may prevent future problems such as phimosis, balanitis, penile cancer, and urinary tract infections. As explained in the introduction to Part II, this procedure is not given a rank among the 100 most common operations because it is not necessarily performed in a hospital.

Surgical removal of the **prepuce** covering the **glans** of the penis

? WHAT CONDITION DOES THE PROCEDURE TREAT?

There are probably no more than three or four clinical conditions requiring circumcision for their prevention or treatment: phimosis, the inability to retract the foreskin; balanitis, an infection of the glans; and penile cancer.[1, 2] The fourth condition, and the one mentioned in the most recent medical literature, is urinary tract infection.[3, 4] Some experts believe that circumcision can reduce the spread of venereal diseases and even prevent AIDS.[5] However, the American Academy of Pediatrics reports that there is no evidence that circumcision decreases the risk of venereal disease.[6] One African study found that in locations where circumcision is practiced, HIV infection was considerably lower than in areas where it is not practiced. While interesting, this study did not establish a definite connection between HIV prevention and circumcision.[7] Circumcision for purely cosmetic or religious reasons technically does not treat any condition, but it may prevent any of these.

? WHAT IS THE PROCEDURE?

Circumcision is simply the cutting or tearing of the foreskin to remove it from the head of the penis. Various techniques have been employed over the centuries to remove the foreskin—some of them unpleasant, such as using a thumbnail or a sharp knife to tear the skin.[8] Today relatively less barbaric procedures are in use. Two of the most widely used techniques utilize the Gomco and Plastibell clamps.[9]

Although circumcisions can be performed on older males, the majority are done on newborn infants. The newborn should be at least 24 to 48 hours old. Before performing a circumcision, the doctor carefully examines the penis to ensure that there are no physical problems such as hypospadias, a condition in which the opening for the **urethra** is on the underside of the penis.

Unfortunately, most physicians still perform routine neonatal circumcisions without anesthesia even though there are effective methods available for reducing pain.[10] Two such methods are local anesthesia, which is given at the surgical site, and regional anesthesia, which numbs the specific region of the body where the surgery is to be performed. One study concluded that local anesthesia was as effective as regional when performing a circumcision,[11] although usually the anesthesia used—when it is used—is regional, such as a dorsal penile nerve block.[12] (The dorsal penile nerve runs down the length of the penis.) The anesthesia takes effect in two to three minutes.

The physician makes a small cut in the foreskin parallel to the penis, and small curved clamps are used to loosen the skin gently from the head of the penis. After the skin is loose, another cut is made in the foreskin all the way back to the corona, which is the ridge where the foreskin attaches to the shaft of the penis. To best understand the procedure from this point, we describe the physical features of the Gomco clamp, which resembles a carpenter's "C" clamp. It is composed of four parts: a bell-shaped cone; a yoke; a flat metal base plate with a hole in one end and a blade; and a nut to tighten the yoke to the base plate. The physician gently inserts the bell-shaped cone between the glans of the penis and the foreskin. The opening in the base plate of the Gomco clamp is placed over the penis and carefully lowered until it rests at the edge of the bell-shaped cone. The nut on the base plate is tightened, crushing the foreskin against the bell and the blade in the base plate. After waiting five minutes for the skin to be crushed and creased, the surgeon uses a scalpel to remove the foreskin from around the base plate and bell-shaped cone. The cone is then removed, and the area is washed with an antiseptic solution. The patient—whether an infant or an older male—is then observed for any signs of bleeding.

The Plastibell clamp is the second most popular method for performing a circumcision. The procedure differs little from the Gomco clamp method except for differences in the bell-shaped cone. The Gomco cone has a smooth edge along the open end, while the Plastibell cone has a groove that surrounds the open end. Once the foreskin is loose and the bell is placed over the glans, the foreskin is secured with a cord that fits into the groove on the bell. The cord is tightened, crushing the foreskin against the bell. The physician trims off the remaining foreskin, and the bell is left in place over the glans. In the three to seven days that follow, the bell falls off, and the procedure is complete.

? WHO PERFORMS THE PROCEDURE?

Anyone with a medical degree and a valid medical license may perform a circumcision—the one exception being one performed for religious reasons. In the Jewish religious community, a rabbi is permitted to perform circumcisions. According to a Utah study, obstetricians perform about 88% of all circumcisions.[13] Other physicians who perform circumcisions are family practitioners and pediatricians.

? WHERE IS THE PROCEDURE PERFORMED?

Most circumcisions are performed in hospitals. However, they may also be performed in a physician's office and, when done for religious purposes, at home. Older boys and men may have the procedure done at an outpatient surgery facility or hospital outpatient department.

? WHAT ARE THE MORTALITY (DEATH) AND MORBIDITY (COMPLICATION) RATES?

A review of the literature reveals that since 1954 there have been three deaths reported for circumcision.[14] With more than one million circumcisions performed a year for the past 39 years, the mortality rate is 0.0000077%. Another report revealed one death from a home circumcision not performed by a physician.[15]

In two studies, the complication rate following circumcision ranged from 0.06% to 0.2%.[16, 17] These complications were limited to bleeding and minor infections.

? WHAT ARE OTHER COMPLICATIONS AND POSSIBLE SIDE EFFECTS?

Another complication—and one that is caused by the doctor—is trauma to the penis. This may be anything from a slight **laceration** to destruction of the penis. An Atlanta hospital reported two cases of infants receiving disfiguring burns caused by **cauterizing** needles. In one case, the penis was so badly damaged that a decision was made to perform a sex-change operation.[18] This is the most severe case reported.

? IS THIS THE MOST APPROPRIATE PROCEDURE FOR THE CONDITION?

If one accepts the medical indications for circumcision, then this procedure is appropriate. The conditions identified earlier—phimosis, balanitis, and penile cancer—do not cure themselves without medical intervention; therefore, circumcision is the appropriate procedure. The exception, however, is circumcision for purely cosmetic value, which cures or resolves nothing.

? ARE THERE ALTERNATIVES TO THIS PROCEDURE?

The only alternative is not to perform a circumcision. A procedure called a dorsal slit, which involves making a small cut in the foreskin, may alleviate phimosis; however, it is not acceptable as a method of complete circumcision.

? WHAT IS CONTROVERSIAL ABOUT THE PROCEDURE?

The issue of whether to circumsize is polarized: The "con" camp argues that males are born with a foreskin as nature intended, so we should not interfere. Furthermore, they say, the baby undergoes needless pain but receives no medical benefit from the procedure. The "pro" camp uses scientific studies to establish a link between circumcision and the prevention of future medical problems.

Some believe that the foreskin harbors bacteria, because it is difficult to clean properly. In fact, some studies have established a link between male urinary tract infections and lack of circumcision.[19]

The issue of anesthesia is another controversy. The "con" group asserts that many circumcisions are done without local anesthesia. This is indeed the case in most hospitals today,[20] as we mentioned earlier. Even if anesthesia is not used, there are other ways to reduce the pain and discomfort of circumcision. One study examined the use of music, recordings of intrauterine sounds, and pacifiers as noninvasive pain-reduction techniques.[21]

Closed Fracture Reduction of the Radius and Ulna (79)

MORTALITY	MORBIDITY	CONTROVERSY
+	+	o

Manipulating and splinting or casting of the forearm to fix broken bones in the arm

? WHAT CONDITION DOES THE PROCEDURE TREAT?

This procedure treats fractures of the **radius** and **ulna**. These two bones comprise the forearm and are critical to hand motion. Their function can be appreciated if you hold your arm out with the elbow just slightly bent and the palm facing down. Grasping the wrist so that it is held flat and parallel to the ground, try to rotate the hand so that the palm is up. It is impossible to turn the hand more than about 30 degrees in either direction as long as the wrist, which contains the ends of the radius and ulna, is held fixed. Releasing the wrist allows the radius and ulna to twist around each other and flip the hand over with almost no motion of the elbow joint.

We need to distinguish between two medical uses of the word *open* in order to understand what follows. Almost invariably the result of trauma, an open fracture is one in which there is an open wound that reaches all the way down to the site of the fracture, with at least part of the bone exposed. A closed fracture is one that does not have such a wound associated with it. An open reduction is a surgical procedure that involves opening of the skin, **fascia**, and other soft tissue to gain access to the site of the fracture. Here, the broken ends are aligned properly, or fixation devices are inserted. Open reductions can be done on both closed and open fractures. Some open reductions can be done through an **arthroscope**. This latter procedure is usually cited as an alternative to the open procedure.

In the case of the radius and ulna, closed fracture reduction aims at fixing breaks in these bones by realigning them without cutting open the arm. In some procedures, however, wires or pins are inserted through the skin to hold the bones in place. It is important to locate and align all breaks; misalignment of the forearm bones may lead to early development of arthritis in the joints between the radius and ulna and the elbow, and the joint between the radius and ulna and the wrist.

? WHAT IS THE PROCEDURE?

The patient is given a local or regional anesthetic. The doctor manipulates the forearm to realign the bones, using his sense of touch, x rays of the break, and perhaps **fluoroscopy**. When the bones are properly aligned and there is no evidence of pinching or pressure on a nerve, the doctor applies a cast or splint to hold the bones in place. Depending upon other injuries and the type of anesthesia given, the patient may be kept in the hospital for a day for observation, sent home when the anesthetic has worn off, or sent home immediately.

? WHO PERFORMS THE PROCEDURE?

This procedure is performed by an orthopedic surgeon or an emergency medicine specialist, and should be done by a board-certified one if at all possible.

? WHERE IS THE PROCEDURE PERFORMED?

This procedure is done in the hospital, the emergency room, or an outpatient clinic or urgent care center.

? WHAT ARE THE MORTALITY (DEATH) AND MORBIDITY (COMPLICATION) RATES?

Any mortality is essentially due to the anesthetic, not the procedure. As with any procedure in which anesthesia is used, death from reaction to the anesthetic drugs, error on the part of the anesthetist, or machine failure is a remote possibility. (See Glossary, p. 309)

Complication rates vary with the exact procedure used, but if closed reduction fails or doesn't work, subsequent open treatment has a complication rate of 50%. However, patient satisfaction is high with open reduction following failed closed reduction, and most people return to their previous occupations.[1]

? WHAT ARE THE OTHER COMPLICATIONS AND POSSIBLE SIDE EFFECTS?

The primary complication is failure to restore the complete range of motion that existed before the break—a common occurrence, although the degree of limitation is usually very slight.

? IS THIS THE MOST APPROPRIATE PROCEDURE FOR THE CONDITION?

A closed reduction is preferable if it can be achieved, but this is not always possible. Some fractures of the arm do not lend themselves to closed reduction techniques because of where they occur on the bones. The bones may be too brittle to use wires, clamps, or screws.

? ARE THERE ALTERNATIVES TO THIS PROCEDURE?

Yes. Placement of wires through the wrist and pins through the fingers to attach to an external alignment device or jig—a preformed plastic tray of molded nylon that keeps bones aligned and prevents rotation while the surgeon is applying pressure to move bones into correct position—is less invasive than open reduction, and can produce good results. If the fracture is a Colles fracture (a fracture of the radius with the ulna intact, and the broken upper end of the radius pulled back towards the shoulder), use of such an alignment jig under x-ray guidance is less painful than closed reduction after local anesthesia, and results in less damage to the soft tissues than reduction without the jig.

The success of any alternative method depends upon: (1) all breaks being identified on the x rays; (2) no free-floating bone fragments; and (3) the ability to line up all the bones in a position that can be held successfully with casts, splints, wires, or pins. If these three conditions are not met, the fracture will not heal properly or will not heal at all, and a later open procedure will be required.

? WHAT IS CONTROVERSIAL ABOUT THE PROCEDURE?

Very little is controversial. The surgical requirements are straightforward and most methods work well most of the time.

Closed Fracture Reduction of the Tibia and Fibula (73)

MORTALITY	MORBIDITY	CONTROVERSY
+	−	o

- Major **COMPLICATIONS** including delayed healing of the bone, clot formation, and bone infections can be expected in 12% of cases.

Repair of broken bones of the lower leg by splinting or casting

? WHAT CONDITION DOES THE PROCEDURE TREAT?

This procedure is used to treat fractures of the two bones of the lower leg that run between the knee and the ankle. These are called the **tibia** and **fibula**. The tibia is the primary weight-bearing bone, and is the only bone that touches both the end of the **femur** and the start of the foot. The fibula runs along the outside of the tibia and acts as a brace. It is connected to the tibia below the knee joint.

See "Closed Fracture Reduction of the Radius and Ulna," p. 130, for a discussion on the two medical uses of the word *open* in order to understand what follows.

A 1990 review article states that closed reduction of tibial fractures should be attempted before open reduction.[1] However, careful selection of patients for the open and closed procedures is needed, because the results of open reduction can be better than those of closed reduction in about 22% of cases.[2]

? WHAT IS THE PROCEDURE?

The exact procedure used depends upon the type of fracture. In most cases the patient is given a general anesthetic and the surgeon aligns the broken ends of the bones using a **fluoroscope**, a specialized x-ray device, as a guide. When the fracture has been aligned properly, a cast or splint is applied. Depending upon the severity of the break, any other injuries, and the age of the patient, the patient may be sent home as soon as the anesthetic has worn off or may be kept in the hospital up to six days.[3]

Because stress on bone encourages the formation of new bone, and because prolonged bed rest increases the risk of **thrombosis** and **thromboembolism**,[4] weight-bearing exercises (basically, assisted walking) and physical therapy are begun as soon as the degree of healing permits.

? WHO PERFORMS THE PROCEDURE?

Complex realignments should be handled only by a board-certified orthopedic surgeon who has had a lot of experience. Simple casts can be applied by general surgeons and family physicians.

? WHERE IS THE PROCEDURE PERFORMED?

Simple casts can be applied in an outpatient surgery facility or well-equipped doctor's office; more complex realignments should be done only in the inpatient or outpatient departments of a hospital.

? WHAT ARE THE MORTALITY (DEATH) AND MORBIDITY (COMPLICATION) RATES?

The mortality rate for this procedure in community hospitals in the U.S. in 1988 was 0.1%.[5] A 1985 Belgian study of 277 patients reports a combined mortality rate for this procedure and **lesions** associated with the fracture of 3.97% and, because the closed procedure failed and the leg had to be amputated, an amputation rate of 2.53%. In a series of cases not graded by severity of open fractures—in other words, no attempt was made to differentiate among minor fractures and more serious fractures that broke the skin—the amputation rate was 3.92%.[6] Deep bone infections occurred in 0.47% of closed fractures and in 5.7% of open fractures.[7] Deep vein thrombosis can be expected in up to 12.9% of cases.[8]

? WHAT ARE THE OTHER COMPLICATIONS AND POSSIBLE SIDE EFFECTS?

Major complications, including delayed healing of the bone, clot formation, and bone infection, can be expected in up to 12% of cases.[9] Deep infection alone can be expected in as many as 10.5% of cases.[10] The mean time between accident and return to work can be as long as 29 weeks for a serious break.[11]

Bone grafting for open fractures that have not joined is successful in about 87% of the cases; amputations will be required in as many as 10.3% of cases.[12] If the bone does not heal and complications set in, the closed reduction has failed, and amputation is the only measure available.

As with any procedure in which anesthesia is used, death from reaction to the anesthetic drugs, error on the part of the anesthetist, or machine failure is a remote possibility. (See Glossary, p. 309)

? IS THIS THE MOST APPROPRIATE PROCEDURE FOR THE CONDITION?

Yes, if the closed reduction can satisfactorily align the bones—otherwise, an open reduction and fixation should be done.

? ARE THERE ALTERNATIVES TO THIS PROCEDURE?

Yes, open reduction is an alternative.

? WHAT IS CONTROVERSIAL ABOUT THE PROCEDURE?

The only major controversy seems to concern whether **intermedullary** nailing (a form of open reduction that involves inserting a metal rod into the canal in the bone that holds the marrow) for tibial fractures should be done more often.[13] The chief advantage is that it prevents the broken bones from rotating, promoting faster healing. The disadvantage is that it takes more skill on the surgeon's part and more time.

Closed Reduction and Internal Fixation of Fracture of the Femur (80)

MORTALITY	MORBIDITY	CONTROVERSY
–	–	o

- The **MORTALITY** rate for this procedure at six weeks is 3.7%, and rises to 10.4% at eight months. The mortality rate for those patients over 65 may reach 25%, depending upon the technique used.

- A **COMPLICATION** rate of 33% is associated with the specific technique used to set the bone.

Repair of a fracture of the **femur** with an **internal fixation** device without use of an incision to expose the site of the break

? WHAT CONDITION DOES THE PROCEDURE TREAT?

This procedure treats breaks in the long bone of the thigh. Although some femur fractures are spontaneous, occurring without obvious trauma in certain diseases or cancerous bone, the great majority result from trauma, in which case a femur fracture is rarely the only injury. The elderly, who generally have other medical problems, are especially prone to hip and thigh fractures.

It is now recognized that **embolization of fat** from the marrow to the lungs, brain, and other organs is a major cause of mortality and morbidity associated with femur fractures. For this reason, current practice places a great deal of emphasis on quick repair of the bone and sealing off of the marrow.[1–3] Because of associated trauma, advanced age, and coexisting disease in many patients, mortality associated with femur fractures tends to be high. In addition, we now know that immobility leads to a rapid decline in functioning, especially in the elderly, and the repair of femur fractures, in most cases, involves at least a short period of immobility.

Fractures can be repaired using a closed procedure in which the limb is straightened, the broken ends aligned, and a cast applied. This is a variation of the "pull-it-straight-and-splint it" method taught in old first aid books. Or the repair can be open. In this case, the surgeon makes an incision through which the bones are examined, aligned, and fixed with some sort of device if necessary. Fixation devices can be internal (that is, wholly inside the limb) or external. For external fixation, thin rods or wires are threaded through the bone from the outside. They connect to an external frame that holds the limb in the correct position, applies traction, or does both. This section concerns fracture repair using variations of the closed, internal-fixation technique.

? WHAT IS THE PROCEDURE?

With the patient under general or spinal anesthesia, the leg with the broken femur is realigned, using a combination of manual traction, placement of wires or pins through the bone to ensure enough straight-line pull to align the broken ends, and **jigs** that hold fixation devices.

Depending upon the type of fracture and the surgeon's preferences, a rod or nail may be placed in the **medullary canal** or wires or screws may be placed across the bone. When the break is properly aligned, the surgeon may elect to treat it with a traction device, a cast, a splint, or a combination of all three. The necessary devices are applied, and the patient is taken to the recovery room and then to her room.

? WHO PERFORMS THE PROCEDURE?

This procedure is done by an orthopedic surgeon.

? WHERE IS THE PROCEDURE PERFORMED?

This procedure is always done in the hospital.

? WHAT ARE THE MORTALITY (DEATH) AND MORBIDITY (COMPLICATION) RATES?

Closed intermedullary nailing (described under "What is the Procedure?") produces a six-week mortality rate of 3.7% and an eight-month rate of 10.4%, with a 2.3% shifting of the bones at the fracture site, a complication that necessitates reoperation.[4] In patients over age 65, use of a sliding plate and screws produces a one-year mortality rate of 25% and a one-year reoperation rate of 25%.[5] Later results with another type of intermedullary nail that locks to prevent rotation of the broken ends of the bone resulted in no mortality and roughly a 33% complication rate.[6]

? WHAT ARE THE OTHER COMPLICATIONS AND POSSIBLE SIDE EFFECTS?

As with all lower limb procedures, **pulmonary embolism** can occur in up to 5% of patients. Closed procedures, which do not involve cutting tissues, seem to produce a lower rate of infection than open procedures, but total mortality and total morbidity for the two procedures are similar.

As with any procedure in which anesthesia is used, death from reaction to the anesthetic drugs, error on the part of the anesthetist, or machine failure is a remote possibility. (See Glossary, p. 309)

? IS THIS THE MOST APPROPRIATE PROCEDURE FOR THE CONDITION?

Obviously, a broken bone must be fixed. This procedure is the most conservative one available, next to simple casting, which is seldom sufficient to deal with a complete break in the thighbone.

? ARE THERE ALTERNATIVES TO THIS PROCEDURE?

An open reduction and internal fixation (see "Open Reduction and Internal Fixation of Fracture of the Femur," p. 185) is an alternative. The open procedure is done when there is any possibility that major complications, such as embolization of fat from marrow to the brain, lungs, and other organs, may arise.

? WHAT IS CONTROVERSIAL ABOUT THE PROCEDURE?

Research into prevention and improved fracture healing suggests that nutrition plays a critical role, and that many elderly patients most subject to hip and femur fractures are malnourished and could benefit greatly from diets supplying extra calcium, protein, vitamins, and calories. One such study showed a 50% reduction in combined mortality and complications.[7]

Cruciate Ligament Repair (75)

MORTALITY	MORBIDITY	CONTROVERSY
+	+	●

- The primary **CONTROVERSY** is whether the procedure should be done at all. There is also the question of medical versus surgical treatment.

Repair of the crisscross **ligaments** at the back of the knee

? WHAT CONDITION DOES THE PROCEDURE TREAT?

The many variations on this procedure are used to treat damage, weakening, or complete destruction of the two crisscross ligaments in the back of the knee. Such problems may be attributable to athletic injuries, trauma, or degenerative disease.

The cruciate ligaments are found at the back of the knee and form an "X," even though the posterior cruciate ligament, which is the one closest to the back of the knee, appears almost vertical in a standing person. Complete tearing of the posterior ligament allows the **tibia** to move too far back relative to the **femur**, and tearing of the other cruciate ligament, the anterior, allows the tibia to move too far forward.

Tearing of both might be thought to produce major problems, but the stability of the knee joint depends mainly upon the collateral ligaments, which are at the sides of the knee, and on the muscle tone of the large muscles of the thigh. If these ligaments and muscles are undamaged, the doctor usually will elect not to treat a torn cruciate ligament or ligaments. Instead, he will apply a cast to hold the knee in a slightly flexed position and send the patient for immediate physical therapy to strengthen the thigh muscle. Recent studies have shown that the large muscle of the calf changes function to support the knee when the anterior cruciate ligament is torn.[1]

Because of the toughness of the cruciate ligaments and their position, however, damage to them is almost always accompanied by some other major damage to the knee, and if repair of other parts is required, the surgeon will generally choose to fix the cruciate ligaments at the same time.[2] However, repair of other knee damage can produce a successful result even if the anterior cruciate ligament is not repaired.[3] Of course, if loss of function and unresolved pain are traced to a torn cruciate ligament, surgery can be attempted to relieve it. Delay in repair is not associated with any loss of function after surgery.[4, 5] Yet another reason for surgery is that it is now understood that unrepaired cruciate ligament damage can sometimes lead to early arthritis.[6]

? WHAT IS THE PROCEDURE?

The knee to be operated on is shaved, scrubbed with soap and antiseptic, and draped. The patient (who lies on his back during the procedure) is given a local or a general anesthetic, depending upon whether or not an **arthroscopic** or an open procedure, which involves a large skin incision, is planned. Despite many variations in technique and myriad materials used to repair or replace the torn ligaments, all procedures involve trimming or removing the torn ligament and fixing the replacement ligament (usually part of the kneecap **ten-don**) to the femur and tibia. Metal screws are often used to fix the replacement.[7]

? WHO PERFORMS THE PROCEDURE?

This procedure should be done only by a board-certified orthopedic surgeon who has extensive experience in ligament repairs and has demonstrated an ability to produce good results. Apparently, there are very large differences in success rates among surgeons.

? WHERE IS THE PROCEDURE PERFORMED?

Some surgeons perform the arthroscopic version of the procedure in outpatient surgery centers. Because of the need for casting or bracing and intensive rehabilitation, however, this procedure is still done mostly in hospitals. The open procedure, because it involves a large skin incision, is always done in the hospital.

? WHAT ARE THE MORTALITY (DEATH) AND MORBIDITY (COMPLICATION) RATES?

Mortality and serious complications are essentially zero. The major problems concern failure of ligament **grafts** and results that are not as good as anticipated.

Use of a thigh tourniquet to control bleeding during the arthroscopic version of the procedure has been shown to cause both nerve and muscle damage.[8] Some techniques for taking a kneecap tendon graft that do not replace the bone lost from the kneecap are associated with fracture of the kneecap after surgery.[9] Formation of abnormal soft tissue within the knee following arthroscopic surgery may require reoperation.[10]

? WHAT ARE THE OTHER COMPLICATIONS AND POSSIBLE SIDE EFFECTS?

A major complication is failure of treatment to provide the level of functioning the patient needs. Conservative treatment, consisting of cleaning out the knee joint with an arthroscope but not repairing the torn anterior cruciate ligament, and otherwise following the conservative treatment described above, produced results that were acceptable for daily living in 97% of a group of amateur athletes. However, only 49% thought that conservative treatment produced a knee that was adequate for their sports. The results of conservative treatment were judged excellent in 11%, good in 32%, fair in 22%, and poor in 35%.[11] Another study found poor results in 54% of young adults.[12] Obviously, conservative treatment can always be tried first, with surgery following if the results are not satisfactory. Studies in rabbits suggest that healing of a partially torn anterior cruciate ligament results in recovery of about 75% of the original strength of the ligament within one year.[13]

Misdiagnosis is also a complication of sorts, as it delays treatment of the real problem. A study of Israeli physicians found that they tended to misdiagnose incomplete anterior cruciate ligament tears as tears of the **meniscus** (another part of the knee) the majority of the time.[14]

The natural cruciate ligaments are stronger than many materials that are used to replace them. Dacron ligament grafts are nonirritating and well tolerated by the body, but can tear with less force than it would take to tear the original ligaments.[15] Eighteen percent of Gore-Tex ligaments fail by the forty-eighth month after surgery.[16] A somewhat strange finding is that natural kneecap ligaments used for replacement fail at an even higher rate than the artificial ones and are not recommended for general use.[17] (A 1990 study of the same technique found excellent results in 98.6% of a group of college athletes after two- to seven-year follow-up.[18] The reasons for the very high success rate with this group are not clear, but may be related to anything from the supplier of the ligament grafts to subtle differences in surgical technique.) Work in 1991 with goats suggests that maintaining the proper orientation of the fibers of the graft—that is, normal anatomical position—is crucial to success; some surgeons may be doing this without reporting it (or being conscious of it), which might account for some of the large differences in reported success rates.[19] Use of gamma ray (high-energy radiation) sterilization of ligament grafts has been found to reduce their strength significantly.[20]

Use of autogenous (from the person's own body) ligament grafts to create supports that are not normally present in the knee (called an iliotibial sling) caused chronic pain and swelling in 40% of the patients who had the procedure and is not recommended for general use.[21] Another study showed that such a sling produced no improvement in overall results even in patients who did not have pain or swelling.[22] On the contrary, a 1990 study found that the use of the iliotibial sling more than doubled the rate of return to sports. The reasons for the difference compared with earlier studies are unclear.[23]

Screws holding grafts in place can break even if the graft holds.[24]

As with any procedure in which anesthesia is used, death from reaction to the anesthetic drugs, error on the part of the anesthetist, or machine failure is a remote possibility. (See Glossary, p. 309)

? IS THIS THE MOST APPROPRIATE PROCEDURE FOR THE CONDITION?

There are so many techniques of nearly equal effectiveness available that the choice is virtually left to the individual surgeon. Emerging as the technique of choice is the use of the kneecap tendon graft with appropriate repair of the bony defects produced by taking the graft.

? ARE THERE ALTERNATIVES TO THIS PROCEDURE?

Nonoperative treatment is the alternative to any surgery. Surgeons are beginning to prefer the arthroscopic technique to the open procedure because it gives them greater access to the joint than the open procedure does. When the open procedure is used, an unacceptably large amount of cutting is required to get to all the places the arthroscope can go.

? WHAT IS CONTROVERSIAL ABOUT THE PROCEDURE?

A 1990 review article concludes that there is almost nothing about repair of the cruciate ligaments that is not controversial, including whether the ligaments have any vital function at all. Another controversy concerns the efficacy of operative versus nonoperative treatment. The author noted that many so-called new research and treatment ideas are recyclings of older approaches.[25] The great variation in results reported from different groups of physicians ostensibly using the same or similar techniques suggests that the operations are not well standardized, or that subtle but important differences in technique are not being communicated clearly in the medical literature.

Dialysis Arteriovenostomy (68)

MORTALITY	MORBIDITY	CONTROVERSY
+	+	o

Surgical creation of a direct union of a vein and artery in the wrist, forearm, or thigh as a site for **hemodialysis**

? WHAT CONDITION DOES THE PROCEDURE TREAT?

This procedure prepares a patient for hemodialysis, a short- or long-term replacement of kidney function for patients with kidney failure resulting from disease or injury (see "Hemodialysis," p. 147). Even with careful control of the temperature and chemistry of the dialysis solutions, the procedure is somewhat stressful for the patient. In addition, it requires the removal of a significant amount of blood, which is run through the dialysis machine, purified, and returned to the body. Arteries and veins can be damaged by continued use of the machine, so a surgically created **shunt** is established between an artery and a vein. The objective is to disrupt the usual pattern of circulation as little as possible and to allow a very rapid outflow and inflow of blood powered largely by the patient's own heart.

? WHAT IS THE PROCEDURE?

At any suitable site—often the wrist,[1] but also the forearm or groin—a vein and artery are located. The patient receives a local anesthetic. The skin is shaved if needed, scrubbed with soap and antiseptic, and draped so that only the area to be operated on is exposed. The skin is cut, and small bleeding vessels are cauterized with an **electrocautery device** if needed. We say "if needed" because local anesthetic solutions containing **vasoconstrictors** may be all that is needed for this procedure. The artery and vein are freed from the surrounding tissues and cut. In order to form a shunt, the cut ends of the artery and vein are sewn together—either directly to each other or to a plastic or fabric **graft** (Gore-Tex shows considerable promise[2])—and a loop is formed. The purpose of creating the loop is to establish a connection between the patient's blood supply and the dialysis machine. The loop that is formed by using a plastic or fabric graft is better tolerated by the patient because the machine is always connected to the same site.

? WHO PERFORMS THE PROCEDURE?

Ideally, this procedure should be done by a vascular surgeon. If the vessels used are large, however, the procedure can be performed by a general surgeon.

? WHERE IS THE PROCEDURE PERFORMED?

This is usually done as an inpatient procedure, simply because people are usually in the hospital when they are placed on dialysis for the first time; nonetheless, the procedure can be done on an outpatient basis in a hospital, in an outpatient surgery center, or in a well-equipped doctor's office.

? WHAT ARE THE MORTALITY (DEATH) AND MORBIDITY (COMPLICATION) RATES?

This is usually minor surgery, with a zero mortality rate and few operative complications. An average of 0.34 procedures per patient per year are required to maintain dialysis access, so that 3.4 operations per patient per decade can be expected.[3] Complications, which typically arise after the graft is in use, include clotting, infection of the entry wound for a **catheter**, and **bacteremia**.

Up to 26.4% of attempts to create a usable shunt can fail. Up to 26% of shunts can be expected to fail within five years of surgery;[4] 56.25% of Dacron grafts are complication-free after nine months.[5]

About 29% of grafts will have had an episode of clotting within nine months.[6] Clotting can occur within 24 hours of surgery in up to 9.6% of cases.[7] Virtually all of the methods for dealing with clots and **stenosis** that have been developed for heart procedures have been applied to dialysis shunts, usually with a relatively high degree of success.[8] Research suggests that clotting, a major problem with shunts, can be avoided by use of an ointment containing hirudin (an anticlotting agent)

applied locally, but the literature does not indicate active pursuit of this possibility.[9]

Occasionally, complications can be devastating. If infection occurs in a groin shunt between femoral vessels (of the thigh), as happens in 16.8% of patients with graft devices in this position, the mortality rate can be as high as 18% and the leg amputation rate 22%.[10]

? WHAT ARE THE OTHER COMPLICATIONS AND POSSIBLE SIDE EFFECTS?

For reasons that are unclear, an arteriovenous shunt can make any existing heart failure worse. Removing or reducing the rate of blood flow in the shunt can help resolve heart failure.[11-14] Damage to the wrist shunt, which can occur with wrist injury, can be avoided with the use of an inexpensive plastic wrist guard.[15] While not strictly a complication, requests that patients squeeze rubber balls to increase blood flow during dialysis are contrary to evidence that blood flow in a wrist shunt is not increased by this activity.[16]

Carpal tunnel syndrome is another possible complication. This condition occurs when a branch of the median nerve in the forearm is compressed at the wrist, thereby causing numbness and tingling and sometimes pain. It develops in 31% to 57% of dialysis patients, even if the shunt is not located in the wrist.[17-20]

One study suggests that shunt failures that occur early in the patient's period of dialysis are caused largely by judgmental or technical errors on the part of the surgeon—such as the failure to use a vein of adequate caliber or the use of a diseased artery incapable of delivering sufficient blood to keep the **fistula** open. Later failures arise from problems inherent in the current method of dialysis.[21] Another study also implicates surgical errors.[22]

? IS THIS THE MOST APPROPRIATE PROCEDURE FOR THE CONDITION?

Both patients and physicians have to reconcile themselves to the conventional wisdom that no dialysis access site is permanent. Because access must be provided, this procedure or some variation of it will always be required.

? ARE THERE ALTERNATIVES TO THIS PROCEDURE?

A catheter can be placed in the **subclavian vein**. A Dacron cuff, placed at the end of the catheter where it enters the subclavian vein, is designed to prevent infection. With the silicone catheter and Dacron cuff—used for short-term dialysis via the subclavian vein—clotting occurred in up to 24.5% of patients and infection occurred in 19.5%.[23] Subclavian catheters may cause narrowing of the vein over time,[24] causing a reduction of blood flow, which may lead to **thrombosis**.

A vitreous, or glassy, carbon connector (something like snap-on clothing) permanently implanted in a fabric graft avoids the pain of needle punctures—which must be done every time someone with a typical shunt undergoes dialysis—and makes it easier to connect the patient to the dialysis machine. However, such a connector has complication rates essentially identical to other forms of shunts.[25]

? WHAT IS CONTROVERSIAL ABOUT THE PROCEDURE?

There is little controversy about the procedure itself, but research into the causes of complications continues.

Dilation and Curettage, Postdelivery (28)

MORTALITY	MORBIDITY	CONTROVERSY
+	+	o

LAY TITLE: D&C

Widening of the mouth of the womb and removal of specific areas of the womb lining for therapeutic purposes following the birth of a baby

In every issue except for appropriateness of the procedure and controversy surrounding it, the information here is identical to diagnostic "Dilation and Curettage" (see p. 65).

? IS THIS THE MOST APPROPRIATE PROCEDURE FOR THE CONDITION?

The postdelivery D&C can still accomplish its purpose of clearing the womb of pieces of tissue that are acting as a source of infection or causing bleeding problems. The doctor performing a D&C, however, is "flying blind." **Hysteroscopy**, which allows the doctor to see the womb through a scope, is medically more rational and likely to result in fewer complications. We have more to say about hysteroscopy below.

? WHAT IS CONTROVERSIAL ABOUT THE PROCEDURE?

The most controversial issue here is whether a D&C should be done at all following birth. Recent articles strongly suggest that the hysteroscope or the suction curette be used whenever possible, and that the classic D&C (postdelivery) be reserved only for women whose cervixes cannot be dilated enough to use the hysteroscope or the suction curette. Of course, if the doctor's initial diagnosis is discovered to be in error—that is, there are no such contents in the womb—the procedure turns into a diagnostic D&C.

Endoscopic Colon Polypectomy (92)

MORTALITY	MORBIDITY	CONTROVERSY
+	+	

- The major **CONTROVERSY** is whether it is appropriate to use this procedure to remove **polyps** embedded deep within the **colon** lining.

Removal of benign or malignant polyps of the colon via a **colonoscope**

? WHAT CONDITION DOES THE PROCEDURE TREAT?

This procedure is used to treat benign or cancerous tumors of the colon that can be removed with a colonoscope. The tumors removed are usually polyps. The exact reason for their growth is unknown, but may be related to irritants in digested food and to a lack of fiber in the diet.

The probability of malignancy increases dramatically with the number of polyps found, reaching 100% in patients with 50 or more polyps. The presence of polyps in the colon can be a clue to malignant or premalignant conditions elsewhere in the body. In one study 11.6% of patients with eight or more colonic polyps were found to have benign stomach polyps—although non-cancerous, such polyps may become malignant and should be removed. The reverse has also been found to be true: Polyps in the stomach can be a clue that there are polyps in the colon.[1] After endoscopic removal of polyps, further colon surgery to treat **lesions** that cannot

be removed with the colonoscope is needed in about 40% of patients with eight or more polyps.[2]

? WHAT IS THE PROCEDURE?

An enema or one of the preparations (such as GoLytely) that cleanse the colon by inducing painless watery diarrhea is usually given the day before the exam and the patient is asked not to eat or drink anything until after the procedure.

A colonoscopic polypectomy is not pleasant if one is awake, but it is possible for the procedure to be done without sedation. So, depending upon the surgeon's preferences and practices, the patient may be lightly or heavily sedated, or given a dose of sedative that is sufficient to induce sleep. The colon has little sensation above the internal anal **sphincter** (one of two sphincters that control defecation), but is sensitive to **dilation** and pulling along its length, which are felt as cramps. If there is no compelling reason not to give sufficient sedation to induce unconsciousness—for example, if the patient has heart disease or difficulty breathing—the doctor should allow the patient this option.

The patient is laid on her left side with the knees drawn up in the classic fetal position. The lubricated colonoscope is inserted through the rectum and snaked up through the colon to the **ileocecal valve**, which is the joint between the large and small intestines. The surgeon or gastroenterologist "drives" the scope around the twists and turns of the intestine by manipulating controls on the eyepiece (or handle, if a TV monitor is used).[3] He then carefully and slowly withdraws the scope, looking for polyps and other lesions of the colon along the way. When a polyp is found, and it appears that it can be completely removed with the scope, an **electrocautery device** or laser beam[4-6] is used to sever the polyp at the stalk. The cautery or laser beam is also used to eradicate the base of the stalk, to ensure that no potentially malignant cells are left. Use of cautery or laser almost always seals off any bleeding vessels.

As each polyp is cut off, it is grasped with a biopsy forceps snaked through one of the channels in the colonoscope. If a polyp is too large to remove through the scope, the polyp is gripped firmly with the biopsy forceps, which run through one of the channels of the scope, and the entire scope is withdrawn with the polyp grasped in the forceps.

When all the polyps that can be seen are removed, the scope is withdrawn. The patient is taken to a recovery area. When the patient has recovered from the sedation and shows no signs of bleeding, she is discharged. Patients who have been given sedation are asked to have someone else drive them home, because their reflexes may be slowed even if they feel fully recovered from the sedation.

? WHO PERFORMS THE PROCEDURE?

This procedure is done by colon-rectal surgeons, gastroenterologists, or family physicians, all of whom should have had special training in the use of the colonoscope.

? WHERE IS THE PROCEDURE PERFORMED?

This surgery can be performed in the inpatient or outpatient departments of a hospital, in an outpatient surgery facility, or in a well-equipped doctor's office.

? WHAT ARE THE MORTALITY (DEATH) AND MORBIDITY (COMPLICATION) RATES?

Now that most surgeons and gastroenterologists performing this no-longer-new procedure are past their learning curve, mortality rates of zero are regularly reported.[7, 8] In a Czech study of patients over age 65, a mortality rate of 1.2% and a total complication rate of 4.7% were reported.[9] The primary complications are **perforation** of the colon (0.34% of patients); excessive bleeding requiring transfusion (0.23% of patients); and physician judgment that a tumor removal is incomplete when it is in fact complete—a misjudgment leading to an unnecessary bowel operation in 0.46% of patients.[10]

Other studies quote complication rates in the range of zero to 1%.[11, 12] Inability to remove the polyp occurs in about 2.33% of patients.[13] In cases in which complications occur, surgical repair is required in about 7% of the cases (0.07% of all cases).[14] A physician who is literally just starting the practice of colonoscopies may have a very high complication rate, but this usually falls dramatically with experience. Failure to detect flat lesions that do not extend far above the surface of the intestine is a further problem, the exact extent of which is unknown.[15, 16]

? WHAT ARE THE OTHER COMPLICATIONS AND POSSIBLE SIDE EFFECTS?

Despite the diagnostic power of the colonoscope, up to 25% of polyps less than 5 millimeters (one-fifth of an inch or less) in size can be missed on colonoscopic exams. Among the many reasons for repeated exams is that the percentage of polyps missed increases as their size decreases; only 5% of polyps larger than 5 mm in diameter are missed by a single endoscopic exam.[17] Smaller ones are often missed, and are not seen until they grow and produce symptoms such as bleeding, which leads to a repeat examination.

A potential complication arising from the procedure is that endoscopic bowel surgery leaves signs (oozing of blood, spasms, large amounts of gas, and abrasions) in the intestine that persist for a short time after surgery and may appear on a **barium enema** study and lead to false diagnosis of other diseases.[18]

? IS THIS THE MOST APPROPRIATE PROCEDURE FOR THE CONDITION?

Yes. Polyps are premalignant and must be removed. This procedure is far less invasive than either an open operation (called a **laparotomy**) or a laparoscopy, which must be used when the surgeon can't reach the polyps with a colonoscope.

? ARE THERE ALTERNATIVES TO THIS PROCEDURE?

The surgeon may elect to remove polyps in the lower part of the colon with a fiber-optic **sigmoidoscope**, a shorter version of the colonoscope that can reach only about 60 cm (about two feet) into the colon. This is much more comfortable for the patient and can be used with no sedation at all, but may lead the surgeon to miss tumors that are higher than two feet into the colon.[19] About 21% of tumors are located beyond the reach of the sigmoidoscope.[20]

? WHAT IS CONTROVERSIAL ABOUT THE PROCEDURE?

See "Endoscopic Large Bowel Examination," p. 69.

Free Skin Graft (94)

MORTALITY	MORBIDITY	CONTROVERSY
+	+	o

Grafting of skin from one location on the body to another to cover wounds where skin is missing, to cover burns, and to aid in the repair of scars

? WHAT CONDITION DOES THE PROCEDURE TREAT?

This procedure is used to cover defects in the skin, to treat burns, and to repair scars. Free-skin **grafts** should be distinguished from free-tissue transfers, in which major losses of soft tissue are repaired by transplanting muscle, **fascia**, fat, and skin—together with associated veins, arteries, and nerves—from one part of the body to another. Strictly speaking, a transplant of skin is limited to the skin only.

The use of the term *transplant* may be a bit confusing here, because the term is used to describe the movement of tissue from one place on the body to another (**autologous transplants**, in which all of the tissue moved belongs to one person) *and* the transfer of tissue from person to person. In this section, the term is used to mean both.

? WHAT IS THE PROCEDURE?

Depending upon the amount of grafting to be done, the condition of the patient, and the preferences of the surgeon and the anesthesiologist, a local, regional, or general anesthetic is administered. The donor site is scrubbed with soap and antiseptic. The sites where the skin is to be placed (the receiving sites) are trimmed of dead tissue and prepared to receive the skin graft. A specialized surgical instrument called a dermatome removes a layer of skin that is about half the total thickness of the skin in depth, from one site on the body. Because of the point of division between the layers that the doctor selects, the donor site is able to regenerate the top layers, and the receiving site is able to regenerate the bottom layers, resulting in healing with minimal scarring at both sites.

The size of the donor site limits the amount of skin removed; obviously, for instance, more skin can be taken from the back than from the calf. The surgeon attempts, within the limits imposed by the patient's natural coloring and hair patterns, to match the donor and recipient sites as well as possible. A new technique for expanding the skin taken for a graft may be used.[1] This technique, as yet unnamed in the medical literature, preserves a more natural appearance in color, texture, and thickness than the usual graft method for facial defects.

The graft is placed over the wound. The corners are lightly sutured to the wound or to undamaged skin surrounding it if possible, and covered with a pressure dressing. Drains or thin nylon threads, which function as wicks to draw off blood and serum, may be inserted.[2] The patient is taken to the recovery room and then to her room. If all goes well, within 36 hours blood vessels will begin to grow from beneath the graft to nourish it.

The graft is checked periodically to make sure that there are no accumulations of blood or serum under it that could inhibit blood vessel growth, and to check that no infection has set in. Transparent bandages may be used to permit constant observation of the graft.[3] If signs of infection are found, intravenous, oral, and **topical** antibiotics may be used.

? WHO PERFORMS THE PROCEDURE?

This procedure can be performed by a general surgeon, but if cosmetic results are important, it is probably best to have a board-certified plastic surgeon do it. In cases of massive skin loss, such as that accompanying severe burns, cosmetic considerations may have to be set aside in order to achieve extensive coverage quickly, to avoid life-threatening fluid loss and infection.

? WHERE IS THE PROCEDURE PERFORMED?

Because of the seriousness of the conditions that typically lead to the need for a skin graft, the procedure is usually performed in a hospital. However, it can be done in an outpatient surgery facility or a well-equipped doctor's office. Free-tissue transplants, which involve muscles, veins, arteries, and nerves in addition to skin, are much more complex than skin grafts, and are generally performed in a hospital.

? WHAT ARE THE MORTALITY (DEATH) AND MORBIDITY (COMPLICATION) RATES?

Mortality from skin grafts, as opposed to mortality arising from the conditions that require them, is essentially zero. The chief complications are infection and failure of the graft to establish an adequate blood supply, either of which can lead to loss of the graft and the necessity of redoing it.

? WHAT ARE THE OTHER COMPLICATIONS AND POSSIBLE SIDE EFFECTS?

Other than possible reactions to medication, there are few (if any) other side effects. Nonetheless, drug reactions can be serious, whatever the drug. One recent study found that 37% of elderly patients have at least one avoidable drug interaction.[4]

As with any procedure in which anesthesia is used, death from reaction to the anesthetic drugs, error on the part of the anesthetist, or machine failure is a remote possibility. (See Glossary, p. 309)

? IS THIS THE MOST APPROPRIATE PROCEDURE FOR THE CONDITION?

Yes, if the amount of skin loss is life-threatening, and if the wound in question will not heal naturally. Even when natural healing of wounds occurs, surgery may produce a much better cosmetic result.

? ARE THERE ALTERNATIVES TO THIS PROCEDURE?

Skin grafts and free-tissue transplants are alternatives to each other. The only other alternative is conservative closure and bandaging of the wound in the hope that healing will occur naturally.

? WHAT IS CONTROVERSIAL ABOUT THE PROCEDURE?

The chief source of controversy is which technique to choose from among the wide variety available for wound closure. For example, full-thickness skin grafts give better cosmetic results at the receiving site than do split-thickness grafts. However, they do not look as good at the donor site, and the patient may regard this as a problem. Similarly, the surgeon very often has to choose between an autologous skin graft and a free-tissue transplant involving tissues from a donor other than the patient.[5] The surgeon must choose the technique that will give the best possible result when all factors are considered, and then must perform that technique flawlessly.[6]

Head and Neck Endarterectomy (33)

MORTALITY	MORBIDITY	CONTROVERSY
–	–	●

- The **MORTALITY** rate is 2.8%, which is more than twice the national average of 1.33%.

- **DAMAGE** to the transcervical nerves of the neck has been reported in 69% of patients, and the incidence of vocal cord palsy is reported at 25%. Vascular headache syndrome is reported in 48% of patients. This severe pain is induced by trauma to the veins in the neck.

- The primary **CONTROVERSY** is the appropriateness of this procedure when the risk of death or complications (such as stroke) is high and the benefits of improved circulation are low.

Removal of blockages in the arteries of the head and neck

? WHAT CONDITION DOES THE PROCEDURE TREAT?

This procedure treats complete or partial blockage of the arteries of the head and neck that carry blood to the brain. Its primary use is in the prevention of stroke, although it is also done for **transient ischemic attacks** that are severe enough to warrant surgery, in the opinion of the patient and the doctor.

? WHAT IS THE PROCEDURE?

The blockage in the arteries is located via angiography (see "Contrast Cerebral Arteriogram," p. 58) and other imaging studies of the vessels in the head and neck. The patient is put under a general anesthetic, and the neck is shaved and scrubbed with soap and antiseptic and draped so that only the area of the incision is exposed. Then the skin is opened to expose the arteries.

There are three common procedures for blockages of the **carotid arteries**; they are discussed as a single procedure below, with important variations indicated. The internal and external carotid arteries run more or less vertically up and down the neck behind the main carotid artery, which runs from the front of the neck to the back of the head at about a 15-degree angle. In head and neck endarterectomy, the artery that needs to be worked on is opened and the blockage is exposed.

The next step varies according to the extent of the blockage, how firmly it is attached to the inside of the artery, how likely it is to shed debris when removed, and how large it is. Depending upon the circumstances, the surgeon may construct a temporary or permanent bypass around the obstruction, using a piece of vein from elsewhere in the body or a Dacron vascular **graft**. If the bypass is permanent, the blocked section of the artery may be left in place or cut away. If the bypass is temporary (that is, lasting only for the duration of the procedure), the surgeon clears the blockage by any of several methods, including using a stream of carbon dioxide to literally blow the obstruction out of the artery.

Sometimes, the incision in the artery cannot be closed because it is too large or the edges are damaged. In this case, a patch is made from a vein that is taken from elsewhere in the body and sewn over the hole. The neck is closed and bandaged. The patient is taken to the recovery room and then to his room.

？ WHO PERFORMS THE PROCEDURE?

This procedure is performed by general surgeons, neurosurgeons, cardiovascular surgeons, and peripheral vascular surgeons. It is best to use a board-certified specialist with a good deal of experience with the procedure.

？ WHERE IS THE PROCEDURE PERFORMED?

This is major surgery that is always performed in the hospital.

？ WHAT ARE THE MORTALITY (DEATH) AND MORBIDITY (COMPLICATION) RATES?

As of 1989, mortality for this procedure in community hospitals was 2.8%.[1] The risk of stroke during an endarterectomy is 1.6%.[2]

Nerve damage resulting from this procedure is apparently much more common than previously thought. One British study found a 25% incidence of vocal cord nerve palsy, or incomplete paralysis, and damage to the transverse cervical nerves of the neck in 69% of patients,[3] although there was some recovery of function over a six-month follow-up period. The same rate of injury to the vocal nerves was found in another study.[4]

Following this procedure, 48% of patients develop vascular headache syndromes which are induced by trauma to the veins in the neck, the pain of which can be severe enough to lead patients to attempt suicide during attacks. The fact that 100% of these patients have the pain on the operated side suggests that the procedure causes hidden injury to the vessels on that side of the head.[5]

？ WHAT ARE THE OTHER COMPLICATIONS AND POSSIBLE SIDE EFFECTS?

Hematomas are a rare but potentially lethal complication of this procedure, because they can produce pressure on the arteries sufficient to cause a stroke. (The rate of hematomas is 1.9%.[6]) They can be treated easily by evacuation, or drainage, with a small incision under a local anesthetic.[7]

Massive swelling of the neck has also been reported.[8]

Airway obstruction requiring emergency treatment can develop in up to 40% of patients who have this procedure following radiation treatment for cancers of the head and neck.[9]

As with any procedure in which anesthesia is used, death from reaction to the anesthetic drugs, error on the part of the anesthetist, or machine failure is a remote possibility. (See Glossary, p. 309)

? IS THIS THE MOST APPROPRIATE PROCEDURE FOR THE CONDITION?

If a patient has already had a stroke, good results can be obtained from using this procedure to increase blood flow within the first five to six hours after the stroke. After this interval, the benefits of the procedure diminish.[10]

? ARE THERE ALTERNATIVES TO THIS PROCEDURE?

The chief alternatives are "watchful waiting" and treatment with **anticoagulant drugs**, including aspirin.

? WHAT IS CONTROVERSIAL ABOUT THE PROCEDURE?

Everything. If ever there was a surgical fad with no logic to back it up, this is it. The performance of this operation increased 613% between 1971 and 1985 with no clear indication of a favorable risk-benefit ratio. The drop in the number of procedures performed after 1985 was judged by the Centers for Disease Control and Prevention to have reduced the overall number of strokes in the country.[11]

The ratio between the risks of stroke and the risks of surgery favor not operating on people with asympto-matic indications of carotid artery **stenosis** (patients have no symptoms but illness is discernible through diagnostic procedures such as x-ray studies) unless they fall into a subgroup with a risk of spontaneous stroke greater than 5%.[12]

Even so, the procedure probably has merit for a subgroup of patients with a high probability of stroke and for those who find the symptoms arising from the blockage disturbing enough to risk surgery.

Hemodialysis (27)

MORTALITY	MORBIDITY	CONTROVERSY
–	–	o

- The average **MORTALITY** for this procedure is 14%, which underscores the fact that some dialysis patients have other serious underlying conditions.

- The **COMPLICATIONS** from dialysis include circulatory problems, heart disease, and stroke. Quality of life issues are also a problem directly related to dialysis, and depression is reported quite often.

LAY TITLE: Kidney dialysis

Use of an artificial kidney machine or of fluid inserted in front of the **peritoneum** to remove waste products and excess minerals from the blood of a person whose kidneys have temporarily or permanently failed

? WHAT CONDITION DOES THE PROCEDURE TREAT?

All forms of dialysis treat failure of the body to rid itself of waste products and/or environmentally acquired toxins (the latter case could occur from a drug overdose, for example). Dialysis can maintain in reasonably good health those patients whose kidneys have failed. It can be lifesaving as a temporary measure in cases of poisoning or temporary kidney failure.

❓ WHAT IS THE PROCEDURE?

All forms of hemodialysis (which we hereafter will call dialysis) rely on a phenomenon called osmosis. A non-technical definition, adequate for our purposes here, is this: Osmosis is the tendency for the concentration of solutions on either side of a semipermeable membrane to equalize over time. There are two forms of dialysis: machine dialysis, using an artificial kidney about the size of a small washing machine; and continuous ambulatory peritoneal dialysis (CAPD), in which dialysis fluid is run into the space behind the peritoneum in the abdominal cavity. In the second form, the rich blood supply and large surface area of the peritoneum allow it to act just like the artificial dialyzer membrane (the filter) in machine dialysis. Because the concentrations of various substances in the dialysis fluid, called the dialysate, are lower than those in the blood, a natural diffusion process occurs by which impurities pass from the blood to the dialysate, thus cleansing the blood of the substances that the malfunctioning kidneys are unable to remove.

Machine dialysis is effected by connecting together a vein and artery of the patient in order to create a site (usually on the wrist, forearm, or groin) where blood can be taken from an artery, pumped through the machine, and returned to a vein. (See "Dialysis Arteriovenostomy," p. 138.) For CAPD, a valve is surgically implanted in the patient's lower abdomen, and fluid is put into the space between the abdominal muscles and the peritoneum and removed at a later time to rid the body of the waste products that have concentrated in it. Although there is a good deal of debate about exactly which patients benefit most from which approach, morbidity and mortality rates are about the same.[1]

Some patients choose peritoneal dialysis because they believe they have more control over when and where to dialyze, and do not feel as if they are tied to a machine. In peritoneal dialysis, however, the person is responsible for mixing the dialysate and monitoring his vital signs.

Frankly, not everyone is a good risk for this mode because other factors—such as age and general health—are not compatible with the requirement that the patient be actively involved in the treatment.

On the other hand, for some people, dialysis treatments at a facility promote a more secure feeling because medical professionals "are in charge." It also means freedom from having to mix the dialysate and introduce the mixture into the abdominal cavity. For many, there are even social aspects to dialysis at a facility: The person gets out of the house and can meet other people who have the same problem. This mode of treatment may greatly relieve the psychological stress of being in kidney failure.

❓ WHO PERFORMS THE PROCEDURE?

Machine dialysis is performed by the staff of an inpatient or outpatient dialysis center; peritoneal dialysis is usually done at home by the patient.

❓ WHERE IS THE PROCEDURE PERFORMED?

See above.

❓ WHAT ARE THE MORTALITY (DEATH) AND MORBIDITY (COMPLICATION) RATES?

As with many other surgeries, mortality rates vary widely with age and other health problems. The bad news is that for all patients on any form of dialysis, the annual mortality rate seems to be about 14% per year.[2] The good news is that, for dialysis patients with no problems other than kidney failure, the survival curves (life-expectancy measures of the probability of death, adjusted for age) are no worse than for the overall population of the United States as of 1990.[3] The key to age-adjusted tables, in this instance, is that (all things being equal) a person on dialysis with proper medical care could enjoy a lifespan equal to that of the general population.

A 1990 study indicates that 90% of dialysis patients without complications survive at least three years of dialysis, for a mortality rate of 10%. In patients in whom complications develop, the three-year survival rate is 60%—for a three-year mortality rate of 40%.[4] For all patients, the one-year survival rate is 73% to 79%—depending upon the condition that produced kidney failure—and the one-year mortality rate is 27% to 21% accordingly.[5] A study of patients using CAPD found 12-, 24-, 36-, and 43-month survival rates of 90% (at 12 months), 80% (at 24 months), 70% (at 36 months), and 70% (at 43 months);[6] mortality appeared to stabilize at 30% after 43 months.

As with many other surgical procedures, mortality rates are lower for younger patients. A study of children on dialysis found survival rates of 100% at six months and 95% at five years for hemodialysis; 92% at six months and five years for those who received kidney transplants from living related donors; and 88% at six months and 85% at five years for kidney transplants from corpses. Thus, the mortality rates at five years were 5% (for hemodialysis), 8% (for kidney transplants from living related donors), and 15% (for kidney transplants from corpses).[7]

Being on dialysis is associated with a higher-than-normal surgical mortality rate. For elective procedures (other than dialysis), the mortality and morbidity rates in a group of dialysis patients over a seven-year period were 6% and 12%, and 47% and 62% for emergency procedures. Even so, appropriate surgical correction of problems—for example, repair of a broken leg, removal of a cataract, or removal of a tumor—can lead to longer survival and a better quality of life.[8]

The mortality rate for dialysis patients is likely to increase substantially in the future because of changes in the patient populations accepted for dialysis. Con-trary to past practice, it is now customary to start extremely ill patients on dialysis. Indeed, one 1990 study found that almost all of the increase in dialysis mortality seen in recent years was attributable to acceptance of sicker patients.[9] The overall mortality rate for dialysis is also highly sensitive to the age distribution of the patients: One-year survival is 95.1% for patients 15 to 24 years of age, but is only 52.5% for patients over the age of 85.[10] Diabetics and whites generally have worse survival rates than other classes of patients. Five-year survival on dialysis for all patients is about 41%.[11]

Morbidity of one sort or another is common in patients on dialysis. As a result of distressing complications (discussed below), voluntary withdrawals from treatment accounted for 9% of all deaths of dialysis patients and 12% of deaths in patients 65 years of age or older in 1988.[12] There is a high correlation between paper-and-pencil scales of patient functioning and the quality of life and probability of death;[13] those who show the lowest quality of life on the paper-and-pencil tests are most likely to die. (A paper-and-pencil test is a questionnaire given in order to determine whether a person has any psychological and physical limitations.)

Much of the short-term morbidity, which may resolve at the end of treatment or shortly thereafter, is related to the inability of dialysis equipment to respond rapidly enough to changes in the patient's blood composition to prevent large and rapid swings in the concentration of water, **electrolytes**, and other substances in the patient's blood. Even when rapid control over one or two elements is possible, only about 50% of patients fit the simple mathematical models that would allow the equipment to be programmed to respond properly.[14]

Common dialysis-associated problems include cramps, low blood pressure, problems with access sites (see "Dialysis Ateriovenostomy," p. 138), and reactions to first use of the dialyzer membrane.[15] Dialysis prescriptions (which are a combination of chemicals in the dialysate, time on the machine, and use of pressure filtration) that reduce the average blood urea nitrogen, or BUN (a measure of waste products in the blood), to as low a level as possible are associated with lower morbidity.[16]

As you might expect, some data suggest that poor nutritional status and low protein intake are associated with higher probability of death while on dialysis. Some doctors prefer to restrict protein intake to control ure-mia, but it appears that this approach can be overdone and can actually contribute to mortality.[17] One study suggests that inadequate protein intake is associated with an 81.8% increase (from 4.4% to 8%) in mortality when dialysis patients were compared with an otherwise-similar group who had adequate protein intake and adequate dialysis.[18] For at least some patients on hemodialysis, malnutrition is clearly the chief cause of morbidity and mortality.[19]

A study conducted by the Institute of Medicine, a branch of the National Academy of Sciences, found indications that mortality among dialysis patients has also been increasing as a result of cuts in federal payments for dialysis: The cuts have led to shorter treatment times and thus to a greater build-up of waste products in the blood of dialysis patients.[20, 21] Treatment times shorter than 3.5 hours per session were associated with an increase in mortality. Another study, however, found that reduction in treatment time from an average of 17 hours to 2.7 hours was not associated with any increase in mortality, provided that concentrations of breakdown products in the blood were kept constant and not allowed to rise with shorter treatments.[22] Another study found no increase in mortality when treatment times were shortened to three hours.[23]

❓ WHAT ARE THE OTHER COMPLICATIONS AND POSSIBLE SIDE EFFECTS?

Other than kidney disease itself, the major cause of morbidity and mortality among dialysis patients is circulatory problems, usually resulting in atherosclerotic heart

disease and stroke.[24, 25] The kidneys have a complicated role in the maintenance of blood pressure and blood chemistry, and it has proven impossible to exert total control over blood pressure in some patients on dialysis. Uncontrolled high blood pressure is associated with a higher rate of heart disease and stroke.

The major cause of morbidity among patients on peritoneal dialysis is infection. Peritonitis can be devastating and carries with it a high mortality rate. Careful attention to sterile technique can reduce the incidence of peritonitis to about one episode per 18 months.[26]

In two cases reported in the medical literature, cerebral edema occurred after patients with the bacterial infection leptospirosis were put on dialysis. This resulted in death for one patient and partial paralysis for the other.[27]

Accumulation of aluminum in bone, which is found in about 50% of dialysis patients,[28, 29] is strongly associated with increased morbidity and mortality. It is unclear whether this is a result of the kidney condition, a doctor-caused problem associated with dialysis (such as the dialysate not being mixed properly to sufficiently filter aluminum, or the use of aluminum-coated tubs for water filtration), or the failure of the procedure to exactly duplicate kidney function.[30] Both dialysis and uremia are associated with bone disorders.[31]

Ascites can also occur, with either dialysis method. This can usually be relieved by a form of dialysis called ultrafiltration or by implanting a shunt that drains peritoneal fluid into a vein via a one-way valve.[32]

As of 1990, about 42% of patients on dialysis showed evidence of infection with hepatitis, even if they did not develop the full-blown disease. It is unclear to what degree this is related to treatment-acquired infection or to the transfer of hepatitis virus antibodies in the many blood transfusions required by dialysis patients.[33]

Psychiatric complications are common in both kidney transplant and dialysis patients—46% of transplant patients and 48% of dialysis patients were found to have at least some evidence of psychiatric problems.[34] Another study found a 33% rate of psychiatric complications among patients undergoing dialysis.[35] Depression while on dialysis is strongly associated with a higher probability of death.[36]

An associated complication of sorts is the labeling by dialysis-unit staff of some patients as sicker, or more problematic. Indeed, one study suggests that, to some extent, such labeling is a self-fulfilling prophecy, because it may lead to poorer care for patients whose conditions are perceived to be worse, even if this perception is inaccurate.[37]

? IS THIS THE MOST APPROPRIATE PROCEDURE FOR THE CONDITION?

The data suggest that there are slight advantages to a kidney transplant over dialysis in terms of survival. Much of the effect may be attributable to a greater sense of health and independence that comes from not being tethered to a machine that must be visited two or three times a week. The supply of donor kidneys has stabilized at a level that permits only about 9000 transplants a year, and 150,000 people are receiving Medicare benefits for end-stage kidney disease. It is realistic to expect that most patients with kidney failure will continue to be maintained on dialysis; about 80% of them will be on machine dialysis and about 20% will be on peritoneal dialysis.[38] Although dialysis may not be the most appropriate procedure, it is the only choice for most patients.

? ARE THERE ALTERNATIVES TO THIS PROCEDURE?

The chief alternative is a kidney transplant.

Based on new discoveries from basic research, we can now reasonably expect within the next 50 to 75 years we will be able to grow kidneys from patient's body cells. This procedure will produce one or two matched kidneys for each patient needing them, and autotransplantation of these specially grown **grafts** will become the standard therapy. Unfortunately, no researcher has come anywhere near being able to grow whole organs from single cells, although the basic mechanisms that govern the body's creation of organs are beginning to be understood.

? WHAT IS CONTROVERSIAL ABOUT THE PROCEDURE?

There has been extensive debate about the practice of reusing dialyzer membranes, or filters, which are sold as single-use items but can easily be sterilized and reused, thus lowering costs to the dialysis facility. The issue is made even more complex because there is evidence that first use and reuse of dialyzers are associated with different, but perhaps equally severe, kinds of complications.

A British study found no increased mortality but did find increased morbidity associated with dialyzer membrane reuse; an American study found decreased mortality and low morbidity.[39] There is also a "first-use syndrome" (usually chills, fever, nausea, vomiting, and mild neurological problems) associated with first use of a dialyzer membrane. Neither reuse nor one-time use affords definite relief from all morbidity.[40]

More broadly, dialysis is what Lewis Thomas, a noted physician and medical writer, called a "halfway technology." It works—sort of—but is expensive and fraught with complications; maintaining the patient is a twilight between good health and fatal disease. The survival of transplanted kidneys has been dramatically improved by cyclosporine, an antirejection drug. Yet cyclosporine itself is toxic to the kidneys and requires constant dosage adjustment to maintain the patient on a razor edge between rejection and drug-induced damage.

The medical literature reveals differences in perspective between the patients as a group and the physicians and staff of dialysis units. Too often, it seems, the sole goal of the medical professionals involved in the care of dialysis patients is reduced to the day's blood chemistry. Other needs, such as adequate nutrition and an acceptable quality of life, are given short shrift. It is not surprising that 9% to 12% of deaths per year result from simple refusal to continue with dialysis. On the other hand, most patients rate their quality of life on dialysis higher than observers do,[41] and for some patients, especially the younger ones, a very high quality of life is possible.

Hemorrhoidectomy (53)

MORTALITY	MORBIDITY	CONTROVERSY
+	+	o

LAY TITLE: Hemorrhoid surgery

Removal of **prolapsed** veins of the rectum

? WHAT CONDITION DOES THE PROCEDURE TREAT?

Hemorrhoids have been the source of many jokes. The condition produces all the psychological jitters that accompany any disturbance in the "intimate" functions of the body, but is usually not serious. Hemorrhoids can be quite painful, however, and the intensity of the pain can also lead patients to assume that the problem is far more serious than it actually is.

? WHAT IS THE PROCEDURE?

Strictly speaking, hemorrhoidectomy means the cutting out of the diseased rectal veins with a scalpel. Of late, the term has been extended to include rubber-band li-

gation of the base of the hemorrhoid. Hemorrhoids can also be dealt with by freezing, injection of a solution that causes the vein to close off, or vigorous **dilation** of the anal canal. All of these procedures may be referred to as hemorrhoidectomies.

Because of the many techniques available, we will discuss each only briefly and summarize, where appropriate, the common elements among them. A local anesthetic is used in most of the techniques. In cases in which surgery is more extensive, a spinal or general anesthetic may be used. The patient is generally placed in a kneeling position with head down and rear in the air across an operating table equipped with a bench for the knees—assuredly a position that significantly compromises one's dignity but is otherwise not too uncomfortable. Most procedures require the insertion of a **speculum** to hold the anal canal open so that the doctor can see what she is doing; some physicians dilate the anal canal quite extensively to expose hidden hemorrhoids.

In the rubber-band ligation technique, each hemorrhoid is grasped with a special instrument that carries a rubber band on the tip. The most exposed part of the hemorrhoid is grasped and pulled into a channel in the instrument. This causes the rubber band on the tip of the instrument to pop free of it and snap around the stalk of the hemorrhoid, thereby cutting off its blood supply. The hemorrhoid quickly shrinks and dies (within a few days), eventually falling off. Some surgeons dress the area with medicated gauze.

In incisional (cutting) techniques, which vary in procedure and are highly controversial, the essential steps are: open the skin, locate the vein, cut it out, and **cauterize** any bleeding vessels. Depending upon the amount of tissue actually removed and the relation of the remaining skin to the underlying mucous tissue of the rectum, skin flaps may be used for repair. The **sphincter** muscle may also be cut with the idea of reducing postoperative pain.

In cryosurgery the hemorrhoids are touched with a

cryoprobe, which is generally cooled by liquid nitrogen. Techniques that limit freezing to small areas are associated with less postoperative pain.

In techniques involving sclerosing (hardening) solution, the vein is located and injected with a chemical which causes inflammation of the vein, producing scar tissue that replaces the soft tissue of the hemorrhoid.

Laser treatment of hemorrhoids is still under development, but has shown considerable promise. In laser treatment, the laser beam both cuts and **coagulates,** destroying the prolapsed veins and stopping bleeding at the same time.

After surgery, the patient is taken to the recovery room and then to her hospital room or home, depending upon the technique used.

? WHO PERFORMS THE PROCEDURE?

All of these procedures can be performed by colon-rectal surgeons. If extensive incisional surgery is required, it is probably best to use a board-certified colon-rectal surgeon.

? WHERE IS THE PROCEDURE PERFORMED?

Only the most technically complex cases of hemorrhoidectomy involving incisional techniques require hospitalization. Laser hemorrhoidectomies have been successful as outpatient surgery, and patients can generally return home immediately afterward.[1]

? WHAT ARE THE MORTALITY (DEATH) AND MORBIDITY (COMPLICATION) RATES?

Mortality is essentially nonexistent for all techniques.

For rubber-band ligation, investigators in one study reported mild to moderate pain in 4.8% of patients; pain severe enough to require restriction of activity in 0.6%, severe bleeding in 1%, and slight bleeding in 3%. Less than one-half of 1% (0.3%) of patients required hospitalization and cauterization for severe bleeding; 99.7% were able to go home immediately after surgery.[2] In another study of rubber-band ligation, 36% of patients described the procedure as "totally painless"; 41% reported only a little pain, and 14% reported severe pain.[3]

Mortality rates of zero and complication rates of 4.5% for acute hemorrhoidal crises (episodes of severe pain, **thrombosis,** or both) in which incisional techniques are used have been reported.[4]

? WHAT ARE THE OTHER COMPLICATIONS AND POSSIBLE SIDE EFFECTS?

Pain, postoperative **urinary retention**, and the need for enemas can occur in 56%, 37%, and 9%, respectively, of patients who have a type of hemorrhoidectomy called the closed Ferguson. (The closed Ferguson is a special suturing technique, a way of sewing the tissue closed after a hemorrhoid has been removed. It's up to the surgeon which of the many available suturing techniques is used.)

While laser treatment dramatically reduces all of these complications, including pain, it does result in delayed wound healing (one to two days' difference) compared with the closed Ferguson.[5]

The anal canal is stretched and the sphincter muscle may be cut to reduce pain after hemorrhoidectomy, but neither measure seems to be very successful. Both are associated with a period of fecal incontinence following the procedure; this incontinence may last from five to 10 weeks, and rarely for up to one year following the surgery.[6, 7] Incidentally, the addition to the patient's diet of a wheat-fiber–based stool bulker after surgery has been shown to reduce pain, length of hospital stay, and problems with incontinence.[8]

Pain associated with freezing of hemorrhoids is about equal to pain from closed surgery. The freezing technique often produces a foul-smelling discharge as the frozen tissue decays. In a survey of patients, 65% preferred the closed operation.[9] Other studies have reported considerable reduction in postoperative pain with the freezing technique.[10] The degree of postoperative pain apparently has a lot to do with the surgeon's technical skill with the cryoprobe.[11]

Urinary retention and painful defecation can occur after almost any incisional technique.[12]

About 7.5% of patients will require re-operation after a closed hemorrhoidectomy.[13]

As with any procedure in which anesthesia is used, death from reaction to the anesthetic drugs, error on the part of the anesthetist, or machine failure is a remote possibility. (See Glossary, p. 309)

? IS THIS THE MOST APPROPRIATE PROCEDURE FOR THE CONDITION?

There was a 20% decrease in the number of hemorrhoidectomies performed between 1978 and 1982, mainly as a result of the use of alternative procedures, many of which are also called hemorrhoidectomies.[14] (Few statistics on numbers of hemorrhoidectomies performed are available after 1982 because the procedure is being done more often in doctors' offices and not in hospitals, which are the only facilities surveyed.) Thrombosed hemorrhoids (affected with clots) and hemorrhoids that cause severe pain should be treated surgically. For other cases, conservative treatment should be tried first.

? ARE THERE ALTERNATIVES TO THIS PROCEDURE?

High-fiber diets and the use of bulk laxatives such as Metamucil (psyllium seed) or Citrucel (methylcellulose) or their generic, low-cost equivalents can treat hemorrhoids satisfactorily in many cases.[15]

? WHAT IS CONTROVERSIAL ABOUT THE PROCEDURE?

Primarily because this is a minor procedure and the anatomy involved is simple in most patients, most surgical approaches are effective. The controversies have more to do with which techniques produce the least pain in the immediate postoperative period, and the greatest patient satisfaction overall. Unfortunately, although there is a great deal of variation in technique, there has been little comparative study of methods.[16]

The Whitehead technique, originally developed in 1882, involves removal of hemorrhoids and the surrounding tissue and reconstruction of the anal canal with skin flaps. It has been harshly criticized as productive of a high rate of serious complications, but one physician at the Mayo clinic has used it since 1963 with zero mortality and a complication rate of 12.2%. The operation may be useful for cases in which both the hemorrhoids and the attached **mucosal** tissue have prolapsed into the anal canal.[17–19]

Incisional Hernia Repair (81)

MORTALITY	MORBIDITY	CONTROVERSY
+	+	o

Repair of a hernia that has occurred through a new surgical wound or an old surgical scar

? WHAT CONDITION DOES THE PROCEDURE TREAT?

This procedure treats a bulging of the contents of a body cavity through a new surgical wound or an old surgical scar. Although incisional hernias can occur anywhere in the body that an incision is made,[1-3] most are in the abdomen. Studies of various surgical techniques and procedures indicate that wound **herniation** occurs in about 0.65% to 7.4% of fresh surgical scars.[4, 5] A 10-year follow-up study indicated that 31% of incisional hernias recur after a first repair and 44% recur after the second repair or any subsequent repair. A study covering the period from 1974 to 1986 showed even worse results: 46% recurrence.[6] Most recurrences happened within the first three years after the initial surgery or hernia repair.[7]

Use of a Marlex (polypropylene) plastic mesh to strengthen the body wall can reduce the recurrence rate to about 8% to 11%.[8, 9] The same can be achieved with microporous expanded Teflon sheets, which do not produce as much irritation as Marlex.[10] Animal studies have shown that use of the Marlex mesh greatly increases the resistance of the abdominal wall to bursting.[11] Marlex can also be used to replace portions of the abdominal wall when there has been massive tissue loss resulting from injury or infection.[12] Other plastics can be used also.[13]

Studies have documented and experience has shown that careful layer-by-layer closure of the abdomen produces far fewer incisional hernias than "mass" closure, in which all layers are closed at once.[14] Although incisional hernias occur more frequently after healing of infected wounds (rather than uninfected wounds), and it has been shown that the wound infection rate can be reduced to zero, use of antibiotics alone does not seem to reduce the risk of incisional hernias.[15] Nor does the use of steel wire sutures reduce the risk of hernia.[16, 17]

Obstructive jaundice, a condition in which liver products collect in the blood because the liver ducts are blocked, increases the risk of developing incisional hernia almost 500%; more than 10% of patients with obstructive jaundice will develop incisional hernias, primarily due to delayed healing.[18, 19]

Wound herniation is closely related to surgical skill. A British study found that herniation was much more common among patients of surgeons-in-training than among patients of surgeons who had completed training.[20] Further, even though patients who require repeat operations may prefer to have incisions made through the old scar for cosmetic reasons—so that only one scar is present—incisions made through old scars have an increased risk of herniation.[21]

? WHAT IS THE PROCEDURE?

The patient is given a local or a spinal anesthetic, depending upon the extent of the work to be done; general anesthesia is used rarely. The area of the hernia is scrubbed with soap and antiseptic and draped with a sterile sheet. The skin is opened, and the **fascia**, muscle, and other tissue layers are opened until the **hernial sac** is located. It is replaced within the abdominal cavity, with care taken not to cause intestinal obstruction.

If the surgeon prefers, a plastic mesh is placed at the bottom of the incision and sutured into position. The various layers are closed separately; the skin is closed using **sutures**, **clips**, or staples. A drain may be left in place. Finally, a bandage is applied, and the patient is taken to the recovery room and then to his room.

? WHO PERFORMS THE PROCEDURE?

This procedure is usually done by general surgeons. Many gynecologists and urologists also know how to do it.

? WHERE IS THE PROCEDURE PERFORMED?

Depending upon the extent of the repair needed, the procedure is done in a hospital or outpatient surgical facility.

? WHAT ARE THE MORTALITY (DEATH) AND MORBIDITY (COMPLICATION) RATES?

Mortality is essentially zero. The only major complication is recurrence, which can occur at rates up to 46%, as noted above. Inadvertent injury to the bowel occurs rarely.

? WHAT ARE THE OTHER COMPLICATIONS AND POSSIBLE SIDE EFFECTS?

Infection rates reported in the literature range from 1.5% to 7%, but a trial of antibiotic use has demonstrated that an infection rate of zero can be achieved.[22]

? IS THIS THE MOST APPROPRIATE PROCEDURE FOR THE CONDITION?

One article we consulted suggests that, because of the high recurrence rate of incisional hernias, conservative treatment be tried, especially in older or seriously ill patients and patients who have only mild discomfort.[23] Conservative treatment consists primarily of providing abdominal support with a **truss**, or wrapping the patient, and monitoring him carefully.

? ARE THERE ALTERNATIVES TO THIS PROCEDURE?

Essentially, the only alternative is careful monitoring of the patient. All hernias are mechanical problems (there is body tissue out of place, which must be put back in its correct position) for which nonsurgical therapy is not effective.

? WHAT IS CONTROVERSIAL ABOUT THE PROCEDURE?

The issue of whether to sew up incisions is one that a layperson would probably think was settled ages ago. Not so. Debates still rage about the type of suture to use and whether mass or layered wound closure is justified. The high recurrence rate of incisional hernias indicates that there is much room for improvement in the techniques of suturing and closure.

The higher incidence of herniation in jaundiced patients is thought to be related to poor nutritional status, but many doctors disagree.[24, 25] Because herniation is related to wound infection, and since it is known that nutritional supplementation reduces the incidence of wound infection following cardiac surgery, exploration of the relationship between herniation and nutritional status seems to be worth investigating.[26]

Intercostal Catheter Insertion (13)

MORTALITY	MORBIDITY	CONTROVERSY
+	+	o

Insertion of a small plastic tube between the ribs into the **pleura** for pain relief or under the pleura for relief of **pneumothorax**

? WHAT CONDITION DOES THE PROCEDURE TREAT?

This procedure is used for relief of pain caused by surgery or a disease such as cancer; to provide local anesthesia for surgery on the chest wall or other parts of the body reached by the nerves of the chest cavity; or as an alternative to the placement of a chest tube for relief of pneumothorax.

? WHAT IS THE PROCEDURE?

Intercostal **catheter** insertion is performed in an almost identical fashion for each of the three above-mentioned uses.

For pain relief, a **trochar** or large-bore needle is inserted between two ribs after a local anesthetic is given to numb the skin. The surgeon or anesthesiologist chooses the ribs based on the anatomy of the nerves within the chest wall, aiming for maximum numbing of the nerves responsible for carrying the pain signals to the brain. After the injection to deaden the area, the catheter is threaded through the incision or needle puncture into the space between the skin and the pleura.

Whether the catheter is being used for pain relief or local anesthesia, intermittent or continuous flows of local anesthetic solutions are run through it.

When used for anesthesia, the catheter is a means of performing an intercostal nerve block, which is powerful enough to serve as anesthesia for some types of breast surgery.[1]

If the goal is to relieve pneumothorax, a catheter with a one-way valve (thereby allowing air to flow out of the chest cavity but not into it) is used. Suctioning or normal efforts to breathe causes air to be rapidly pumped out through the catheter, restoring the partial vacuum in the chest cavity, which is needed to help the lungs expand normally.

Deadening a particular set of nerves at various levels in the chest wall in order to relieve pain is a procedure that also can be used to diagnose the source of flank pain.[2] (The flank is the side of the body between the rib cage and the pelvis.) The procedure also may be useful in the treatment of spinal reflex pain syndrome, a condition in which the transmission of reflex motor signals to the spine causes pain.[3]

Why is pain relief for the chest wall so important? One reason is that breathing is painful after any surgery on the chest cavity (including cardiac, lung, **trachea** surgery; **esophagus** surgery; **adrenal gland** surgery);[4] some types of kidney surgery for portions of the kidney lying above the bottom of the rib cage;[5] surgical approaches that go through the rib cage to reach high-lying kidney stones;[6] and gallbladder surgery that uses an incision just below the rib cage (subcostal incision).[7] Bones, muscles, and tissues that have been cut slide across each other every time a breath is taken.

Because many of the most powerful analgesics have a tendency to suppress breathing, it is often self-defeating to use one of these to stop the pain that interferes with breathing. Catheters are used if a continuous or intermittent **infusion** of anesthetic is planned. Otherwise, for one-time administration, a needle is used.

If breathing is impaired following an operation, the consequences can range from trivial and transient (in healthy, fit people who have a relatively high pain tolerance) to potentially fatal (in physically debilitated people). The most serious consequence of impaired breathing is impaired gas exchange, which reduces the amount of oxygen flowing through the bloodstream to the tissues. Because cells need oxygen to produce the energy required to build new tissues, impaired gas exchange delays recovery from surgery and impedes overall healing. Again, in a young, fit, healthy person, this may make half a day's difference in healing. In an elderly person who comes to surgery with some lung impairments (perhaps resulting from many years of smoking), pain on breathing can lead to atelectasis (absence of gas from all or part of a lung), which can lead to pneumonia.

Even with modern antibiotic treatments, pneumonia can be deadly in debilitated patients, and should be avoided if at all possible.

Pulmonary complication rates as high as 57% have been reported as a result of impaired breathing caused by postoperative pain.[8] Therefore, any effort to improve breathing after surgery is a good idea.

Administering local anesthetic (usually bupivicaine hydrocholide, marketed under the brand names Marcaine and Sensorcaine) through an intercostal catheter to deaden the muscles of the chest wall, and thereby make breathing easier, seemed like a good idea when it was conceived. The practice has since become widespread.[9] Research shows that gas exchange—a measure of efficiency of breathing—is better immediately following surgery in patients who have intercostal blocks.[10–12] Other studies have found that while patients subjectively report less pain and better breathing, objective measures of body function do not show such improvement.[13]

Clinical trials that measure only subjective pain accounts, or objective measures of pain such as patient requests for additional painkillers, almost universally report that intercostal nerve blocks reduce postoperative pain[14] and are also useful for chronic pain in nerves supplying the thorax.[15] However, some researchers have found no improved relief of patients' pain after gallbladder surgery using the subcostal incision,[16] and others found no relief after general thoracic operations.[17] The rate of pulmonary complications after gallbladder surgery dropped from 11% to 6% when intercostal nerve blocks were used, according to one study.[18] Reduced complication rates after lung surgery have also been noted when intercostal nerve blocks were used;[19] the same results were found for **renal** surgery and surgery for testicular cancer that has metastasized, or spread beyond the original site,[20, 21] and generally for upper abdominal surgery.[22] Because the effect of a single injection seems to last only about six hours,[23] use of a catheter would seem to be rational for avoiding lung complications. It also seems to be good for pain relief after operations on the appendix[24] and after incisions in the lower back for kidney surgery.[25] There is some evidence that ultrasound applied at the same sites as the intercostal catheters can produce the same effects.[26] If developed and thoroughly researched, this might be a noninvasive alternative.

Intercostal catheter insertion also has been used as anesthesia for minor breast surgery.[27]

? WHO PERFORMS THE PROCEDURE?

This procedure is usually performed by a thoracic surgeon, and on rare occasions by an anesthesiologist or a physician specializing in pain control.

? WHERE IS THE PROCEDURE PERFORMED?

Intercostal catheter insertion is simple and can be performed anywhere. Because it is generally used following major thoracic surgery for relief of pain or for the potentially life-threatening condition of pneumothorax, it is usually performed in a hospital. The catheter can be inserted in the operating room before the patient awakes from surgery, in the recovery room if it is noted that pain is causing breathing difficulties, or in the emergency room as an emergency procedure to treat pneumothorax.

? WHAT ARE THE MORTALITY (DEATH) AND MORBIDITY (COMPLICATION) RATES?

Because the procedure is minimally invasive if performed correctly, the mortality rate is essentially zero and reported morbidity is under 1%. The chief problem is pneumothorax, which has complication rates ranging from zero[28–33] to under 1%,[34] to 2.33%,[35] to 3.45%.[36]

According to one study, however, pneumothoraxes detectable only on x ray occurred in 25% of patients with intercostal catheters.[37] This may indicate that pneumothorax is quite common but that most pneumothoraxes are so minor that they produce no symptoms.

Although the procedure seems generally safe, it is uncertain why there are very few reports of complications in the literature. This may mean that the procedure is in fact safe, but might reflect the possibility that complications associated with intercostal catheter insertion have not been adequately studied.

❓ WHAT ARE THE OTHER COMPLICATIONS AND POSSIBLE SIDE EFFECTS?

The only major complication is pneumothorax, which, paradoxically, can be dealt with by the insertion of yet another catheter with a one-way valve. Pneumothorax occurs if the needle or trochar used to insert the catheter penetrates the pleura and allows air to enter the chest cavity when the surgeon creates the opening for the catheter. Abnormal anatomy in the patient's chest cavity or patient movement while the procedure is being done may sometimes cause this, but it is usually the fault of the surgeon performing the procedure.

Hypotension,[38] loss of feeling or sensation in the upper spine (called upper spinal anesthesia),[39] and total spinal anesthesia are rare complications. (It would seem to take strenuous effort to aim for the space between the skin over the ribs and the pleura and wind up with the catheter in the spinal canal, but it has been suggested as an explanation for this complication.[40] A more likely possibility, based on an anatomical study using dye, is that the anesthetic spreads around the back to reach the spinal nerves.[41, 42]) The reports on these complications are anecdotal—that is, reports of experience outside of formal, controlled research studies—and data on rates are not available. Oddly, most reports concerning hypotension relate to attempts to perform the nerve block in the operating room under direct vision, rather than "blind," or through-the-skin, attempts,[43] which seem to have a lower incidence of this complication.

One case of respiratory failure in a patient with chronic lung disease has been reported.[44] Again, this may be because this complication is in fact quite rare or because the matter has not been adequately studied.

Bupivacaine, the injectable anesthetic most commonly used for the procedure, may increase the effects of **beta-blockers** in people with heart failure, and this could be a problem in some cases.[45]

❓ IS THIS THE MOST APPROPRIATE PROCEDURE FOR THE CONDITION?

The weight of studies seems to suggest that although intercostal catheter insertion is certainly not a necessary procedure (in the sense that patients get well without it), it may reduce postoperative lung and breathing complications and improve comfort—and for a small number of patients may make the difference between life and death. Two studies warn that it should be avoided because of possible complications: one recommends against the procedure because it found no improved pain relief and because pneumothorax is a theoretical possibility,[46] the other is against the procedure because two serious complications were observed.[47] On the other hand, several studies demonstrate reduced hospital stays with the use of intercostal catheters. Because complications of any sort increase the longer a person stays in the hospital, use of this procedure to shorten hospital stays may reduce overall complications.

❓ ARE THERE ALTERNATIVES TO THIS PROCEDURE?

Clearly, use of painkillers that do not suppress breathing is one alternative;[48] another is intensified efforts with respiratory therapy, even though these may make patients more uncomfortable in the absence of extra pain relief. For pneumothorax, the alternative is insertion of a larger and stiffer chest tube with underwater drainage—one that uses a water trap to ensure that air flows only out of the chest cavity and not back in. Again on the basis of sparse literature, this does not seem to be more effective than a catheter with a one-way valve and is probably more uncomfortable for the patient.

Injection of morphine directly into the spinal canal, a relatively new technique used in surgery of the lower body (essentially below the **diaphragm**), seems to give better relief without suppressing respiration.[49] But the technique has the same hazards as any injection between the **vertebrae**. (See "Myelogram with Contrast Enhancement," p. 89, and "Intervertebral Disk Excision," p. 160.)

Freezing of the intercostal nerves has been used as an alternative. In this procedure—called cryoanesthesia or cryotherapy—a probe cooled with ether or some other quick-evaporating substance is applied to the intercostal nerve. One study found that relief was comparable to that obtained with bupivacaine;[50] another found that some permanent loss of sensation along the rib cage may result. The latter point may be either a blessing or a minor problem from the person's perspective. Use of cryotherapy for flank pain following herpes infection is apparently not effective.[51]

❔ WHAT IS CONTROVERSIAL ABOUT THE PROCEDURE?

The majority of studies that we could locate found this procedure to be beneficial and essentially harmless. One important controlled trial found the intercostal catheter procedure for pain relief to be much superior to the use of morphine,[52] and two others found it to be associated with significant improvements in postoperative lung function.[53, 54] A minority of studies, usually those that describe serious complications, recommend against it. At the same time, it can reduce high postoperative com-

plication rates. If one has a keen sense of the harm that surgery can do and of the possible seriousness of pulmonary complications, a balancing of the risks involved (from a lay standpoint) seems to favor the use of this procedure.

Intervertebral Disk Excision (7)

MORTALITY	MORBIDITY	CONTROVERSY
+	+	●

● The use of this procedure is **CONTROVERSIAL** because it may not be appropriate in all cases of lower back pain.

Removal of all or part of the fibrous disk found between the **vertebrae**; may be accompanied by a spinal fusion of two or more vertebrae

❔ WHAT CONDITION DOES THE PROCEDURE TREAT?

Between each of the vertebrae lies a disk of varying thickness, consisting of a tough, fibrous capsule (annulus fibrosus) and an inner, jellylike cushioning substance (nucleus pulposus). The term *jelly doughnut* has been used by some to describe the disk—it's apt. The function of the disk is to prevent the bones of the spine from grinding together and to provide flexibility to bend and twist the neck and torso. When the disk is distorted or ruptures, it presses on the nerve roots emerging between the vertebrae, or on the spinal cord itself. The pain can be mild to excruciating. The jellylike substance inside the disk is irritating to the nerve roots and the spinal cord. In very serious cases, paralysis can result if the condition is left untreated. Usually, there is some degree of limitation of movement, if only because the pain limits range of motion. Irritation of the roots of the sciatic nerve, which runs down each thigh, is common, and results in pain on attempt to raise the leg when it is held straight, or unbent.

As with hernias elsewhere in the body, any bulging or rupture of an intervertebral disk would seem to be a mechanical problem with a relatively straightforward mechanical solution—since the jellylike substance extrudes from between the vertebrae and pushes out—but matters turn out to be not so simple in practice. The available treatments for **herniated, or ruptured, disks** are widely regarded as unsatisfactory: One surgeon likens them to using a cannon when a peashooter would do the job. Pain caused by postsurgical scarring around the spinal cord and nerves is an unresolved problem; there is no satisfactory membrane that can be used to shield the cord and nerves from the bone; exercise (which repositions the bones and takes pressure off the spine) and psychological counseling (to help the person deal with the pain) actually do nothing to resolve the mechanical problem of the "slipped disk" but seem to be more effective than surgery; finally, the surgeon's ultimate weapon—fusion of the vertebrae—often fails to resolve pain.[1]

? WHAT IS THE PROCEDURE?

In the classical procedure—sometimes called laminectomy—the patient is anesthetized with a general anesthetic and laid on his stomach on the operating table. The region of the back to be operated on is shaved if needed. The back is then scrubbed with soap and antiseptic and draped so that only the portion to be operated on is exposed. The back is opened, and all or part of the disk is cut away from the vertebrae. If, in the surgeon's judgment, it is necessary to fuse two or more of the vertebrae to make the spine stable in the absence of the disk, bone is taken from a donor site on the hipbone or the bony "wing," called the process, that lies at the rear of each vertebra. Parts of the excised disk may be used together with the bone **graft**.[2] Patients generally require some physical therapy for rehabilitation after the procedure.

? WHO PERFORMS THE PROCEDURE?

This procedure is done by orthopedic surgeons and neurosurgeons. Anyone doing this operation should be board-certified in one specialty or the other, and ideally should do *at least* 100 operations per year.

? WHERE IS THE PROCEDURE PERFORMED?

This surgery is always done in a hospital or in a back clinic that has inpatient facilities.

? WHAT ARE THE MORTALITY (DEATH) AND MORBIDITY (COMPLICATION) RATES?

Mortality from this procedure in community hospitals was 0.1% in 1988; the average length of hospital stay was 8.9 days. Mortality rates of zero have been reported.[3] Increased pain occurs in about 3.3% of the cases.[4] The rates of most other complications are under 2%.[5] Complications include defective bladder function arising from impaired nerve signal transmission (a condition called neurogenic bladder, in which nerve damage results in incontinence), which reached 60% in one report.[6]

The chief concern with this procedure is unrelieved, worsened, or recurrent pain, which may arise from scarring inside and outside the membrane that covers the spine, called the dura. Recent studies using **MRI scans** suggest that scarring is the cause of unrelieved or recurrent pain in about one-sixth of the cases that do not have "excellent" results. In various studies, results that were "excellent or good" ranged from 73.5% to 95%, with an average of 84.4%. "Poor" results ranged from 5% to 26.5%, with an average of 29.1%—almost a third. One study suggests that removal of the disk from the front of the spine rather than the rear avoids possible further nerve-root irritation and produces "excellent" results in 90.9% of cases.[7] This approach is technically more difficult than the posterior approach and carries a somewhat greater risk of cord damage.

? WHAT ARE THE OTHER COMPLICATIONS AND POSSIBLE SIDE EFFECTS?

Damage to veins and arteries near the spine has rarely been reported; no deaths are reported in association with it.[8]

Allergic reactions to chymopapain, a chemical used in the alternative procedure of **chemonucleolysis** can be fatal; in fact, one death has been reported from the skin test used to determine whether or not patients are allergic.[9]

As with any procedure in which anesthesia is used, death from reaction to the anesthetic drugs, error on the part of the anesthetist, or machine failure is a remote possibility. (See Glossary, p. 309)

? IS THIS THE MOST APPROPRIATE PROCEDURE FOR THE CONDITION?

It is probably safe to say that there is no wholly appropriate procedure for this condition. The traditional laminectomy, chemonucleolysis, and percutaneous diskectomy (removal of disk fragments through a small hole drilled into the vertebrae) all result in a substantial minority of patients who have no or incomplete relief of pain or increased pain. The complete cure rate for laminectomy is only about 50%.[10] As with many other procedures, it is possible to try the more conservative procedures first—these being exercise and counseling, rest, heat, and muscle relaxants[11]—chemonucleolysis, and percutaneous diskectomy, then follow them with laminectomy and/or fusion. The reverse is not true, so the more conservative procedures should be tried first

unless there is some compelling reason to believe that they will not work.

? ARE THERE ALTERNATIVES TO THIS PROCEDURE?

See the preceding section. Computer control of the percutaneous diskectomy may offer significant improvement in results: The surgeon uses a robot arm, which controls the positioning of the needle that drills the hole into the vertebrae. The computer is more precise in placing the drill than is the human hand. However, as of late 1991, no controlled trials had been reported.[12]

About 13% of patients having percutaneous diskectomy in a recent trial had unsatisfactory results and required repeat surgical procedures.[13] As for chemonucleolysis, an American Medical Association (AMA) panel has recommended that it be judged neither safe nor effective in certain circumstances that cannot be detected reliably. In other words, the AMA regards it as neither safe nor effective for any case.[14]

It is important to note that when the damage to the disk is caused by a gunshot wound, early laminectomy is appropriate, to avoid scarring and spinal **abscess** formation.[15]

? WHAT IS CONTROVERSIAL ABOUT THE PROCEDURE?

As increasing amounts of data are gathered on the effects of alternative treatments, the traditional laminectomy looks progressively worse. The most common cause of failure is surgeons' recommendation of the operation for the wrong patients. Assuredly, there is a range of disorders, apart from a ruptured disk, that are associated with low back pain and for which (when all conservative efforts have failed) surgical treatment should be offered. The decisive factor is to clarify, as best as possible, the cause of the pain before resorting to surgical intervention. Unfortunately, in many cases the real cause of low back pain still cannot be determined with certainty.[16]

Joint Replacement Revision (48)

MORTALITY	MORBIDITY	CONTROVERSY
+	−	o

- The major **COMPLICATION** for this procedure is risk of infection, which is reported to be between 12% and 17%.

Revision of the replacement of a natural joint—for example, hip, knee, ankle, shoulder, elbow, or wrist—with a **prosthesis**, or artificial body part

❓ WHAT CONDITION DOES THE PROCEDURE TREAT?

This procedure treats any of a wide variety of conditions that create problems with artificial joints. These include loosening of the prosthesis (or manufactured body part) within the bones to which it is attached, infection, dislocation of the joint, bone loss, and fracture.

❓ WHAT IS THE PROCEDURE?

Essentially, revision procedures are identical to the original operations, except that removal of old cement and infected bone and bone grafting are often included. (See "Total Hip Replacement," p. 252, and "Total Knee Replacement," p. 257.)

❓ WHO PERFORMS THE PROCEDURE?

This procedure is performed by orthopedic surgeons.

❓ WHERE IS THE PROCEDURE PERFORMED?

This is major surgery that is always performed in the inpatient department of a hospital.

❓ WHAT ARE THE MORTALITY (DEATH) AND MORBIDITY (COMPLICATION) RATES?

Mortality and morbidity vary widely depending upon the joint replacement being revised, the age of the patient, the problem for which the revision is being done, and any other diseases that may be present. All lower limb surgery is subject to the complication of clotting and **thrombosis**, which can be fatal. Mortality for first-time replacement operations ranges from 0.5% to 0.8%.[1,2]

The rate of failure of total hip replacements for reasons other than infection is about 1.7% per year; by the twelfth year after surgery, 20% will have failed.[3] The strength of the bone-glue-joint bond in first revisions is only about 21% of that obtained in original operations, and the strength of the second revision can be as much as 93% lower than the original operation.[4] Ideally, the bond between the bone, glue, and artificial joint should be equal—the entire replacement should hold together as one unit. In any revision, residual glue on the bone or artificial joint weakens the bond, so with subsequent revisions the opportunity for obtaining a strong bond decreases. In the case of artificial joints that are cemented into place, failure rates between 17% and 60% have been reported.[5]

The outcome of first revisions of hip replacements is generally regarded as good; the outcome of second attempts at revision is generally regarded as poor.[6] (A good outcome means that the bond between the bone and the replacement joint is such that the replacement doesn't move around or cause pain.)

The major complication rate in first hip replacement revisions can be as high as 25%.[7] Another study reports complication rates up to 22% for first revisions of hip replacements.[8] The rate of infection after first hip replacement revisions without existing infection can be as high as 12%, and after revisions with infections, can reach 17%.[9] About 13% of first hip replacements revisions in infected hips fail.[10] A relatively recent report (1990) of a long-term follow-up of patients shows good or excellent results in around 45% of patients.[11] Another series shows an 80% success rate in infected hips when the healing rates for first and second revisions are combined.[12] It has also recently been shown that an infection rate of zero can be achieved.[13]

Early (1981) reports on knee replacements indicate a failure rate of 13.5% and only fair or poor results in 52% of revisions.[14] (The terms *fair* and *poor* refer to outcomes, such as whether there is pain upon walking, and whether the replacement joint fits properly.) Revision of infected knee joint replacements can have a failure rate as high as 42.9%.[15, 16] As of 1990, about 33% of patients who have revisions to knee replacements will not be able to walk without crutches or a walker; some cannot walk at all.[17]

The need for revision of artificial elbow replacements is apparently rather rare, but when a revision is needed, the results are good in only a little more than half of the patients.[18]

? WHAT ARE THE OTHER COMPLICATIONS AND POSSIBLE SIDE EFFECTS?

The extent to which the replacement revision is successful varies widely with the factors cited above, and from study to study. Patients who have revisions to total hip replacements because of loosening of the artificial parts tend to be slightly more dependent upon a cane and report slightly more pain than those whose replacements do not require revision.[19]

Fracture of the the long bone of the thigh occurs during surgery in about 6.3% of revisions of total hip replacements. If this fracture occurs, 40% of the patients do not regain satisfactory hip function.[20]

About 6.7% of patients show some damage to the sciatic nerve of the thigh during surgery. This can be detected, and largely avoided, by continuous electronic monitoring of the sciatic nerve during surgery.[21]

As with any procedure in which anesthesia is used, death from reaction to the anesthetic drugs, error on the part of the anesthetist, or machine failure is a remote possibility. (See Glossary, p. 309)

? IS THIS THE MOST APPROPRIATE PROCEDURE FOR THE CONDITION?

Yes, if the patient can tolerate the procedure and needs the mobility that an artificial joint can provide. The surgeon must determine whether there is sufficient viable bone to anchor the replacement joint before deciding to perform the operation. If replacement does not appear possible, other alternatives—such as **arthrodesis** or amputation—may have to be considered. In all cases, it is important to determine what went wrong the first time (mechanical wear, infection, bone death, or some other problem) and take steps to make sure that it does not happen again.

? ARE THERE ALTERNATIVES TO THIS PROCEDURE?

Use of antibiotic-containing cement helps reduce the rate of infections in both first procedures and revisions.[22–24]

? WHAT IS CONTROVERSIAL ABOUT THE PROCEDURE?

A significant debate concerns the use of cementless versus cemented prostheses. Cement wears down eventually, it generates heat as it sets, and its application causes brief circulatory and respiratory reactions in many patients. Cementless prostheses are not associated with these problems, but they do not adhere as tightly to bone as do the cemented ones, at least in the initial months of wear.

Most surgeons today use the various prostheses available and use cementless or cemented procedures based on the patient's age and lifestyle, the amount of damage to the bone that has resulted from arthritis or trauma, and how good a fit they achieve with the artificial components after trimming the bones. Undoubtedly, doctors are influenced by those people selling the prosthetic parts, but there is a growing trend to try to fit the parts to the patient, rather than the other way around.

A 1984 article predicted that revisions of total hip replacements would "overwhelm" operating rooms in the 1990s; it further indicated the need for the development of surgical instruments and tools that would make the operation easier on both the patient and the surgeon. Although there has been considerable research into the design of joint replacements themselves, little has been done in the area of **jigs** and instrumentation to make revision surgery easier on both the patient and the surgeon.[25, 26]

Relatively recent (1989) results indicate that of the various hipbone replacement joints available, the press-to-fit type with titanium fins is superior to others in fixation to the bone and avoidance of bone destruction. The increasing use of bone grafting is also raising the success rate of hip and knee replacement revisions.[27, 28] The surgeon takes a piece of bone from another part of the patient's body—or from another person or a cadaver—and attaches it to an area, such as the hip or knee, where bone is destroyed or deficient.

Left Hemicolectomy (71)

MORTALITY	MORBIDITY	CONTROVERSY
–	–	o

- The operative **MORTALITY** rate of 6.2% reflects the fact that the patient's condition is usually serious when the procedure is performed.
- **INFECTION** is a major complication of any abdominal surgery, as well as **adhesions** and postoperative bleeding.

Removal of the left (descending) half of the **colon**

? WHAT CONDITION DOES THE PROCEDURE TREAT?

A left hemicolectomy is performed for cancer of the colon; for trauma to the colon (e.g., gunshot wounds) that is too damaging to permit repair; for **Crohn's disease** and ulcerative colitis, which are two bowel diseases of unknown origin that lead to destruction of the intestinal wall and formation of scar tissue; for uncontrollable bleeding from the left side of the colon; for severe diverticular disease (a condition characterized by the formation of small outpouchings from the colon, it is more common in the aged and may result from lack of fiber in the diet); for left-sided pelvic tumors or masses that require removal; and for radiation injury to the bowel, which follows radiation treatment for cancer or other conditions.

The colon, or large intestine, sits at the front of the abdominal cavity in a position like an upside-down letter "U." On the right, it connects with the end of the small intestine, the **terminal ileum**. Just past the **ileocecal valve**, the large intestine balloons out to about three times the diameter of the small intestine. It runs up the right side of the body to just below the liver—most people think it is lower in the body—and then across with its bottom about even with the navel. It runs down the left side of the abdominal cavity before making the

"S"-shaped turns that has given the name **sigmoid co-lon** (from the Greek letter sigma, which looks something like an angular English S).

The main job of the colon is to remove water from the digested food passed on by the small intestines. It also reabsorbs bile salts so that the body can use them again. Because it receives the end products of digestion and also has to deal with the intestinal flora—over 500 different species of bacteria that inhabit the colon and weigh about as much as one of the major organs of the body—it has a chemical feast to contend with and is often the site of benign tumors, precancerous tumors, and cancer. The incidence of colon cancer is around 10 cases per one million people in the under-age-40 population and increases with advancing age thereafter.[1] There is some evidence that the risk is increased by heavy beer consumption and decreased by the use of **non-steroidal anti-inflammatory drugs** such as aspirin and ibuprofen.[2, 3]

? WHAT IS THE PROCEDURE?

The patient is put under general anesthesia and the surgeon places a tube down the patient's windpipe. The abdomen, which will have been shaved the night before, is washed with soap and antiseptic, and draped so that only the planned area of the incision is exposed. An incision is made with a scalpel about a half inch to the left of the navel and is carried to about three inches below the navel and one inch above it. The fat, **fascia**, muscles, and **peritoneum** are opened one by one, with small bleeding vessels being **ligated** along the way. The **transverse colon**, which is the portion of the colon that runs across the middle of the abdomen, is located just above the middle of the incision. The small intestines and the **omentum** (a fatty "apron" that hangs down from the bottom of the stomach and seems to have the role of plugging intestinal leaks and walling off

abscesses[4]) are pushed up towards the **diaphragm** with moist gauze pads.

The left colon is located and, beginning at the bottom of the incision, is cut free of the fascia that supports it. The dissection is continued with scissors up to the level of the gastrocolic **ligament**, which supports the colon and stomach. The ligament is cut and tied off. The splenocolic ligament, which supports the spleen and colon, is clamped and severed, and the left colon is pulled down.

If there is a tumor, or if the colon is connected to the spleen by **adhesions**, the surgeon will probably extend the incision upward, or make a transverse incision converting the shape of the incision to a "T" so that she can fully expose the spleen. The spleen is the hub of the **lymphatic system** and has a rich blood supply. Bleeding from a damaged spleen can be impossible to control, and removal of the spleen may be necessary. The surgeon will be very careful to avoid damaging it while freeing the splenic flexure of the colon—the right-angle bend right under the spleen—if at all possible.

If the operation is for cancer, the omentum is removed also to ensure that any cancer cells that have spread to it are removed, and to eliminate some lymph drainage that could spread cancer. It is detached by cutting along its border with the stomach. For other purposes, the surgeon may use part of the omentum to provide "patches" for **lesions** in the part of the colon that is to be retained.

The surgeon then opens the fascia covering the rectum with a scissors, reaches in, and frees the sigmoid colon by blunt, or finger, dissection. He cuts away the remainder of the colon from the membrane that supports it and supplies blood to it—the mesocolon. Then he ligates the arteries and veins running to the mesocolon from the portion of colon to be removed. The mobilized portion is placed into a plastic bag and laid on the upper abdomen of the patient: Before the cancerous portion of the colon is cut away, there is preparatory work to be done.

In surgery for cancer, there is extensive dissection of the lymph nodes that drain the portion of the colon containing the tumor. The surgeon has to seek a balance here between the complications that may result from wider dissection and the risk of leaving cancer cells behind. (The use of chemotherapy following colon cancer surgery has shown potential to reduce recurrence, but very specific treatment regimens are required to produce a good result.)

The portion of the colon containing the tumor is cut away, beginning at about the middle of the transverse colon and ending at the sigmoid colon. Many surgeons ligate the area of the tumor to avoid spreading cancer cells.

As soon as the sigmoid colon is cut, the surgical site is declared contaminated (exposed to bacteria in the colon) and covered with a red sheet; care is taken not to spread bacteria. The transverse colon is brought down and sewed or stapled to the sigmoid colon, using any one of a number of techniques. This artificial juncture is called the **anastomosis**. When the surgeon is satisfied with the anastomosis, she sews the cut **mesentery** back together and lays the intestines back in the abdomen. If the greater omentum has been retained, it is laid back over the intestines as well. Any packing material is removed, and the various layers of the intestinal wall are closed separately. A dressing is applied, and the patient is taken to the recovery room. Either in the recovery room or in the operating room, a **nasogastric tube** will be inserted through the nose to remove the stomach secretions—about a quart a day—until it is clear that the intestines can handle them. The pathologist will examine the removed intestine for cancer or other diseases.

? WHO PERFORMS THE PROCEDURE?

This procedure is performed by a general surgeon.

? WHERE IS THE PROCEDURE PERFORMED?

This is a major procedure that must be performed in a hospital.

? WHAT ARE THE MORTALITY (DEATH) AND MORBIDITY (COMPLICATION) RATES?

This is not a trivial procedure. Mortality is low in patients who are being operated on under ideal conditions. However, the diseases or injuries that require removal of the left colon have often weakened the patient prior to any operation. Consequently, the surgeon may be confronted with the need to operate on a patient in very bad state of health.

Operative mortality rates of around 6.2% are reported in the literature.[5] Complications with the anastomosis, the point where the intestines are rejoined, range around 4%.

? WHAT ARE THE OTHER COMPLICATIONS AND POSSIBLE SIDE EFFECTS?

As with any abdominal procedure, infections, formation of **adhesions**, and postoperative bleeding may occur. The anastomosis may fail to heal in patients whose nutritional status is poor or who have widespread cancer. **Hyperalimentation** may help speed healing, especially in patients with radiation injury to the bowel or Crohn's colitis.[6] There is some evidence that intravenous feeding with solutions of branched-chain amino acids (types of the building blocks of protein that have "Y" shapes in their molecular structure) is helpful in fighting severe infections.[7]

Diarrhea after the operation is a potential problem, but it can be controlled by avoiding foods that produce diarrhea, use of antidiarrheal drugs such as Imodium and Lomotil, and eating more water-soluble fiber or taking over-the-counter drugs containing water-soluble fiber, such as Metamucil, Citrucel, and Fiberall.

As with any procedure in which anesthesia is used, death from reaction to the anesthetic drugs, error on the part of the anesthetist, or machine failure is a remote possibility. (See Glossary, p. 309)

? IS THIS THE MOST APPROPRIATE PROCEDURE FOR THE CONDITION?

For cancer located in the left colon that cannot be treated through **colonoscopic** removal of the lesion or the more conservative procedure of removing only the segment containing the tumor, this is the best alternative. Bowel that is gangrenous or dead must be removed, and this is the appropriate procedure if the bowel to be removed is in the left half of the colon. The same applies to radiation injury to the bowel.

Trauma to the bowel may permit a more conservative approach involving removal of multiple small segments, but there is some evidence that the more anastomoses required, the greater the risk. Strictureplasty, which removes only the portions of the bowel that are narrowed in Crohn's disease, can be used also, but the same caution applies.

Research is now being done on immune system modulation therapy—which stimulates the person's own immune system to fight the cancer. If effective, this type of treatment may lead to reduction of the scope of surgery for bowel cancer, to less radical procedures, and to reduction of the number of procedures performed.

? ARE THERE ALTERNATIVES TO THIS PROCEDURE?

One alternative is segmental resection, or cutting away, of the portion containing the tumor. This is done for cases in which the cancer is confined to the left colon. The procedure has proven to have lower mortality and morbidity rates than left hemicolectomy, and the five-year cancer-free survival rates are as good or better than those achieved with left hemicolectomy.[8, 9] If the tumor is high in the left colon, an extended right hemicolectomy can be performed. This procedure simply extends the amount of colon removed from the **ileum** to a point past the tumor on the left side.[10–12]

? WHAT IS CONTROVERSIAL ABOUT THE PROCEDURE?

Points of controversy are limited to technical details of the procedure, usually regarding the best ways to handle tumor masses and ligate vessels so as not to seed tumor cells in other parts of the abdomen during the operation. The structures handled—the abdominal organs—are relatively large, so the risk of damage to a tiny, delicate structure does not enter into the picture. While each surgeon has his own way of preparing the end of the intestines, these variations in technique are not the object of a good deal of controversy.

Ligation and Stripping of Varicose Veins of the Legs (96)

MORTALITY	MORBIDITY	CONTROVERSY
+	+	o

The **ligation** and removal of damaged veins in the legs to avoid clotting, circulatory problems, and ulceration, or to improve cosmetic appearance

❔ WHAT CONDITION DOES THE PROCEDURE TREAT?

Veins have valves (comprised of tiny flaps called leaflets) every few inches, which open in only one direction—toward the heart—in order to prevent the backflow of blood. This design reduces the work of the circulatory system, which returns blood to the heart, but also makes the valves subject to damage if there is too much back-pressure against the leaflets that make up the valves in the veins. Back-pressure can result from pregnancy, prolonged standing, or other conditions that increase the pressure in the leg veins. If the valves are destroyed, sections of the veins between intact valves bulge, twist, and can ulcerate through the skin, producing sores often difficult to heal. An eczemalike condition—characterized by itching, scaling, and small, oozing blisters—can also appear over the veins. In addition, veins in this condition often are regarded as unsightly. This factor, rather than pain or clotting, is frequently the primary reason that people seek treatment.

❔ WHAT IS THE PROCEDURE?

With the patient under general or local anesthesia,[1] the area of the leg with the varicose veins is shaved and scrubbed with soap and antiseptic. An incision is made in the thigh to expose the origin of the **saphenous vein,** which is then tied off. The vein is cut and then removed with any one of a number of instruments, most of which cause the vein to turn inside out as it is pulled up or down. With the vein successfully removed, tributary veins that have ulcerated, are associated with skin ulcers, or are particularly visible are ligated and stripped. The deeper vein supply of the leg and the remaining veins closer to the skin surface take over the task of returning blood to the heart.

In **sclerotherapy,** an irritating solution is injected into the varicose vein causing inflammation and the formation of scar tissue, which closes off the vein; sclero-therapy can also be used with, or as an alternative to, ligation. A combination of surgical removal of the long saphenous vein and sclerotherapy of tributaries is also possible.[2]

❔ WHO PERFORMS THE PROCEDURE?

This procedure is usually done by a vascular surgeon; some plastic surgeons handle superficial veins that present only cosmetic problems.

❔ WHERE IS THE PROCEDURE PERFORMED?

Injection therapy of superficial veins can be done in a doctor's office or outpatient surgery center. Depending upon the extent of the work needed and the risk of **thrombosis,** ligation and stripping can be done as an inpatient or outpatient procedure. Ligation and stripping combined with repair is done as an inpatient procedure.

❔ WHAT ARE THE MORTALITY (DEATH) AND MORBIDITY (COMPLICATION) RATES?

In severe cases, wound infection can occur in up to 7% of patients and **necrosis** in up to 12%. These usually heal without further surgery.[3] **Lesions** of, or injury to, the saphenous nerve can be expected in 39% of patients who have the entire saphenous vein removed and 5% of those who have only the groin-to-knee portion removed.[4] Apparently, the surgeon can avoid nerve damage entirely if he strips the vein downward rather than upward; given the human anatomy, in such a technique the vein pulls away from the nerve without damage. If stripped from the bottom up, however, the vein tears off the small branches of the nerve.[5]

A rare but devastating complication occurs when the surgeon mistakes the arteries for the veins and strips out the entire arterial system of the leg. On occasion, however, the mistake has been corrected by replacing the stripped arteries with the varicose veins.[6]

? WHAT ARE THE OTHER COMPLICATIONS AND POSSIBLE SIDE EFFECTS?

Damage to the **femoral artery** during removal of the saphenous vein has been reported. Such damage is often further complicated by delayed recognition that the injury has occurred.[7, 8] Provided corrective surgery is done as soon as the arterial injury is recognized, it is usually possible to avoid permanent damage even with late recognition. Nonfatal but clinically detectable **pulmonary embolism**—that is, complete or partial blockage of a lung artery by a clot originating in or near the operated vein—can be expected in up to 0.39% of patients.[9] Studies of reoperations for varicose veins generally show that the first procedure didn't work because of failure to ligate the cut vessels at the proper location, or failure to trace and cut off all of the **collateral vessels**.[10]

Impotence has been reported by patients in whom the blood supply of the penis is derived from the external pudendal artery, which is often ligated during vein stripping, rather than the internal pudendal artery, the normal source. (Both the internal and external pudendal arteries are located in the groin.) This can be avoided by not operating on either of the arteries during the vein stripping;[11, 12] it is rarely necessary to disturb either artery.

As with any procedure in which anesthesia is used, death from reaction to the anesthetic drugs, error on the part of the anesthetist, or machine failure is a remote possibility. (See Glossary, p. 309)

? IS THIS THE MOST APPROPRIATE PROCEDURE FOR THE CONDITION?

The literature suggests that superficial varicose veins that are only a cosmetic problem for the patient can best be treated with compression (support) stockings, a walking exercise program,[13] and sclerotherapy, if necessary. Surgery should be reserved for incompetent veins—those in which valvular control or venous return to the heart is completely compromised, thus allowing reverse flow—or ulceration.[14–16]

The literature also suggests that incompetent veins be identified with **ultrasound**: If only incompetent veins are stripped, both the scope of the operation and the incidence of complications can be reduced.[17]

? ARE THERE ALTERNATIVES TO THIS PROCEDURE?

Open surgery and sclerotherapy are alternatives to each other. Conservative treatment with compression stockings, exercise, and periodic leg elevation is also possible.

Plication is another alternative, although it has some controversy attached to it. (See discussion below.)

? WHAT IS CONTROVERSIAL ABOUT THE PROCEDURE?

Because cosmetic factors produce such a high demand for varicose vein surgery, research on alternative surgeries and careful diagnostic methods is seldom done. If cosmetic considerations are set aside, it is often possible to eliminate backward flow in the saphenous vein by a technique called plication, in which the vein is exposed and tissue, such as muscle in the vicinity of the varicose vein, is wrapped around it to cause a slight constriction. When the person walks, the muscle tightens, thus closing off the vein and forcing it to act like a valve. This eliminates the circulatory problems but does not produce immediate cosmetic improvement. As a result, and because the degree of improvement depends upon the amount of leg exercise done, surgeons generally do not perform this procedure, which is an otherwise valuable technique.

Lobectomy of Lung (86)

MORTALITY	MORBIDITY	CONTROVERSY
+	+	●

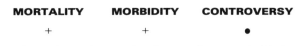

- Lobectomies require more time than complete removal of the lung and do preserve breathing function. The **CONTROVERSY** is whether the complete lung should be removed in all cases of lung cancer.

Removal of one of the three divisions of the lungs

? WHAT CONDITION DOES THE PROCEDURE TREAT?

The tip of the upper lobe of each lung projects into the neck above the **clavicle**. The bottom of the lower lobe is just about at the bottom of the tenth rib, which is the lowest rib that can be felt with the hands just below the **sternum**; the other ribs are attached only to the spine and "float" in front. The middle lobe lies in between. Lobectomy is the removal of one of these three lobes.

This procedure is primarily used to treat various forms of lung cancer. However, it can also be used to treat intractable tuberculosis, which is rare, and other infections in a lung lobe;[1, 2] benign tumors that interfere with lung function; uncontrollable **pulmonary** hypertension, which is high blood pressure limited to the vessels of the lungs;[3] uncontrollable bleeding in a lung;[4] lung problems present at birth;[5] and collapse of a lobe of a lung that cannot be reexpanded.[6]

? WHAT IS THE PROCEDURE?

Although forms of anesthesia other than general anesthesia are technically possible, this operation is almost invariably done under general anesthesia. The sense of panic that accompanies enforced alterations in breathing makes it very difficult for even the most self-controlled patient to cooperate while awake with procedures involving the lungs. (When **intubated**, the person momentarily panics, so the anesthetist uses mechanical means to keep the person breathing.) While the patient is under general anesthesia, the anesthetist is able to administer inhalation anesthesia through only one lung. She can use the inflatable cuffs on the tubes used to administer anesthesia gases to effectively seal off the lung (or lobe of the lung) that is being worked on.

A number of approaches are possible in lung surgery, and there are many different techniques for operating on each lobe. What we describe here is the simple removal of the right upper lobe, without the need for a surgical alteration of the **bronchi**: The anesthetized patient is placed on her left side, and her skin, which is shaved before surgery if necessary, is scrubbed with soap and antiseptic. The patient is draped so that only the area where the incision will be made is exposed. The surgeon makes an incision at the level of the nipple, between the fourth and fifth or the fifth and sixth ribs, depending upon his preference.

The ribs may be simply pulled apart or cut away, depending upon the surgeon's preferences and the technical difficulty of the procedure. The **pleura** is cut away with scissors, and the veins and arteries leading to the upper lobe that are visible at this point are **ligated** with sutures and cut. The lower and middle lobes of the lung are pulled apart and the **pleura** covering the major interlobar fissure, which is the line between the two largest lobes of the lung, is cut with scissors.

The lung is extremely elastic; it shrinks about two-thirds in size when the chest cavity is opened and the partial vacuum that assists in breathing is lost. The lung adapts well to the loss of a lobe,[7] and survival with only two lobes of one lung has been reported.[8]

Pulling the two lobes farther apart further exposes the **fissure** between the upper and middle lobes. The upper and middle lobes are then pulled as far apart as possible and the normal separation between the two lobes is completed with scissors and scalpel. Veins or arteries that bleed are either ligated or sealed with an **electrocautery device**.

The portion of the bronchial tree leading to the upper lobe is exposed and ligated between the right main bronchus and the lobe. It is cut and sewn together to form an airtight seal. The severed upper lobe is rolled out of the chest, and any last blood vessels or other structures attached to it are severed. To provide suction, which will help the lungs stay expanded, and drainage, the wound is closed in layers around two tubes that are placed in or near it. The patient is taken to the recovery room, where respiratory assistance is provided if needed, and then to his room. Local anesthetic may be administered via a **catheter** placed between the ribs to reduce pain and aid breathing. (The bronchi and lungs themselves have no pain or touch receptors, but can communicate inflammation, such as that occurring in a severe cold or pneumonia, as a sort of burning sensation.)

? WHO PERFORMS THE PROCEDURE?

This procedure used to be in the province of the general surgeon and, indeed, general surgeons may still perform it in remote areas. However, it is now almost always done by a thoracic surgeon in areas where specialty surgeons are available.

? WHERE IS THE PROCEDURE PERFORMED?

This is major surgery that should be performed only on an inpatient basis in a hospital.

? WHAT ARE THE MORTALITY (DEATH) AND MORBIDITY (COMPLICATION) RATES?

Operative mortality rates of around 1% have been reported, along with low complication rates. The most common complication is **stenosis**, or narrowing, of the bronchi, which can result from recurrence of tumor (6% of patients) or scar formation (2% of patients).[9] Combined operative and postoperative mortality of 8% for cancer patients has been reported.[10] Mortality rates as high as 19% and complication rates as high as 59% have been reported for lung cancer patients who already had problems with lung function when they were operated on.[11] A Soviet study reported 5.9% operative mortality and 6.5% postoperative complication rates.[12] Other studies report zero mortality and a 10% major complication rate in lung cancer patients.[13] As is the case with most surgeries, reports that occur more recently in the medical literature show lower mortality and complication rates. To some extent, this is attributable to improvements in surgical technique, as well as to limited time for follow-up.

? WHAT ARE THE OTHER COMPLICATIONS AND POSSIBLE SIDE EFFECTS?

Because the surgeon has to reconstruct the connection between the lung and the bronchus in many lobectomy procedures, air leaks can occur at the joint and the lung may collapse, completely or partially.[14] Experimental work in dogs suggests that the speed and degree of healing is dramatically affected by different surgical techniques, and that the preservation of adequate blood supply to the bronchi is especially critical.[15]

Twisting of the middle lobe around the bronchus after removal of the upper lobe has been reported.[16]

As with any procedure in which anesthesia is used, death from reaction to the anesthetic drugs, error on the part of the anesthetist, or machine failure is a remote possibility. (See Glossary, p. 309)

❓ IS THIS THE MOST APPROPRIATE PROCEDURE FOR THE CONDITION?

Whether a surgeon has to perform a lobectomy or remove the entire lung depends upon a number of factors, including the location of the cancer and the extent of its spread. **CT scans** are not particularly helpful in determining which operation will be necessary before surgery.[17] A lobectomy can always be converted to a removal of the entire lung if the spread of the tumor or complications that develop during the operation require it.[18] Hence, it seems that this more conservative procedure is generally the most appropriate if: (1) the lobe has to be removed to stop the spread of cancer or intractable infection; and (2) removal of the entire lung is not clearly indicated.

❓ ARE THERE ALTERNATIVES TO THIS PROCEDURE?

Wedge resection—removal of less than the entire lobe of the lung—had zero mortality compared with 5% mortality associated with lobectomy in a study of Veterans Administration patients diagnosed with lung cancer; five-year survival rates were 26% for wedge resection and 25% for lobectomy. Wedge resection is an alternative for patients with limited disease that has not yet spread beyond the original site.[19]

Radiation therapy may be another alternative some day, because animal studies have indicated that it is possible to avoid spread of radioactivity to other parts of the body: Experiments with dogs have demonstrated that microscopic bits of plastic treated with the radioactive element phosphorous-32 can be injected into a single lobe of the lung and 94% of the radioactivity remains there. The radioactivity of the spheres then destroys the tissue. In one study, complete destruction of the injected lobe was reported after 12 months, indicating that such a procedure may be an alternative for humans in whom lobe operations are impossible or very risky.[20] As the radioactivity of the spheres decays, the phosphorous-32 becomes nonradioactive phosphorous, a natural element of the body. This method may be used to treat benign or malignant tumors, as well as lung **abscess.**

❓ WHAT IS CONTROVERSIAL ABOUT THE PROCEDURE?

Lobectomies may be technically more difficult for the surgeon and thus require more operating time than removal of the entire lung in a procedure called a pneumonectomy. Therefore, similar to the argument among surgeons over complete removal of a cancerous breast versus lumpectomy, some controversy surrounds the choice of lobectomy versus complete lung removal.[21] Survival data for lobectomy and pneumonectomy are comparable in most recent studies, and lobectomy offers better preservation of lung function. A matter of debate among surgeons is how important preservation of lung function is, when compared with complete lung removal—which is technically easier for the surgeon, has a lower complication rate, and has similar survival rates for cancer patients.[22]

From the patient's standpoint, preserving part of the affected lung may mean the difference between a perfectly normal existence and one of being tied to an oxygen supply. The loss in vital capacity, defined as the largest volume of air that can be exhaled after the largest possible inhalation, is cut by 15% following a lobectomy and 35% to 40% following the complete removal of a lung.[23] Clearly, assessment of probable lung function after surgery should play a large role in the choice of lobectomy or complete removal of the lung.[24, 25]

Five-year survival following lobectomy for squamous cell carcinoma is 71% when the hilar lymph nodes—the lymph nodes near the depression in the lung where the bronchus enters—are not involved, and is 17% when they are. This finding tends to favor lobectomy over pneumonectomy; nonetheless, other procedures are still performed.[26]

Local Destruction of Ovarian Lesion (62)

MORTALITY	MORBIDITY	CONTROVERSY
+	+	o

Destruction of a **lesion** on the ovary without removal of the intact ovary

? WHAT CONDITION DOES THE PROCEDURE TREAT?

Similar to the other female reproductive organs, the ovaries are subject to a variety of benign and malignant tumors. The current medical recommendations stress complete removal of ovaries that have malignant tumors, and preservation of ovaries that have benign tumors or cysts. The rationale for preservation is the recognition that estrogen plays a large part in protecting even postmenopausal women from bone loss and heart disease.

? WHAT IS THE PROCEDURE?

This procedure can be done either via an abdominal incision (called an open procedure) or with a **laparoscope**.[1] In either case, a general anesthetic is used. The patient's lower abdomen is shaved and scrubbed with soap and antiseptic.

For the **open procedure**, an incision is made between the pubis and the navel, and the fat, **fascia**, muscle, and **peritoneum** are opened separately. Bleeding vessels are **cauterized** or tied off. The ovary is located and examined, and a tissue sample may be taken for immediate examination to determine if the ovary is cancerous. If so, it is removed. If the ovary is not found to be cancerous, the surgeon determines how much functional ovarian tissue can be preserved, and may remove the ovary if the amount is too small. If the ovary can be preserved, the benign tumor or cyst is cut away with a scalpel, or destroyed with an **electrocautery device** or laser beam. If necessary, the ovary is sutured shut to cover the hole left by the removal of the tumor or cyst. The peritoneum, muscle, fascia, and skin are closed in separate layers with **sutures**, staples, or **clips**.

In the laparoscopic procedure, the surgeon may use instruments or a laser beam shone through a fiber-optic pipe, which is a bendable "wire" of glass that carries light, to destroy the lesion or remove the ovary.

After surgery, the patient is taken to the recovery room and then to her room. Patients who have had the laparoscopic procedure may be allowed to go home as soon as it is clear that they have recovered from the anesthetic and that there is no bleeding from the ovary; patients who have the open procedure may have to stay in the hospital for several days.

? WHO PERFORMS THE PROCEDURE?

This procedure is performed by general surgeons or obstetrician-gynecologists.

? WHERE IS THE PROCEDURE PERFORMED?

Open procedures are always performed on an inpatient basis in a hospital. Depending on the scope of the work done, some laparoscopic procedures are performed as outpatient procedures and others are performed as inpatient procedures with a stay of less than a day.

? WHAT ARE THE MORTALITY (DEATH) AND MORBIDITY (COMPLICATION) RATES?

The death rate for this procedure is essentially zero; most of the deaths and complications relate to anesthesia. As with any procedure in which anesthesia is used, death from reaction to the anesthetic drugs, error on the part of the anesthetist, or machine failure is a remote possibility. (See Glossary, p. 309)

? WHAT ARE THE OTHER COMPLICATIONS AND POSSIBLE SIDE EFFECTS?

There are few side effects and complications other than failure to remove all the diseased tissue. This can lead to recurrence of malignancy or to the **ovarian remnant syndrome**.

? IS THIS THE MOST APPROPRIATE PROCEDURE FOR THE CONDITION?

Generally speaking, this is the least invasive procedure possible for destroying ovarian lesions that are causing problems. Some lesions can be treated medically, and it is even possible to observe others carefully rather than operating immediately.[2] Tumors that are suspected to be malignant should be biopsied as soon as possible and removed if found to be malignant.

? ARE THERE ALTERNATIVES TO THIS PROCEDURE?

See above.

? WHAT IS CONTROVERSIAL ABOUT THE PROCEDURE?

There is little controversy about this procedure, because it is one of the more conservative ways of approaching ovarian problems and is far less invasive than either a bilateral ovary-and-tube removal (see "Bilateral Salpingo-Oophorectomy or Salpingo-Ovariectomy," p. 116) or a hysterectomy and ovary-tube operation (see "Total Abdominal Hysterectomy," p. 243).

Local Destruction of Skin Lesion (65)

MORTALITY	MORBIDITY	CONTROVERSY
+	+	o

Destruction of **lesions** of the skin by various methods

? WHAT CONDITION DOES THE PROCEDURE TREAT?

Skin lesions are caused by a wide variety of diseases, so many methods are available to treat them. Skin lesions are removed for three major reasons—concern about appearance, concern about irritation of the lesions by clothing, and concern that a lesion is malignant or may become so.

? WHAT IS THE PROCEDURE?

The exact method chosen depends upon the lesion, its size and location, the doctor's preferences, and whether the lesion is malignant or benign. Most methods are performed either with no anesthesia or with local anesthesia, depending upon the amount of pain produced by the technique chosen.

The general recommendation for most benign lesions is to remove only the lesion itself and leave the underlying skin and tissue intact. For malignant or premalignant lesions, cutting of a wide area of skin and tissue at the base of the lesion—a technique called wide excision—is recommended.

Some special skin conditions that should be monitored include actinic keratoses, which are overgrowths of the horny outer layer of the skin caused by sun exposure; these can be removed by alternating application of the anticancer drug fluorouracil and triamcinolone acetate, a relative of cortisone, which is used to reduce the irritation caused by the fluorouracil.[1] Patches of dilated blood vessels, called telangiectasias, can be destroyed with an argon laser,[2] and warts can be removed with a carbon dioxide laser.

Application of liquid nitrogen in a widely used technique called cryotherapy destroys lesions by freezing them. Any portion of the lesion that remains after the frozen skin has healed can be removed with a scalpel.[3]

Other methods for treating skin lesions include: a technique called curettement or shave biopsy, in which a **curette** is used to shave away the lesion in layers until normal skin is reached; cutting of stalked lesions with a surgical scissors; removal of the lesion and surrounding skin by a biopsy punch, which works just like a paper punch; destruction by a heated needle or high-frequency current; and wide excision.

The aim of treatment of skin lesions is to destroy the entire lesion and produce minimal scarring. This latter objective is difficult to achieve in many dark-skinned persons who are predisposed to form keloids, tough masses of fibrous tissue that grow from scars. Keloids can be triggered by skin damage as minute as that caused by a pimple, and can grow to become disfiguring. The trick to removing keloids is to make sure that they don't grow back. The most effective method available to remove keloids is layer by layer, with a laser beam under local anesthetic. This procedure is followed by injections of anti-inflammatory drugs such as triamcinolone.

? WHO PERFORMS THE PROCEDURE?

This procedure is within the competence of many family physicians and general surgeons. Small lesions are usually removed by a dermatologist. If the lesion is large or complex or there are multiple lesions covering a large area, it is best to have a board-certified plastic surgeon do the work.

? WHERE IS THE PROCEDURE PERFORMED?

This procedure is usually performed in a doctor's office or outpatient surgery facility. Treatment of large lesions may require a brief hospital stay.

? WHAT ARE THE MORTALITY (DEATH) AND MORBIDITY (COMPLICATION) RATES?

Deaths from skin lesion removal are essentially zero.

The only major complications are failures of two goals that are occasionally in conflict: failure to produce an acceptable cosmetic result and failure to remove all of a malignant or premalignant lesion. Removal of malignant and premalignant lesions is critical and any melanoma present (a dangerous form of skin cancer) that has spread is essentially incurable. Because of this, it may be desirable to have a plastic surgeon do a combined lesion removal and reconstruction—that is, if the lesion that has to be removed is large and disfigurement might result from the surgery.

? WHAT ARE THE OTHER COMPLICATIONS AND POSSIBLE SIDE EFFECTS?

When cryotherapy is used to destroy lesions of the hands, it is possible for a portion of the bone and bone-forming tissues to be destroyed also. In children, this can result in stunted growth of the fingers.[4]

? IS THIS THE MOST APPROPRIATE PROCEDURE FOR THE CONDITION?

It depends upon whether the lesion is benign or malignant. Malignant lesions should be removed, and the methods discussed above are about the most conservative available. Benign lesions do not have to be removed, and irritation from clothing may be dealt with by covering the lesions with a gauze pad while clothing is worn. Removal of lesions on the face and other exposed portions of the body can be of great help to self-image if the lesions cause the patient to feel self-conscious.

? ARE THERE ALTERNATIVES TO THIS PROCEDURE?

All of the procedures discussed above are alternatives to each other.

? WHAT IS CONTROVERSIAL ABOUT THE PROCEDURE?

There are few controversies in this area, other than those concerning the use of new vitamin A derivatives called retinoids (such as Retin-A) for treatment of skin manifestations of aging (wrinkles, "age spots," and so on).

Representatives of the Food and Drug Administration testified before Congress in mid-1991 that retinoids are potent compounds whose long-term side effects are unknown and that their use for signs of aging was not approved.

Low-Forceps Delivery with Episiotomy (9)

MORTALITY	MORBIDITY	CONTROVERSY
+	+	●

- The major **CONTROVERSY** is the further medicalization of birth through the active intervention of the physician. Studies have shown very little improvement in maternal and infant mortality and morbidity as a result of **forceps** delivery.

Use of instrument to deliver baby stuck low in the vagina, plus a surgical incision to enlarge the vaginal opening

? WHAT CONDITION DOES THE PROCEDURE TREAT?

This procedure is used when a baby's head is already deep into the vagina during a birth and labor stops completely, the mother is in danger or exhausted, or the infant develops indications of sudden distress requiring immediate delivery. Forceps are also used to rotate the baby from a face-up to a face-down position if necessary and to manipulate the infant if there is an indication that its shoulders are in a position to become wedged in the birth canal. This latter use is rather rare.

Most childbirths go well, but the size of a baby's head is approximately the maximum that the female anatomy will permit, and it is not surprising that complete or partial tears of the **perineum** occur occasionally during delivery. A surgical cut in the perineum, called an **episiotomy**—which is done (theoretically) to prevent a large tear—seems to prevent some kinds of tears and increase the chance of others. (We have more to say about episiotomy below.)

? WHAT IS THE PROCEDURE?

Frankly speaking, this procedure lacks elegance. It is a rather old one thought to have stood the test of time. An instrument that looks like an enlarged version of salad tongs is taken apart, and each side is slid into the vagina and pushed beside the baby's head. The handles of the forceps are put back together, and the doctor starts pulling, and simultaneously rotating the baby if it is not in the face-down position.

Because the use of forceps has the potential to tear the vaginal opening, an episiotomy is done. An episiotomy is simply an incision, made with a surgical scissors, from the vaginal opening into the tissue of the pelvic floor, called the perineum, to avoid a natural tear. The cut may be made directly down towards the anus or off to one side.

With the top of the infant's head securely in the forceps, the baby is pulled out of the vagina, the forceps are removed, and delivery is finished normally.

Forceps need not be applied within the birth canal alone. They can be used when the baby is low in the birth canal and the widest part of its body is out of the uterus, and contractions of the uterus, which can be stimulated with drugs or natural release of oxytocin by nipple stimulation, are of progressively less help in moving the birth along. If the mother is dangerously exhausted or the fetus suffers distress, the physician assists delivery with forceps. There are also alternatives to the forceps, which we discuss later.

The distinctions between low-forceps and mid-forceps deliveries have been in question for some time. In 1988 the American College of Obstetricians and Gynecologists revised and clarified the classifications of forceps deliveries.[1] Because of this change, the catalog of complications in this section also includes those attributable to mid-forceps deliveries. (Basically, a low-forceps delivery is done when the head is clearly visible in the birth canal; anything else is mid- or high-forceps, depending upon the position of the head in the canal.[2]) You should keep in mind that if the rates quoted below for mid-forceps deliveries in fact refer to deliveries that would now be called "low," they fairly represent the low-forceps complication rate. If they are all representative of what are now called "mid-forceps" deliveries, it is logical to expect the same sorts of complications, but at lower rates and in less severe forms.

? WHO PERFORMS THE PROCEDURE?

This procedure is performed by an obstetrician-gynecologist or family or general practitioner who delivers babies. Because studies indicate that junior hospital staff produce much more maternal pelvic trauma when using forceps than do senior hospital staff,[3] you should discuss with your doctor—well before the delivery date—his philosophy of forceps use, and how many forceps deliveries he has done and with what results. To ensure that there is a written record of the discussion, it may be useful to write a letter to the doctor about agreements made, prior to labor and delivery, regarding the birth process and your preferences in medical interventions. (The doctor may or may not note the agreements in your chart.) Also, make sure that any agreements with the doctor about forceps use are in writing.

? WHERE IS THE PROCEDURE PERFORMED?

This procedure can be performed anywhere it is needed and the doctor has the proper instruments. Usually, it is performed in a hospital or birthing center.

? WHAT ARE THE MORTALITY (DEATH) AND MORBIDITY (COMPLICATION) RATES?

Without detailed autopsy studies, it is hard to distinguish the mortality rate associated with any particular manipulation late in delivery with the mortality rate of delivery itself. The mortality rate for all forceps deliveries with episiotomies for community hospitals in the U.S. in 1989 was less than 0.1%.[4] Maternal mortality rates associated with the procedure reported in the literature have declined from .55% in the 1940s to zero in the 1980s.[5] One study of mid-forceps deliveries found maternal mortality so low that maternal mortality resulting from forceps delivery should not, in the opinion of the investigators, be studied any longer.[6]

The chief complication of forceps deliveries for the mother is damage to the vagina, the vaginal opening, and the tissues of the pelvic floor. A good deal of the medical literature on forceps deliveries consists of studies comparing forceps and vacuum extraction—a useful analysis showing how bad forceps deliveries can be. (A vacuum delivery is basically done with a suction cup of metal or plastic attached to an instrument similar to a household vacuum cleaner. See "Vacuum Extraction Delivery with Episiotomy," p. 285.)

As one might expect, third- and fourth-degree perineal lacerations and vaginal and cervical lacerations were found to be fewer with vacuum extractions as opposed to forceps deliveries.[7] (The most serious kind, a fourth-degree tear, runs all the way through the perineum and causes complete separation of all tissue layers. For further information on degrees of lacerations, see "Repair of Obstetric Laceration," p. 208.) Even though the procedure appears barbaric, maternal morbidity is lower with forceps deliveries than with cesarean sections.[8]

"Significant" maternal soft tissue trauma was found in 48.9% of mothers delivered with low forceps versus 21.6% of those delivered with the Mityvac vacuum system in one study.[9] Maternal fever occurred in 48% of cesarean births but in only 6% of vacuum extraction births. The same study found that vaginal and cervical lacerations occurred in 48% of forceps deliveries but only in 18% of vacuum deliveries, and maternal anemia occurred in 30% of mothers who had cesareans versus 4% of those who delivered with the vacuum extractor.[10]

A 15-year study of one hospital shows that forceps deliveries dropped from 47.5% to 12.0% and vaginal breech deliveries decreased from 86% to 35%.[11] Instead, cesarean sections were done, and spinal anesthesia was used in 90%. (Arguably, substitution of cesarean sections increased the rate of maternal deaths, because the mortality rate for forceps deliveries is lower than that for cesarean sections.)

Apparently, it takes time to learn to use forceps gently. In one study, use of Kielland's forceps (one of the many types of forceps used for delivery) by junior staff resulted in significantly greater rates of maternal and cervical lacerations and hemorrhage.[12]

What about the baby? A study of Norwegian military recruits found that males delivered by forceps had significantly higher IQs at age 18 than those who were delivered by a vacuum extractor.[13] This finding may be an **artifact**, however. More significantly, there was no excess morbidity or mortality in either the forceps or the vacuum group, and the same result was found in a British study.[14] A two-year follow-up study of infants delivered by mid-forceps and infants delivered by cesarean section found no significant difference in abnormal outcomes in development.[15] These same findings were duplicated in a study of six years' worth of mid-forceps deliveries between 1976 and 1982.[16]

A higher rate of respiratory disorders has been found in infants who were delivered under general anesthesia, as compared with those who were delivered under other forms; this would argue for use of procedures that do not require general anesthesia, but even cesarean sections can be done with regional anesthesia. A 1990 comparison of mid-forceps or vacuum extraction with cesarean sections at a California hospital found decreased maternal morbidity and increased infant morbidity for the vacuum extractions.[17] Another 1990 study, also from a California hospital, found reduced morbidity for both mother and infant in mid-forceps deliveries as opposed to cesarean sections. The difference could be accounted for by differing levels of capabilities in the hospitals and physicians, or by more difficult births at one of the institutions. Another single-institution study found that infant morbidity declined as fewer forceps deliveries and more cesarean sections were done.[18] The study notes the fact that more babies are injured during forceps deliveries than during cesarean sections.

A Viennese study found that an infant mortality rate of 2.8% was associated with the use of forceps, compared with a mortality rate of 0.95% associated with vacuum extraction.[19] The incidence of skull fractures in newborns was found to be essentially identical for spontaneous vaginal and vacuum delivery births.[20]

A study of forceps versus the Kobayashi vacuum extractor (named after the doctor who invented it) found that infants delivered with the vacuum extractor had a higher risk of **cephalhematoma**. There was no difference in major morbidity between the forceps and vacuum extraction groups.[21] Forceps deliveries cause **hematomas** of the scalp in 5.1% to 6% of deliveries done with them, versus 22.9% with vacuum extraction.[22, 23] Another study found the incidence of neurological injuries to the infant to be essentially the same for vacuum extraction and forceps deliveries.[24] A 1987 comparison of vacuum and mid-forceps deliveries found that cephalhematoma was more common with forceps than with the vacuum.[25]

The use of Kielland's forceps (yet another variation on forceps, named after the doctor who invented them) was associated with an infant mortality rate of 3.49%, a 23.3% rate of **transient neurological deficits** and abnormal behavior that resolved quickly, and a 15.1% incidence of birth trauma. **Subgaleal hematomas**—

which form between the brain and a band of fibrous tissue that forms the cap of the skull in newborns—have a mortality rate of 22.8%. Fifty-two percent of the cases of subgaleal hematomas reported in a 1980 review of the literature were associated with vacuum deliveries, compared with 11% occurring after mid-forceps deliveries, 28% following normal vaginal deliveries, and 8.9% following cesarean section.[26]

Normal births are stressful for the infant too; this should be kept in mind in thinking about various modes of delivery. A study of the incidence of retinal hemorrhage (bleeding of the membrane at the back of the eye) found that infants born by cesarean section had a 2.6% incidence, those delivered by forceps had a 25% incidence, and those born without intervention had an incidence of 38%.[27] Broken bones have been reported following delivery of the infant by forceps, vacuum extraction, and cesarean section.[28] The incidence of broken collarbones in spontaneous vaginal deliveries is around 1.25%.[29]

? WHAT ARE THE OTHER COMPLICATIONS AND POSSIBLE SIDE EFFECTS?

Rupture of Descemet's or Duddell's membrane (the French and British disagree over who saw it first), which is the lining between the back of the cornea and the deeper structures of the eye, can occur, as can other eye damage, if the forceps grab the infant's head over or too near the eye. This results in **astigmatism**, **myopia**, and **amblyopia**. All of these can be corrected either by glasses, contact lenses, or treatment usually consisting of putting a patch on the good eye to force the lazy eye back to work.[30] It is possible for a permanent corneal **lesion** that cannot be corrected to be produced as well.[31] The loss of an eye in a forceps delivery has also been reported.[32]

A case of spinal cord transection (cutting of the spinal cord in two) and brain stem damage in a forceps delivery was reported in 1984. The infant died 60 days after delivery.[33]

A 1990 study, which reported on follow-ups of mid-forceps and spontaneous vaginal deliveries at four to seven years, found that 5.77% of a group delivered with forceps had had seizures, versus 2.69% of a group delivered without intervention. The difference was considered statistically significant.[34]

A 1989 study that examined problems of facial growth and dental development among forceps and spontaneous vaginal deliveries found no indication that forceps deliveries produced any permanent problems.[35] Facial paralysis caused by nerve damage was found in 0.08% of infants in one study, the investigators of which insist that a particular design of forceps, called Theirry forceps, can avoid it.[36]

? IS THIS THE MOST APPROPRIATE PROCEDURE FOR THE CONDITION?

Forceps deliveries, vacuum extractions, and cesarean sections "compete" for usage among doctors. Examination of the studies from 1975 to the present indicates that both forceps deliveries and vacuum extractions are becoming safer, and the mortality rate from cesarean sections is six times that of vaginal deliveries now. Because both infant and maternal mortality, as opposed to morbidity, are quite low, the question of appropriateness turns on the likely amount of damage to the mother and the baby, versus the risk of not doing a given procedure. Yet who decides? Many, if not most, women no longer regard childbirth as open season for scalpel and scissors, regardless of what the doctor thinks.

We believe that the sum of the evidence indicates that just about anything that can be done with a forceps can be done with a vacuum extractor. Vacuum extractors produce less trauma to the mother, do not require the stretching of the vaginal canal that forceps do, and allow the infant to rotate to the easiest position for delivery.

They do produce scalp trauma, but this is serious in only a few cases. An infant mortality rate of 0.6% and no maternal mortality have been reported.[37] The risk of scalp trauma can be lessened by the use of plastic rather than metal cups.[38]

? ARE THERE ALTERNATIVES TO THIS PROCEDURE?

There is some disagreement about the aggregate benefit of obstetrical manipulations, and the suggestion that, overall, these procedures may do more harm than good (see below). One alternative, already discussed above, is the vacuum extraction.

Cesarean section is an alternative if the infant is not most of the way out of the womb. It is rare for the infant to be so low in the birth canal that a forceps or vacuum delivery cannot be done. In addition, the maternal mortality rate for cesarean section is six to 20 times higher than the vaginal delivery rate, with the better ratios coming in more recent studies.[39]

Of course, unassisted birth is an option. The present climate of litigation rewards the doctor who cuts, not the doctor who waits, but it is certainly reasonable for parents to insist that the doctor wait until there is clear evidence of continuing fetal distress before using any surgical means. A 1983 study of low-forceps versus spontaneous vaginal deliveries of low-birthweight infants found that the use of forceps did not improve survival,[40] so the benefit is questionable in any case.

? WHAT IS CONTROVERSIAL ABOUT THE PROCEDURE?

The doctor can choose from a wide variety of forceps, some of which cause more trauma to mother and baby than others. The medical literature cites many discussions about the various types. Laufe forceps are designed to hold the infant's head firmly without putting too much pressure on the skull. In one study, use of Laufe forceps (as opposed to Barnes forceps, another variation) was associated with lower infant complications: 62% of infants delivered with Barnes forceps had evidence of neonatal morbidity; 41.3% of the infants delivered with Laufe forceps had complications.[41]

The biggest question is whether all of the "medicalization" of birth—transforming it from a natural, albeit very uncomfortable, process, into a disease—and the further "gadgetization" of the process have contributed anything at all to the decline in maternal mortality that has been observed in this century. A comparison of Holland, where home births are the norm, and Denmark, where hospitals are the usual location, found essentially identical infant mortality rates.[42] One study concluded that obstetrical medical intervention (as distinct from medical measures to improve maternal health prior to birth and general public health measures) has nothing whatsoever to do with the improvements in maternal and infant mortality and morbidity that have been seen.[43] If that conclusion is true, then the painful conclusion that must follow is that obstetrical manipulations impose wholly unnecessary mortality, morbidity, and expense. The cited study concludes that maternal and infant morbidity would have declined even further without obstetrical intervention.

Even if we accept the legitimacy of continued intervention in the case of clear doubts about the aggregate benefits of the procedures, an associated question is the scientific foundation of the practices that are used. A study of European countries found that operative delivery rates (rates of cesarean sections, forceps deliveries, and vacuum extractions combined) varied from 6% to 24% and the rate of artificial induction of labor ranged from 12% to 36%. No obvious health benefit other than a very slight reduction in infant mortality rates was found, with most of the variation in infant mortality rates being accounted for by other factors.[44]

If conducted, a **meta-analysis** would most likely indicate that the one group to clearly benefit from increased obstetrical intervention is high-risk infants.

Overall, it would seem best to let nature take its course until it is quite clear that labor will not proceed normally, then to use the vacuum extractor, followed by more invasive approaches only when both a trial of natural labor and vacuum extraction have failed.

Medical Induction of Labor (34)

MORTALITY	MORBIDITY	CONTROVERSY
+	+	o

LAY TITLE: Inducing labor

Starting or strengthening labor by the use of chemicals injected and/or applied to the **cervix**

❓ WHAT CONDITION DOES THE PROCEDURE TREAT?

This procedure is used when a pregnant woman is overdue for delivery or when delivery is progressing too slowly. It is also used for cases of **eclampsia** and **preeclampsia**, serious complications of late pregnancy that cannot be controlled other than by inducing labor. The maternal mortality rate for eclampsia is 10% to 15%.[1, 2]

The process of birth is extremely complex and involves a host of physical and chemical interactions. For example, natural destruction of **collagen** in the cervix prepares it for widening to allow the baby to pass through it. The breaking of the amniotic sac and loss of "water" sensitizes the uterus to the influence of oxytocin, a substance naturally found in the body that starts and strengthens contractions of the uterus.[3]

Medical induction of labor is considered to be surgery because it can involve surgical breaking of the amniotic sac to help labor start. Medical personnel may "paint" the cervix with gels containing **prostaglandins**, which encourage the cervix to "ripen" and dilate more easily.

? WHAT IS THE PROCEDURE?

If the amniotic sac has not broken, the doctor will insert a **speculum** into the vagina and pass a sharp instrument through the cervix to break the amniotic sac—a procedure called amniotomy. The cervix may be painted with prostaglandin gel at the same time. Oxytocin is given through an intravenous line, usually inserted in the hand or arm. Otherwise, labor proceeds as it would if it were not induced.

? WHO PERFORMS THE PROCEDURE?

This procedure is performed by obstetrician-gynecologists and general or family practitioners who deliver babies.

? WHERE IS THE PROCEDURE PERFORMED?

This surgery can be performed in a hospital or a birthing center.

? WHAT ARE THE MORTALITY (DEATH) AND MORBIDITY (COMPLICATION) RATES?

Morbidity and mortality are the same as for uninduced labor with the exception of labor induced for eclampsia; the higher mortality in that case is attributable to the eclampsia, not to the induction of labor. In women who have had previous cesarean sections and have what is called a trial of labor in anticipation of a vaginal delivery, the maternal death rate can be as low as zero and the fetal death rate as low as 0.22%.[4] If a repeat cesarean is needed, the maternal death rate is about 0.15% and the fetal death rate about 0.2%.[5]

Painting of the cervix with prostaglandin gel causes hyperstimulation of the uterus (when the uterus is over-stimulated to a point where the intense and rapid contractions pose a danger to the fetus) or fetal distress in under 1% of cases. Drugs called **beta-blockers** can be used to reverse the effect of the prostaglandin gels if hyperstimulation or fetal distress occurs.[6, 7]

? WHAT ARE THE OTHER COMPLICATIONS AND POSSIBLE SIDE EFFECTS?

There are no other complications, beyond those associated with normal labor and delivery. If anesthesia is given, death may occur from rare anesthetic-related complications. As with any procedure in which anesthesia is used, death from reaction to the anesthetic drugs, error on the part of the anesthetist, or machine failure is a remote possibility. (See Glossary, p. 309)

? IS THIS THE MOST APPROPRIATE PROCEDURE FOR THE CONDITION?

In cases of eclampsia, medical induction of labor is one of the therapeutic alternatives available if the infant is sufficiently mature (26 to 28 weeks) or the mother's life is in danger. For overdue deliveries, the procedure is appropriate because infant mortality rises as the mother gets further and further past her due date. Other indications are a matter of judgment for the physician and woman.

? ARE THERE ALTERNATIVES TO THIS PROCEDURE?

For eclampsia, magnesium sulfate injections, fluid and sodium restrictions, drugs to reduce blood pressure, and close monitoring may be sufficient. Aspirin may help to avoid a repeat occurrence if the first episode can be controlled. Most physicians favor induction of labor as soon as the fetus can survive outside the womb, because of the high maternal mortality rate associated with eclampsia.[8]

❓ WHAT IS CONTROVERSIAL ABOUT THE PROCEDURE?

Essentially very little about this procedure is controversial. If eclampsia occurs, the doctor usually delivers the baby at once.

Nephroureterectomy (83)

MORTALITY	MORBIDITY	CONTROVERSY
+	+	o

Removal of a kidney and all or part of a **ureter**

❓ WHAT CONDITION DOES THE PROCEDURE TREAT?

This procedure can be done for any kidney condition that cannot be successfully treated surgically or medically, such as intractable infections and severe injury to the kidney. It is usually performed for malignant tumors of the kidney that cannot be treated with chemotherapy or radiation.

❓ WHAT IS THE PROCEDURE?

With the patient under general anesthesia, the back is shaved, scrubbed with soap and antiseptic, and draped with a sterile sheet so that only the region to be operated on is exposed. The skin, **fascia**, and muscle are opened in layers, and the affected kidney is exposed. The veins and arteries leading to it are **ligated** one by one and then cut. The ureter is also **ligated** and cut. Some patients may have already undergone surgery to divert the flow of urine around a cancerous blockage. If this is the case, the specially constructed channel is tied off and removed, to ensure that any cancer cells that have spread are also removed. The kidney is freed from its attachments and lifted out of the body. The muscle, fascia, and skin are closed in layers. The patient is taken to the recovery room and then to his room.

❓ WHO PERFORMS THE PROCEDURE?

This procedure should be performed only by a board-certified urologist, preferably one with a good deal of experience in surgical oncology, the treatment of cancer by surgery. The operation is not technically difficult, but the care the surgeon takes to remove all potentially cancerous tissue can make a major difference in survival.

❓ WHERE IS THE PROCEDURE PERFORMED?

This is major surgery that should be performed only on an inpatient basis in the hospital.

❓ WHAT ARE THE MORTALITY (DEATH) AND MORBIDITY (COMPLICATION) RATES?

No mortality from the procedure itself has been reported in the literature in the period from 1975 to 1991, and it is routinely referred to as carrying a zero risk of mortality.[1] A rarely performed, complex procedure for kidney cancer—called **pyelocystostomy**—of which nephroureterectomy is the first step, has a reported mortality rate of 25%.[2]

? WHAT ARE THE OTHER COMPLICATIONS AND POSSIBLE SIDE EFFECTS?

As with any procedure in which anesthesia is used, death from reaction to the anesthetic drugs, error on the part of the anesthetist, or machine failure is a remote possibility. (See Glossary, p. 309)

? IS THIS THE MOST APPROPRIATE PROCEDURE FOR THE CONDITION?

The main indication for this operation is kidney cancer. Studies have repeatedly shown that procedures less radical than removal of the entire kidney and ureter carry an increased risk of recurrence of the cancer. Because this operation has essentially no mortality and low morbidity, and because less radical surgery carries a greater risk that the cancer will recur, it seems to be an appropriate procedure.

? ARE THERE ALTERNATIVES TO THIS PROCEDURE?

The less radical alternatives to this procedure, which attempt to preserve portions of the kidney, seem to have worse results when cancer is the reason for the operation. At present there appear to be no better alternatives.

? WHAT IS CONTROVERSIAL ABOUT THE PROCEDURE?

The only controversy is whether to remove a portion of the bladder along with the ureter leading from the cancerous kidney. Because the cancerous kidney could spread tumor cells throughout the entire bladder, removal of only a portion of the bladder seems to make little sense. (Survival without a bladder is possible, using a ureterostomy, a bag which collects urine outside the body much as a colostomy collects solid waste.) But such a course of action may contribute slightly to cancer-free survival. The issue has not been well studied.

Open Reduction and Internal Fixation of Fracture of the Femur (16)

MORTALITY	MORBIDITY	CONTROVERSY
–	–	•

- The national **MORTALITY** rate for this procedure is 4.5%.

- **COMPLICATIONS** are reported to occur in 26% to 46% of cases. The chief complication is failure to heal. Nonunion of bone is reported in 33% of cases.

- The fixation method used to mend the bone is the main **CONTROVERSY**.

Repair of a broken leg with an **internal fixation device**

? WHAT CONDITION DOES THE PROCEDURE TREAT?

See "Closed Reduction and Internal Fixation of Fracture of the Femur," p. 133.

To understand what follows, see "Closed Fracture Reduction of the Radius and Ulna," p. 130, for a discussion on two medical uses of the word *open*.

Fixation devices can be internal (wholly inside the limb) or external. External fixation devices employ thin, threaded rods or wires, which are run through the bone from the outside to connect to an external frame. The external frame holds the limb in the correct position, applies traction, or does both.

In this section, we discuss fracture repair using variations of the open, internal-fixation technique.

❓ WHAT IS THE PROCEDURE?

With the patient under general or spinal anesthesia, the surgeon makes an incision into the thigh with the broken **femur** to examine the fracture. If it is a **comminuted fracture**, the surgeon determines which pieces can be reunited; the ones that cannot are removed and may be used for bone **grafts**. Depending on the type of fracture and the surgeon's preferences, a rod or nail may be placed in the **medullary canal**. Wires or screws may be placed across the bone, or metal plates with screws may be used on each side of a fracture.

When the location or nature of the break makes a good repair unlikely, a total hip replacement may be done. (See "Total Hip Replacement," p. 252.)

Once the fracture is repaired, the muscles, **fascia**, and skin are closed in layers with **sutures** and **clips** or staples. The leg is bandaged, and the patient is taken to the recovery room, and then to his room.

❓ WHO PERFORMS THE PROCEDURE?

This procedure is done by an orthopedic surgeon.

❓ WHERE IS THE PROCEDURE PERFORMED?

This procedure is done at general hospitals and at specialty hospitals for orthopedic injuries.

❓ WHAT ARE THE MORTALITY (DEATH) AND MORBIDITY (COMPLICATION) RATES?

In-hospital mortality rates for this procedure in community hospitals in the U.S. were 4.5% in 1989.[1] **Perioperative mortality** rates reported in the medical literature range from zero to 21%.[2] Mortality rates have been steadily improving over the last two decades.

Representative studies of complications found rates of 26% to 46%,[3] and 35.6%.[4] Infection is a relatively common problem; rates as high as 28% have been reported,[5] although rates as low as 3% can be achieved.

❓ WHAT ARE THE OTHER COMPLICATIONS AND POSSIBLE SIDE EFFECTS?

The chief complication, which is better described as complete failure of the procedure, is failure of the broken bone ends to join. Rates of nonunion reported in various studies range from zero[6] to 33%.[7] Other complications include rotation of the broken pieces relative to one another around a fixation device. The result of this rotation is that the anatomical position of the lower leg relative to the upper leg is altered, so that the foot turns inward or outward more than it should. The effects of this on the ability of the patient to walk and on the appearance of the limb may be serious enough to require reoperation.

As with any procedure in which anesthesia is used, death from reaction to the anesthetic drugs, error on the part of the anesthetist, or machine failure is a remote possibility. (See Glossary, p. 309)

❓ IS THIS THE MOST APPROPRIATE PROCEDURE FOR THE CONDITION?

Obviously, a broken bone must be fixed. If a closed reduction and casting are not feasible, the surgeon must perform an open reduction with external or internal fixation. As with virtually all procedures in which tubes, wires, or rods without flanges are run into the body from the outside, external fixation devices create a channel for infection. Theoretically then, internal fixation ought to be the preferred procedure. In reality, the results with internal fixation are not as good as those with external fixation.[8]

Because devices and operative technique used vary widely, it is difficult to say exactly which procedure is the most appropriate. The wide range of success rates reported in the literature should rule out some procedures, such as those that provide little if any protection against incorrect rotation of the broken bone segments.

Research into prevention and improved fracture healing suggests that nutrition plays a critical role. Studies have shown that many elderly patients most subject to hip and femur fractures have malnutrition and can benefit greatly from diets that supply extra calcium, protein, vitamins, and calories. One such study showed that elderly patients who were given supplemental nutrition had a 50% reduction in combined mortality and complications, compared with a similar group not given nutritional supplements.[9]

? ARE THERE ALTERNATIVES TO THIS PROCEDURE?

If **embolization of fat** from marrow to the brain, lungs, and other organs were not a problem, one could argue that any fracture likely to heal with closed reduction and casting should be treated with that method first. Unfortunately, this major problem demands rapid, definitive treatment, so there are at present no real alternatives.

? WHAT IS CONTROVERSIAL ABOUT THE PROCEDURE?

Success rates with various fixation devices and techniques for applying them vary widely. When a total hip replacement is required, the surgeon has two choices: The first is a cemented procedure, in which a type of Super Glue is used to fix the bone to the artificial hip.

The second is a cementless procedure, in which the bone is carved to press-fit the artificial hip joint, which has a specially textured surface into which bone theoretically will grow. Unfortunately, natural bone growth into the prosthesis does not always occur in many older patients. Many surgeons now favor a mixture of cement and cementless techniques depending upon the exact character of the break, the patient's age, and other factors —such as whether infections develop; whether the proper antibiotic has been used; whether physical therapy is appropriate; and whether the patient is willing or able to follow instructions.

Open Reduction and Internal Fixation of Fracture of the Radius and Ulna (72)

MORTALITY	MORBIDITY	CONTROVERSY
+	+	o

Opening of the forearm to fix broken bones

? WHAT CONDITION DOES THE PROCEDURE TREAT?

To understand what follows, see "Closed Fracture Reduction of the Radius and Ulna," p. 130, for a discussion of two medical uses of the word *open*.

In this case open fracture reduction aims at fixing breaks in the forearm bones and realigning the bones by cutting open the arm and by placing wires or pins to hold the bones in place. It is important to locate and align all breaks: The joints between the radius and ulna and the elbow, and the radius and ulna and the wrist, are very prone to early development of arthritis resulting from misalignment.

? WHAT IS THE PROCEDURE?

The patient is given a general or regional anesthetic. The forearm is shaved, scrubbed with soap and antiseptic, and draped so that only the area of the planned incision is exposed. The usual approach is from the top surface, but it is also possible to work from the bottom of the forearm (called the volar aspect) if this is easier for the surgeon. The skin, fat, **fascia**, and muscle are opened. Bleeding vessels are tied off and **cauterized**; great care is taken to avoid damage to the nerves that supply the hand, although these already may have been damaged in the accident that caused the break.

Free fragments of bone are located and placed in the proper position. If they are too shattered to be put back into place, they are removed. Depending upon the location and type of the break, either wires, pins, screws, or metal plates are used to hold the bones in the proper alignment. The surgeon takes great care to ensure that the ends of the bones are not pushed up or pulled back; this would interfere with normal motion or allow excessive motion. When the surgeon is satisfied with the result, she closes the muscle, fascia, fat, and skin in layers. Then the arm is bandaged and splinted. The patient is taken to the recovery room and then to his room.

? WHO PERFORMS THE PROCEDURE?

This procedure is performed by an orthopedic surgeon, and should be done by a board-certified one if at all possible.

? WHERE IS THE PROCEDURE PERFORMED?

This procedure is done in the hospital. Depending upon the extent of the break, response to anesthetic, and hospital policies, the patient may be released after less than a full day in the hospital.

? WHAT ARE THE MORTALITY (DEATH) AND MORBIDITY (COMPLICATION) RATES?

Any mortality is essentially attributable to the anesthetic, not to the procedure. As with any procedure in which anesthesia is used, death from reaction to the anesthetic drugs, error on the part of the anesthetist, or machine failure is a remote possibility. (See Glossary, p. 309)

Complication rates vary with the exact procedure used, but open reduction performed after failure of closed reduction (see "Closed Fracture Reduction of the Radius and Ulna," p. 130) has a complication rate of 50%. Patient satisfaction is high, however, and most return to their previous occupations.[1]

? WHAT ARE THE OTHER COMPLICATIONS AND POSSIBLE SIDE EFFECTS?

An infection rate of zero has been achieved.[2] The chief complication is failure to restore the complete range of motion that existed before the break—a common occurrence, although the degree of limitation is usually very slight.

? IS THIS THE MOST APPROPRIATE PROCEDURE FOR THE CONDITION?

A closed reduction is preferable if it can be achieved, but this is not always possible.

? ARE THERE ALTERNATIVES TO THIS PROCEDURE?

See "Closed Fracture Reduction of the Radius and Ulna," p. 130.

? WHAT IS CONTROVERSIAL ABOUT THE PROCEDURE?

See "Closed Fracture Reduction of the Radius and Ulna," p. 130.

Open Reduction and Internal Fixation of Fracture of the Tibia and Fibula (22)

MORTALITY	MORBIDITY	CONTROVERSY
+	–	o

- Major COMPLICATIONS, including delayed healing of the bone, clot formation, and bone infection, can be expected in up to 12% of cases.

Repair of broken bones of the lower leg by the insertion of a device to hold the broken bones together

? WHAT CONDITION DOES THE PROCEDURE TREAT?

For a description of what this procedure treats, see "Closed Fracture Reduction of the Tibia and Fibula," p. 132.

To understand what follows, see "Closed Fracture Reduction of the Radius and Ulna," p. 130, for a discussion on the two medical uses of the word *open*.

? WHAT IS THE PROCEDURE?

The procedure used depends upon the type of fracture, and the fixation device used to stabilize it. Certain devices can be placed through the use of an **arthroscope**, a small telescope that allows the surgeon to look into, and manipulate, bones and joints through a small incision. Some surgeons favor the use of wires run through holes drilled in the bone. Wires allow a great deal of flexibility in how the fracture is repaired, do not seriously disrupt the blood supply to the bone, and can be safely left in place permanently.[1]

Other surgeons routinely ream out the **medullary canal** when inserting a nail to hold the fracture together. Some surgeons recommend that this be done only when the patient has narrow canals, or when nails are inserted into the lower third of the **tibia**. Reaming of the canal is associated with a higher incidence of complications.[2]

We describe the general procedure here not the variations. The patient is placed under general anesthesia. The leg containing the broken bone is positioned to allow the surgeon easy access to the fracture. If the fracture is a closed one on which an open reduction will be done, the leg is shaved and scrubbed with soap and antiseptic. If the wound is open, it is cleansed around the edges and irrigated with a solution of saline or antibiotics.

The surgeon opens the leg, or expands the existing open wound, using a scalpel, an **electrocautery device**, **forceps**, **retractors**, and **skin hooks**. Bleeding vessels are **ligated** or **cauterized**. When the wound has been opened sufficiently to allow easy access to the fracture site or sites, the broken bones are gently realigned. Broken fragments are removed, and bone **grafts** are made if necessary; parts of the fractured bone, bone taken from elsewhere in the body, or donor bone may be used. When the break is caused by bone cancer, part of the shaft of the tibia or **fibula** may be replaced with a metal **prosthesis**.

The repair of the bone is completed with wires,

screws, metal plates, nails, staples, or other instruments of the surgeon's choice; bone cement may be used to hold some of these in place. The wound is closed in layers. If it is necessary to achieve soft tissue coverage of a wound that has severely damaged the tissues overlying the break, then skin, fat, and muscle from elsewhere in the body can be used to close the wound. After the wound is closed, a cast may be applied. The patient is taken to the recovery room and then to her room.

Because stress on bone encourages the formation of new bone, and because prolonged bed rest increases the risk of **thrombosis** and **thromboembolism**,[3] weight-bearing exercise and physical therapy are begun as soon as the degree of healing permits.

? WHO PERFORMS THE PROCEDURE?

This procedure should be done only by a board-certified orthopedic surgeon who has performed 100 or more procedures with the type of internal fixation device he intends to use.

? WHERE IS THE PROCEDURE PERFORMED?

Open reduction is major surgery that carries a high risk of thrombosis and thromboembolism and should only be done on an inpatient basis in a hospital.

? WHAT ARE THE MORTALITY (DEATH) AND MORBIDITY (COMPLICATION) RATES?

See "Closed Fracture Reduction of the Tibia and Fibula," p. 132.

? WHAT ARE THE OTHER COMPLICATIONS AND POSSIBLE SIDE EFFECTS?

See "Closed Fracture Reduction of the Tibia and Fibula," p. 132.

In severe open fractures of types III and IIIa (those definitely requiring open reduction and internal fixation),[4] the rate of amputation can be as high as 13.9%, deep bone infections can be as high as 19.4%, and failure of the bones to form a union can be as high as 8.33%. Depending upon whether complete soft tissue coverage of the break is achieved early or late in the course of treatment, problems with healing of the soft tissue wound can be expected in 20.8% and 83.3% of cases, respectively.[5] (Another study, which did not cite open fractures by type, also reported a complication rate of about 20% with early soft tissue coverage.[6]) Severe fractures of the tibia just above the ankle joint have unsatisfactory results in about 25% of the cases.[7]

When the fracture is severe enough to require a limb-lengthening procedure, the total complication rate can be as high as 92%, but complications apparently do not result in failure to achieve the degree of lengthening desired.[8] Limb-lengthening involves adding a piece of bone, usually from a **cadaver**, in the space where damaged bone has been removed. There are two conditions in which limb-lengthening might be called for: when a fracture heals but bone loss was sufficient to cause one leg to be shorter than the other; and when an artificial hip or knee has been implanted and there is some shrinkage in the length of the leg. The other option is to wear a built-up shoe.

As with any procedure in which anesthesia is used, death from reaction to the anesthetic drugs, error on the part of the anesthetist, or machine failure is a remote possibility. (See Glossary, p. 309)

? IS THIS THE MOST APPROPRIATE PROCEDURE FOR THE CONDITION?

Yes, if a closed reduction has failed or is not possible.

? ARE THERE ALTERNATIVES TO THIS PROCEDURE?

Yes, one alternative is closed reduction and casting, but it is not always successful.

? WHAT IS CONTROVERSIAL ABOUT THE PROCEDURE?

See "Closed Fracture Reduction of the Tibia and Fibula," p. 132.

Partial Small Bowel Resection (67)

MORTALITY	MORBIDITY	CONTROVERSY
+	+	o

Removal of a part of the **small intestine**

? WHAT CONDITION DOES THE PROCEDURE TREAT?

Small bowel resection is performed in cases of trauma to the small intestines (for example, that resulting from car accidents, stabbings, and gunshot wounds); benign and malignant tumors; **Crohn's disease**; death of bowel caused by loss of blood supply; **necrotizing enterocolitis**;[1] intestinal obstruction or blockage; and pseudo-obstruction due to damage to the nerve supply of the bowel—in the latter, a person has the feeling of an obstruction but there is no physical blockage.[2]

? WHAT IS THE PROCEDURE?

The site of the problem in the small bowel is located via some combination of scans—x ray, **CT scan**, and **MRI scan**—clinical signs and symptoms, and possible exploration of the extreme upper and lower ends of the small intestines with fiber-optic **endoscopes** inserted through the mouth or anus. The surgeon chooses a site of incision that gives the best exposure to the problem area. The patient is given a general or spinal anesthetic, and the abdomen is shaved and scrubbed with soap and antiseptic.

The skin, fat, **fascia**, muscle, and **peritoneum** are cut and **retracted**. Bleeding vessels are tied off or **cauterized**. When the problem area is located, the small intestine is freed from the supporting tissue (called the **mesentery**), clamped above and below it, and severed between the two clamps. The cut ends are joined if possible; if this is not immediately possible, the surgeon performs one or more permanent or temporary **ileostomies**.

If the intestine has been damaged by trauma or **perforated** as a result of cancer or **inflammatory bowel disease**, the abdominal cavity may be irrigated with saline alone or in combination with antibiotics to clear out clots, fragments of tissue, and intestinal contents. The tissues of the body wall are closed in layers, using **sutures** or **clips**, and bandaged. One or more drain tubes may be left in place. A **nasogastric tube** is usually put in place, and connected to a suction pump to keep stomach secretions and bile from damaging the healing intestines, and a **catheter** is usually placed in the bladder to measure output. The patient is taken to the recovery room and then to his room. The tubes will be removed when normal bowel sounds and functions return.

? WHO PERFORMS THE PROCEDURE?

This operation is usually performed by general surgeons.

? WHERE IS THE PROCEDURE PERFORMED?

This is major surgery that is always done on an inpatient basis in a hospital.

? WHAT ARE THE MORTALITY (DEATH) AND MORBIDITY (COMPLICATION) RATES?

Mortality varies greatly with the underlying condition, age of the patient, and amount of intestine removed. Mortality and complication rates of zero have been reported for removal of small cancers of the small intestine.[3]

On the other hand, massive small-intestine resection (defined as average loss of 91% of bowel) required because of **bowel infarction** had a reported mortality rate of 46% in a group of men whose average age was 64.[4] Mortality rates of 60% have been reported when 89% of the bowel is lost.[5] Long-term follow-up of pediatric patients with massive bowel resection shows a long-term mortality rate of 48%.[6]

? WHAT ARE THE OTHER COMPLICATIONS AND POSSIBLE SIDE EFFECTS?

Most resections remove so little of the small intestine that there are few, if any, noticeable changes in digestion. When much of the small bowel is removed, however, the patient is unable to absorb sufficient calories and nutrients. Nearly all nutrient absorption takes place in the small intestine; the large intestine essentially recycles water, minerals, and bile.

Investigations in both humans and animals have shown that, when part of the small bowel is removed, the small intestine compensates rather heroically by increasing the size of its absorptive structures and making other adaptations.[7, 8] There is a limit to the rate at which absorption can be increased, however, so eventually there is some loss of ability to digest food. Many patients who have had large portions of the small bowel removed (more than 75% or so) cannot tolerate any fats. Such patients may suffer from diarrhea and abdominal discomfort, and may be unable to absorb enough food to allow them to perform even light tasks.[9–11] Also, some drugs may be poorly absorbed, thereby making treatment of the results of the resection even more difficult.[12] Absorption of certain critical amino acids may be reduced.[13] In one study, all patients who had lost two-thirds or more of the small intestine and whose diets were not carefully supplemented were found to be in a state of subclinical malnutrition, which is a form of malnutrition that does not result in symptoms of the disease but can be detected by laboratory tests.[14]

Long-term intravenous feeding called **total parenteral nutrition (TPN)** is not an acceptable solution to the loss of the small bowel[15] for several reasons: The small intestine plays a role in regulation of excretion of calcium by the kidneys, and long-term TPN leads to loss of bone.[16–18] Liver damage can also occur and may be severe enough to require liver transplantation.[19]

Even when oral feeding is resumed, other problems may occur, including kidney stones, gallstones, bone fractures caused by mineral loss,[20] delayed growth, and delayed or absent puberty.[21]

Whether a return to oral feeding is possible depends upon the length of remaining small intestine. The critical breaking point seems to be between 20 and 30 cm of remaining bowel—roughly between eight and 12 inches. Although adults with less than 20 cm of remaining intestine may return to eating solid foods, children with less than 20 cm remaining can rarely return to oral feeding; those with more than 30 cm nearly always can.[22]

The output of ileostomies—substances and secretions such as gastric juices, stomach acid, bile, and enzymes—is very high and largely liquid, and failure to replace the fluid loss can lead to dehydration, particularly in the elderly.[23]

Pseudo-obstruction of the small intestine can occur after massive intestinal resection for Crohn's disease. Because of pain and vomiting brought about by both the residual Crohn's disease and by continuing partial obstruction, TPN may be required even if adequate bowel is left.[24]

As with any procedure in which anesthesia is used, death from reaction to the anesthetic drugs, error on the part of the anesthetist, or machine failure is a remote possibility. (See Glossary, p. 309)

? IS THIS THE MOST APPROPRIATE PROCEDURE FOR THE CONDITION?

Present surgical wisdom aims at preserving as much small intestine as possible. It is unlikely that a well-trained modern surgeon will enthusiastically remove much of the bowel.[25] One technique for reducing the loss of bowel and, therefore, absorptive surface is side-to-side **anastomosis**. In this procedure, the **stricture**, caused by Crohn's disease, is surgically removed from the intestine. Then another surgical opening is made on the wall of the intestine directly across from the original stricture. The two openings are brought together and sutured. Because only the local site of the stricture is removed, rather than a large section of bowel, the absorptive surface is preserved. The disease may reappear at another site in the intestinal tract, however, requiring further surgery. This anastomosis does not prolong

disease-free intervals, and the disease is likely to recur.[26]

There are some indications that this procedure is underused in patients who develop small-bowel obstruction after operations for colon cancer. In the great majority of patients, the obstructions turn out to be **adhesions**, which can be released easily. Obstructions are usually not caused by malignancy.[27]

? ARE THERE ALTERNATIVES TO THIS PROCEDURE?

A technique studied in monkeys uses a transplanted portion of the colon—which is flipped so that its **peristaltic** waves run back towards the stomach and partially recycle food in the small intestine. These special reverse-transplants have shown considerable success in increasing nutrient absorption and lessening diarrhea in the monkeys. The technique has been used in humans, but not extensively.[28] It may become standard practice one day, depending upon the results of clinical trials.[29, 30]

? WHAT IS CONTROVERSIAL ABOUT THE PROCEDURE?

Nutrition, a generally neglected aspect of surgical practice, is very important to patient recovery. Very recent work has demonstrated that short-chain fatty acids—special types of fat absorbed by the small intestine—are the preferred "food" of the bowel. Supplementation of intravenous feeding with them helps people compensate for the loss of the small intestine.[31] Studies in rats have shown that both intravenous and oral feeding are needed in the immediate postoperative period, because food is the stimulant for growth factors that help the bowel adapt to partial loss. During this period, however, nutrient absorption from food is poor, so intravenous feeding is also required.[32]

Although many studies clearly indicate that malabsorption results from extensive small-bowel resection, each new publication carries a tone of surprise in reporting the discovery of another form of malnutrition in patients who have had this procedure. Supplementation with minerals, vitamins, and amino acids is cheap and can be accomplished entirely with over-the-counter products. Yet if it is true that the average American elects to eat a diet that does not provide all the necessary nutrients in the recommended amounts, then this should be especially true of people who are avoiding foods that cause pain or discomfort. So you might expect that doctors would pay particular attention to the diets of patients who have bowel diseases or have had portions of bowel removed. Unfortunately, they seldom do.

If you have bowel disease, you should actively solicit your doctor's advice on nutrition. At the very least, discuss vitamin, protein, and mineral supplementation with your doctor.

Percutaneous Transluminal Coronary Angioplasty (12)

MORTALITY	MORBIDITY	CONTROVERSY
–	–	●

- The **MORTALITY** ranges from 0.2% to 8.5%.

- Significant **BLEEDING** is reported in 2% to 3% of cases, and 1% to 5% of patients experience a heart attack during the procedure. Tearing of the vessel was also reported in 3% of the cases.

- The main **CONTROVERSY** centers around the question of who is the ideal candidate for **angioplasty**. Although the procedure is safer than an open procedure such as bypass, the results have not been as good as surgeons had hoped.

LAY TITLE: **Balloon angioplasty**

Crushing of **plaque** in an artery with an inflatable balloon inserted into the artery through a **catheter** threaded through the **femoral** or **brachial artery**

? WHAT CONDITION DOES THE PROCEDURE TREAT?

This procedure treats what is now the leading cause of death in the United States and much of the developed world—**coronary artery** disease. For further discussion of coronary artery disease, see "Combined Right and Left Cardiac Catheterization," p. 50.

? WHAT IS THE PROCEDURE?

The patient is sedated, and a small incision is made in the femoral or brachial artery under local anesthesia. If **angiographic** studies were not previously done, a catheter carrying a **contrast medium** is threaded through the artery, the dye injected, and studies performed. A catheter tipped with a balloon is threaded through the artery and into one of the arteries supplying blood to the heart. The tip of the catheter is positioned at the center of a narrowed section of artery. The balloon at the end of the catheter is inflated for as long as the surgeon thinks necessary, but inflation is stopped if electronic monitoring and patient protests indicate that the patient is not tolerating the procedure. PTCA briefly blocks the flow of blood and can produce a "mini-heart attack" if the balloon is left inflated too long. Repeat x rays may be done following the balloon inflation to check the extent to which the vessel is opened. If the procedure damages the artery, if the patient has a heart attack while it is being performed, or if another major cardiac problem develops, the patient may be taken to the operating room for an emergency coronary artery **bypass surgery** (see "Aortocoronary Bypass," p. 105).

? WHO PERFORMS THE PROCEDURE?

The procedure is performed by a cardiovascular surgeon or an invasive cardiologist.

? WHERE IS THE PROCEDURE PERFORMED?

This surgery always requires an inpatient hospital stay; usually only the larger hospitals have all the personnel and equipment needed to perform the surgery and provide monitoring afterwards. A 1990 British study indicates that mortality rates under 1% can be obtained for carefully selected patients in facilities that are not equipped for emergency coronary artery bypass surgery, provided that patients can be readily transported to a facility that can perform such surgery.[1]

? WHAT ARE THE MORTALITY (DEATH) AND MORBIDITY (COMPLICATION) RATES?

Mortality for this procedure has steadily fallen since it was first done, and the current (1984 to 1991) literature reflects operative mortality rates of 5%,[2] 0.8% to 3.8%,[3] 0.7% to 0.9%,[4] 1%,[5] 7.2% (for patients operated on during or after a heart attack, 43% of whom had single-vessel disease),[6] and 0.2% to 8.5%.[7] One-year survival rates of 95%, and one-year heart attack rates of 3%, are typical for patients who undergo PCTA.[8, 9] It is not possible to disentangle results for single-vessel disease in all studies reviewed, but the mortality rate is lower when fewer vessels are treated. One study cites a mortality rate of 1.9% per vessel treated with PCTA.[10]

As for complications, rates of under 2% for **perioperative** heart attack and emergency bypass surgery and 12% for **acute reocclusion** of the vessel are achievable.[11, 12] Significant bleeding can be expected in 2% to 3% of patients.[13] Heart attack during the procedure occurs in about 1% to 5% of patients. A 1984 study from the National Heart, Lung, and Blood Institute cites occurrence of coronary artery dissection (essentially, a tearing apart of the artery) in 3%; vessel **occlusion** in 1%; prolonged chest pain in 1%; and artery spasm in 1%, noting that these rates declined as surgeons gained experience.[14] Cardiac rupture, which in-

volves massive tearing of the wall of the heart and profuse bleeding in the chest, is a rare event.

Remarkably, there is only one study of a group of 26 patients who died following PTCA.[15] Unfortunately, we don't know what percentage of the total number of patients having PTCA these patients represent. The study findings for 21 of the 26 patients who died within three weeks of operation showed demonstrable cardiac complications in 19 patients: clots formed from platelets in 10 patients (48%); coronary artery disintegration was seen in 17 patients (81%); blood clots that had moved from the site where they formed to other parts of the body were noted in 13 patients (62%); **atheroemboli** were found in seven patients (33%); and heart attacks occurred in 17 patients (81%). An increased incidence of clots formed from **fibrin** platelets in the heart and coronary vessels was noted when compared with a non-PTCA cardiac autopsy population (five of 53 patients).[16]

? WHAT ARE THE OTHER COMPLICATIONS AND POSSIBLE SIDE EFFECTS?

Groin **hematomas** at the point where the catheter is inserted, and two heart rhythm disturbances—**atrial fibrillation** and **left bundle branch block**—were reported in under 1% of elderly patients in one study.[17] Rates are probably lower in younger patients.

Repair of the artery used for the catheterization, even in experienced hands, is required in 1% to 3% of the cases.[18]

? IS THIS THE MOST APPROPRIATE PROCEDURE FOR THE CONDITION?

Based on current knowledge, PTCA is the most appropriate procedure if you have single-vessel disease. It can also be attempted on a patient who is a candidate for bypass surgery, because bypass surgery can always be performed if PTCA fails. The final decision should rest with the patient and her doctor.

The disturbing aspect of coronary artery disease is that, given our current knowledge about its causes and history, almost no one needs to face a PTCA. Appropriate diet and exercise can slow the progress of **atherosclerosis** or prevent it entirely; there is recent evidence that a rigidly vegetarian, low-fat diet can reverse it. There are new drugs that block cholesterol production, speed up the liver's removal of cholesterol from the bloodstream, or both.

Both PTCA and coronary artery bypass surgery, moreover, have problems with reocclusion of the arteries operated on if significant dietary and exercise changes are not made. Clearly, the best choice is an active program of prevention. PTCA is the appropriate choice only if medical (nonsurgical) management does not produce an acceptable work performance and quality of life.

? ARE THERE ALTERNATIVES TO THIS PROCEDURE?

As mentioned above, prevention and medical management are all alternatives to this procedure. A number of new techniques, including **laser angioplasty**, are in research and development stages. All of these techniques carry risks, are expensive, and cause discomfort that is entirely avoidable for the great majority of people.

A 1989 study comparing coronary artery bypass with PTCA found hospital mortality rates to be just about even at 0.4% and 0.5%, respectively. In-hospital heart attack rates were 1.7% and 5.1%, respectively, or about three times higher for angioplasty patients. Projected five-year survival rates are slightly better for PTCA patients than for bypass patients (96.3% and 92.3%, respectively). However, PTCA patients had a five-year heart attack rate of 11.9%, nearly double the rate of 5.4% for bypass patients. Less than 1% of bypass pa-

tients required a subsequent angioplasty, compared with 25% of angioplasty patients. Only 1.2% of bypass patients required a second procedure, but 15% of angioplasty patients required a bypass operation. The bottom line seems to be that PTCA patients have a higher five-year survival rate but have slightly higher risk of heart attack.[19]

? WHAT IS CONTROVERSIAL ABOUT THE PROCEDURE?

It is almost impossible to comment definitively on either this procedure or its alternatives: results are improving, new and refined techniques are being developed, and not enough time has gone by since the procedures were initially performed. By very careful selection of patients for studies, it is possible to obtain excellent results. This observation does not necessarily imply intellectual dishonesty, just a desire of investigators to put the best clinical foot forward. The trouble is that the ideal candidate for either coronary artery bypass surgery or PTCA is not representative of the entire patient population. In the usual tradition of "treat the disease and ignore the patient," studies have focused on the easily measured physiological parameters such as percentage of **occlusion** and **ejection fraction**, rather than the overall quality of life of the patients, although more attention is gradually being paid to that aspect.

The classic balloon procedure and laser and "roto-rooter" variations on it were developed as an alternative to coronary artery bypass surgery. Because of the serious nature of bypass surgery and the relatively high (though rapidly decreasing) morbidity associated with it, PTCA was developed as, it was hoped, a kinder, gentler procedure. The theory, based on what was then known about plaque in heart arteries, was that the plaque could be crushed against the vessel wall to increase the inner diameter of **lumen** of the artery (a **transluminal** procedure). As with bypass surgery, the results are mixed. Although results in many studies are good, and attendant morbidity is less than that with CABG (coronary artery bypass graft; see "Aortocoronary Bypass," p. 105), the results are not as good as surgeons had hoped they would be.

Much of the reason for this seems to lie in plaques and the factors that govern their transformations after PTCA—specifically the fact plaque formation is more complex than originally thought. There is evidence that at least some slight injury is needed to start plaque formation; otherwise, one would expect to find plaques spread uniformly throughout the arteries. Adding to the complexity are the interactions among the various layers of the vessel wall, the clotting factors in the blood, cholesterol, and the body's fat-disposal system. Depending upon how they interact, plaques may behave differently at different stages in their formation.

At any rate, PTCA itself certainly imposes at least minor injury on the vessel wall. Experiments with expandable metal **stents** placed in arteries after PTCA show that many stents are soon overgrown with plaques. The formation of plaques may simply be what injured artery walls do in human beings with high cholesterol levels. If so, almost any form of surgery would have worse results than prevention. Although it is too early to tell, and one authority has noted that "our knowledge of lipid [fat] metabolism in humans turns over completely every 10 years," the drift of present studies is in the direction of prevention.

The best course is to prevent coronary artery disease by appropriate diet, exercise, lifestyle (for example, refraining from smoking, and avoiding chronic stress), and use of medications. There is strong evidence that we know how to do this. The next best course is medical treatment. If such treatment produces an acceptable quality of life, surgery is not indicated. If surgery is indicated, PTCA may work. Otherwise, CABG is available.

Peritoneal Adhesiolysis (35)

MORTALITY	MORBIDITY	CONTROVERSY
+	+	o

Destruction of abnormal tissue connections inside the abdomen that result from inflammatory diseases, injury, or prior surgery

? WHAT CONDITION DOES THE PROCEDURE TREAT?

Although inflammation is part of the normal healing response, inflammation in the abdominal cavity can lead to the formation of abnormal structures called **adhesions**. Pain usually results. Many of the abdominal organs have few classic pain receptors, but do register stretching and tugging in unusual directions as intense pain.

This procedure is most commonly performed to treat infertility, which can occur when adhesions attach themselves to the **fallopian tubes**. Even microscopic adhesions can interfere with the movement of the egg through the fallopian tubes by creating small kinks that block the path of the egg. If the egg is unable to complete the journey from the ovary, through the fallopian tube, and to the uterus, it cannot be fertilized; the result is the inability to become pregnant.[1] Death may occur if an adhesion causes intestinal obstruction or results in a tear in the intestine.

Unfortunately, destruction of the adhesions results in more inflammation, which in turn can cause new adhesions to form. Extensive research is underway to find the best way to treat adhesions in the abdomen and adhesions from the abdomen to the **peritoneum**.

? WHAT IS THE PROCEDURE?

Techniques vary with the location of the adhesions and the problem. One is to disturb the adhesions as little as possible, simply cut them, and then use rubber or Teflon sponges to keep them from re-forming. This technique prevents contact between the inflamed surfaces.[2] Microsurgery using **electrocautery** to cut adhesions has a better result with infertility than traditional procedures, which involve more extensive cutting.[3] Use of lasers seems to produce slightly better results than mechanical cutting.[4]

Microsurgery and **laser microsurgery** are being used increasingly for infertility surgery: Surgeons have recognized that rough tissue handling alone can cause adhesions to form. Also, all adhesions, even microscopic ones, may have to be removed before the ovaries and fallopian tubes can function properly. The **laparoscope**, a mini-telescope that can be inserted through a small incision near the navel, is also being used more frequently for these procedures. The general philosophy is to open the abdomen only if less invasive means do not allow all the adhesions to be cut.

To illustrate, consider a laparoscopic procedure: The patient is given a general anesthetic and a small region around the navel is shaved and scrubbed. A puncture is made with a **trochar**, and the laparoscope is inserted. The abdomen is inflated with carbon dioxide (CO_2) to separate the organs, and the adhesions are located and cut with a laser beam aimed through a fiber-optic channel on the laparoscope. When all the adhesions have been located and cut with the laser beam, the surgeon may remove the CO_2 and wash out the abdomen with Hyskon (dextran sulfate dissolved in a dextrose [sugar] solution), which has been shown to reduce adhesion formation. The solution is suctioned off through a catheter and the incision is closed with a Band-Aid, or with a single **suture** and a Band-Aid. The patient is taken to the recovery room and then to her room, or sent home, depending on the extent of the surgery.

? WHO PERFORMS THE PROCEDURE?

This procedure is done by general and gynecological surgeons, as well as infertility specialists.

? WHERE IS THE PROCEDURE PERFORMED?

The procedure is performed on an inpatient or outpatient basis in a hospital, in an outpatient surgery facility, or in a well-equipped doctor's office.

? WHAT ARE THE MORTALITY (DEATH) AND MORBIDITY (COMPLICATION) RATES?

Mortality is essentially related only to the anesthetics used. As with any procedure in which anesthesia is used, death from reaction to the anesthetic drugs, error on the part of the anesthetist, or machine failure is a remote possibility. (See Glossary, p. 309)

? WHAT ARE THE OTHER COMPLICATIONS AND POSSIBLE SIDE EFFECTS?

Besides failure of the operation to correct pain or infertility, the only other major complication is infection, which is relatively rare. Prior to operation, only about 17% of women with adhesions affecting the uterus and ovaries can conceive; afterwards, 87% can.[5]

? IS THIS THE MOST APPROPRIATE PROCEDURE FOR THE CONDITION?

Yes, because virtually all alternatives involve opening the abdomen.

? ARE THERE ALTERNATIVES TO THIS PROCEDURE?

Essentially, the only alternative is an open-abdomen operation.

? WHAT IS CONTROVERSIAL ABOUT THE PROCEDURE?

There is not so much controversy as there is an appreciation of progress. Animal studies indicate that a 5% solution of polyethylene glycol, poured into the abdominal cavity before it is closed, inhibits new adhesion formation; the technique is beginning to be used in humans.

Placement of Central Venous Catheter (23)

MORTALITY	MORBIDITY	CONTROVERSY
+	+	o

Placement of a **catheter** into the **central venous system** of the body, specifically the **superior vena cava**, as opposed to the **peripheral venous system**

? WHAT CONDITION DOES THE PROCEDURE TREAT?

A central venous catheter is placed in one of the veins near the surface of the body and threaded through it until it enters the superior vena cava, which carries blood returning to the heart into the **right atrium**.

Central venous catheters are used to deliver chemotherapeutic drugs in cancer patients; to deliver any drug that is highly irritating to the smaller veins in the arms and legs; to provide large volumes of fluid for near-total or total feeding by vein; to diagnose heart and circulatory problems; to provide kidney dialysis treatments (see "Hemodialysis," p. 147); and to monitor heart and lung performance in critically ill patients. The procedure "treats" few of them definitively; it is not the curative operation for any of the aforementioned conditions. On the other hand, therapy provided through this procedure can be life-saving.

Most people are familiar with the intravenous needle, which is stuck into a vein in the hand or the shallow depression on the inside of the forearm, just below the elbow joint (called the **antecubital fossa**). These are not the only places where catheters can be inserted into the veins—any vein can be used, even those only reachable by surgical dissection (a "cutdown") or by penetrating overlying tissues with a long needle. (In Samuel Shem's medical novel *The House of God,* one of the laws learned by first-year medical residents is, "There's no place in the human body that can't be reached by a number 16 needle and a good strong arm.")

For most purposes, the veins used for central venous catheter placement are the **subclavian vein** and the **internal jugular vein**.

Many of the drugs used for cancer chemotherapy, many of the solutions used for intravenous feeding for extended periods, and some other medications are extremely irritating to the smaller veins in the hands and arms. Aside from the pain caused, which very few patients are willing to tolerate, the irritation can cause leakage into the surrounding tissues, localized swelling, and eventual **sclerosis** of the vein. Furthermore, the tissues of the wall of the vein can scar and close it off entirely. When larger veins are used—such as with this procedure—the various solutions are rapidly diluted by the larger flow of blood, and are sent out into the body in diluted form faster than they can be through a peripheral vein; this allows for rapid administration of drugs with minimal irritation of the venous system.

WHAT IS THE PROCEDURE?

Depending on the vein used and the preference of the surgeon, the patient may be lying in bed or seated in a chair. A small region of skin is shaved, if necessary, and washed with an antiseptic solution. The skin—and usually the patient's head—is draped so that only the place where the needle will be inserted in exposed. A local anesthetic is injected into the skin, and a large, hollow needle with a sharp stylet is inserted into the vein. The stylet is withdrawn, and if the color and flow characteristics of the blood (that is, if the blood is dark and not spurting) indicate that the needle has entered the vein, the catheter is threaded through the **lumen** of the needle until it reaches the vena cava. The surgeon depends on his knowledge of anatomy and the size of the patient to know how far to insert it. If the procedure is done well, it is nearly painless; the chief sensation, felt only when the needle or catheter is moving, is pressure. The catheter is anchored with adhesive tape (some surgeons prefer to fasten it to the skin with a single **suture**), and the whole area is thickly bandaged. (The catheter is left in place as long as necessary for the purpose intended; lengths of time vary from procedure to procedure.)

WHO PERFORMS THE PROCEDURE?

This procedure can be done by any physician. Depending upon the policies of the facility or office, physician's assistants, nurse-practitioners, or nurses may do it instead.

WHERE IS THE PROCEDURE PERFORMED?

This operation is usually done as an inpatient hospital procedure, if only because the need for it usually first becomes apparent there. It also can be done in a walk-in clinic or in a doctor's office.

WHAT ARE THE MORTALITY (DEATH) AND MORBIDITY (COMPLICATION) RATES?

In our review of the medical literature, we were surprised to find only one article that covered the morbidity and mortality of this procedure in depth. In a study of central venous catheterization for dialysis, morbidity consisted of inadequate flow of intravenous fluid in 7.6%, accidental withdrawal of the catheter in 5.6%, and infection (specifically, **bacteremia**) in 5.1%, with a total overall complication rate of 27.2%. Accidental withdrawal was more than twice as common (10.8% vs. 4.3%) when the catheter was placed in the internal jugular vein, as opposed to the subclavian vein.[1]

Mortality is quite low—between zero and 0.125%—and in two of the six cases reported in the literature mortality was attributable to **septicemia**; accidental **perforation** of the vessel wall and/or heart in three of the six cases; and **air embolism** in one case. If one gets septicemia, the mortality rate ranges from 6.0% to 58.1%, depending upon the infecting organism and the health of the patient before the procedure.[2, 3]

WHAT ARE THE OTHER COMPLICATIONS AND POSSIBLE SIDE EFFECTS?

Other complications and side effects generally result from the medications used and not from the catheter itself. Local infection at the site of insertion, without general bloodstream infection, also occurs. Damage to the phrenic nerve (which runs from the brain to the diaphragm), resulting in paralysis of the diaphragm and asphyxiation if the patient is not placed on a respirator, is a rare complication of internal jugular vein catheterization.[4]

? IS THIS THE MOST APPROPRIATE PROCEDURE FOR THE CONDITION?

Because this procedure is used primarily for the delivery of drugs and for high-volume or long-duration intravenous feeding, the question really is whether those treatments are appropriate. This is one of the few procedures that may not be used enough, because there is clear evidence that many cancer patients do not receive the latest recommended chemotherapy. (The U.S. Department of Health and Human Services [HHS] operates a service called "Physicians Data Query" for oncologists to learn the latest cancer treatments; therefore, HHS can tell by the number of inquiries that not enough oncologists are using the service.) Similarly, **hyperalimentation,** a feeding procedure that uses a central venous catheter to provide nutrients to patients who cannot take an adequate diet orally, may be underutilized.

? ARE THERE ALTERNATIVES TO THIS PROCEDURE?

No, not if the intravenous therapy is really needed and if the solution is too irritating for peripheral veins.

? WHAT IS CONTROVERSIAL ABOUT THE PROCEDURE?

This procedure is controversial only in contrast with another: namely, intra-arterial (within the artery) placement of a Swan-Ganz catheter. One study suggests that monitoring with a central venous line is more effective than monitoring with a Swan-Ganz catheter, which is run through the heart and into one of the pulmonary arteries.[5] Not only is the Swan-Ganz catheter more painful in its placement—arteries can "feel" whereas veins cannot, it exposes the patient to a higher-risk procedure, only to obtain the same results and useful information as the central venous catheter would yield.

Removal of Tube and Ectopic Pregnancy (63)

MORTALITY	MORBIDITY	CONTROVERSY
+	+	o

- The **COMPLICATION** rate for this procedure is very low; the chief concern expressed by surgeons in the literature is their ability to remove the entire ectopic pregnancy while maintaining the ability of the woman to have a normal pregnancy in the future.

Removal of a **fallopian tube** in which a fertilized egg has implanted itself

? WHAT CONDITION DOES THE PROCEDURE TREAT?

An ectopic (Greek for "away from the place") pregnancy is any pregnancy that occurs with the fetus outside, rather than inside, the womb. The most common site of implantation of the fetus in an ectopic pregnancy is in one of the fallopian tubes. The usual surgical treatment of this life-threatening condition is removal of the fallopian tube in which the ectopic pregnancy occurred. Either the open technique, which involves cutting into the abdomen, or **laparoscopy** can preserve the fallopian tubes so that further attempts at pregnancy are possible.[1]

The incidence of ectopic pregnancies has been increasing so rapidly that it has been called a "surgical epidemic."[2] The primary reason appears to be an increasing incidence of infection of the fallopian tubes with the microscopic *Chlamydia* organism, which is responsible for several human diseases, including some sexually transmitted disease. There are other risk factors as well,[3] which will be described in the pages that follow.

Pelvic inflammatory disease (PID), an infection of the pelvic organs (the uterus, fallopian tubes, and ovaries), which is a risk factor for ectopic pregnancies, now occurs in 12.5% of 15- to 19-year-olds, and the rate is rising. If current trends continue, 50% of women who were

15 years of age in 1970 will have had at least one episode of PID by the year 2000.[4] Consequently, the rate of ectopic pregnancies can be expected to rise in the future.

Failure of a sterilization procedure that uses **electrocoagulation** to close a fallopian tube occurs in about 0.5% of such procedures; 20% to 25% of women in whom electrocoagulation fails will have an ectopic pregnancy.[5] Because the tube is not blocked completely, the fertilized egg is able to travel down the tube until it encounters a blockage. There, it implants itself and begins to grow.

The causes of all ectopic pregnancies are not known, but they are more common in women who have had induced or elective (as opposed to spontaneous) abortions or any abdominal surgery. Other risk factors include previous ectopic pregnancy, current intrauterine device use, prior fallopian tube surgery, previous pelvic inflammatory disease, and prior history of infertility. In women being treated for infertility via **gamete intrafallopian transfer (GIFT)**, which places an egg fertilized outside the body into the fallopian tubes and who have pelvic **adhesions** resulting from prior surgery or unknown causes, the rate of ectopic pregnancy is 7.2% per attempt at implantation and 18.3% per case of clinical pregnancy achieved.[6]

Prior surgery on the fallopian tubes is an apparent major risk factor: 3% to 20% of women who have had fallopian tube surgery will have an ectopic pregnancy. However, the greater the success of the tubal surgery in fully restoring the normal function of the tubes, the lower the chance of an ectopic pregnancy.[7]

Cases of implantation of the fetus in the scar from a previous cesarean section, and implantation in rather than onto the wall of the uterus (the normal course), have been reported, but are rare.[8] Ninety-eight percent of all ectopic pregnancies occur in the fallopian tubes.[9]

An ectopic pregnancy is a problem because the growth of the fetus damages and eventually ruptures the fallopian tube. Hemorrhage usually accompanies both ruptured and unruptured ectopic pregnancies and can be severe enough to lead to shock. In some cases the rate of blood loss is so high that blood transfusions must be given under pressure to keep the woman alive.[10] Even if there is no immediate hemorrhage severe enough to send the woman to a doctor or hospital, the accumulated blood in the abdomen puts her at risk for **peritonitis**, for which the mortality rate ranges between 12% to 57%, depending on the causative organism (usually a bacterium or, very rarely, a virus), the treatment given, and other factors.[11–14] Improved antibiotics have lowered the mortality rate, but it still remains high.

An ectopic pregnancy is a surgical emergency, and the appearance of the symptoms can be dramatic. Abdominal pain is the most common symptom, along with **amenorrhea**, vaginal bleeding, nausea, vomiting, fainting spells, and dizziness. Pain can radiate along a nerve pathway to areas other than the site of actual injury or disease. In ectopic pregnancies that cause bleeding in the abdomen, the pain often appears in the shoulder. Physicians should be alert for shoulder pain in women who are known to be, or who may be, pregnant; it can be a sign of a ruptured ectopic pregnancy, one that has broken through the walls of the fallopian tubes.[15–17]

Surgery to restore reproductive function after an ectopic pregnancy can be done with lasers or with an **electrocautery device**. Rates of pregnancy following laser surgery are slightly higher (53.3%) than the rates after electrocautery surgery, but the difference is not statistically significant.[18]

When a woman has had one tube removed, it is possible for her to conceive if her remaining fallopian tube is functioning normally. Obviously, fertility is increased if both tubes can be retained, which is an alternative to removal of the tube. Such conservative surgery to preserve both tubes has led to fertilization in 58.2% to 71.8% of women, normal deliveries in 48% to 49.2%, and a repeat ectopic pregnancy in 10% to 16%.[19, 20] Even if the tube that is not removed is diseased or abnormal—if the woman only had one fallopian tube at surgery—in vitro fertilization (IVF), in which an egg is fertilized in a dish and implanted in the uterus, results in pregnancy at least 40.7% of the time.[21]

? WHAT IS THE PROCEDURE?

Removal of a tube in which there is an ectopic pregnancy can be done in several ways: The surgeon can make an opening in the abdomen (called an **open procedure**); through the navel, with a small instrument called a **laparoscope**; or through the upper part of the vagina, with an instrument called a **culdoscope**. The aim of the recently developed conservative surgeries (in this case, laparoscopy and culdoscopy) is to preserve the tube and maintain fertility as well as to avoid the extra cost and time associated with an abdominal incision.

In the classic open tube removal procedure, the woman is given a spinal or general anesthetic. If she is still hemorrhaging at the time of surgery, or has begun to do so while in the hospital, she will be given blood transfusions. If the surgeon thinks it is safe, the anesthesiologist will give drugs to lower the woman's blood pressure to aid the surgeon in locating and ligating or **cauterizing** sites of bleeding. Once bleeding is controlled, drugs will be used to return the blood pressure to normal (if it is very low), or it may be allowed to rise naturally. In either case, the anesthesiologist should watch blood pressure closely.

The abdomen is washed with soap and antiseptic, and draped so that only the area of the incision is exposed. The skin, fat, **fascia,** muscles, and **peritoneum** are opened in layers. Bleeding vessels are **ligated** or cauterized with an **electrocautery device** as the operation proceeds. The fallopian tube with the ectopic pregnancy is located and removed. The stump of the fallopian tube attached to the uterus is cauterized or **sutured** shut, or both, and any blood clots are removed. If there has been extensive bleeding, the surgeon may wash out the exposed portion of the abdomen with sterile saline to flush out clots. The saline solution is removed with suction

tubes. The abdomen is closed with the tissues **sutured** in layers, and a dressing applied. The woman is then taken to the recovery room.

For the laparoscopic procedure, the woman is given a general anesthetic and placed on her back on the operating table. Things proceed as described above, but there is no large incision in the abdomen. Instead, very small incisions are made in the navel and elsewhere in the abdomen where the surgeon will need to insert instruments. The incisions are usually small enough to cover with a Band-Aid. The laparoscope, a rigid tube with lights, lenses, and a camera—if the surgeon wants to use a TV screen rather than the scope's eyepiece— are inserted into the navel. Carbon dioxide is used to inflate the abdomen and spread the organs apart to provide an adequate view. Instruments needed to perform the surgery, such as forceps, a laser beam, or an electrocautery device, are inserted through the other incisions. The fallopian tube is located and cut off, and its stump is sutured, cauterized, or both, at the point where it joins the ovary. The instruments are withdrawn, the gas is released from the abdomen, and the woman is taken to the recovery room.

In cases in which the woman is discovered to have only one salvageable ovary and one salvageable fallopian tube, and they are on opposite sides, it is possible to move the functioning ovary over to the same side as the functioning tube so that a normal pregnancy is possible.[22] This is a technique acknowledged to be relatively simple.

The culdoscopic procedure is much the same as the open procedure, except that the surgeon places the woman in the **lithotomy position** and makes an incision in the top part of the vagina above the place where the cervix enters, a region called the cul-de-sac—hence culdoscopy. This approach is seldom used, but may avoid an abdominal incision, particularly if the surgeon is confident of being able to control bleeding through the small incision.[23] However, the surgeon may feel that the open procedure or a laparoscopic procedure gives her better vision and control than the culdoscopic approach.

? WHO PERFORMS THE PROCEDURE?

This procedure is done by an obstetrician-gynecologist or a general surgeon. Either one who does laparoscopic or laser procedures should have special additional training.

? WHERE IS THE PROCEDURE PERFORMED?

Because of the condition of the woman, this surgery is performed in the inpatient department of a hospital, even though operations equivalent to the laparoscopic procedure can be done in an outpatient surgery facility or a clinic with a laparoscopy suite.

? WHAT ARE THE MORTALITY (DEATH) AND MORBIDITY (COMPLICATION) RATES?

The mortality rate associated with this procedure is 1% to 2%,[24] even when some quoted morbidity figures (for example, infection) seem high. Zero mortality and a 2% complication rate have been reported for the laparoscopic procedure.[25] Complication rates of zero to 2% have been reported.[26, 27]

The chief concern mentioned in the literature is whether the surgeon can remove the entire pregnancy and maintain the ability of the woman to have a normal pregnancy in the future. For this reason—as we mentioned earlier—conservative alternatives to the procedure have been developed and are being refined.

Earlier detection of ectopic pregnancy (through **ultrasound** studies or laparoscopic examination) has reduced rates of morbidity and mortality.[28] Infection can occur in up to 22% of women, but may cause no symptoms and may be detectable only by bacterial culture.[29]

Bleeding as a major complication has been reported in 2.53% of laparoscopically treated ectopic pregnancies, with a mortality of zero and no hospital stay longer than 24 hours.[30]

In ectopic pregnancies treated with laparoscopy, reoperation required because of failure to remove the entire pregnancy the first time occurs in up to 5.12% of cases. Rates of pregnancy inside the womb (following microsurgery to correct tubal defects) are variable, but have been reported to be as low as 19.4%.[31]

? WHAT ARE THE OTHER COMPLICATIONS AND POSSIBLE SIDE EFFECTS?

Depending upon the degree of scarring of the fallopian tubes, and the functioning of the other tube if only one was removed, fertility may be impaired. Among women who want to get pregnant again after an ectopic pregnancy, success rates (as measured by objective evidence of pregnancy) vary from 61% to 100%. Both the rate of fertilizations and the rate of pregnancies carried to term have been reported to be around 90%,[32] with 10.9% of the pregnancies failing because of a repeat ectopic pregnancy.[33]

Adhesions, which can interfere with the chances of future pregnancy, occur by the eighth day after surgery in more than 50% of women operated on for ectopic pregnancy. They can be repaired by laparoscopy and tend not to recur following such surgery.[34]

While removal of the ovaries is not, strictly speaking, a part of this procedure, ovarian damage in a woman who has only one functioning ovary will make estrogen supplements necessary. If the woman takes the drug assiduously, her survival rate is as good as that for women with intact ovaries.[35] True, hormone replacement therapy is controversial—the use of replacement estrogens is believed to increase the incidence of breast cancer. However, studies of this question have given equivocal results. Current research strongly suggests that the combined effect in reducing bone loss and heart disease (a major and growing problem in women) more than outweighs any risk of breast cancer that might be associated with hormone replacement therapy.

A complication of the ectopic pregnancy itself is hemolytic uremic syndrome. This condition is characterized by anemia, bleeding, and kidney failure, and has been reported following the successful removal of an ectopic pregnancy.[36]

Endometriosis is a condition in which tissue from the uterine lining somehow escapes the uterus and becomes implanted on pelvic organs, usually causing pain. There is a small chance following this procedure that this endometrial tissue can become entrapped in scar tissue, but this is relatively rare.[37]

In women treated with the laparoscope, possible complications include a bulging of the navel where the laparoscope was inserted, cardiac arrest, and electrical burns of the abdominal viscera, usually the **small intestine**.[38]

Puncture of the womb is a rare complication. So is the need to convert a closed operation, as laparoscopy is, to an open procedure, such as laparotomy, to finish it.[39]

The operation, if done through the vagina, is carried out on the stirrup table with the woman in the lithotomy position. If the procedure is lengthy and the woman is not shifted to relieve pressure on various parts of the body, permanent nerve damage can occur.[40]

Ovarian remnant syndrome, which is characterized primarily by pelvic pain, can occur when a surgeon is removing both tubes and ovaries and fails to remove all of an ovary. Because the doctor thinks that the ovaries are gone, the woman's pain is dismissed as psychosomatic, and she is either ignored or referred to a psychiatrist. Although relatively rare, ovarian remnant syndrome may progress to tissue damage requiring bowel and bladder surgery.[41] **Necrotizing fasciitis**, in which the tough tissue containing the muscles is de-

stroyed, with destruction spreading to the overlying and underlying tissues, is a rare but absolutely devastating complication. In some cases, loss of the full thickness of the abdominal wall occurs and multiple reconstructive surgeries are required.[42]

Formation of a **fistula** occurs in about 1.9% of women.[43] It is also possible for the tube to recanalize, affording an unbroken route from the ovary to the uterus, which may cause another ectopic pregnancy.[44]

Studies in monkeys indicate that there are no hormonal changes following removal of one or both tubes if the ovaries are left intact.[45]

As with any procedure in which anesthesia is used, death from reaction to the anesthetic drugs, error on the part of the anesthetist, or machine failure is a remote possibility. (See Glossary, p. 309)

? IS THIS THE MOST APPROPRIATE PROCEDURE FOR THE CONDITION?

Yes. Ectopic pregnancy is a life-threatening condition that causes severe pain, and can only be treated surgically. Hence, the question is not the appropriateness of surgical treatment, but rather which procedure will be least invasive. Generally, this is laparoscopy, but an open procedure may be needed if there is widespread bleeding (for example, if the fallopian tube has burst).

? ARE THERE ALTERNATIVES TO THIS PROCEDURE?

Having three ways to remove a tube is complex enough; alternatives to the standard tube removal are also available, and all can be done with an open procedure or a laparoscope. Open procedures are being done much less frequently these days, and are usually reserved for in cases in which the surgeon cannot achieve control of bleeding through the scope.

Research into conservative measures that save the fallopian tube by opening it, removing the ectopic fetus, and allowing the cut to heal with or without sutures suggests that fertility can be preserved if the surgery is done properly. It is possible to save the tube in about 75% of such cases.[46] Rates of intrauterine pregnancy and repeat ectopic pregnancies are both higher with this procedure than with performing the classic practice of removing the tube.[47] Women who want to become pregnant again should ask for the more conservative procedure described above, called salpingostomy, rather than salpingectomy, which is the complete removal of a tube.

Laparoscopic surgery is an alternative to the open procedure, just as the open procedure is an alternative to laparoscopy.[48] Tube removal or tube-sparing surgery can be done either way.

Surgery though a laparoscope can use lasers or electrocautery devices for cutting tissue, stopping blood loss, and destroying excess tissue. Use of the new, highly specialized Neodymium-Aluminum-Yttrium-Garnet (Nd:YAG) laser with conical sapphire lenses to concentrate the light has shown good promise in preserving the fallopian tubes while destroying the ectopic pregnancy. In a recent study of the performance of this laser, 88% of the women had unblocked, or open, tubes when assessed by x ray or diagnostic laparoscopy ("second-look surgery") following the laser operation.[49]

? WHAT IS CONTROVERSIAL ABOUT THE PROCEDURE?

It is not uncommon for surgeons to remove the appendix when a tubal removal or removal of an ectopic pregnancy is done, ostensibly to avoid future problems with appendicitis. Although controversial, this appears to be a safe practice.[50]

Arguments about the relative merits of using laser surgery versus **electrocoagulation** to close a fallopian tube will continue for some years to come. Current research indicates that lasers produce better results but

are associated with a slightly higher rate of complications.[51]

Repair of Cystocele or Rectocele (97)

MORTALITY	MORBIDITY	CONTROVERSY
+	−	o

- Thirty-four percent of patients report some postoperative **COMPLICATION**, of which 12.5% were attributed to postoperative urinary retention.

Repair of a **herniation** of the bladder or the rectum into the vaginal vault

? WHAT CONDITION DOES THE PROCEDURE TREAT?

A cystocele or rectocele is a bulging of the bladder or rectum, respectively, into the vaginal vault. A normal female pelvis viewed in cross-section has straight vaginal walls; a cystocele or rectocele causes a bulge of the bladder or rectum into the space normally occupied by the vaginal vault. This can make intercourse painful or impossible. A large rectocele contributes to hemorrhoid formation and can require insertion of a finger into the vagina to straighten the rectal canal to make passing stool possible.[1] An equivalent condition in men, in which the cystocele bulges into the scrotal canal, has been reported, but the condition is almost totally confined to women.[2, 3]

A cystocele or rectocele often results from injury during childbirth—weakened pelvic muscles and cartilage following childbirth are common—but can also arise from loosening of the tissues that comes from aging.

Other than pain and inconvenience associated with either condition, a large cystocele can lead to kinking of the **ureters** and a condition called **hydronephrosis**.

The problem usually disappears when the cystocele is repaired.[4]

WHAT IS THE PROCEDURE?

There are several techniques for repairing cystoceles and rectoceles. All of them involve strengthening the muscular walls between the vagina and the bladder or rectum. Techniques include cutting out the weakened section and suturing the cut closed;[5] this can be done through the vagina or through an incision in the lower abdomen. A rectocele can be repaired either through the vagina or through the anus.[6]

Depending upon the technique, general or local anesthesia is used.[7] If an abdominal incision is used, the skin is shaved and washed with soap and antiseptic, and the patient is draped so that only the area of the incision is exposed. More commonly, a **speculum** is inserted into the vagina or the rectum and the surgeon operates through this, without a skin incision. Some approaches combine repairs through a skin incision and through a speculum. For example, the bladder is repaired through a skin incision, and the vaginal wall is repaired with the use of a speculum.

An incisionless technique (through the vagina) involves capturing the excess tissue in a "running suture" that cuts off blood flow. The excess tissue dies and is sloughed off, and healing occurs along what would have been the incision line in a traditional repair.[8]

WHO PERFORMS THE PROCEDURE?

The procedure can be performed by a general surgeon, an obstetrician-gynecologist, a urologist, or a colon-rectal surgeon. Because of the occasional difficulty of repairs of the rectum, rectoceles are probably best treated by a colon-rectal surgeon. As always, a board-certified surgeon is preferable.

WHERE IS THE PROCEDURE PERFORMED?

Depending upon the technique and the type of anesthesia used, this procedure can be done in the inpatient or outpatient department of a hospital, or in an outpatient surgery center. If a general anesthetic is used, surgery should be performed in a hospital.

WHAT ARE THE MORTALITY (DEATH) AND MORBIDITY (COMPLICATION) RATES?

A large study of transanal and transvaginal (procedures done through the anal and through the vaginal openings, respectively) rectocele repair shows zero mortality and a complication rate of 34%, of which 12.5% was postoperative **urinary retention**. Patients who had had a transvaginal repair reported a much greater incidence of persistent rectal pain than those who had had the transanal repair. Overall, 80% of patients reported improvement.[9]

Infection rates vary depending upon the technique used, and range from zero to 5.6%.[10]

The classic procedure can lead to **stress incontinence**. This can be avoided if the surgeon uses a technique that straightens the urethra and avoids pressure on the bladder.[11]

WHAT ARE THE OTHER COMPLICATIONS AND POSSIBLE SIDE EFFECTS?

Persistent pain, vaginal tightness, sexual dysfunction, occasional rectal bleeding, constipation, and incontinence of urine are reported with all techniques in various degrees. The literature indicates that techniques that most completely restore the normal anatomic positions of the bladder, vagina, and rectum have the best results.

As with any procedure in which anesthesia is used, death from reaction to the anesthetic drugs, error on the part of the anesthetist, or machine failure is a remote possibility. (See Glossary, p. 309)

? IS THIS THE MOST APPROPRIATE PROCEDURE FOR THE CONDITION?

Because of the variety of techniques used, it is difficult to select any one as invariably the best. The range of techniques was developed to deal with different degrees of deformity and associated complications. Ideally, the surgeon should select the technique that will give the best result with each patient, rather than always relying on the same method regardless of the patient's condition.

? ARE THERE ALTERNATIVES TO THIS PROCEDURE?

A cystocele or rectocele is a mechanical problem that can be corrected only by surgery. Of course, the patient may choose to live with the symptoms if they are not too severe.

? WHAT IS CONTROVERSIAL ABOUT THE PROCEDURE?

Essentially, the technique used is the only controversy. One study notes that poor results in rectocele surgery may result from failure to evaluate the patient for all possible rectal diseases, because of the assumption that all of the reported problems stem from the rectocele.

Repair of Obstetric Laceration (5)

MORTALITY	MORBIDITY	CONTROVERSY
+	+	o

Repair of tears to the soft tissue of the pelvis following childbirth

? WHAT CONDITION DOES THE PROCEDURE TREAT?

Most childbirths go well, but the size of a baby's head is approximately the maximum that the female anatomy will permit, and it is not surprising that complete or partial tears of the **perineum** occur occasionally during delivery. A surgical cut in the perineum, called an **episiotomy**—which is done (theoretically) to prevent a large tear—seems to prevent some kinds of tears and increase the chance of others.

In part, obstetrical tears arise from one of the flaws in nature's design of the human species. The tissues of the floor of the pelvis are not as elastic as the tissue of the vagina. When a baby's head emerges from the birth canal, the tissues of the perineum often tear. If the person delivering the baby uses **forceps** or if there is some other problem with labor, a tear may be caused.

There is strong evidence that perineal tears are **iatrogenic**, or doctor-caused, problems. The position most convenient for the doctor, is that in which the woman is on her back with her feet up in stirrups. This is probably the worst possible anatomic position in which to deliver a baby. One study showed that only 0.9% of first-time mothers who did not have an episiotomy or deliver in the "stirrups" position had deep perineal **lacerations**. In contrast, such lacerations occurred in 27.9% of women who had both an episiotomy and delivered with their feet in stirrups. No correlation with age or the use of a midwife or a doctor as the delivery attendant was found; in short, the procedure is at fault.[1]

An episiotomy (see "Low-Forceps Delivery with Episiotomy," p. 177), a cut made in the soft tissues of the perineum, runs from the edge of the vagina as far into the tissues as needed to make an opening the doctor thinks is large enough. Episiotomies are highly debated among medical personnel involved with childbirth. Many argue that episiotomies reduce the risk of damage to the mother's bladder or rectum, and that the planned, straight-cut episiotomy heals more readily than a natural tear. Critics of the procedure contend that many women have unnecessary episiotomies. Indeed, there is great variation among hospitals in the use of episiotomies, without significant differences in frequency of perineal lacerations.[2]

? WHAT IS THE PROCEDURE?

Whether the laceration is the result of an episiotomy, an episiotomy that tore during childbirth, or a natural tear, it still must be repaired. This is done with a few stitches for small tears.

Obstetric lacerations are graded in four degrees, according to the extent of the tear. (Bear in mind throughout this discussion that tissue is three-dimensional—it has length, width, and depth.) In first-degree tears, none of the tissue is torn all the way through to the underlying **fascia** and muscle. In addition to skin and mucous membrane, second-degree tears involve the fascia and muscles of the perineal area but not the rectal **sphincter**. Third-degree tears extend through the skin, mucous membrane, and perineal area, and also involve the rectal sphincter. In fourth-degree tears, all layers are completely separated, extending through the rectal mucosa to expose the rectal **lumen**. In other words, in lesser-degree tears, some tissue of some of the layers remains connected, so that the soft tissue surrounding the vagina is at least partially intact—in a fourth-degree tear, it isn't.

? WHO PERFORMS THE PROCEDURE?

The procedure is performed by obstetrician-gynecologists, family practitioners who deliver babies, and occasionally by general surgeons. The repair of simple tears is within the competence of any physician.

? WHERE IS THE PROCEDURE PERFORMED?

The surgery is performed wherever the baby is born, if the location is suitable. (If, for example, the baby is born in a taxi, the mother will be moved to a hospital operating room or minor procedure room for the laceration repair.)

? WHAT ARE THE MORTALITY (DEATH) AND MORBIDITY (COMPLICATION) RATES?

The mortality rate from this procedure is zero. Any mortality arises from the events of childbirth, not the repair of the tear. The one exception is the most serious lacerations, graded as third or fourth degree. A 1989 study found that the use of episiotomies reduced the incidence of first- and second-degree lacerations, but increased the incidence of third- and fourth-degree ones.[3] The chief complications generally associated with an episiotomy are damage to the rectal and bladder sphincters, and infection.

? WHAT ARE THE OTHER COMPLICATIONS AND POSSIBLE SIDE EFFECTS?

There may be some loss of sensation in the perineum, which can lead to a loss of sexual pleasure. This is caused by cutting and tearing of nerves during the episiotomy. In many people, all of the nerves grow back, but this cannot be guaranteed in every case.

? IS THIS THE MOST APPROPRIATE PROCEDURE FOR THE CONDITION?

Obviously, if the perineum is torn to a degree that does not permit natural healing—that is, if the edges of the wound are not properly aligned—a repair is necessary.

? ARE THERE ALTERNATIVES TO THIS PROCEDURE?

If there is a laceration of the perineum too large to heal naturally, then there is no alternative. The only alternative to the episiotomy is not to do one unless and until it is clearly indicated.

? WHAT IS CONTROVERSIAL ABOUT THE PROCEDURE?

The procedure itself is not controversial in terms of safety; rather, controversy surrounds the care with which episiotomy is performed. As we mentioned earlier, results suggest that at least some of the more severe tears are iatrogenic—that is, doctor-caused—and would not have been as severe, or would not have occurred at all, if an episiotomy had not been done. There is some irony here, because the purpose of the episiotomy is to *prevent* severe tearing of tissue. If the use of episiotomies significantly increases the incidence of major tears (as it has been demonstrated to do), that purpose has not been met, at least for some women. The use of episiotomies is a judgment call: If the doctor successfully weighs the size of the baby's head against the degree of relaxation of vaginal tissue, and makes the cut in the proper depth or at the proper position, there will be either no tear or a lesser tear than would have occurred without the episiotomy. If she doesn't, the situation is made worse, not better. The statistical evidence suggests that this latter scenario happens more often.

Repair of Obstetric Laceration of the Rectum and Anus (50)

MORTALITY	MORBIDITY	CONTROVERSY
+	+	o

Repair of damage to the rectum and anus (anorectal region) occurring during childbirth

? WHAT CONDITION DOES THE PROCEDURE TREAT?

For information on **perineal** tears and episiotomies, see "Repair of Obstetric Laceration," p. 208.

Measurements of rectal pressure revealed hidden rectal injury in almost half of women who had had an episiotomy, despite the fact that neither the physician nor the patient thought that any injury had occurred.[1]

? WHAT IS THE PROCEDURE?

The technique varies according to the extent of injury and whether or not nerve damage is present. In cases in which the tear does not extend through all the tissue layers, the torn muscles and tissues are either overlapped or brought back together and sewn in place. Overlapping of the muscle layers, rather than simple closure of the tear, seems to give better long-term results.

Obstetric lacerations are graded in four degrees, according to the extent of the tear. (Bear in mind throughout this discussion that tissue is three-dimensional—it has length, width, and depth.) In first-degree tears, none of the tissue is torn all the way through to the underlying **fascia** and muscle. In addition to skin and mucous membrane, second-degree tears involve the fascia and muscles of the perineal area but not the rectal **sphincter**. Third-degree tears extend through the skin, mucous membrane, and perineal area, and also involve the rectal sphincter. In fourth-degree tears, all layers are completely separated, extending through the rectal mucosa to expose the rectal **lumen.** In other words, in lesser-degree tears, some tissue of some of the layers remains connected, so that the soft tissue surrounding the vagina is at least partially intact. This is not true of a fourth-degree tear.

For tears that extend through all tissue layers and have essentially destroyed the rectum, the colon is separated from the rectum through an abdominal incision, and a temporary **colostomy** is performed. The rectal stump is sewn shut on the inside, and the damage to the rectum is repaired using the **muscle overlap technique**. When the rectum is healed, the abdomen is re-opened, the rectal stump is opened, and the colon is reconnected. Both the new incision for the second stage of the repair and the colostomy are sewn shut.

When there is nerve damage, the torn nerve is located and repaired with sutures if possible, or with a nerve **graft** taken from elsewhere in the body. Depending upon the degree of damage and the way in which the nerve is torn, the work required can range from simple to very complicated.

Ideally, this procedure is done as soon as possible after delivery, to avoid the stress of additional surgery and anesthesia. However, the surgeon may choose to wait a few days and do the repair before the woman leaves the hospital.

A spinal or general anesthetic is used, depending upon the extent of the work to be done.

? WHO PERFORMS THE PROCEDURE?

This procedure is best performed by a board-certified colon-rectal surgeon.

? WHERE IS THE PROCEDURE PERFORMED?

This is an inpatient procedure that is always performed in the hospital.

? WHAT ARE THE MORTALITY (DEATH) AND MORBIDITY (COMPLICATION) RATES?

The standard technique for total tearing of the rectum and anus—a temporary colostomy and surgical closure of the wound, followed by reversal of the colostomy—has zero mortality and restores complete rectal continence in 78% of patients. It is partially successful in another 13%. The complication rate is 28.7%,[2] which is accounted for primarily by major damage to the nerves supplying the rectum.

Repair of the pelvic floor is not normally part of the operation, but one study has shown that 60% of women with rectal tears have damage to the pudendal nerve, located in the floor of the pelvis. This indicates that the surgeon should carefully check for damage to the pelvic floor and repair any that is found.[3] Repair of the nerve damage is relatively easy, provided that the damage is recognized.[4, 5]

? WHAT ARE THE OTHER COMPLICATIONS AND POSSIBLE SIDE EFFECTS?

In one study, 42% of women who had repairs of complete tears of the **perineum** in the anorectal region reported problems with incontinence of gas and stool (inability to control the release of gas and feces), even after repairs that were deemed successful.[6]

As with any procedure in which anesthesia is used, death from reaction to the anesthetic drugs, error on the part of the anesthetist, or machine failure is a remote possibility. (See Glossary, p. 309)

? IS THIS THE MOST APPROPRIATE PROCEDURE FOR THE CONDITION?

Yes, keeping in mind the need to look for and repair nerve damage.

? ARE THERE ALTERNATIVES TO THIS PROCEDURE?

This is a mechanical problem for which no nonsurgical treatment is available.

? WHAT IS CONTROVERSIAL ABOUT THE PROCEDURE?

The only thing really controversial about the procedure is the extent to which inappropriate medical intervention in the process of childbirth is the cause of the injury it attempts to repair. The most recent evidence suggests that nearly all these injuries are the result of current obstetrical practices, including episiotomies and stirrups.

Repair of Vessel (70)

MORTALITY	MORBIDITY	CONTROVERSY
+	+	o

Repair of a blood vessel damaged through disease or injury

? WHAT CONDITION DOES THE PROCEDURE TREAT?

This procedure is used to repair blood vessels that have been damaged by disease or injury, such as a gunshot wound, an auto accident, or a broken bone.

The body is adept at repairing damage to small vessels, but not good at all at repairing large veins or arteries. Failure to adequately repair damaged vessels (or microscopic ones that are responsible for blood supply to a critical area of an organ) can lead to the loss of a limb or an organ.

? WHAT IS THE PROCEDURE?

Depending upon the extent of the repair and other diseases or injuries, the patient is given a local, regional, or general anesthetic. The skin overlying the vessel to be operated on is shaved and scrubbed with soap and antiseptic. Often the surgeon will be able to repair the vessel through a cut that is the result of an accident or other trauma. In cases in which there is not an existing opening that gives access to the vessel, the surgeon makes an incision to reach it, by cutting through the skin, **fascia**, and muscle. Bleeding vessels are **ligated** or **cauterized**.

Large vessels that are big enough to be operated on with the naked eye are clamped and sewn back together. If part of the vessel has been lost, a replacement part of Dacron or **Silastic** may be used to replace it. Silastic **stents** are also used in microsurgery—when the vessels are too small to be repaired with unaided vision and an operative microscope must be used—to make sure that small vessels stay open once they are repaired. Success rates of 100% have been achieved in microsurgery both with and without stents.[1]

Use of vessels from **cadavers** to replace damaged vessels is gaining in popularity, but the extent to which rejection of the transplanted vessel might be a problem is not known. Studies in dogs indicate that rejection can be severe and lead to at least a 67% failure rate of donor vessels; however, use of the immunosuppressant azathioprine (brand name Imuran) has increased the success rate to 89%. However, use of Imuran may promote the growth of cancers that are already present by interfering with the body's ability to destroy cancer cells.[2]

? WHO PERFORMS THE PROCEDURE?

Repair of large vessels is within the competence of general surgeons. Microsurgical repair of blood vessels should be performed by a vascular surgeon with special training in microsurgery.

? WHERE IS THE PROCEDURE PERFORMED?

Depending upon the procedure, the extent of the repair, and the patient's other injuries or conditions, this procedure can be done in the outpatient or inpatient departments of a hospital, an outpatient surgery facility, or a well-equipped doctor's office.

? WHAT ARE THE MORTALITY (DEATH) AND MORBIDITY (COMPLICATION) RATES?

There is essentially no mortality resulting from vessel repair itself. The chief complication is failure of the repair. A 1989 study of microsurgical repairs of leg vessels indicated that **patency**—the condition of being wide open—fell steadily during the first 90 days, from a high of 86.1% immediately after surgery to a low of 68.4% after 5.4 months; further, there seemed to be little change in patency after the first 90 days.[3] This suggests that the final failure (that is, loss of patency) rate is in the range of 32% of microsurgical repairs attempted, and this figure is probably lower with larger vessels.

The surgical folk wisdom that it is important to **suture** all layers of the vessel wall (to avoid plugging of the vessel by flaps of the innermost layers) has not been proven in animal studies.[4] The conventional technique of suturing all layers seemed to produce a higher long-term patency rate.

? WHAT ARE THE OTHER COMPLICATIONS AND POSSIBLE SIDE EFFECTS?

Gangrene and loss of limbs can occur after unsuccessful repairs that are not diagnosed and corrected.

As with any procedure in which anesthesia is used, death from reaction to the anesthetic drugs, error on the part of the anesthetist, or machine failure is a remote possibility. (See Glossary, p. 309)

? IS THIS THE MOST APPROPRIATE PROCEDURE FOR THE CONDITION?

Particularly in cases where a limb might otherwise be lost, it is reasonable to attempt vessel repair. If vessel repair fails, amputation can always be done.

? ARE THERE ALTERNATIVES TO THIS PROCEDURE?

Essentially no. Blood supply is critical and large vessels that are completely severed do not heal themselves.

? WHAT IS CONTROVERSIAL ABOUT THE PROCEDURE?

There is little controversy surrounding the procedure. New techniques are being researched.

Revision of Vascular Procedure (69)

MORTALITY	MORBIDITY	CONTROVERSY
–	–	o

- The reported **MORTALITY** rate for this procedure is difficult to estimate because the procedure itself does not necessarily cause death. Emergency vascular repairs carry mortality rates as high as 50%.

- **INFECTIONS** are a major problem with all vascular procedures. One study discovered that 79% of replacement grafts contained bacteria. Wound complications are another risk of this procedure.

Reoperation on a vessel for a repair or other surgery that did not work the first time

? WHAT CONDITION DOES THE PROCEDURE TREAT?

This procedure is used to redo repairs and replacement **grafts** of blood vessels that have been damaged by disease or injury, such asa gunshot wound, an auto accident, or a broken bone.

The body is adept at repairing damage to small vessels, but not good at all at repairing large veins or arteries. Failure to adequately repair damaged vessels (or microscopic ones that are responsible for blood supply to a critical area of an organ) can lead to the loss of the limb or the organ.

? WHAT IS THE PROCEDURE?

Depending upon the extent of the repair and other diseases or injuries, the patient is given a local, regional, or general anesthetic. The skin overlying the vessel to be operated on is shaved and scrubbed with soap and antiseptic. The surgeon makes an incision to reach it, cutting through the skin, **fascia,** and muscle to get to the vessel needing repair. Bleeding vessels are **ligated** or **cauterized**.

See "Repair of Vessel," p. 212.

? WHO PERFORMS THE PROCEDURE?

When a previous vessel repair has failed and a reoperation is necessary, it is best handled by a board-certified vascular surgeon.

? WHERE IS THE PROCEDURE PERFORMED?

Depending upon the procedure, the extent of the repair, and the patient's other injuries or conditions, this procedure can be done on an outpatient or inpatient basis in a hospital, in an outpatient surgery center, or in a well-equipped doctor's office.

? WHAT ARE THE MORTALITY (DEATH) AND MORBIDITY (COMPLICATION) RATES?

A recent Japanese study warns, "Since vascular disease is always progressive and a perfect vascular **prosthesis** has yet to be developed, postoperative complications are almost inevitable." Further, the study indicates that about 8.4% of patients with initially successful repairs will have late graft (replacement blood vessel) failure.[1] Some vascular procedures have a reoperation rate as high as 75%.[2] A Hungarian study of **revisions** following cardiovascular surgery shows a mortality rate of 12.5% and a failure rate of 17.5%.[3]

Mortality is hard to estimate for this, actually a catch-all group of procedures. Doctors bill insurers for services under procedure codes. Some procedures that are infrequently performed or are so variable that they defy more detailed classification are lumped together, like this one: It applies to any revision to any prior vascular procedure, if the revision is not clearly described by a separate code.

In vascular repairs and reconstructions, and re-operations for them, death rarely results directly from the repair, but instead results from failure to reestablish adequate blood flow to the organ or limb in question. Universally, in terms of morbidity and mortality, the results for second and later operations are worse than for initial operations, and emergency procedures invariably carry a high mortality.

Take, for instance, a late complication of vascular reconstruction—formation of a **pseudoaneurysm** at the suture line. The mortality rate for reoperation for this complication is 2.08% when the procedure is done electively, and 50% for emergency procedures. The authors of the study cited recommend early operation, for obvious reasons.[4]

The need for revision because of bleeding after surgery ranges from 2.8% to 4.2%, depending upon the operative site. There are significantly more complications, mainly infections, if the reoperation is done more than 48 hours after the first procedure.[5]

A 1989 study of microsurgical repairs of leg vessels indicated that **patency** (how open or unobstructed the vessel is) fell steadily during the first 90 days from a high of 86.1% right after surgery to a low of 68.4% after 5.4 months; further, there seemed to be little change in patency after the first 90 days.[6] This suggests that the final failure of patency rate is in the range of 32% of microsurgical repairs attempted, and this figure is probably lower with larger vessels.

The surgical folk wisdom that it is important to **suture** all layers of the vessel wall to avoid plugging by flaps of the innermost layer has not been proven in animal studies.[7] However, the conventional technique of suturing all layers seems to produce a higher long-term patency rate.

? WHAT ARE THE OTHER COMPLICATIONS AND POSSIBLE SIDE EFFECTS?

In one study bacteria were cultured from 79% of grafts that were removed during the revision procedure. **Subclinical infection** may be a reason for graft failure.[8] The rate of deep infection following vessel reconstruction is about 1.2%.[9]

Vascular procedures are often done in attempts to prevent loss of a leg resulting from inadequate blood flow. If the first procedure fails, and one or more attempts at reconstructing the blood vessel(s) are required, it can be much harder for the surgeon to perform a successful below-the-knee amputation if it is needed later. This is because an adequate flow of blood to the stump is needed for postoperative healing.[10]

Wound complications occur in up to 62.5% of patients who have had revised vascular procedures in the groin area. In the attempt to repair or replace the vessel that preceded the revision procedure, use of the **sartorius muscle**, located in the groin/hip region, to cover the graft reduces later complications significantly.[11]

As with any procedure in which anesthesia is used, death from reaction to the anesthetic drugs, error on the part of the anesthetist, or machine failure is a remote possibility. (See Glossary, p. 309)

? IS THIS THE MOST APPROPRIATE PROCEDURE FOR THE CONDITION?

Yes, particularly in cases where a limb might otherwise be lost, it is reasonable to attempt vessel repair many times. If it fails, amputation can always be done, although arguably it is not an ideal solution.

? ARE THERE ALTERNATIVES TO THIS PROCEDURE?

Percutaneous atherectomy, a procedure that involves removal of a clot from a vessel through the skin, has been used to treat some obstructed grafts, with a major complication rate of 7.1% and a mortality rate of 0.89%.[12] Blood supply is critical and damaged large vessels rarely heal themselves, so there is generally a need for some sort of surgical intervention in the case of graft failures.

? WHAT IS CONTROVERSIAL ABOUT THE PROCEDURE?

There is little that is controversial about the procedure, which is undertaken only when a prior attempt has obviously failed. New techniques are being researched.

Right Hemicolectomy (46)

MORTALITY	MORBIDITY	CONTROVERSY
–	–	o

- The **MORTALITY** rate for this procedure is 5.7% to 12.5% in cancer patients. Emergency procedures have a reported mortality of 29%.
- **INFECTION**, formation of **adhesions**, and postoperative bleeding are associated with right hemicolectomy.

Removal of the right (ascending) half of the **colon**

? WHAT CONDITION DOES THE PROCEDURE TREAT?

A right hemicolectomy is performed for cancer of the colon; for trauma to the colon (from gunshot wounds, for example) that is too damaging to permit repair; for **Crohn's disease** and **ulcerative colitis**, two bowel diseases of unknown origin that lead to destruction of the intestinal wall and formation of scar tissue; for uncontrollable bleeding from the left side of the colon; for severe **diverticulitis** (which is more common in the aged and possibly resulting from a lack of fiber in the diet); for right-sided pelvic tumors or masses which require removal; and for radiation injury to the bowel, which follows the use of radiation for cancer or other conditions.

For a description of the colon and its anatomy and function, see "Left Hemicolectomy," p. 165.

? WHAT IS THE PROCEDURE?

The patient is put under general anesthesia with a tube placed down the windpipe. The abdomen, which will have been shaved the night before, is washed with soap and antiseptic, and draped so that only the planned area of the incision is exposed. An incision is made with a scalpel about one-half inch to the right of the navel and is continued to about three inches above the navel and one inch below. The fat, **fascia**, muscles, and **peritoneum** are opened one by one, and small bleeding vessels tied off or **cauterized** along the way. The **transverse colon** is located just above the middle of the incision. The small intestines and the **omentum** (a fatty "apron" that hangs down from the bottom of the stomach and seems to have the role of plugging intestinal leaks and walling off **abscesses**[1]) are pushed up toward the **diaphragm** with moist gauze pads.

The right colon is located and, beginning just above the appendix, is cut free of the fascia that supports it. The dissection is continued with scissors, or by tearing the membrane with a finger (called blunt dissection). The rationale for using the finger is to avoid damaging the critical structures behind the right colon—the right **ureter**, the **inferior vena cava**, and a portion of the **duodenum**—which could be injured by scalpel or scissors. If the operation is for cancer, the omentum is also removed to make sure that any cancer cells that may have spread to it are removed, and to eliminate some lymph drainage that could spread cancer. For other purposes, the surgeon may use part of the omentum to provide "patches" for **lesions** in the colon to be retained.

The colon is encircled by rubber tubes or tapes and pulled up and to the right, freeing it from all the surrounding structures except the **mesentery**, a large membrane that, among other things, supports the blood supply to the intestines. Arteries and veins feeding the portion of the bowel that is to be removed are identified, **ligated**, and cut. The colon and small intestine to be retained are held in noncrushing clamps, and the colon and portion of the small intestine to be removed (usually eight to 10 inches of the **ileum**) are cut and removed. The small and large intestines are sewn together at a joint called the **anastomosis,** using any one of a number of techniques—perhaps the most complex and time-consuming is placing a number of outside-in stitches in the portions of the intestines to be reconnected. Staples may be used as well. There are a number of closure techniques available. Surgical staplers seem to cut a good deal of time from the procedure, which otherwise involves a great deal of careful stitching of the intestines.[2]

When the surgeon is satisfied with the anastomosis, he sews back together the cut mesentery and lays the intestines back in the abdomen. If the greater omentum has been retained, it is laid back over the intestines as well. Any packing is removed, and the various layers of the intestinal wall are closed separately. A dressing is applied, and the patient is taken to the recovery room. Either in the recovery room or in the operating room, a **nasogastric tube** will be inserted through the nose to remove the stomach secretions—about a quart a day—until it is clear that the intestines can handle them. The pathologist will examine the removed intestine for cancer or other diseases.

❓ WHO PERFORMS THE PROCEDURE?

This procedure is performed by a general surgeon.

❓ WHERE IS THE PROCEDURE PERFORMED?

This is a major procedure that must be performed in a hospital.

❓ WHAT ARE THE MORTALITY (DEATH) AND MORBIDITY (COMPLICATION) RATES?

This is not a trivial procedure. Mortality is low in patients operated on under ideal conditions, but the diseases or injuries that require removal of the right colon frequently leave such people in poor health.

Operative mortality rates ranging from 5.7% to 12.5% in cancer patients have been reported.[3, 4] Mortality and complication rates of 7% have been reported in another study.[5] Complications with the anastomosis range around 4%. Mortality in patients being treated for radiation injury to the colon can be as high as 14%.[6] For patients receiving emergency right hemicolectomies for trauma, the mortality rate has been reported as high as 29% and the complication rate 11%.[7]

❓ WHAT ARE THE OTHER COMPLICATIONS AND POSSIBLE SIDE EFFECTS?

As with any abdominal procedure, infections, formation of **adhesions,** and postoperative bleeding may occur. The anastomosis may fail to heal in patients whose nutritional status is poor or who have widespread cancer. **Hyperalimentation** may help speed healing, especially in patients with radiation injury to the bowel or Crohn's disease.[8] There is some evidence that intravenous feeding with solutions of branched-chain amino acids (types of the building blocks of protein that have "Y" shapes in their molecular structure) is helpful in fighting severe infections.[9]

As with any procedure in which anesthesia is used, death from reaction to the anesthetic drugs, error on the part of the anesthetist, or machine failure is a remote possibility. (See Glossary, p. 309)

? IS THIS THE MOST APPROPRIATE PROCEDURE FOR THE CONDITION?

See "Left Hemicolectomy," p. 165.

? ARE THERE ALTERNATIVES TO THIS PROCEDURE?

At present, there are few alternatives. Diversion colostomies, which route the flow of food around diseased sections of bowel, have proven far less satisfactory than removal of the affected bowel. The latter is the more prudent course in dealing with real or potential malignancy in any case. The patient is likely to be more comfortable with complete removal, because bowel deprived of short-chain fatty acids derived from foods becomes irritated and inflamed.

? WHAT IS CONTROVERSIAL ABOUT THE PROCEDURE?

See "Left Hemicolectomy," p. 165.

Rotator Cuff Repair (89)

MORTALITY	MORBIDITY	CONTROVERSY
+	+	o

- Although few **COMPLICATIONS** are associated with the operation itself, reports of less than satisfactory outcomes range from 3% to 29%. Many factors, including delay of treatment, appear to affect this rate.

Surgical repair of damage to the soft tissues of the shoulder joint

? WHAT CONDITION DOES THE PROCEDURE TREAT?

This procedure treats injuries to the soft tissues—muscles, **ligaments**, and **tendons**, plus the membranes lining the joints—that make up the rotator cuff. The rotator cuff holds the ball of the shoulder's ball-and-socket joint in the **glenoid cavity** on the shoulder blade.

The anatomy of the shoulder joint is deceptive. If you feel your shoulder, the upper bone of the arm (**humerus**) appears to attach to the end of the collarbone (**clavicle**), but this is an illusion created by coverage of the upper part of the joint by the **deltoid muscle**. The "ball" of the ball-and-socket shoulder is much farther back on the shoulder than it appears to be from the outside, and actually fits into a depression on the front part of the shoulder blade called the glenoid cavity.

Four muscles—the **supraspinatus**, the **infraspinatus**, the **teres minor**, and the **subcapsularis**—hold the shoulder joint together on the top and sides, in cooperation with a few other muscles and many tendons. This is not at all obvious, because the muscles that do the work are covered by the deltoid at the back and side and by the large chest muscle that runs from the clavicle to just below the nipple (**pectoralis major**) in the front.

The shoulder is one of nature's Rube Goldberg devices. As the author of an anatomy text for medical students puts it, the stability of the joint has been sacrificed to achieve its wide range of motion.[1] There is far less support from below the shoulder joint than at the top, back, and sides; this means that the entire joint can be ripped partially or completely apart by a hard downward pull, or by any other motion that has the effect of forcing the humerus down out of the glenoid cavity.

The result is a rotator cuff tear, a source of much consternation to athlete and couch potato alike. These tears seldom heal naturally with good results, and either **arthroscopic** or **open surgery** (that requiring an incision) is usually indicated.

Surgery is necessary to restore mobility to the joint:

After a tear, pain limits mobility; as a result of combined immobilization and irritation of the joint, **adhesions** form within seven to 10 days. The adhesions are so severe within three weeks that the joint may be completely immobile—hence, the term "frozen shoulder."

? WHAT IS THE PROCEDURE?

This procedure can be performed either as an open procedure or through a small surgical interjoint telescope called an arthroscope. Current medical practice is tending towards repairing tears arthroscopically, and reserving the open procedure for cases in which the surgeon cannot grasp, trim, staple, **suture**, rivet,[2] or pin everything that needs repair through the **arthroscope**. In short, an open procedure is used if the damage cannot be repaired through the arthroscope or one of the "brute force" maneuvers characteristic of orthopedic surgery, such as stretching a muscle to get the tendon back into proper position. Freeze-dried **cadaver** transplants can be used effectively in cuff repair,[3] as can Dacron tendon **grafts**. (A freeze-dried **cadaver** transplant is a tendon or ligament that has been taken from a dead person and freeze-dried in a process that involves placing the tissue in a vacuum and letting the water content "boil off" at room temperature. The process does far less damage than many other means of preservation. When the tissue is transplanted, it absorbs water from the saline solution it is soaked in before the procedure and from the fluid in the joint, regaining its original flexibility and stretch properties.) If it is known from x rays, diagnostic arthroscopy, or the nature of the symptoms that the procedure must be an open one, then the usual approach is through the middle of the deltoid muscle, which gives the surgeon access to the front, top, and back of the joint.

In the more common arthroscopic procedure, the patient's chest, shoulders, and back are shaved if necessary and, with the patient under general anesthesia, the skin over the shoulder is washed with soap and antiseptic, and the arthroscope is introduced through a small incision (usually less than an inch long). Bleeding is controlled with an **electrocautery device** or the **ligation** of a vessel, if needed. If access and leverage are sufficient through the arthroscope, the surgeon can irrigate the joint to remove tissue fragments, shave roughened bones and tendons, reattach tendons to bones and muscles, suture and staple torn tissues, and generally do everything that is required to repair the joint.

When the repairs are finished, the wound—open or arthroscopic—is closed with sutures and bandaged. The patient is usually given an arm sling that holds the joint in an anatomically correct position and allows only limited movement; sometimes a shoulder cast is used. **Anti-inflammatory medications** block or slow the formation of adhesions. Vigorous physical therapy is started as soon as the extent of healing permits it.

? WHO PERFORMS THE PROCEDURE?

This procedure should be done only by a board-certified orthopedic surgeon who has extensive experience in shoulder injuries and a statistically good record of results. Even with the best surgical care, complete recovery from this injury cannot be guaranteed, and poor surgical skill dramatically increases the odds of a poor result. If the procedure will be done arthroscopically, the surgeon should have additional training in use of the arthroscope.

? WHERE IS THE PROCEDURE PERFORMED?

Depending upon the extent of the tear, this surgery can be performed on an inpatient or outpatient basis in a hospital, or in a sports medicine clinic or outpatient surgery clinic. The facility should either have, or have connections with, a good physical therapy department or group.

? WHAT ARE THE MORTALITY (DEATH) AND MORBIDITY (COMPLICATION) RATES?

We were unable to locate any reports of mortality arising from rotator cuff repair (as opposed to mortality associated with anesthesia for it) in the medical literature since 1975.

The chief "complication" is failure of the procedure to produce a satisfactory result. This happens 3%[4] to 29%[5] of the time.

Studies suggest that, for the most complete recovery of shoulder function, the operation should be performed within three weeks from the time of injury.[6] Some joint deformity can be expected in about 10% of the cases repaired with a Dacron graft, even if function is satisfactory.[7] Some loss of strength can be expected in up to about 70% of repairs.[8]

? WHAT ARE THE OTHER COMPLICATIONS AND POSSIBLE SIDE EFFECTS?

Arthritis can be a late complication of some repair techniques (in the cited study, an average of 13.2 years after the repair); although some (37%) may require reoperation,[9] virtually all cases can be treated successfully. Damage to the origin of the deltoid muscle may occur, requiring reoperation.[10] Second and third operations are likely to give poor functional results, even though about three-fourths of these operations result in the reduction of pain.[11] In a rupture of the cuff, the tendon of the supraspinatus muscle in the upper back may snap back, and surgery on the supraspinatus muscle may be required to avoid excessive tension on the tendon. This is actually a result of a type of injury and not an operative complication, but failure to recognize the necessity for it may lead to a poor result.[12]

Damage to the spinal accessory nerve has been reported, with successful microsurgical repair in 43% of patients, partial success in 43%, and failure in 14%.[13]

As with any procedure in which anesthesia is used, death from reaction to the anesthetic drugs, error on the part of the anesthetist, or machine failure is a remote possibility. (See Glossary, p. 309)

? IS THIS THE MOST APPROPRIATE PROCEDURE FOR THE CONDITION?

Given the tendency of rotator cuff damage to progress to restricted motion, and possibly to frozen shoulder if left untreated, early repair is the only realistic option for anything other than small tears. For very small tears, a reasonable policy is one of "watchful waiting," to assess healing and development of problems.

? ARE THERE ALTERNATIVES TO THIS PROCEDURE?

The arthroscopic and open procedures are alternatives to each other, but there is no alternative to surgical treatment for anything other than minor tears.

? WHAT IS CONTROVERSIAL ABOUT THE PROCEDURE?

The chief sources of controversy concern ways to reduce the high percentage of unsatisfactory results. So far there have been no dramatic advances other than the arthroscope. Use of **carbon-filament grafts**, which have enormous strength compared with other **prosthetic** replacements, have not been successful to date.[14]

Septoplasty (99)

MORTALITY	MORBIDITY	CONTROVERSY
+	+	o

Repair or revision of the **septum** between the two nostrils

? WHAT CONDITION DOES THE PROCEDURE TREAT?

Septoplasties are surgical **revisions,** or reoperations, of the wall between the two nostrils, performed to improve breathing, relieve nasal obstructions, remove benign and malignant tumors, and reconstruct the septum after extensive surgery or accidents. A septoplasty may also be required as part of a rhinoplasty (commonly referred to as a "nose job"), which is usually done for cosmetic purposes.

? WHAT IS THE PROCEDURE?

Under a general anesthetic, a **speculum** is inserted into the nostril on which the surgeon is working. An incision is made in the tissue covering the septum. Depending upon the degree of deformity and the location, either the **cartilage** near the tip of the nose or the nasal spine bone (near the skull) is shaved or trimmed, or broken, carved, and repositioned. Major bleeding vessels are closed with **sutures** or **electrocautery**, or an attempt is made to stop all bleeding with fine sutures and electrocautery if the **microsurgery** is used.

Generally, the surgeon can do all that is necessary by working through the nostril that is most obstructed. Very rarely, work on both sides of the septum is required (for example, when there is abnormal growth of bone that requires complicated reshaping near the union of the skull and nasal spine). As soon as the septum is properly positioned and bleeding has been controlled, vaseline-coated gauze packing or plastic splints are used to hold the septum in place while it heals. The patient is taken to the recovery room and then to his room.

Use of gauze packing is associated with significantly more postoperative discomfort than splints, and its removal may be painful. Gauze can be removed when there is enough healing to prevent bleeding upon its removal. How soon it is removed depends upon the surgeon, but rarely is it left in as long as a week.

? WHO PERFORMS THE PROCEDURE?

Both otolaryngologists and plastic surgeons can perform this procedure. If breathing problems or repair of a broken nose in the absence of serious damage to the overlying skin is the reason for surgery, it is probably best to have it done by an otolaryngologist. If cosmetic repairs are needed, if skin surgery is required in addition to the septoplasty, or if septoplasty is being combined with a rhinoplasty, it is probably best to have the procedure done by a plastic surgeon. In any case, it is best to use a board-certified specialist.

? WHERE IS THE PROCEDURE PERFORMED?

If the surgeon has to use gauze packing, this procedure is usually performed in the inpatient department of a hospital. If it is possible to avoid packing, the procedure can be done in the outpatient department of a hospital, an outpatient surgery center, or a well-equipped doctor's office. Aside from serious complications, the only reason for hospitalization is pain control, and the chief cause of severe pain is packing.

? WHAT ARE THE MORTALITY (DEATH) AND MORBIDITY (COMPLICATION) RATES?

Mortality from this relatively minor procedure is essentially zero, and more likely to be related to allergic reactions to the drugs used (anesthetics, antibiotics, or **vasoconstrictors**) than to the procedure itself. In a five- to nine-year follow-up study, 63% to 69% of patients expressed satisfaction with the results of septoplasty or an alternative procedure called **submucosal resection**, which involves similar techniques. Ten percent of patients reported problems with crusting, which can be dealt with by gentle and careful removal of the crusts that form following the procedure.[1, 2]

Patient satisfaction with the procedure is perhaps not the best measure of results, because objective measurements of airway flow correlate only weakly with the patient's sense of the degree to which breathing is easier. Large measurable changes in airflow can produce only a small sense of relief.[3-6] Subjective patient satisfaction following the procedure is highly correlated with the technical skill of the surgeon as perceived by his colleagues, suggesting that better surgical technique can achieve better results, which are felt by the patient but not measured by objective tests currently in use. Of course, it is possible that the more technically skilled surgeons have better bedside manners,[7] but the persistence of perceived differences after several years seems to underscore that more than bedside manner is involved.

Use of a technique that avoids nasal packing produced complication rates of 0.98%. The complications seen were one **perforation** of the septum and one **hematoma**.[8]

? WHAT ARE THE OTHER COMPLICATIONS AND POSSIBLE SIDE EFFECTS?

Septoplasties are not followed by infections to an unusual extent. The defense mechanisms of the nasal passages, which have to deal with airborne bacteria and viruses, may help to avoid them. If infections occur and spread to the cartilage and bone (the nasal spine), they can be problematic.[9, 10] However, **toxic shock syndrome**, a rare but potentially fatal infection and reaction to toxins produced by bacteria, has been reported following septoplasties in which either gauze packing or plastic nasal splints were used following surgery.[11, 12]

Complications seem to be associated more with the use of gauze packing than with the surgery itself. Packing expands as it absorbs blood and exerts pressure on healing tissues, which reduces the blood supply and may delay healing. In addition, blood-soaked packing at close to body temperature is a fine growth medium for bacteria. Microsurgical techniques that locate and **ligate** bleeding vessels[13] and the use of biological glues to seal vessels are two means of avoiding the problems associated with packing.[14] Patients should probably ask the surgeon whether she plans to use packing and why, and what alternatives might be considered. Even if the surgeon does not plan to use packing, it may be necessary if bleeding cannot be controlled, but it should be left in no longer than necessary.

Damage to the nasopalatine nerve can occur if much of the surgery has to be done in the front of the nose —a complication that can usually, but not always, be avoided by proper technique. Damage to this nerve results in pain, numbness, tingling, or a combination of all three, as well as diminished sensation in the upper part of the nose.[15, 16]

Complications tend to develop if any of the air pockets that surround the nasal structures in the skull (**sinuses**) are opacified (completely filled with something other than air or fluid) or completely fluid-filled, as shown on a sinus x ray. Air and fluid are transparent to x rays and show up as dark on x-ray film, which is a negative; a completely opacified sinus, filled with pus or inflamed tissue, or both, shows up as a bright spot.) Some sinus problems can be dealt with by inserting drainage tubes or otherwise clearing out the sinuses as part of the septoplasty procedure. In 4% of patients, however, the seriousness of possible complications—chiefly infection and delayed healing—indicates that surgery should be postponed until the sinus problem has been cleared up. However, 96% of patients can have either the septoplasty or septoplasty plus sinus drainage as part of a single procedure without problems.[17]

In children between the ages of six and 12 years, there is a tendency for cartilage and bone to regenerate after surgery, which may require a second operation. Because this is the result of a natural process of healing following surgery, nothing can be done to prevent it. This phenomenon has not been noted in adults.[18]

Acoustic studies of the nasal passages have shown that swelling of the nasal **mucosa**—in this case, the outermost layer of tissue that lines the sinus cavities and the nose—while not a complication strictly speaking, contributes much more to blockage of breathing in the upper part of the nose than do deformities of the septum. This is because even in the normal nose, the passages narrow dramatically from the nostrils to the entry of the nasal passages into the skull. Patients whose main problem is swelling of the mucosa in the upper part of the nose may not experience the relief they expect from septoplasty, even if they have septal problems as well as allergies. Therefore, for the surgery to produce a good result, the doctor must assess what factors might be contributing to obstructed breathing. She must treat any allergic problems that may be present, in addition to addressing problems with the septum.[19, 20]

Cosmetic deformities may result from septum surgery. Although these are correctable by plastic surgery, careful surgical technique and attention to the shape of the septum can usually avoid them.[21]

As with any procedure in which anesthesia is used, death from reaction to the anesthetic drugs, error on the part of the anesthetist, or machine failure is a remote possibility. (See Glossary, p. 309)

? IS THIS THE MOST APPROPRIATE PROCEDURE FOR THE CONDITION?

If there is genuine obstruction of breathing or a need to repair a broken nose or cosmetic deformity that is associated with a problem with the septum, this procedure is appropriate. As we explained earlier, there is some question about the merits of performing the procedure in children.

? ARE THERE ALTERNATIVES TO THIS PROCEDURE?

When septal problems and allergies or persistent sinus infections occur together, treatment of the allergy or the sinus infection may give the patient sufficient relief, so that surgery is not needed. The choice depends upon the patient's subjective feeling of relief, and should be left to the patient. Allergies or chronic sinus infections that add to a septal problem should be treated even if the patient opts for surgery. If you require this type of surgery and a plastic surgeon is doing the surgery, it would be useful for you to see an allergy specialist or otolaryngologist for treatment of allergies or chronic sinus infections.

If there are no associated allergies or chronic sinus infections, the patient has a mechanical problem with the structure of the nose. Like most other mechanical problems with the body, there is really no nonsurgical alternative, assuming a correction is required to give a degree of relief that will satisfy the patient. Significant improvements in the ease of breathing after this surgery, however, can be measured by instruments but often are not noticeable to the patient. It is important for you to ask the doctor how much measurable improvement has occurred and how it compares with the normal "easy breathing" expected for a person of your age and gender.

? WHAT IS CONTROVERSIAL ABOUT THE PROCEDURE?

The only significant controversy concerns how early in life the operation can be performed without causing problems with the normal growth of the nose. Distortions in the growing nose caused by a septoplasty performed too early can be repaired by further surgery. This involves subjecting a child to another operation, however. The general recommendation is to try to treat problems nonsurgically (with medications that relieve congestion and ease breathing, such as antihistamines and decongestants) until the growth of the nose is complete, unless breathing problems are severe enough to make the operation worth the risk of later problems.[22] Studies with cats, however, suggest that the fear of growth distortion may be unfounded; the degree of applicability to humans is unclear.[23]

Shoulder Arthroplasty (74)

MORTALITY	MORBIDITY	CONTROVERSY
+	+	o

LAY TITLE: Surgical creation of an artificial shoulder joint

Resurfacing, repair, or replacement of the shoulder joint

? WHAT CONDITION DOES THE PROCEDURE TREAT?

This procedure treats arthritis of the shoulder and injuries to, or deformities of, the shoulder joint, which produce pain or limitations of motion or function. These include **rheumatoid arthritis**, **osteoarthritis**, posttraumatic arthritis (any form of arthritis that appears following trauma), **rotator cuff arthropathy**,

avascular **necrosis**, failed shoulder **prosthesis**, and **congenital** dislocation.[1]

For a discussion of the anatomy of the shoulder joint, see "Rotator Cuff Repair," p. 218.

It is very easy to design a joint that is more stable than the natural shoulder joint. It is virtually impossible to design a stable artificial joint that has the same range of motion as the anatomical joint.[2] Relief of pain and recovery of a large range of motion are possible, however.[3]

? WHAT IS THE PROCEDURE?

Technology in this area is still evolving, as with joint replacement in general.[4] Total shoulder replacement was described as "frankly experimental" as late as 1983.[5] When the musculature of the shoulder is defective for one reason or another (because of a congenital deformity, gunshot wound, or auto accident, for example), modifications of the artificial parts can replace some of the function of the muscle in holding the shoulder joint together, at the expense of some loss of motion (because inflexible metal and plastic are being used to replace flexible muscles and tendons).[6] Either the head of the **humerus**, the **glenoid cavity**, or both, can be replaced with artificial parts (which may be all metal or partly metal).[7]

The patient's chest, shoulders, and back are shaved if necessary. With the patient under general anesthesia, the skin over the shoulder is washed with soap and antiseptic. The incision site is draped and the surgeon begins the process of disassembling the shoulder joint.

Bleeding is controlled with an **electrocautery device** or the **ligation** of vessels if needed. In addition to exposing, resurfacing, or replacing the glenoid cavity and the top of the humerus, the surgeon will also remove tissue fragments, shave roughened bones and tendons, reattach tendons to bones and muscles, **suture** and staple torn tissues, and generally do everything that can be done, provided access and leverage are sufficient. When the repairs are finished, the incision is sutured shut and bandaged. The patient is usually given an arm sling that holds the joint in an anatomically correct position and allows only limited movement; sometimes a shoulder cast is used. Vigorous physical therapy is started as soon as the extent of healing permits it.

? WHO PERFORMS THE PROCEDURE?

This procedure should be done only by a board-certified orthopedic surgeon who has extensive experience in treating shoulder injuries and a statistically good record of results. Even with the best surgical care, complete recovery from this injury cannot be guaranteed, and poor surgical skill dramatically increases the odds of a poor result.

? WHERE IS THE PROCEDURE PERFORMED?

This is major surgery that is always done on an inpatient basis in a hospital.

? WHAT ARE THE MORTALITY (DEATH) AND MORBIDITY (COMPLICATION) RATES?

Mortality is related primarily to anesthesia, not to the procedure. As with any procedure in which anesthesia is used, death from reaction to the anesthetic drugs, error on the part of the anesthetist, or machine failure is a remote possibility. (See Glossary, p. 309)

Complications requiring reoperation can occur in up to 7% to 9% of patients.[8, 9] Accidental fracture of the humerus, the glenoid cavity, or both, can occur during

surgery in up to 6.2% of patients.[10] Overall complication rates as high as 16.9% have been reported.[11]

After 11 years, 27% of shoulder replacements will have failed and will require repair or additional surgery.[12] Relief of pain may be inadequate in 10% to 20% of patients.

Mechanical failure seems to be rarer in shoulder replacements than in artificial hips. The most common problems are loosening of the glenoid cavity component;[13] in some series of patients, this complication has been held to under 1% by careful surgical technique.[14]

? WHAT ARE THE OTHER COMPLICATIONS AND POSSIBLE SIDE EFFECTS?

Damage to the shoulder joint during conservative surgery—attempts to resurface (or plane off and make smooth) the glenoid cavity—may force a total shoulder replacement.[15]

For reasons that are not clearly understood, shoulder replacements are prone to trigger the formation of bone in areas of the shoulder where there should be none—more so than with knee or hip replacements. Formation of ectopic, or out-of-position, bone is quite frequent but does not cause significant problems in most patients. The chief difficulty is limitation of the range of motion, which can be treated by surgically trimming the excess bone if the limitations are unacceptable.[16]

Infection and nerve damage rates of zero have been achieved.[17]

? IS THIS THE MOST APPROPRIATE PROCEDURE FOR THE CONDITION?

Yes, if more conservative repair techniques (see the alternative procedures discussed below) have not corrected the problem.

? ARE THERE ALTERNATIVES TO THIS PROCEDURE?

A procedure called **shoulder arthrodesis**, which entails a partial fixation of the shoulder joint, is much less acceptable than a functioning artificial shoulder, but may be the only available option if infection or failure of a shoulder replacement makes another try impossible.[18]

Resurfacing of the glenoid cavity and replacement of only the glenoid cavity with an artificial component are possible alternatives, but pain relief with both seems to be less than with total shoulder replacement.[19, 20]

A useful way to think about the various alternatives, which applies to a number of other procedures as well, is this: It is generally possible to try a more radical operation if a conservative one fails; the reverse is almost never true. If resurfacing of the glenoid cavity does not give a good result, a total shoulder replacement is still possible. This logic may be a useful guide for both the patient and the surgeon, unless the patient's health makes a single, definitive operation absolutely essential.

? WHAT IS CONTROVERSIAL ABOUT THE PROCEDURE?

There is little that is controversial about this procedure. Because it does not appear to have developed the enthusiastic following that other joint replacements have, it seems not to be abused. The literature suggests that other, more conservative procedures are usually tried first, but exact data are hard to find. The chief controversy concerns the definite inferiority of the artificial replacements to the natural shoulder. It does not seem likely that an artificial joint that gives the same range of motion as the natural shoulder will be developed in the near future, but many patients are willing to trade some restriction of motion for pain relief.

Sigmoidectomy (42)

MORTALITY	MORBIDITY	CONTROVERSY
+	+	o

Removal of the **sigmoid colon**

? WHAT CONDITION DOES THE PROCEDURE TREAT?

Sigmoidectomies are performed to treat cancer of the sigmoid colon; benign tumors of the sigmoid colon; **sigmoid volvulus**; **diverticulitis**; giant cysts of the sigmoid (actually, a form of outpouchings that fill with gas); obstruction of the sigmoid colon; **prolapse of the rectum**;[1] inflammatory bowel diseases (**Crohn's disease** and **ulcerative colitis**); polyposis (multiple **polyps**) of the sigmoid colon; scleroderma of the colon (spread of fibrous tissue into the colon wall);[2] and a **fistula** between the sigmoid colon and the bladder.[3]

? WHAT IS THE PROCEDURE?

The patient is given a general anesthetic, unless heart or lung complications make a spinal anesthetic and sedation necessary. The patient's lower abdomen is shaved and washed with soap and antiseptic, and draped so that only the portion between the navel and the pubis is exposed. A vertical incision is made between the navel and the pubis; some surgeons prefer a horizontal incision along a line just above the pubis. The skin, **fascia**, and muscles are cut in layers, and bleeding vessels are **ligated** or **cauterized**. The sigmoid colon is located, and freed from its supporting structures by scalpel and blunt (finger) dissection. When the diseased portion of the sigmoid has been freed, it is clamped at both ends and cut between the two clamps. The removed portion is sent for examination by the pathologist.

If the patient's condition permits, the cut ends of the healthy colon and the portion of the rectum that is left attached to the anal opening (called the rectal stump) are sutured together, restoring the continuity of the large intestine. Sometimes, because of inflammation resulting from Crohn's disease, ulcerative colitis, or damage to the bowel from poison or parasites, a **suture** line between pieces of intestine cannot be counted on to heal. In those cases, a temporary **colostomy** is needed, an opening is made in the abdomen and the cut end of the colon is pushed through it and sutured to the skin outside. The cut portion of the rectal stump is temporarily sutured closed. The large intestine can be reconstructed later, by closing the colostomy opening in the skin, bringing the colon end back inside the body, removing the sutures from the rectal stump, and connecting the colon and the rectal stump just as is done in the one-stage procedure.

The various layers over the colon (muscle, **fascia**, and skin) are closed with sutures. Staples may also be used. The patient is taken to the recovery room and then to her room. Most patients will have a **nasogastric tube** for the first several days after the operation to keep the body's usual secretion of gastric juices (about a quart a day) out of the lower intestine. The tube is removed when it is clear that the bowel is functioning again and the internal connections have had time to heal. The patient is started on a liquid diet and gradually returned to solid food.

? WHO PERFORMS THE PROCEDURE?

This procedure can be done by general surgeons or colon-rectal surgeons. The medical literature suggests that there is a large variety of operations for rectal prolapse and that only a few surgeons are expert in a wide range of them.[4] If this procedure is needed as part of the repair of a rectal prolapse, you should be sure to use a board-certified colon-rectal surgeon with a lot of experience in surgery for prolapse, or a general surgeon who is using a common technique.

? WHERE IS THE PROCEDURE PERFORMED?

This surgery is always performed on an inpatient basis in a hospital.

? WHAT ARE THE MORTALITY (DEATH) AND MORBIDITY (COMPLICATION) RATES?

Mortality rates for sigmoidectomies can be as low as zero for elective cases in which bowel preparation (enemas and antibiotics to sterilize the colon to prevent infection) has been adequate and as high as 43.5% in emergency cases in which adequate preparation could not be done.[5-7] Complication rates of 28.3% have been reported.[8] Another study reports zero mortality and a complication rate of 15%.[9]

? WHAT ARE THE OTHER COMPLICATIONS AND POSSIBLE SIDE EFFECTS?

Both fecal incontinence (inability to hold stool) and constipation have been reported following surgery for rectal prolapse.[10]

Misdiagnosis is a "complication" of sorts. **Barium enema** examinations tend to produce high **false-negative** and **false-positive diagnoses** for cancer and polyps, and a colonoscopy, if possible, is likely to result in a more accurate diagnosis.[11, 12] (See "Endoscopic Large Bowel Examination," p. 69.) In the elderly, the classic signs and symptoms of various different intestinal diseases are muted; as a result, it is very easy for the doctor to confuse **ischemic bowel disease**, cancer, benign tumors, inflammatory bowel disease, and diverticulitis with each other unless definitive tests are done. For this reason, it would be better if elderly patients do not object to complete bowel work-ups, as unpleasant as they may seem.[13, 14]

As with any procedure in which anesthesia is used, death from reaction to the anesthetic drugs, error on the part of the anesthetist, or machine failure is a remote possibility. (See Glossary, p. 309)

? IS THIS THE MOST APPROPRIATE PROCEDURE FOR THE CONDITION?

Most conditions affecting the sigmoid colon are either life-threatening, painful, or embarrassing, so most patients ask for a therapy that will produce as complete a cure as possible. "Watchful waiting," though, is an acceptable alternative in many cases, depending upon what the affliction is. For example, Crohn's disease and ulcerative colitis can go into remission with intensive treatment with steroids such as cortisone, with the antibiotic metronidazole, or with newer anti-inflammatory medications such as Dipentum. If drug treatment is successful, it is reasonable to wait to see if the condition flares up again before deciding to operate, especially since the loss of the rectum and the use of a colostomy bag can be emotionally devastating.

In other cases, such as cancer, it is important that the diseased sigmoid be removed as soon as possible. On the other hand, doctors generally do not recommend surgery for diverticulitis that can be controlled with medication and diet.

? ARE THERE ALTERNATIVES TO THIS PROCEDURE?

Sigmoidectomy is an alternative to more radical operations, in which even more of the intestines are removed, and is very often the most conservative procedure that can be performed.

? WHAT IS CONTROVERSIAL ABOUT THE PROCEDURE?

There is little argument that nonemergency operations, when possible, are easier on both the patient and the surgeon than emergency surgery. This is particularly true because adequate bowel preparation allows the surgeon to work with an intestine that is not contaminated by fecal matter, so the chance of infection is reduced. The challenge for the patient's primary doctor and the surgeon lies in determining when it is safe to delay surgery and when it is not. The trend in the literature seems to be towards delay if at all possible.[15–18] Cases of sigmoid volvulus showed a mortality rate of 43.5% for emergency surgery versus 6.6% for delayed operation in one study; mortality was 50% for patients over age 65 when **peritonitis** occurred following surgery.[19, 20]

Acute bowel obstruction—that cannot be relieved by insertion of a tube for decompression, in which the blockage is relieved and the fecal matter flows normally—and swelling of the muscular wall of the intestine (called **toxic megacolon**) seem to be conditions in which delaying operation is unwise. Any bowel obstruction is potentially a disaster, especially if the bowel bursts inside the body. In all other cases, an attempt at adequate bowel preparation seems to be worth trying. The judgment in individual cases, of course, has to be left to the patient and the doctors. Two studies recommend immediate operation for volvulus of the sigmoid colon, but not for volvulus in other portions of the colon.[21, 22]

Surgeons try to preserve as much bowel as possible to avoid the syndromes that are associated with loss of intestine—such as vitamin deficiencies, electrolyte imbalances, failure to thrive in children, and possible heart rhythm disturbances in adults. In cases involving the sigmoid colon, which is a small portion of the total bowel and has only a small role in the absorption of water and nutrients, complete removal of the damaged segment rather than attempts to salvage it carry less risk of morbidity and mortality.[23, 24]

Contrary to earlier thinking, it is now believed that a low-fiber diet is of no benefit in the treatment of diverticula of the sigmoid colon. It is becoming increasingly clear, however, that adequate fiber intake carries less risk of heart attack and cancer of the large intestine.

Skin Lesion Incision and Destruction (41)

MORTALITY	MORBIDITY	CONTROVERSY
+	+	o

Destruction of **lesions** of the skin by various methods after an initial attempt does not produce complete removal

? WHAT CONDITION DOES THE PROCEDURE TREAT?

Skin lesions are removed for three main reasons—concern about appearance, concern about irritation of the lesions by clothing, and concern that a lesion is malignant or may become so. One type of skin cancer, melanoma, is very aggressive and can be fatal if it spreads to other organs. This particular procedure is used when an initial attempt at destruction of a lesion fails, or the lesion is so large that it must be removed in stages.

? WHAT IS THE PROCEDURE?

When one of the various approaches for removal or destruction of a lesion (see "Local Destruction of Skin Lesion," p. 175) has failed, the lesion is removed by cutting out with a scalpel the area of skin on which it is located. The cutting procedure may be combined with a repeat performance of one or more of the lesion-destruction methods discussed in "Local Destruction of Skin Lesion." Everything else about this procedure is identical.

Skin Suture (36)

MORTALITY	MORBIDITY	CONTROVERSY
+	+	o

LAY TITLE: *Stitches*

Sewing up a wound or incision in the skin

? WHAT CONDITION DOES THE PROCEDURE TREAT?

This procedure treats wounds of the skin or skin incisions that are too deep, wide, or long to heal with bandaging alone.

? WHAT IS THE PROCEDURE?

There are many variations on the fundamental and simple technique. The skin to be **sutured** is numbed with an injectable local anesthetic. A threaded curved needle is grasped with a needle holder and passed through one side of the wound or incision, then the other. Tension on the suture is used to draw the lips of the wound together; a knot is tied, the end of the suture farthest from the needle is cut, and the next suture is placed. This process is continued until the wound is closed. Sutures placed in this way are called interrupted sutures. Sutures can also be placed in a continuous line, the way cloth is normally sewn. However, many doctors believe that the interrupted-suture technique gives better control on the tension at each point in the wound.

To produce minimal scarring, the surgeon places the sutures so that the lips of the wound are pulled slightly upward, and uses suture materials that are nonirritating. To produce closure that will scar only slightly, it is also important to remove dead tissue from the edges of the wounds and trim the edges, if needed.

? WHO PERFORMS THE PROCEDURE?

This procedure is within the competence of any physician, but is usually performed on an outpatient basis in hospital emergency rooms. Of course, all surgeons use suture techniques to close skin after operations.

? WHERE IS THE PROCEDURE PERFORMED?

The procedure is done on an inpatient or outpatient basis in a hospital, in an outpatient surgery facility, or in a well-equipped doctor's office.

? WHAT ARE THE MORTALITY (DEATH) AND MORBIDITY (COMPLICATION) RATES?

There is no mortality and no morbidity other than infection and unacceptable scarring, which can be revised by a plastic surgeon.

? WHAT ARE THE OTHER COMPLICATIONS AND POSSIBLE SIDE EFFECTS?

There are none.

? IS THIS THE MOST APPROPRIATE PROCEDURE FOR THE CONDITION?

Suturing is so innocuous that it seems unreasonable not to use it when there is a chance that the wound will not heal properly with bandaging alone.

? ARE THERE ALTERNATIVES TO THIS PROCEDURE?

Yes. A 1989 study showed that automatic skin staplers, commonly used for surgical wound closure for many years, are as effective as sutures in closing wounds and produce cosmetic results that are as good as those produced by sutures, and at a lower cost.[1, 2] Skin closure tapes can also be used.[3]

About two-thirds of children tolerate suturing well under local anesthesia; the remaining third are generally physically restrained rather than given general anesthesia.[4]

? WHAT IS CONTROVERSIAL ABOUT THE PROCEDURE?

Animal studies show that zinc is very important in forming a strong scar. Zinc supplementation can clearly aid wound healing.[5]

Surgical Repair of Indirect Inguinal Hernia (45)/ Direct Inguinal Hernia (57)/ Unilateral Inguinal Hernia (84)

MORTALITY	MORBIDITY	CONTROVERSY
+	+	●

- The **CONTROVERSIES** surrounding this procedure are: use of a barrier method to close the tear; use of antibiotics at the time of surgery; nonuse of drains because of the potential for infection; use of **clips** instead of **sutures**; and cutting of the **cremaster muscle** to avoid tension on the wound.

Direct Inguinal Hernia: Surgical repair of a tear in the abdominal wall that allows a loop of intestine to protrude

Indirect Inguinal Hernia: Surgical repair of a tear in the abdominal wall that allows a loop of intestine to slip through the pelvic floor and into the **inguinal canal**.

Inguinal hernias are divided into two classes: direct and indirect. The hernia is called direct when a loop of the intestine emerges through a gap or tear in the muscles of the abdominal wall between the deepest lying artery (the epigastric artery) and the abdominal muscles. The hernia is called indirect when a loop of the intestine slips through a gap or tear in the muscles of the pelvic floor and drops through the inguinal canal and into the scrotum in men—or into the analogous area to the left or right of the vagina in women.

The procedure "Surgical Repair of Unilateral Inguinal Hernia" is just like treatment of direct or indirect hernia, but the term is used for billing purposes when the surgeon fails to specify the hernia as direct or indirect. Its inclusion in the most frequently performed procedures is attributable to a quirk of reimbursement.

❓ WHAT CONDITION DOES THE PROCEDURE TREAT?

This procedure treats a condition in which a defect in the **fascia** allows a portion of the intestine to slip through the pelvic floor and into the inguinal canal, which is the passage through which the testes descend from the abdomen into the scrotum in men and where the round ligament of the uterus leaves the abdomen to connect with the **labium majus** in women.

The hernia can usually, but not always, be felt beneath the skin of the groin. A hernia is a problem because the intestine within the **hernial sac** can be twisted and/or cut off from its blood supply, which can lead to intestinal obstruction and **gangrene** of the bowel, both quite unpleasant conditions with high mortality.[1-7] In addition, pain, tingling, and numbness above the site of the hernia may be present, even if a hernial sac cannot be felt.

The inguinal canal contains two rings of fibrous tissue through which, on both the right and left sides, pass the spermatic cord which supports the testicle, the **vas deferens,** and blood vessels. The canal is present in females, but in a shortened form. Some women experience hernias from time to time; however, because of structural differences in the pelvis, inguinal hernias do not occur as frequently in women. More women than men develop abdominal hernias. Because the testicles in men descend from the abdomen, the muscle structure is weaker due to the opening to the inguinal canal. The fascia through which the inguinal **herniation** typically occurs forms part of the floor of the pelvis. Both hernias and the defects in the fascia or musculature through which herniation later occurs may be **congenital** or acquired as the result of an injury or excessive strain.

Strengthening the major back and abdominal muscles, which work together to support the structures in the groin area, and exhibiting proper lifting techniques can reduce the risk of hernia. However, evidence[8, 9] suggests that most hernias occur through a congenital or acquired defect and are not the result of a single episode of strain.

To get a sense of the location, place both hands on the low abdomen with the thumbs on the navel and the index fingers just touching the line where the pubic hair thickens suddenly (for males, the index fingers should be resting at the base of the penis). Direct inguinal hernias occur low, between the little fingers and the prominent tip of the hipbone; indirect inguinal hernias occur in the groin at about the location to which the little fingers are pointing.

? WHAT IS THE PROCEDURE?

There are various techniques for performing the operation, virtually every one of which was developed as an attempt to deal with the problem of hernial recurrence. Even today, it is acknowledged that there is no fully satisfactory operation for this condition,[10] but changes in techniques in the last 20 years have led to major improvements. However, experts still debate whether to use muscle tissue (taken from the site of the incision) to reinforce the defective fascia, whether to try to restore the anatomy exactly as it was before the hernia or to do something to make the area stronger by reinforcing the repair with steel sutures or some artificial material and if so, with what, and how patients should be cared for postoperatively.

A "generic" explanation of the operation should not obscure the fact that relatively minor differences in technique have major effects on the infection rate,[11] the rate of complications in the immediate postoperative period, and the rate of recurrence.[12-25] Here, broadly speaking, is how the procedure goes: The patient is prepared for the operation with preoperative sedatives. Any kind of anesthetic—general, spinal, local, or some combination of the three—may be used, depending upon the preferences of the surgeon and the anesthetist. (The most common anesthesia is regional unless the patient is uncooperative or cannot stand the discomfort of the procedure.) The area where the surgeon plans to make the incision is shaved, washed with antiseptic, and draped so that only the area where the incision will be made is exposed. The surgeon makes an incision in the groin (some favor making the incision in the skin fold between the thigh and the trunk of the body, to avoid a visible scar[26]), and cuts through the fascia, fat, and muscle overlying the hernial sac.

She then gently moves the bowel back into place if necessary, cuts off any loose **peritoneum**, and **ligates** or sutures the remaining "stump" of peritoneum, which is then allowed to slip back underneath the muscles. The opening in the fascia that allowed the hernia to occur is located and either stitched closed or covered with mesh. Most surgeons avoid the use of muscle tissue to close the defect and either use nearby fascia or a plastic mesh to patch it, because muscle tissue has a jelly-like consistency when relaxed, is hard to sew, and tears easily. Once the defect has been repaired, the various layers that have been cut (muscle, fascia, and skin) are sutured separately and the surgical wound is stitched, clipped, or stapled shut.

? WHO PERFORMS THE PROCEDURE?

This procedure is usually done by a general surgeon, but may be well within the competence of gynecologists and urologists who wish to perform it.

? WHERE IS THE PROCEDURE PERFORMED?

One of the major trends in hernia surgery over the past two decades has been an emphasis on getting out of bed early in the postoperative course (called "early ambulation")—which has been found to be suitable for most patients—and on outpatient, or same-day, surgery. At present, hernia repairs are being performed in hospitals, well-equipped walk-in clinics, outpatient surgery facilities, and some well-equipped doctors' offices.

? WHAT ARE THE MORTALITY (DEATH) AND MORBIDITY (COMPLICATION) RATES?

The mortality rate at community hospitals in the U.S. was 0.1% in 1988. Mortality rates ranging from zero to 16.5% have been reported, with the great majority clustering in the low end of the range.[27-32] As is usually the case, mortality rises with patient age, and is higher in emergency surgery than in elective surgery.

? WHAT ARE THE OTHER COMPLICATIONS AND POSSIBLE SIDE EFFECTS?

All surgery, including hernia repair, carries a risk of excessive bleeding and wound infection. Overall morbidity for this procedure reported in various studies ranges from zero to 58%, with most studies clustering at the low end of the range, and the highest rate—58%—occurring in a group of elderly patients undergoing emergency operations.[33-44]

The chief concern with hernia repairs is recurrence. Studies report recurrence rates from zero to around 30% with various periods of follow-up—ranging from a month to several years, depending on the study.[45-60]

Urinary retention, which may necessitate temporary catheterization of the bladder (the insertion of a **catheter** into the bladder for the purpose of draining urine), occurs in around 6% of patients. We should mention that most studies do not report such a complication, and instead lump it together with other morbidity.[61] Infection rates ranged from zero to just under 16% in a number of studies.[62-64] One case of **toxic shock syndrome** attributed to infection of a hernia operation wound has been reported (the patient lived).[65]

As with any procedure in which anesthesia is used, death from reaction to the anesthetic drugs, error on the part of the anesthetist, or machine failure is a remote possibility. (See Glossary, p. 309)

? IS THIS THE MOST APPROPRIATE PROCEDURE FOR THE CONDITION?

Because of the wide variety of techniques in hernia repair, one has to know exactly what the surgeon proposes to do in order to judge whether the procedure is most appropriate. There is no absolute "standard" technique. Based on the very good results obtained with Teflon mesh in operations for recurrent hernias, it seems reasonable to use it universally for first hernia repairs, but most surgeons appear to think that they can produce a successful closure with tissue-suturing alone. In the majority of cases, they are correct, but it is disappointing that they have not paid more attention to the risk of recurrence and developed a completely effective procedure for definitive repair. This appears to be one of the very few areas in surgery in which less conservative approaches might produce better results overall.

? ARE THERE ALTERNATIVES TO THIS PROCEDURE?

An inguinal hernia is a mechanical problem,[66] as was observed in the year 1598 by Ambroise Paré, the French surgeon who accidentally discovered that gunshot wounds healed better if one didn't pour boiling oil into them. Because it is a mechanical problem, involving part of the body being in an abnormal place, only a mechanical (surgical) correction will work. This is as true today as it was in Paré's time. There is simply no medical (drug) treatment for a mechanical problem. Thus, if a hernia is symptomatic and causing distress, a hernia operation is appropriate. Even a **truss**, which keeps the hernia from protruding, is a surgical appliance because it is a mechanical device much like the wires, pins, and rods used to repair fractured bones.

? WHAT IS CONTROVERSIAL ABOUT THE PROCEDURE?

The most recent medical literature on this subject suggests an evolving body of knowledge indicating that: (1) some sort of barrier material (plastic mesh, a Teflon patch, or a plastic "plug") should be used to close the **fascia** and muscle defects in recurrent hernias;[67, 68] (2) antibiotics should be given at the time of surgery to reduce the risk of infection;[69] (3) drains (which are a potential source of infection) should not be used, but the surgical wound should be completely closed[70] unless complications require suction drainage;[71] (4) clips are as effective as sutures and that the removal of clips is less painful to the patient than suture removal;[72] and (5) the cremaster muscle of the groin should be cut to avoid tension on the wound. (The cremaster muscle in the upper thigh exerts tension on the wound which slows healing; by cutting this muscle, tension is released and the wound heals better and faster.)

Recent evidence suggests that a Teflon mesh is less irritating than Marlex mesh for wound reinforcement. The fascia grows into the Teflon, producing a reinforced normal fascia. The Marlex mesh, though effective, produces internal scarring.[73]

Temporary Pacemaker System Insertion (95)

MORTALITY	MORBIDITY	CONTROVERSY
+	+	•

- The primary **CONTROVERSY** is the use of the temporary pacemaker system during coronary angiography because it reportedly causes additional problems.

Insertion of wiring and devices for temporary control of heart rate and rhythm

? WHAT CONDITION DOES THE PROCEDURE TREAT?

A temporary pacemaker is used when there is a need to control for a short time the rate at which the entire heart, or part of the heart such as the **auricles** or **ventricles**, beats. Temporary pacemakers are commonly used after cardiac surgery, when there is a tendency for heart rates to be abnormally slow,[1] and during anesthesia, when a normal heartbeat cannot be maintained.[2, 3] They are also used when a permanent pacemaker fails.[4] Inserted under the skin on the chest wall, a permanent pacemaker provides an artificial, regular impulse when any one of various heart disorders results in an irregular or absent natural impulse in the heart.

? WHAT IS THE PROCEDURE?

The patient is under local anesthesia, plus sedation, if necessary. The exact procedure depends upon the type of device used. Wires can be inserted through veins,[5, 6] usually the subclavian vein, which runs under the collarbone; through the chest wall to reach the heart; or through a **catheter** with a pacing electrode (the electrical contact that delivers the shock to the heart, which causes the paced beat), which can be placed down the **esophagus**.

? WHO PERFORMS THE PROCEDURE?

Depending upon the circumstances, this procedure can be performed by an internist or family physician (with special training in pacemaker selection, insertion, and operation[7, 8]), a cardiologist, a cardiac surgeon, an anesthesiologist, or a cardiac care nurse.[9]

? WHERE IS THE PROCEDURE PERFORMED?

Because of the circumstances in which temporary pacemakers are used, this procedure is usually performed in a hospital, but it can be done wherever the necessary equipment is available, such as in an outpatient surgery center or a well-equipped doctor's office.

? WHAT ARE THE MORTALITY (DEATH) AND MORBIDITY (COMPLICATION) RATES?

We could find no reports of mortality attributable to the use of a temporary pacemaker other than rare reports of unrecognized failure of the pacemaker system. Such failure is caused by the combination of a faulty device and failure of the physician or nurse to recognize the problem. If recognized, the problem can be corrected immediately by changing the pacemaker or, if the failure results from a dead battery, by replacing the battery.[10] One recent British study reported a 46.7% mortality rate in those receiving temporary pacemakers; most of these deaths were attributable to heart rhythm disturbances associated with pacemaker insertion. Most of these patients had had severe heart attacks, however, so the extent to which mortality should be attributed directly to the use of the pacemaker is unclear.[11] In short, one cannot assume that the patient would have lived had the pacemaker not been used.

Minor malfunctions of temporary pacemaker systems seem to be quite common; in one study alone they were found in up to 37% of temporary pacemakers. In the same study, 20% of patients had complications that ranged from too rapid a heartbeat during pacemaker wire insertion, to fever and **phlebitis**.[12] The mortality rate associated with these complications was zero. A similar study showed an overall complication rate of 18%, a major complication rate of 7%, and a mortality rate of zero.[13] Another study reports serious complication rate of zero.[14]

If the **femoral vein** is used for insertion of the pacemaker wires, clotting, which can be fatal, occurs in up to 55% of patients, with 5% showing clinical signs of **thrombosis**. Use of other insertion sites reduces, but does not completely avoid, this complication.[15–17]

? WHAT ARE THE OTHER COMPLICATIONS AND POSSIBLE SIDE EFFECTS?

When patients undergo coronary angiography (see "Left Cardiac Catheterization," p. 88) with a pacing wire in the **right ventricle**, there is a 300% increase in the rate of heart rhythm disturbances. The surgeon can prevent this by temporarily withdrawing the wire into the right **atrium** or the **vena cava**.[18]

If a pacing wire pierces the heart (albeit a rare event), it can lead to collection of blood in the membrane covering the heart, a condition called **cardiac tamponade**, which interferes with the heartbeat.[19] Damage to bypass **grafts** during removal of pacemaker wires has been reported.[20]

? IS THIS THE MOST APPROPRIATE PROCEDURE FOR THE CONDITION?

Research on the proper **indications** for the use of temporary pacemakers is ongoing. These devices clearly should not be used routinely in all situations in which mild, temporary, and harmless changes in heart rhythm can be expected as a result of surgery, disease, or medication. Studies indicate that routine pacemaker use during diagnostic heart catheterization and balloon angioplasty (see "Percutaneous Transluminal Coronary Angioplasty," p. 194) is both unnecessary and extremely expensive. However, these same studies showed that rhythm disturbances during balloon valvuloplasty (a procedure that involves the opening of a narrowed heart valve with a balloon attached to a catheter) were common enough, and the use of a temporary pacemaker cheap enough, to make routine use desirable.[21–23]

? ARE THERE ALTERNATIVES TO THIS PROCEDURE?

Yes. Noninvasive transcutaneous, or through-the-skin, pacing (control of the heartbeat)—in which the pacing signal is sent through the skin via electrodes on the chest—has been successful in 94% to 100% of patients, depending upon the device and techniques used.[24, 25] However, there have been reports of electrical shocks from transcutaneous pacemakers. The discomfort from the shocks, according to patients' descriptions, ranges from none to extreme discomfort, depending upon the individual. About 16% to 20% of patients find transcutaneous pacing too uncomfortable to endure; in those cases a temporary pacemaker can be inserted through a vein.

? WHAT IS CONTROVERSIAL ABOUT THE PROCEDURE?

There now seems to be general agreement that routine use of a temporary pacemaker during coronary angiography causes more problems than it solves. Research on the appropriateness of other uses continues.

Toe Amputation (77)

MORTALITY	MORBIDITY	CONTROVERSY
+	+	o

Surgical removal of one or more toes (with possible use of the toes to replace fingers lost to trauma)

? WHAT CONDITION DOES THE PROCEDURE TREAT?

Amputation of the toe is used to treat: (1) diabetic vascular problems that destroy the blood supply of a toe;[1] (2) loss of the thumb, by replacing it with the amputated big toe;[2-4] (3) loss of a finger other than the thumb, by replacing it with the amputated second toe[5, 6] (although the toe is smaller than the finger, it's the only movable part of the body that's remotely close in shape and size and has the nerve and muscle structure to be functional if transplanted to the hand); (4) partial at-wrist amputation of the hand, by replacing it with a toe, usually the big one, in order to make a sort of claw, which has more gripping ability than a stump;[7] (5) treatment of congenital defects or traumatic injuries to the hand short of the loss of an entire finger;[8] (6) "blue toe syndrome," an indication of clots in the venous system migrating downward in the body (it is used if limb salvage surgery to restore circulation is unsuccessful and the toe becomes gangrenous or otherwise dangerously diseased); (7) osteosarcoma (a rare type of bone cancer) of the toe (there is one case reported in the literature);[9] (8) other cancers of the toes;[10, 11] (9) pain in the toe that cannot be managed by other means.[12] Amputations may also follow failed attempts at surgery of the toes.[13]

? WHAT IS THE PROCEDURE?

The foot is washed with soap and antiseptic, and the patient is given a local, spinal, or general anesthetic, depending upon the extent of the surgery that is planned. The foot is draped so that only the toes to be worked on are exposed. The surgeon cuts away sufficient skin to make flaps to cover the wound (he may obtain these flaps from other parts of the body if there is a malignant tumor in or on the toe). The skin, **fascia**, and muscles are cut away in layers to expose the bone; bleeding vessels are **ligated**. The bone is sawed through and the toe is removed. Bone wax is applied to the remaining bone to stop bleeding, if necessary.

The surgeon may use a portion of the amputated toe's flesh to provide padding over the stump of the toe that was removed. The skin flaps are closed over the wound and the wound is bandaged. The patient is taken to the recovery room.

If a hand reconstruction is involved, the hand is washed and draped to expose only the area to be worked on. The existing finger or portion of the finger to be replaced is removed in the same manner as for the toe amputation. A metal pin, run through the center of the bone, may be used to stabilize the union between the toe and the body of the hand or wrist (attachment is made directly to the wrist in cases of complete hand amputation). The arteries, veins, and nerves that can be clearly seen with the naked eye are carefully **sutured** together to ensure an adequate blood supply and sensation and motor function. The surgeon then uses high-power magnifying glasses, magnifying goggles, or an operating microscope to suture together the arteries, veins, and nerves that cannot be worked on without magnification. When the surgeon believes that an adequate blood and nerve supply is assured, she closes the skin, using flaps from elsewhere on the body if necessary, and the wound is bandaged. (Common donor sites are the buttocks and the top of the thighs.) The patient is taken to the recovery room. Particularly with transplants to the hand, a good deal of physical therapy will have to be endured as soon as the hand has healed enough to allow it. Little if any physical therapy is needed for the loss of one or two toes, even the big toe. The reason is that, when we walk, the push off is done with the entire front of the foot and not the big toe.

WHO PERFORMS THE PROCEDURE?

Simple removal of the toe can be done by a general surgeon, an orthopedic surgeon, or any physician who practices minor surgery. Replacement of the thumb and fingers with amputated toes is a delicate procedure that requires high skill and experience in the fields of orthopedic surgery, vascular surgery, neurosurgery, and microsurgery. It should be done only by a physician who specializes in limb transplants and reattachments, by a hand surgeon, or by an orthopedic surgeon for whom such cases make up a good deal of his practice. If such a person is not available, a team of surgeons—an orthopedic surgeon, a vascular surgeon, a neurosurgeon, and a microsurgical specialist—can do it.

The complexity arises from the need to produce a transplanted toe that functions as close to the way a finger functions as possible. Since this procedure—replacement of the thumb and fingers with amputated toes—is not common, it is unrealistic to look for a surgeon who has done a large volume. However, good results probably come from using a surgeon who has done several dozen such operations. If the surgeon is not an artist, she can do everything but the skin surgery and have a plastic surgeon do the skin closure and any skin transplants that are needed to minimize scarring and blend skin tone.

WHERE IS THE PROCEDURE PERFORMED?

This surgery can be done in an outpatient surgery clinic, the outpatient or inpatient departments of a hospital, or in some hand surgeons' offices if the facilities are elaborately equipped for surgery. Because of the special skills involved, the procedure is most likely to be done in a large, university-affiliated hospital.

WHAT ARE THE MORTALITY (DEATH) AND MORBIDITY (COMPLICATION) RATES?

Following any vascular surgery or attempts at limb transplant or reattachment, a complication which can set in is a combination of the loss of blood supply and infection, resulting in tissue death and amputation of the transplanted toe.[14] Simple amputation of the toes doubtless goes back beyond the beginning of recorded history. On the other hand, successful use of the toe as a replacement thumb is a relatively new procedure. Although the procedure is not likely to be the immediate cause of a death, **iatrogenic** (doctor-caused) morbidity associated with the procedure may be fatal. For example, you may die of a hospital-acquired infection if the germs are resistant to all antibiotics, if you have an immune system compromise such as AIDS, or if you have had past heavy use of anti-inflammatory steroid drugs.

We could locate no reports of death in the National Library of Medicine's Medline database for any years after 1974. Significant morbidity appears to be related to the underlying causes (the **etiology,** in medical jargon) of the need for toe amputation—diabetes, cancer, or trauma—rather than to the amputation of the toe itself.

? WHAT ARE THE OTHER COMPLICATIONS AND POSSIBLE SIDE EFFECTS?

The second toe gradually assumes the role of the big toe in the pushing off portion of a footstep after the big toe has been amputated. In diabetic persons the forces associated with this new role can result in **necrosis** in the second toe. Because a diabetic has a greater chance of having circulatory problems than a nondiabetic, especially in the feet, as the second toe begins to absorb the full impact of walking, it becomes more susceptible to developing a sore spot and then, possibly, tissue death. This can be prevented by custom-made orthotics (in this case, shoe inserts).[15]

Athletes are likely to find performance in running compromised by the loss of the big toe, but the loss is unlikely to cause any difficulty in nonathletic endeavors.[16]

As with any procedure in which anesthesia is used, death from reaction to the anesthetic drugs, error on the part of the anesthetist, or machine failure is a remote possibility. (See Glossary, p. 309)

? IS THIS THE MOST APPROPRIATE PROCEDURE FOR THE CONDITION?

A functioning thumb is the key to a fully functioning hand, and, as no wholly satisfactory thumb **prostheses** (artificial thumbs) exist as yet, use of the big toe in place of the thumb is a reasonable alternative. True, there are potential problems with this procedure, but they relate mostly to getting the nerves to regenerate.

Gangrenous tissue carries a great risk to the patient, with mortality rates from 9.1% to 74%, depending upon the site and extent of the infection and the treatment given;[17, 18] therefore, amputation of gangrenous toes seems prudent.

? ARE THERE ALTERNATIVES TO THIS PROCEDURE?

If the desired outcome is a functioning thumb, there is no alternative at present. The patient may elect not to have other fingers replaced. For vascular conditions leading to **ischemia** to the toes, **vasodilator** drugs and closer control of diabetes should be tried before surgery.

? WHAT IS CONTROVERSIAL ABOUT THE PROCEDURE?

There seems to be no particular controversy about this procedure.

Tonsillectomy (52)

MORTALITY	MORBIDITY	CONTROVERSY
+	+	●

• The main **CONTROVERSY** is whether this procedure is appropriate.

Removal of lymph nodes at the back of the throat that, when swollen as a result of infection, can cause various problems such as recurrent infections

? WHAT CONDITION DOES THE PROCEDURE TREAT?

Lymph nodes of the throat, tonsils are located at the back of the throat (one on either side). Tonsillectomies are performed for swelling of the tonsils that interferes with breathing or hearing by blocking the mouth (which contains one end of the eustachian tubes that are essential for hearing); **peritonsillar abscess** (also known as quinsy); acute infections of the tonsils; **sleep apnea** caused by swollen tonsils obstructing the airway;[1, 2] cancer of the tonsils (a relatively rare occurrence);[3] and repeated ear, throat, and upper respiratory tract infections.[4] Tonsillectomy, adenoidectomy, and combined tonsillectomy and adenoidectomy are three separate procedures, and there is a different rationale for performing each.[5, 6] (For a discussion of tonsillectomy with adenoidectomy, see "Tonsillectomy and Adenoidectomy," p. 241.)

The tonsils have an important role in the immune system, especially in children below age eight. Current recommendations are to perform only a one-sided tonsillectomy, if at all possible, so that functioning tonsillar tissue can be preserved. Complete tonsillectomy for repeatedly swollen tonsils is done only after age 12.[7]

Current speculation on the role of the tonsils suggests that they evolved to protect the upper throat and air passages by secreting immune system compounds into saliva and concentrating white blood cells to attack entering bacteria. As with many other bodily systems, one is simultaneously impressed with how well the tonsils work—assuming their function has been correctly identified—and how badly they are designed.[8]

Loss of the tonsils does not appear to compromise the immune system, largely because the lymphoid tissue (any tissue in the lymphatic system, which is concerned primarily with fighting infection) in the oral **mucosa** (in the mouth) can take over the function. If this were not the case, immune system deficiencies following re- moval of the tonsils would probably be seen. As it is, there is only a brief reduction of resistance to polio, which is of no consequence when most children are vaccinated against it.[9] The tonsils seem to be a mainstay of resistance to polio, but the body's immune system can adapt to their loss. Parents should be sure that a child who has had one or both tonsils removed is current on polio immunization and any boosters that are needed (which depends upon the vaccine used).

? WHAT IS THE PROCEDURE?

General anesthesia is used, primarily because of the usually young age of the patients and the need for the surgeon to work deep in the mouth, where gag reflexes and panic caused by brief intermittent airway obstruction make it hard to work, even on a sedated patient. Several techniques are used. The tonsils may be grasped with a clamp and peeled away from the back of the mouth by finger dissection, a probe may be used for the same purpose, or a combination of blunt dissection (using a finger or instrument to peel the tonsils away from the underlying tissue) and cutting may be used. A cold-wire snare (simply cuts the tissue automatically) or hot-wire tonsil snare (uses a heated, sharp wire that cuts and **cauterizes** at the same time) can also be used. Bleeding is controlled by **ligating** the bleeding vessels or by an **electrocautery device** in severe cases.

Once the procedure is complete, the patient is taken to the recovery room, and if no complications are discovered by the time the anesthetic has worn off completely, he is sent home.

? WHO PERFORMS THE PROCEDURE?

This procedure can be done by an otolaryngologist (ear, nose, and throat specialist), or by a general surgeon or pediatric surgeon. Complicated problems—for example, benign or malignant tumors of the tonsils, infection or ulceration of the tonsils that has spread to surrounding tissue, or an extremely narrow airway—are best handled by a board-certified otolaryngologist.

? WHERE IS THE PROCEDURE PERFORMED?

Most such procedures are done on an outpatient basis now, although in 1988 the average length of stay for those treated as inpatients was reported to be 1.2 days.[10]

? WHAT ARE THE MORTALITY (DEATH) AND MORBIDITY (COMPLICATION) RATES?

In 1988 a large sample of community hospitals in the U.S. reported no deaths in 93,198 tonsillectomies-adenoidectomies.[11] A 1983 estimate of mortality placed it at about 0.006%, or one in every 16,700 procedures.[12]

A 1990 study of 3340 outpatient tonsillectomies found a rate of major complications—including severe hemorrhage, severe nausea, anesthetic complications, and dehydration—of 1.5%. In the same study, 0.5% of patients required hospitalization for complications, and 0.15% of patients had complications that would have been detected during a 48-hour postoperative hospital stay.[13]

Even in developing counties, blunt dissection tonsillectomy and general anesthesia can have a mortality rate of zero.[14] In developed countries, deaths are attributed to anesthesia, not to the procedure itself.[15]

As with any procedure in which anesthesia is used, death from reaction to the anesthetic drugs, error on the part of the anesthetist, or machine failure is a remote possibility. (See Glossary, p. 309)

? WHAT ARE THE OTHER COMPLICATIONS AND POSSIBLE SIDE EFFECTS?

Treating unnecessary surgery as a "complication," we believe that it is worth noting that in a 1978 study only 32% of tonsillectomies met even lenient guidelines for surgery.[16] The authors of that study suggest that stringent review would dramatically reduce the incidence of tonsillectomy.

? IS THIS THE MOST APPROPRIATE PROCEDURE FOR THE CONDITION?

Because tonsillectomy has been advocated for many conditions, the answer to this question depends upon what the condition is and what the proposed procedure is. Clearly, tonsillectomy is required for cor pulmonale (right-sided heart failure due to obstruction of the airway) caused by swollen tonsils, cancer of the tonsils, and benign tumors of the tonsils that produce obstruction, but all three of these conditions are rare.[17]

Repeated upper respiratory tract infections that are associated with systemic rheumatic or kidney disease are also strong reasons for tonsillectomy. Two to four colds a year as a child seem to be the price we pay for increased immunity to colds in adulthood. The tonsils are an important part of the childhood immune system that creates the broader adult immunity, and removal of them simply to reduce the annual number of colds is ill-advised at best.

Because sleep apnea in children is at least theoretically associated with failure to thrive—a failure to maintain a growth pattern that is normal for the child's probable adult height and weight—tonsillectomy to correct this is probably advisable.

? ARE THERE ALTERNATIVES TO THIS PROCEDURE?

Treatment with antibiotics and drainage of pus from infected tonsils are effective alternatives to tonsillectomy in many patients.[18] Unless the tonsils shrink appreciably after medical treatment and drainage, alternatives to tonsillectomy may not relieve obstructive sleep apnea.

? WHAT IS CONTROVERSIAL ABOUT THE PROCEDURE?

Just about everything. There is widespread disagreement about tonsillectomy, with some doctors scorning indications for the operation that others regard as "absolute."[19] More than a decade ago, researchers were seriously questioning whether there were any valid **indications** for tonsillectomy.[20] In 1985, tonsillectomy was regarded by one author as an "unproven" therapy for recurrent sore throat.[21] A 1988 review article recommended tonsillectomy only when a trial of adequate antibiotic therapy targeted at a broad range of bacterial species had failed.[22]

A review of various techniques indicated that blunt dissection, control of bleeding with the **ligation** of vessels, and the nonuse of postoperative antibiotics resulted in the lowest morbidity in children.[23] Giving surgeons feedback about the rate at which they and their colleagues perform tonsillectomies has resulted in reductions of an average of 46% in the number performed.[24] The feedback may be given by the hospital's internal quality control staff; by outside consultants hired by the hospital; or by a state agency such as the department of health or a cost-containment council.

Tonsillectomy and Adenoidectomy (11)

MORTALITY	MORBIDITY	CONTROVERSY
+	+	●

- The main **CONTROVERSY** is whether this procedure is appropriate.

Removal of lymph nodes at the back and top of the throat that, when swollen due to repeated infections, can cause various problems such as recurrent infections

? WHAT CONDITION DOES THE PROCEDURE TREAT?

Lymph nodes of the throat, tonsils are located at the back of the throat (one on either side). Tonsillectomies are performed for swelling of the tonsils that interferes with breathing or hearing by blocking the mouth (which contains one end of the eustachian tubes that are essential for hearing); **peritonsillar abscess** (also known as quinsy); acute infections of the tonsils; **sleep apnea** due to swollen tonsils obstructing the airway;[1, 2] cancer of the tonsils (a relatively rare occurrence);[3] and repeated ear, throat, and upper respiratory tract infections.[4] Tonsillectomy, adenoidectomy, and combined tonsillectomy and adenoidectomy are three separate procedures, each with a different rationale.[5, 6] (For a discussion of tonsillectomy only, see "Tonsillectomy," p. 238.)

The tonsils and adenoids are part of the lymphoid tissue system of the body, which is heavily involved in immune defenses against invading bacteria and viruses. The palatine tonsils, which are the ones that are usually called tonsils, lie on either side of the extreme back of the mouth, at the top of the throat. The pharyngeal tonsils, which are called the adenoids when they get large enough to be troublesome, are actually inside the nose right under the sphenoid **sinus**, which is deep in the head behind the eyes.

There are two ways to locate the pharyngeal tonsils, or adenoids: First, insert an angled dental mirror (with the mirror surface pointing up) into the mouth all the way to the back of the throat, passing under the uvula (the soft "tail" of the palate that can be seen hanging down from the rear of the roof of the mouth); when the mirror bumps against the back of the throat, the spongy things that are reflected in the mirror are the adenoids, assuming that they haven't been removed. The second way, which is very difficult to do if one has a normal gag reflex, is to reach back into the mouth with a finger or tongue blade and press the uvula up until it touches the back of the throat; when the uvula is straight toward the back of the head, the finger or tongue will be pointing right at the adenoids.

The tonsils and adenoids have an important role in the immune system, especially in children younger than eight years of age. Current recommendations are to perform a one-sided tonsillectomy (rather than remove both tonsils) for obstructive symptoms if at all possible so that functioning tonsillar tissue can be preserved. Complete tonsillectomy is done only after age 12.[7] Current speculation on the role of the tonsils suggests that they evolved to protect the upper throat and air passages by secreting immune-system compounds into saliva and concentrating white blood cells to attack entering bacteria. As with many other bodily systems, one is simultaneously impressed with how well the tonsils work, assuming that their function has been correctly identified, and how badly they are designed.[8]

Loss of the tonsils does not appear to compromise the immune system, largely because the lymphoid tissue (any tissue in the lymphatic system, which is concerned primarily with fighting infection) in the oral **mucosa** (in the mouth) can take over the function. If this were not the case, immune-system deficiencies following removal of the tonsils would probably be seen. As it is,

there is only a brief reduction of resistance to polio, which is of no consequence when most children are vaccinated against it.[9] The tonsils seem to be a mainstay of resistance to polio, but the body's immune system can adapt to their loss. Parents should be sure that a child who has had one or both tonsils removed is current on polio immunization and any boosters that are needed (this depends upon the vaccine used).

There was a great deal of concern in the past about hearing loss and facial deformity arising from swollen adenoids that obstruct the upper airway and the eustachian tubes, which run from inside the ear to the roof of the mouth. However, eustachian tube obstruction is less of a problem than previously believed. Now the only accepted indication for adenoidectomy is upper-airway obstruction,[10] the major concern being sleep apnea, which disrupts the normal sleep pattern.[11]

Another concern is the effect that airway obstruction has on the development of the face in the growing child. It has been shown by experimentally plugging the upper airway in monkeys and by observations of human children with obstructed upper airways that so-called mouth breathers have longer and narrower faces and more receding jaws than nose breathers. It is not clear whether correcting the upper airway obstruction reverses this process once it has begun. Therefore, physicians are urged to be cautious in advising parents that adenoidectomy will resolve such facial developmental abnormalities.[12, 13]

Obstruction of the airways by swollen adenoids can lead to partial or complete loss of the sense of smell; if the adenoids are removed, the sense of smell will be restored. Strangely, when smell is lost as a result of obstruction of the nostrils by the nasal **septum**, repair of the septum does not reliably restore the sense of smell.[14]

Although recurrent ear infections were once the primary indication for adenoidectomy, a 1990 study showed that the procedure had no effect on objective hearing tests in patients with recurrent ear infections.[15] Hence, the procedure is not needed to protect against hearing loss.

For a discussion of the remaining issues, see "Tonsillectomy," p. 238.

Total Abdominal Hysterectomy (3)

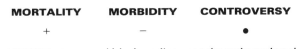

MORTALITY	MORBIDITY	CONTROVERSY
+	−	●

- **MORBIDITY** rates vary widely depending upon the study conducted. Anywhere from 6.6% to 46.3% of cases report morbidity, most of which seems related to laceration of the ureters and bladder.

- The **CONTROVERSY** surrounding this procedure primarily concerns appropriateness, because less radical surgical and medical treatment are available.

LAY TITLE: Hysterectomy

Removal of the uterus through an incision low in the abdomen. This procedure involves removal of the uterus and is to be distinguished from hysterectomy that includes removal of the ovaries and tubes, technically called a hysterectomy and salpingo-oopherectomy.

? WHAT CONDITION DOES THE PROCEDURE TREAT?

Physicians agree on only two indications for hysterectomies of any type: cancer, and obstetrical emergencies in which the uterus is too damaged to be repaired or in which there is uncontrollable bleeding. Cancer and obstetrical emergencies account for only about 10% of the hysterectomies performed. The other 90% lie in the broad area of "female trouble," which consists of excessive menstrual bleeding, uterine myomas (formerly called fibroid tumors, these are benign tumors of the muscular wall of the uterus), uterine **prolapse** (bulging of the uterus into the vagina), and **endometriosis**. Nonsurgical treatment, surgery less radical than a hysterectomy, or both are available for all these conditions.

The logic of the medical profession for virtually every other condition that offers the choice of medical (drug) treatment and minimal-to-radical surgery is to attempt medical treatment first. If medical treatment fails, minimal surgery is performed. Radical surgery is reserved for conditions that cannot be handled medically or with minor surgery. The rationale behind these nearly universal recommendations is: medical treatment always leaves the option of later surgery, whereas the opposite is not true—the organ may no longer be present for medical treatment if surgery comes first; complication rates and mortality from surgery are higher than for medical treatment in almost all conditions; and the risks of surgery rise as procedures become more radical. Why this logic has not been followed in the case of hysterectomies would make a fascinating sociological study, which we cannot pursue here.

? WHAT IS THE PROCEDURE?

The patient's genitalia are shaved before she enters the surgical suite. General anesthesia is used. With the patient under the anesthetic, the body is washed with soap and antiseptic and draped so that only the area to be operated on is exposed. In what follows, we describe one standard technique—there are many variations.

A **catheter** is placed in the bladder to facilitate drainage. An incision is made to the left of the navel, running from the navel to the start of the pubic hair. The skin, subcutaneous fat, and abdominal muscles are cut in layers; bleeding vessels are **cauterized** or **ligated**. The deep epigastric artery and vein, located near the stomach, are ligated and severed. The **peritoneum** is opened with scalpel and scissors. The **small intestine** is pushed out of the way with moist gauze. The peritoneal covering of the bladder, which is contiguous with that covering the uterus, is cut away with scalpel and scissors.

The **fallopian tubes**, which run from the ovaries to the uterus, and the **ligaments** that hold the uterus in position are located and severed. The uterus is held with **forceps** on the ends of the cut ligaments. The exposed bladder is then pushed away from the upper front of the **cervix** with moist gauze held in a clamp.

This is the point at which damage to the **ureters**, which connect the kidney to the bladder, is likely to occur. Such damage is the bane of this operation, and results from the surgeon grabbing at the infundibulo-pelvic ligament, which runs along the ureters, without first carefully identifying the ureter and separating the ureter from the ligament so that the ligament and not the ureter is cut. After the ligament has been identified and separated from the ureter, it is doubly or triply clamped, and it and the connecting tissue are ligated and severed. One by one, the tissue connecting the uterus to the body is severed and gradually lifted away from the body, until the uterus is connected only at the upper portion of the vagina.

Sutures are placed in the upper portion of the vaginal vault to maintain the upper portion of the vagina in position; tension is supplied by the doctors and nurses acting as surgical assistants. The uterus is cut away from the vagina at the level of the **cervix**, which is removed with the uterus. The vagina is supported by incorporating one or more of the severed ligaments that had supported the uterus into the stitching that closes the top of the vaginal vault. Some surgeons do not do this, believing that a simple closure of the vaginal vault incorporating only the cardinal ligament—which runs along the top of the vagina and holds it in place—is more comfortable and creates less tension on the ovaries than the more elaborate repairs. The peritoneum is closed over the bladder and the stump of the vaginal vault, and the muscle, fat, and skin are closed in layers.

? WHO PERFORMS THE PROCEDURE?

This procedure is done by obstetrician-gynecologists and general surgeons.

? WHERE IS THE PROCEDURE PERFORMED?

The procedure is done in a hospital.

? WHAT ARE THE MORTALITY (DEATH) AND MORBIDITY (COMPLICATION) RATES?

The mortality rate in community hospitals in the U.S. in 1989 was 0.1%. The literature reports rates of 0.06%[1] to 10.5%,[2] depending upon the country and the reasons for which the procedure was performed. The vast majority of quoted rates are well under 1%. In a 1979 to 1980 nationwide study examining data from hospitals participating in the Commission on Professional and Hospital Activities, the mortality rate for vaginal hysterectomies was 0.038%. The mortality for total abdominal hysterectomies was 0.15%—almost four times as high. Mortality rates rose with age and were twice as high for black women.[3] (In general, black women have less access to adequate medical care and so may have other complicating illnesses.)

Reported morbidity rates range downward from a high of 46.3% in one German study.[4] Most morbidity seems related to **lacerations** of the ureter or bladder and to infections. Preoperative use of antibiotics has a large positive effect on morbidity.

Morbidity rates for vaginal hysterectomy and abdominal hysterectomy groups were similar (24.21%), with a 48% rate of complications in patients operated on for cancer.[5] Other studies report morbidity rates as low as 6.6%[6] and as high as 41.07%.[7]

In a German study, the complication rate for the abdominal hysterectomy was almost twice as high as for vaginal hysterectomy (19.1% versus 9.6%), and total mortality for the abdominal procedure was five times as high as the vaginal procedure (1.7% versus 0.37%).[8]

Leaving the ovaries and tubes in place after either a vaginal or abdominal hysterectomy is associated with a low rate of complications. In a study of 2132 women who had had hysterectomies, 0.66% required further gynecological surgery; there were two deaths (0.09%), both from cancer.[9]

Catheters in the bladder are routinely used after gynecologic surgery (and are left in place from one to two days, or even a week, after surgery) to ensure proper urinary drainage. Either a **Foley catheter** (inserted through the **urethra**) or a suprapubic catheter, inserted into the bladder through the skin between the pubic bone and the top of the vaginal lips, may be used. Both are associated with high rates of infection, blockage, and bleeding from the bladder. Many patients find the suprapubic catheter more acceptable than the Foley catheter, despite the need for the skin puncture, because, if its diameter is large enough to stretch the bladder **sphincter**,[10] the Foley catheter can induce a sensation of constantly having to void. Infection rates with the Foley catheter can be as high as 67.1%, versus 20.9% for the suprapubic catheter.[11]

Women frequently report a change in sexual responsiveness and ability to enjoy intercourse following hysterectomy. Until recently, this complaint has been dismissed by many in the medical profession as simply the products of an inflamed female imagination. The official position of the American College of Obstetricians and Gynecologists was that "neither the production of hormones nor a woman's ability to have satisfying sexual relations is affected. . . ."[12] Concerning this potential complication, you need to distinguish carefully between hysterectomy that includes removal of the ovaries—which clearly causes dramatic hormonal changes—and hysterectomy that leaves the ovaries in place, a procedure that preserves the normal female hormonal balance but may alter pelvic and vaginal sensations, which play a large role in women's sexual responsiveness.

In a 1983 German study that focused on sexual responsiveness and female self-image, 56% of women under age 45 and 69% of women over age 45 reported no changes in their sex lives as a result of hysterectomy. However, these women reported significant changes in their self-image. Clearly, for about 44% of women under age 45 and one-third of women over age 45, the procedure does produce a perceived alteration in sexual response.[13] A 1989 German study found significant changes in sexual behavior and responsiveness even if the ovaries were left in place, and recommended hormone therapy for changes in sexual responsiveness even for women with intact ovaries.[14] Because sexual response has a very large mental component, both alterations in subjective perception and objective physical changes can produce objective changes in sexual response; neither are under the control of the patient to any significant degree. Surgery anywhere on the body frequently leads to diminished sensation, at least for a period following surgery, because most of the nerves that are cut are not individually reconnected.

? WHAT ARE THE OTHER COMPLICATIONS AND POSSIBLE SIDE EFFECTS?

The urge to void frequently is a complication associated more often with vaginal hysterectomies than with abdominal ones, according to one study.[15] For women who prior to surgery had complaints of a sensation of residual urine in the bladder after voiding, vaginal hysterectomy produced better results than total abdominal hysterectomy.[16]

A study of complications of vaginal and abdominal hysterectomy between 1978 and 1981 showed that women having vaginal hysterectomies had fewer infections, less bleeding, less fever, and shorter hospital stays than women who had the abdominal operation.[17]

Complications following vaginal and abdominal hysterectomy can include enterocele (a **herniation** of the vagina into the pelvic cavity) and complete and incomplete prolapse of the vaginal vault. These complications can be treated with low operative morbidity (other than fever) by sewing the residual vaginal cuff to the sacrospinous ligament (between the base of the pelvis and the bottom of the spine), a procedure that can be done through the vagina and does not require an abdominal incision. This produced complete resolution of the prolapse in 90% of the patients treated. Slightly more than 14% (14.1%) had laxity of the vaginal walls without symptoms, 12.67% had vaginal **stenosis** or stress incontinence—which is the inability to hold urine while coughing or laughing—5.63% developed a **cystocele**, and 4.22% had recurrent vaginal prolapse. (Numbers add to more than 100% because some patients fell into multiple categories.[18]) A further modification of the surgical technique apparently can completely prevent prolapse.[19]

A procedure that essentially closes off the vagina has been recommended for the avoidance of vaginal prolapse and stress incontinence in elderly, nonsexually active women who have stress incontinence.[20] Completely aside from the fact that vaginal prolapse appears to be associated with ineffective operative technique in the first place, the same result can be achieved with the purchase of a box of adult diapers.

As a late consequence of hysterectomy, **fistulas** have been observed between the **colon** and the vagina. The authors of the study note that the eruptions of pus when the cul-de-sac (the blind pouch between the vagina and the neck of the cervix, which is reduced to a single, open pouch via most hysterectomy techniques) was opened were "volcanic" and propose naming the disease the "Io Syndrome" after the most eruptive body in the solar system. The illness is life-threatening, but can be treated with surgery and antibiotics.[21]

The first, and only, case of an enormous pararenal **hematoma** (in the region of the kidney), which stretched from the vaginal stump to the kidney, was reported in 1987. The portion of the hematoma near the vaginal stump was seen by **ultrasound**, but only a **CT scan** revealed the full extent. Such hematomas can be treated with surgery, but can be devastating if they became a focus of infection.[22]

Pulmonary embolism is a potentially fatal complication of any surgery in the lower body. The rate of embolism in vaginal hysterectomies is about one-fifth that of abdominal hysterectomies (0.3% versus 1.7%).[23] Abdominoplastic surgery (cosmetic operations on the abdomen, such as "tummy tucks") performed at the same time as a number of different gynecological operations were associated with significantly greater blood loss and increased incidence of pulmonary embolism. This is an important finding, since embolisms can be fatal.[24] There are situations in which combining procedures reduces morbidity and mortality, but this is apparently not one of them.

Urinary retention can follow almost any surgery, but is especially common after operations on the abdomen and pelvis. In a highly detailed 1987 study from Germany, the frequency of urinary tract problems following vaginal hysterectomy was between one-half to one-fifth of that following abdominal hysterectomy, with the sole exception of retention of urine in an amount greater than 10% of maximum bladder capacity, for which the rate was 24.2% after vaginal surgery and 13.2% after abdominal hysterectomies.[25] Insertion of a solution of **prostaglandin** F2, a compound produced naturally by the body, into the bladder was significantly more effective than salt water in overcoming urinary retention.[26] A similar result was found with the related compound prostaglandin E2.[27] Prostaglandins were first identified in the prostate gland of men (hence the name). They exert a number of physiological effects, including the stimulation of contraction in smooth muscle tissue such as that found in the bladder.

Damage to ureters, which lie close to the paracervical ligaments that support the uterus, arises from the belief that the paracervical ligaments must be ligated before they are cut, in order to prevent excess bleeding. This is a part of both the standard vaginal and standard open procedures, but is obviously more difficult to perform vaginally. In both procedures, ligation and division of the paracervical ligaments may result in accidental ligation and cutting of the ureter, the repair of which requires relatively delicate corrective surgery. Described in the literature is a variation on the standard operation, which does not involve ligation of the paracervical ligaments. This procedure reduced ureteral damage to 0.03%, and reduced the need for further surgery to control bleeding to 0.02%.[28] Apparently, the paracervical ligaments are not as prone to bleeding as had been thought.

There are no other significant complications besides the anesthesia risks and thromboembolic complications that attend all surgery. As with any procedure in which anesthesia is used, death from reaction to the anesthetic drugs, error on the part of the anesthetist, or machine failure is a remote possibility. (See Glossary, p. 309)

? IS THIS THE MOST APPROPRIATE PROCEDURE FOR THE CONDITION?

As already noted, the only conditions on which clear medical agreement for hysterectomy exists are cancer and obstetrical emergencies. Few decision-support models (devices for making better medical decisions based on accumulated outcome data) appear in the literature, but a cost-benefit analysis[29] suggests that cancer prevention is a faulty rationale for hysterectomy. "Quality of life" considerations often play a role in the decision to use this procedure, but the medical profession has clearly failed to inform women adequately about pos-

sible effects of hysterectomy on mood, sexual enjoyment, and lasting postoperative discomfort. As with nearly all procedures for nonmalignant conditions, nothing is lost by trying more conservative therapies first and operating only if they fail.

? ARE THERE ALTERNATIVES TO THIS PROCEDURE?

Laser surgery and removal of **myomas** without removal of the entire uterus have been developed and are being increasingly used.

? WHAT IS CONTROVERSIAL ABOUT THE PROCEDURE?

Almost everything. As noted above, all of the **indications** for this procedure other than cancer and obstetrical emergencies are controversial; beyond these, there is only general agreement that it should not be used for sterilization. New research, especially on the role of the uterus in sexual functioning, is leading to a complete rethinking of the unique medical "logic" that has been applied to this procedure. In general, if the indication is not cancer or obstetrical emergency, medical treatment and less radical surgical treatment (such as excision of fibroid tumors from the uterus, rather than removal of the uterus itself) should be tried first. A hysterectomy should be resorted to only if symptoms are intolerable, and if the operative risks and potential disruption of sexual response are worth having the procedure done. Those decisions are best left up to the patient.

Total Cholecystectomy (2)

MORTALITY	MORBIDITY	CONTROVERSY
+	+	o

Gallbladder removal

? WHAT CONDITION DOES THE PROCEDURE TREAT?

This procedure is used to treat gallstones, acute sterile inflammation of the gallbladder, acute infections of the gallbladder that do not respond to antibiotics, and benign and malignant tumors of the gallbladder.

The gallbladder is a small sac that hangs below the liver and stores bile until it is needed in the digestive process. (Bile is produced by the liver and helps the intestines break down and digest fats of all types.)

Because of the high concentration of various chemicals in the bile, gallstones may be formed. Many gallstones are formed from cholesterol. (Cholesterol, although implicated in heart disease, is a key constituent of cell walls and hormones and is absolutely necessary for life. The liver produces about 70% of the total cholesterol in the bloodstream; a fatty diet and consequent excess weight seem to tip the balance enough to cause stone formation. Stones can be formed from other constituents of the bile, even in the presence of normal cholesterol levels. The exact process of stone formation is unknown; inflammation and infections appear to play a role.

After removal of the gallbladder, bile produced by the liver drains into the small intestines in a steady stream. Although the bile retains its digestive function, the amounts present in the small intestines after a fatty meal may be less than would have been present if the gallbladder were still intact.

The three conditions noted above are connected: The presence of stones seems to make the gallbladder more prone to inflammation and infection, and these conditions seem to lead to more stone formation. Chronic inflammation and irritation of the gallbladder, in turn, encourage tumor formation to some degree. The pain produced by gallstones is called biliary colic; inflammation of the gallbladder is called cholecystitis.

? WHAT IS THE PROCEDURE?

A number of techniques, all variations on the same theme, can be used for the total cholecystectomy. Normally, a general anesthetic is used. At least three different incisions may be used—one running just below the ribs on the right side of the body, one running from the right side of the **sternum** down to the right side of the navel, and a third along a roughly horizontal line on the right side of the body halfway between the navel and the sternum. (These are known, respectively, as the right paramedian muscle-retracting lateral incision, the right subcostal, and the right transverse incision.) Experts generally hold that the subcostal incision affords the surgeon the best access to the gallbladder, whereas the right paramedian is much more comfortable for the recovering patient.

The skin is shaved and washed with a disinfectant solution, and the patient is draped so that only the area to be operated on is exposed. Once the chosen incision is made, the underlying structures, such as the muscles and the **peritoneum**, are cut, and any bleeding that occurs is controlled. The surgeon may, if she chooses, push her hand between the liver and the **diaphragm** to rotate the gallbladder and bring it into better view. Using moist gauze pads, the stomach is pushed up and away to the patient's left and held there, and the transverse (middle) part of the **colon** and the beginning of the small intestine below the stomach are covered and pushed slightly down and to the right if necessary.

The margins of the wound are **retracted** enough (by the surgical assistants—doctors, nurses, and/or physicians' assistants) to give the surgeon access to the gallbladder and the **ligaments** that hold it in position. The first of these is cut, giving access to the bile ducts and the veins and arteries that supply the gallbladder and the liver. These structures are hard to repair if damaged, so great care is used to ensure that they are properly identified, kept out of the way, and not cut too short.

Two clamps are placed on the cystic artery, which supplies the gallbladder, and on the cystic duct that drains bile from the gallbladder into the **small intestine**, and these are cut in two and tied off. During this process, care is taken not to put the cystic artery under too much tension, as it is hard to repair if torn. Once the duct and artery are cut and tied off, they are tied off again, to avoid the possibility of hemorrhage or bile leakage.

The opening of the gallbladder is clamped to avoid leakage, and is then gradually freed from the peritoneum that covers it by a combination of sharp (scalpel and scissors) and blunt (finger) dissections until it can be brought out onto the sterile drape covering the patient. The final connections between the gallbladder and the interior of the abdomen are not cut until the surgeon has inspected the bottom of the liver and **ligated** or **cauterized** any small bleeding points. The peritoneum is partially closed over the liver, the last connections with the gallbladder are severed, and the peritoneum is closed. A soft rubber drain is placed in the wound, and the muscle and skin layers are sutured or stapled separately.

Some further variations in technique concern drainage of acutely inflamed gallbladders, intraoperative x rays of the bile ducts to make sure that all stones are removed before the incision is closed, and rerouting of the drain—from its normal route under the side of the liver, to out the right flank under the ribs. Some surgeons believe that acutely inflamed gallbladders should be punctured and suctioned before their removal is attempted, to avoid spreading irritants or infectious material into the surgical wound. Others think that the tension on the walls of the gallbladder makes its removal easier. **Intraoperative cholangiography** is done to make sure that no stones have been missed; however, this x ray is gradually becoming less common with the arrival of transcutaneous ("through-the-skin") procedures for stone removal.

Another variation in the procedure concerns the method by which some surgeons route the drain. Rather than through the operative incision, some surgeons prefer to route the drain out through a fresh stab wound made from inside the abdominal cavity with a **trochar.** Many surgeons believe that the presence of a drain in the healing wound weakens the scar or leaves a depression below skin level (an unhappy cosmetic result), or both. The drain is removed when any observed leakage of bile from the wound has stopped.

While the assistants are closing the surgical incision, the operating surgeon opens the gallbladder (by now lying in a tray on a stand well away from the operating table) and counts the stones for the operative report. The average size of a stone is roughly one-quarter inch, and the number of stones recovered may range from fewer than 10 to hundreds.

? WHO PERFORMS THE PROCEDURE?

This procedure is usually done by a general surgeon.

? WHERE IS THE PROCEDURE PERFORMED?

This operation is usually done as an inpatient hospital procedure.

WHAT ARE THE MORTALITY (DEATH) AND MORBIDITY (COMPLICATION) RATES?

The overall death rate for total cholecystectomies is 1.2%, but rates as high as 6% and as low as 0.5% have been reported in some studies.[1, 2] Complications include hemorrhage, leakage of bile, infectious **peritonitis**, **bile peritonitis**, and wound infection that does not go deep enough to infect the peritoneum, as well as anesthetic and general surgical risks.

As with any procedure in which anesthesia is used, death from reaction to the anesthetic drugs, error on the part of the anesthetist, or machine failure is a remote possibility. (See Glossary, p. 309)

The rate of minor technical and postoperative complications ranges from 1.1% to 6.1% and from 2% to 8.1%, depending upon the series and patient group.[3] In one study that involved emergency operations on elderly patients with gangrenous gallbladders, the mortality rate was 19%.[4] When the procedure is needed for treatment of gallbladder problems that develop as postoperative complications of other surgery, the mortality rate can be as high as 47%.[5] Very aggressive surgery combining removal of the gallbladder and portions of the liver for cancer has had a mortality rate of zero in studies with carefully selected patients.[6] It is important to note that these mortality rates are roughly quadrupled if **common bile duct** exploration for stones is combined with gallbladder removal. No one knows for certain why mortality rates for the combined procedure are so high, but they may be attributable to duct damage that is not visible to the surgeon. Such exploration should be done only as a last resort, when cholangiography is not available to the surgeon.

WHAT ARE THE OTHER COMPLICATIONS AND POSSIBLE SIDE EFFECTS?

Of course, the operation alters the pattern of digestion—how long food stays in the stomach and the small intestine and how much gas and cramping are produced. As a result, digestion of a fatty meal may not be as rapid or efficient as it was before. Tolerance for fatty foods may be reduced. The symptoms for which the surgery was conducted are resolved in about 90% of the cases.[7]

IS THIS THE MOST APPROPRIATE PROCEDURE FOR THE CONDITION?

In otherwise healthy patients and even in patients with cancer, cholecystectomy can offer a mortality rate of zero and relief of symptoms in 90% of cases. Nonetheless, as in all operations in which the abdomen is entered, the procedure is potentially risky. Cholecystotomy—making an incision in the gallbladder, removing the stones, draining it, and leaving it in place—has been around for about a century and is used when the surgeon thinks that the standard operation (complete removal of the gallbladder) will pose too great a risk.

ARE THERE ALTERNATIVES TO THIS PROCEDURE?

Recently, several alternatives have been developed. The first is the mini-cholecystotomy,[8] in which the patient is under local anesthesia and the gallbladder is reached and opened by a radiologist through a small incision. A radiologist removes the stones with the aid of a fluoroscope, which enables him to see where the stones are in relation to the various instruments. The mini-cholecystotomy has been used quite successfully in high-risk patients, such as those who cannot tolerate general anesthesia.

Another alternative is endoscopic sphincterotomy. In this procedure, a gastroenterologist passes a flexible scope through the mouth, through the **esophagus** and stomach, and into the **duodenum**, where bile enters. From there she cuts open the **sphincter** that constricts the gallbladder opening and holds in the bile. If failure of the stones to pass through to the small intestine was caused by a narrow sphincter, this procedure can allow removal of the stones. The procedure also works well for many small stones or "sludge" in the gallbladder, as well as for stones lodged in the cystic duct, the duct from the gallbladder and pancreas to the small intestine. In one study, endoscopic sphincterotomy brought relief to 97% of patients without demonstrated gallstones, a situation in which the person has pain but x rays do not show stones.[9] However, the procedure does no good for stones that are too big to pass through the widened sphincter.

Drugs can be used to dissolve cholesterol gallstones. The only one in use at present is ursodiol (brand name Actigall) (ursodeoxycholic acid), which is found in small quantities in the bile of people and some species of bears.[10] Through a number of chemical actions in the body, ursodiol switches the chemical environment in the gallbladder from cholesterol-precipitating to cholesterol-dissolving. Eighty-one percent of patients whose largest stones were no more than 5 mm in size (about one-fifth of an inch) had complete dissolution of all stones. Those with calcified stones (in which calcium compounds either enclose cholesterol stones or are combined with them) and those with stones larger than 20 mm (about three-quarters of an inch) had essentially no stone dissolution. The known drawbacks of ursodiol, at the time this is being written, are diarrhea and the price, which runs around $1.85 to $2.00 per pill, making the cost for a complete year approximately $1500.

Lithotripsy, the shattering of gallstones by sound waves, has been gaining a lot of attention lately. In this procedure, the patient is given a general anesthetic and placed in a water bath. The patient's position is adjusted by a remote-controlled sling until the gallstones are at the focus of shock waves generated by a spark gap (a miniature bolt of lightning, in essence) at the bottom of the tub. If the procedure is successful, the gallstones are shattered into a fine sand that can be painlessly passed in stool. In theory, there is little if any damage to the rest of the body because only the stones are at the focus of the shock wave. In practice, most patients have some mild bleeding, bruising, or tenderness, which usually does not require further treatment. The limitation of this procedure is that it only works on stones that are hard and rigid enough to be shattered by the shock waves.

A newer alternative is the laparoscopic cholecystectomy. In this procedure, a trochar is inserted into the navel, and the abdomen is inflated with carbon dioxide to separate the organs. Another small incision is made in the right flank just below the usual location of the gallbladder, and a **laparoscope**—a rigid or flexible fiberoptic instrument with lenses, laser or **electrocautery** channels, a channel for biopsy and grasping **forceps**, and channels for gas and suction—is inserted. As in the open procedure—the cholecystectomy—the gallbladder and the ducts running from it are located and separated, the ducts, arteries, and veins are clipped or ligated, and the gallbladder is cut away from the underside of the liver, grasped with the scope, and removed.

Reports of this procedure are highly enthusiastic, show very low complication rates, and indicate that some patients can return to heavy manual labor within a week after the procedure, versus the usual six weeks after the open procedure. As you might expect from the relative size of the wounds, postoperative pain is much less than with the open procedure. Mortality rates reported are all zero,[11] and complication rates run from zero[12] to 1.6%[13] to 2.88%.[14] A **prospective**, or forward-looking, as opposed to **retrospective study** of the results of diagnostic laparotomy, a technically similar procedure, suggests that these results may be better than those that will be seen with wider experience. The prospective study showed complication rates of 7.4% and a mortality rate of 0.49%, both much higher than those previously reported in the literature.

Percutaneous cholecystotomy, in which the gallbladder is drained through a small incision or large needle puncture using x-ray guidance, is also a possibility in some cases. The reported complication rate in a 1990 study was 13.2%, with 5.2% serious complications (such as bile peritonitis).[15]

? WHAT IS CONTROVERSIAL ABOUT THE PROCEDURE?

Clearly, gallbladder surgery is becoming less traumatic. Furthermore, the laparoscopic procedure will eventually replace the open procedure where it is technically feasible. (**Adhesions** from previous surgery, unexpected hemorrhage, severe infection or inflammation, instrument failure, and accidental damage to the ducts can make it necessary to stop an attempted laparoscopic removal and use the open procedure.)

Among surgeons, the major controversy over the laparoscopic procedure concerns the relative merits of laser light versus electrocautery. The laser offers better precision; electrocautery seems to be better at controlling bleeding and allows for a slightly quicker operation (about 40 minutes as compared with about 90 for the laparoscopic procedure, although this varies with the proficiency of the surgeon).

Total Hip Replacement (37)

MORTALITY	MORBIDITY	CONTROVERSY
+	–	●

- The **MORBIDITY** following hip replacement surgery is highly age-dependent. The older the patient, the greater the risk of complications following surgery. The general complication rate is 20%.
- The **CONTROVERSY** involves the use of cementless versus cemented **prostheses**.

Replacement of the hip socket and upper portion of the **femur** with metal and plastic prosthetic parts

? WHAT CONDITION DOES THE PROCEDURE TREAT?

This procedure is used to treat **rheumatoid arthritis** and **osteoarthritis** of the hip that cannot be controlled with medication; benign and malignant tumors of the hip or thigh bones; and fractures of the hip or thigh that cannot be handled with a more conservative procedure (such as insertion of metal screws, plates, or nails) or that do not heal satisfactorily.

The first attempted total hip replacement was in 1890,[1] and although interest was revived in the 1920s and the 1950s, it was not until 1960 when the English surgeon John Charnley first used bone cement to attach the components to the bones that the operation began to be widely used.[2]

? WHAT IS THE PROCEDURE?

The patient is given a general or spinal anesthetic and the hip to be operated on is washed with soap and antiseptic. A tourniquet may be wrapped around the thigh to control bleeding, and an incision is made that is long enough to permit complete exposure of the hip joint. The skin, fat, **fascia**, and muscle are cut open, bleeding vessels are **cauterized** or tied off, and the lips of the incision are pulled apart (**retracted**) to give the surgeon access to the joint. The **ligaments** holding the hip together are cut and trimmed away. Using a hammer, chisel, files, and drills, the hip socket is trimmed back until the opening is large enough to hold the artificial hip socket (prosthesis), which is made of metals (such as Vitallium and chrome and titanium alloys) well-tolerated by the body and lined on the inside with high-density polyethylene (a type of plastic).

When sufficient trimming is done, the surgeon attempts to fit the hip portion of the prosthesis in place. If needed, further trimming is done until the prosthesis fits properly. If a cementless procedure is used, the artificial hip socket is pressed into the pelvis until it locks into place. If cement (usually methyl methacrylate, a variation of Super Glue) is used, it is applied before the final fitting of the artificial socket.

The top of the femur is cut away, and the canal running down the center of the bone, called the **medullary canal**, is cleaned or reamed out. When the surgeon regards the medulla as fully cleaned out, she places the femoral part of the prosthesis (which contains the "ball" of the joint) into the canal, then checks for fit with the hip socket and for proper alignment of the bones and correct length of the leg. If cement is used, it is applied before the final fitting. (A proper fit is one that is not loose and that duplicates as closely as possible the workings of the natural hip joint.)

When the fit is as good as can be achieved, the ligaments of the hip joint are reattached over the prosthesis, and the muscle, fascia, and skin are closed in layers. If there is a chance that a **hematoma** may form, plastic suction tubes are inserted in the operative wound. (These drains remain in the wound until the doctor observes no further discharge of blood from the incision. In younger patients this may take a day or two, and up to a week in older patients.) The patient is taken to the recovery room, then to her room after recovering from the anesthetic. There she is given **inhalation therapy**, physical therapy, and drugs for the prevention of blood clots in the lower limbs. Walking is attempted within one or two days after surgery. If it is needed, physical therapy may be continued after discharge for up to a month for older patients and up to two weeks for younger patients.

? WHO PERFORMS THE PROCEDURE?

Total hip replacements should be performed only by board-certified orthopedic surgeons who have done many of them. Here, as with most other surgeries, the results achieved by hospitals and individual physicians improve as the number of procedures done increases.[3] Generally, surgeons and institutions in areas with the highest number of cases will have the best outcomes, but many do not reach the volumes at which research indicates the best results are achieved.[4]

? WHERE IS THE PROCEDURE PERFORMED?

This is major, complex surgery with a high potential for fatal complications, and should be performed only in a hospital where a large number of such surgeries are performed. Operating rooms equipped with rapid air exchange and filtration systems that can change the air up to 300 times per hour have been shown to reduce the chance of infection.[5]

? WHAT ARE THE MORTALITY (DEATH) AND MORBIDITY (COMPLICATION) RATES?

As is the case with most operations, morbidity and mortality rates were fairly high while this procedure was being perfected, but have now fallen appreciably, with a mortality rate of about 0.5% to 1.5%, and a complication rate of about 20%.

A 1980 study of patients with an average age of 80 years reported a mortality rate of 4% and a morbidity rate of 77%. Another study found a mortality rate of 5.7% in the period 1967–1975.[6] A 1990 German study showed a mortality rate of 1.6% and a fatal **pulmonary embolism** rate of 1.85%.[7] A pulmonary embolism is a blood clot or other obstruction—such as air, fat, or bone marrow—that travels through the blood vessels to the lung and stops all or part of a lung from receiving oxygen-depleted blood from the heart or returning oxygenated blood to it. The severity can range from trivial to fatal, depending upon the size and location of the obstruction. Pulmonary embolism is a relatively common problem after major lower limb surgery.[8–12] **Air embolism** is a variety of embolism arising from free air in the circulatory system; rather than resulting from a clot, blockage is attributable to inability to move the air. The consequences of air embolism, as with embolism caused by clots, can range from trivial to fatal. One small study found air embolism, diagnosed by a change in continuously monitored heart sounds, in 83% of total hip replacement patients. It was possible to use a **catheter** to recover free air from the **right atrium** in two-thirds of them.[13] In another study, flushing the opened femoral shaft with carbon dioxide gas was found to completely prevent air embolism.[14]

The range of morbidity and mortality rates worldwide is attributable to variations in patient populations and technique, and is probably illustrative of variations that occur among surgeons at different hospitals in the U.S. A German investigation reported in 1990 a mortality rate of 0.43% in a group of patients who were 60 years of age or older.[15] A 1986 French study reported a mortality rate of 1%.[16] In a group of elderly Canadians studied, the one-month mortality rate was about 8%.[17] A 1989 German study revealed that **intraoperative** complications occurred in 2% of patients, postoperative complications related to the surgery occurred in 19.8% of patients, and unrelated complications occurred in 36.8%.[18] A 1982 French study reported mortality

rates of 1.73% and complications of 10.9% (stroke, 3.6%; loosening of the artificial component without infection, 3%; postoperative hip dislocations, 2.47%; and an infection rate of 1.28%).[19] A 1989 study found a surprisingly high mortality rate—11.54%—and two near-fatal episodes (or 3.9%) of **hypotension** during the implantation of cemented hip replacement parts.[20] A 1985 Canadian study reported a complication rate of 25%, with complications interfering with the functioning of the hip replacement in 4.5%.[21] In 1990, Dutch investigators reported a three-month mortality rate of 24.3% for hip fractures, and found that only 60% of patients were able to return home after surgical treatment of various kinds.[22]

Mortality rates in excess of those generally observed for hip replacement surgery appear to be limited to the first six months following surgery, according to one study.[23] Another study found that the higher mortality rate was limited to the first year following surgery for women but continued past the first year for men. The exact reasons for this are unclear; however, it was noted in the findings that men had a tendency to form blood clots.[24]

The mortality rate from pulmonary embolism is at least 2%, and the incidence of deep venous **thrombosis**, which is clot formation in the vessels of the lower leg closest to the bone, is 50%.[25] If pulmonary embolism occurs, the mortality rate is about 10%.[26] A study of patients receiving medication for embolism prevention after total hip replacements found that deep vein thrombosis occurred in 14.1%, in spite of the treatment.[27] One study using **transesophageal echocardiography** revealed that embolization of air occurred in 92.3% of patients who did not have a vent hole drilled in the femur before insertion of the femoral part of the hip prosthesis, but in only 30.8% of those who had a vent hole drilled.[28] In another echocardiographic study, patients had an average of 1.9 echocardiographically detectable embolisms during hip replacement surgery.[29] Yet another study found that deep vein thrombosis, a precursor of embolism, occurred in 52% of patients given general anesthesia but only 29% of patients given spinal anesthesia.[30]

Infection is a relatively rare problem, but can be devastating if it occurs.[31] Use of bone cement mixed with the antibiotic gentamicin has been shown to reduce recurrence of infection to 3.8% at a follow-up of two-and-a-half years.[32] Another study found an infection rate of 0.56%—which it noted was "very low"—a loosening rate of 9.8%, and other complications in 6.8% of patients.[33] If infection occurs, it can be treated successfully with antibiotics in approximately 91% of patients, with minor to major surgery to refine the bone/prosthesis joints, or with removal of the hip prosthesis and replacement at a later time, if the patient's condition permits.[34]

Loosening of the parts of the prosthesis remains a major unsolved problem.[35, 36] A 1989 study with follow-up at five and seven years found loosening of some component (pelvic or femoral) in 12.5% of cases.[37] Loosening may require reoperation, depending upon its severity, whether there is associated pain, and whether it interferes with the patient's activities. A study using cemented parts and use of bone **grafts**, rather than cement, to fill gaps found a loosening rate of only 5%.[38]

Heterotrophic ossification, or bone growing into the flesh surrounding the prosthesis, occurs in 70% of patients with hip replacements, and progresses to an extent that causes pain in 2% to 5% of cases. It is usually not a problem unless it causes pain or range-of-motion limitations, and can be treated successfully with low-dose radiation,[39] **nonsteroidal anti-inflammatory drugs** such as ibuprofen, or both.[40–42]

Another possible complication, extrusion of cement from the bone during the procedure, which can further irritate already damaged tissues, can be prevented with the use of cement dams.[43] (These are metal or plastic shields that prevent the cement from coming in contact with the surrounding tissue.)

One particularly meticulous study of complications associated with a cementless prosthesis found that 1.12% of cases had leg lengthening as a result of an overly large femoral part; 1.12% of cases had loosening attributable to a part that was too small; 1.76% of cases had some damage to the thigh bone during surgery; 12.06% had excess bone growth; 3.23% had **thromboembolisms**; and 1.76% developed pneumonia. Use of the drug ethane-1-hydroxy-1, 1-diphosphonate (EHDP) reduced the incidence of excess bone growth from 28% to 12% over the period studied.[44]

A total hip replacement may become loose, wear out, or cause bone erosion, requiring reoperation to repair the connections between the bone and the replacement or complete removal and replacement of the prosthesis. Results of studies of the need for **revision** or replacement vary greatly, as to the duration of the study over the period 1960–1991, the type of prosthesis used, the length of time over which the patient's condition was followed, whether cement was used, and patient age. One study found a need for replacement in 1.7% of patients per year.[45] Others reported reoperation rates ranging between 0.8% and 12%, with the lower rates found in later studies. Some of the reported improvement may be attributable simply to the simple fact that the newer implants have not yet had time to wear out or erode the bone.[46–50]

? WHAT ARE THE OTHER COMPLICATIONS AND POSSIBLE SIDE EFFECTS?

Because the surgical wound is large, the area operated on has a rich blood supply, and because the handling of tissue during the operation is unavoidably rough, significant bleeding during and after the operation is common. Because the donated blood supply is subject to contamination with the HIV (AIDS) virus even with careful testing, the medical community has sought ways to reduce bleeding, and thereby reduce the need for transfusions. Powdered **collagen** sprinkled around the operative site has been shown to significantly reduce bleeding,[51] as has inducement of hypotension by the use of drugs during surgery.[52, 53]

Venous complications of one sort or another (such as tearing, clotting, infection, or destruction of the vein's valves) occurred in 10% of cases in an early series of patients;[54] such complications are occasionally fatal.[55]

Rough handling can result in **iatrogenic** fractures of the femur—in other words, the surgeons are being too rough when performing the procedure or implanting the new joint—in up to 22.2% of patients, with an average of 0.2 fractures per procedure performed in one series.[56] Other series report rates under 1%.[57] One study found a fracture rate of 6.3% in reoperations,[58] and the Mayo Clinic found the same fracture rate in one of its series of initial operations.[59]

Rough handling, especially overzealous retraction of the surgical wound, can result in a wide range of vascular problems, many of which can cause pulmonary embolism. The heat given off by the cement when setting can damage veins and arteries near it and result in thromboembolism from this source alone.[60]

Acute inflammation of the gallbladder, a condition called cholecystitis, follows orthopedic surgery in a small percentage of cases. Its symptoms are obscure and differ from the usual way that acute cholecystitis appears in patients who have not had orthopedic surgery. If caught early, it can be successfully treated with drugs or surgery, but can be fatal if not recognized.[61]

Use of hydrogen peroxide to clean the femoral channel has resulted in deaths; however, its use is not common.[62]

A 1989 German study of elderly patients being operated on under spinal anesthesia found complication rates of 6.5% for hypotension; 7.42% for unacceptable variations in heart rate; 1.08% for shock; respiratory arrest in 0.09% of patients; and intraoperative pulmonary embolism in 0.12%.[63]

Damage to the nerves in the area of the operation is possible. If the large nerve that runs down the back of the leg is damaged, complete recovery without further surgery can be expected in only 58% of cases.[64]

Hematomas that occur after the procedure are treated with suction drainage. As a result of treatment for primary hematomas, secondary hematomas can occur because of the high-pressure suction used in some systems; however, the use of low-pressure, closed-drainage systems can reduce this occurrence to under 1%.[65] (A medical suction device is a vacuum cleaner that sucks up fluids, and some have high-speed motors that create a high vacuum and evacuate fluids very quickly. Because of the amount of suction created, it is possible to suck up and pinch tissue, thereby creating a blood blister.)

Cracks in the femoral bone that do not extend all the way through and are therefore not visible to the naked eye or with the use of x rays may occur during the operation when a cementless femoral part is used, and may cause significant pain that has no clear diagnosis when the patient attempts to walk after surgery.[66]

Hypertension during surgery, which in theory could present a risk of stroke during the operation, was found in 11% of patients in whom a tourniquet was used to control bleeding during the operation, versus 1% of those operated on without the use of a tourniquet.[67]

The spread of bone cement into the tissues of the pelvis is usually regarded as harmless, but occasionally can lead to devastating complications, including pain during sexual intercourse (dyspareunia).[68]

As with any procedure in which anesthesia is used, death from a reaction to the anesthetic drugs, error on the part of the anesthetist, or machine failure is a remote possibility. (See Glossary, p. 309)

❓ IS THIS THE MOST APPROPRIATE PROCEDURE FOR THE CONDITION?

Yes, if medical therapy does not produce a satisfactory result. Patients need to be aware that, based on the combination of surgeon, hospital, any preexisting medical problems they may have, and prosthetic parts chosen, the results can range from superb recovery, to catastrophic complications, to fatalities. Patient and physician reports of the percent of cases with good to excellent results vary from 9% to 94%.[69-82]

❓ ARE THERE ALTERNATIVES TO THIS PROCEDURE?

Alternatives include reliance on nonsurgical treatment alone, such as drug treatment for arthritis. It is also possible to replace only the head of the femur with a prosthesis, but good to excellent results were achieved in only slightly more than half the cases reported in one study.[83] Replacement of the femoral head alone was found by another group of investigators to be quite unsatisfactory, and the authors concluded that this procedure might even be contraindicated.[84] These authors found that following replacement of the femoral head alone the hip socket will erode with continual wear and tear. Another study, however, found relatively good results with femoral head replacement alone, although 16.7% of the patients had continuing postoperative pain at average follow-up of 21 months.[85]

It is probably safe to say that most total hip replacement patients have decided that continued nonsurgical treatment is not satisfactory, although the physician may have some influence on the choice to have the surgery at a particular time.

❓ WHAT IS CONTROVERSIAL ABOUT THE PROCEDURE?

A significant debate concerns the use of cementless versus cemented prostheses. Cement eventually wears, it generates heat as it sets, and its application causes brief circulatory and respiratory reactions in many patients. Such problems are avoided with the cementless type, but these do not adhere as tightly to bone as do the cemented ones, at least in the initial months of wear.

When the cementless versions were developed, it was hoped that a combination of surface texture and materials would induce the bone to grow into and around the prosthetic parts. This has proven to be true for the artificial hip socket, but false for the femoral part. Most surgeons base their choice of prosthesis upon the patient's age and lifestyle, the amount of bone damage that has resulted from arthritis or trauma, and how good a fit they achieve with the artificial components after trimming the bones. Undoubtedly, doctors are influenced by sellers of prosthetic parts, but there is a growing trend to try to fit the parts to the patient, rather than the other way around.

Total Knee Replacement (24)

MORTALITY	MORBIDITY	CONTROVERSY
+	+	●

- The **CONTROVERSY** involves the replacement of a single component of the knee with an artificial material. The question is whether only part of the structure should be replaced or whether it is better to replace the entire joint.

Replacement of the knee with an artificial joint

? WHAT CONDITION DOES THE PROCEDURE TREAT?

The usual indications for total knee replacement are severe **rheumatoid arthritis** or **osteoarthritis** that does not respond to medical treatment, or trauma that damages the knee joint beyond repair. Even though bone is weakened in both forms of arthritis, it is uncommon for bone to be weakened to a degree that would make joint replacement impossible.[1] Severe juvenile rheumatoid arthritis that leads to continuous pain and loss of function despite medical treatment can be treated with total knee replacement, even though the bones may still be growing.[2] The procedure can also replace joints destroyed by cancerous and noncancerous tumors.[3]

? WHAT IS THE PROCEDURE?

Artificial replacements for one damaged surface of an arthritic or traumatized joint have been evolving slowly since the mid-1930s, but effective total joint replacement for both the knee and the hip was not possible until a discovery in the mid-1960s by a British physician named John Charnley. He found that bone has a high tolerance for acrylic cements (variations on Super Glue) and will bond with them. Compared with the older and more conservative procedures (such as replacing only the damaged surfaces, replaning joints, or removing membranes), results of total joint replacement have been so good that they have replaced almost all of the older techniques.[4]

Assuming that there is no damage to the **ligaments** and **tendons** of the knee and that all are salvageable, here is how the procedure is typically done: The patient's leg is shaved on the night or the morning before surgery. She is taken to the operating room, where a general anesthetic is administered. The knee is opened and the joint examined to determine the amount of bone damage. Based on x-ray measurements taken before sur-

gery, the correctly sized **prosthesis** that will permit removal of all damaged bone and ensure good stability is selected. The various ligaments are freed from their attachments to the bone surfaces that will be removed. The end of the **femur** and the top of the **tibia** are cut off with a bone saw. The canal in the center of the bone is reamed deep enough to allow insertion of the prosthesis to a depth that will preserve the normal length of the leg. If a cemented procedure is used, cement is applied to the artificial parts before they are inserted into the bone for the final time; otherwise, they are pressed into place. (Cementless, or "press-to-fit," procedures are done this way.) The knee joint is carefully reassembled with as little disruption of the ligaments as possible; the ligaments that had to be removed from bony surfaces are reattached. The joint is put in a cast and the patient is taken to the recovery room.

? WHO PERFORMS THE PROCEDURE?

This procedure should be done only by a board-certified orthopedic surgeon who performs a large number of such operations each year.

? WHERE IS THE PROCEDURE PERFORMED?

This is a hospital inpatient procedure.

? WHAT ARE THE MORTALITY (DEATH) AND MORBIDITY (COMPLICATION) RATES?

The mortality rate in community hospitals in 1989 was 0.6%.[5] Complications are of much greater concern than mortality in total knee replacements. The one extensive general review of mortality and morbidity that we could locate found mortality rates, reoperation rates, and complications rates as follows:

Two knees performed during the same operation: 5.5%, 2.4%, 9.3%.

Two knees performed during the same hospitalization: 0.9%, 4.8%, 7.0%.

Two knees performed in separate hospitalizations: 3.8%, 8.5%, 12.0%.

One knee: 7.0%, 5.6%, 11.0%.

Despite the wide range, none of these differences was statistically significant.[6] (This means that the results found are as likely to be due to chance as to real differences.)

Appreciation of what can go wrong with a knee replacement requires some knowledge of the way the normal knee functions. The knee is the largest and most complex joint in the body, and the motions of the joint are complex. Examination of a skeleton shows that the bones actually involved in the joint are the femur, the tibia, and the **patella**; the **fibula** braces the tibia but does not extend all the way to the level of the knee joint. The combination of the femur, tibia, and the ligaments and muscles that surround them function almost exactly like the universal joints in the drive shaft of a rear-wheel-drive car; the knee can swing back and forth in one plane and rotate in another at the same time.

This unusual function (for a joint), combined with the ability of the joint to lock in extension, allows for the many complex and graceful maneuvers that one sees in athletes and dancers. The kneecap is a sesamoid (that is, ovoid and flat like a sesame seed) bone that lies wholly within the tendon that connects the **quadriceps** to the tibia, and permits the motion by which the leg is straightened and locked.[7] What the kneecap does is obscure. At one time it may have served to strengthen the kneecap tendon, which holds the thigh and calf bones together. Its main function in modern man seems to be to erode the tendons and ligaments when it gets the slightest bit out of proper alignment with the femur!

Artificial knee joints are an attempt to replace the sliding surfaces of the end of the femur and the top of the tibia with artificial surfaces. In most procedures, ligaments and tendons that are healthy are preserved if possible, and the kneecap and the kneecap tendon are usually not replaced. Ligaments that are too damaged to be used can be replaced with artificial components.[8] (Gore-Tex, for example, is a material that gives good results.[9]) The result, if the kneecap does not move up and down on the artificial femoral (thigh) part of the artificial knee in the same way it did on the normal bone, can be rapid erosion of the ligaments and tendons. Increasingly, the medical practice during the procedure is to resurface the kneecap if necessary to ensure normal tracking.[10]

Our review of knee replacement failures requiring re-operation found the major complications to be infection; mechanical failure of the components; problems when the leg is straightened or extended; fractures of the bones near the artificial components; and healing problems with the skin.[11] A 1989 study revealed that the most common problems appearing to require **revision** of the joint replacement are kneecap and patellar-femoral tendon problems. The study suggests that medical measures such as anti-inflammatory medications, exercises, and bracing of the knee be tried before revision surgery is chosen.[12]

Success rates, the inverse of complication rates, vary with the underlying condition and the extent of damage caused by it. A review of follow-up studies for the first 20 years of total joint replacement with artificial joint components concludes that the complications of infection, early loosening, and breakage of the components have been controlled, and that now the major complication is late loosening of the components, without infection.[13] Mechanical failure is often associated with malpositioning of the components by the surgeon.[14] The rate of good to excellent results has been as high as 97.4% with some devices.[15]

Following particularly complex knee replacements for rheumatoid arthritis, 86% of patients had either no pain or pain only upon changes in barometric pressure or the weather; the remaining 14% had continuing pain.

Eighty-eight percent of patients had markedly increased walking ability following surgery; 12% did not.[16] In another series, 85% of patients had significant pain relief, 15% did not; the failures were attributed to various postoperative complications.[17] A 1979 series reports pain relief in 85% of patients, with a 2% rate of component loosening and a 3% rate of deep infection.[18] Infections can require removal of the artificial joint, creation of a fused joint, and lengthy (one- to two-year) regimens of antibiotics.[19]

Revision surgery for failed knee replacements reportedly produces good to excellent results in 76% of cases. Loosening of one or both components occurred in 6% of the cases; **hematomas** occurred in 2% of the cases; and cement fractures that resulted in loose pieces having to be removed occurred in 2% of the cases. The rate of deep infection (that is, near the bone) in the series reported was zero.[20] Septic arthritis—triggering of additional arthritic responses by infection—is a rare complication and can be treated with antibiotics and drainage.[21]

The principal early (anywhere from one month to one year following knee replacement) and late (eight to 10 years following surgery) complications are: loosening of the components; failure to relieve pain and problems with walking; failure of soft tissue to heal; and deep infection.

As is true with nearly all surgeries, the rate of complications falls as experience is gained, and the later series report better results than the earlier ones. This may reflect shorter follow-up times, actual improvements in the results obtained, or a combination of both. A four- to 10-year follow-up study of the Attenborough knee, one of the earlier types of artificial joints, found that 65% of patients had no problems with pain, walking, or loosening of the component at six years; 35% had one or more of these problems. Twenty percent of the prostheses required revision because of loosening and another 7.5% had x-ray evidence of loosening. Deep infection occurred in 3.5%. Problems with wound healing after surgery were common, and there was a 20% complication rate following the initial knee replacements.[22]

Mechanical failure (i.e., failure of the artificial joint itself as a result of, for example, improper manufacturing) rates and times from surgery to first mechanical failure vary greatly among designs: One showed 73% mechanical failure at three years, but this is an extreme example.[23] Another design, the Minns knee, had a mechanical failure rate of 4.8% at 4.5 years.[24]

As with virtually all lower-body surgery, thromboembolic problems (which involve migration of clots, bone marrow, or fat and blockage of veins and arteries) can occur.[25]

? WHAT ARE THE OTHER COMPLICATIONS AND POSSIBLE SIDE EFFECTS?

Infection is nearly always a significant problem if it occurs deep within a joint after surgery. In severe cases, surgical removal of the infected tissue and bone (a process called debridement), revision of the infected bone, replacement of the artificial components, and planned stiffening of the joint to provide support (a procedure called **arthrodesis**) may be required.[26] Rates of infection in early series ranged as high as 8%.[27]

Fungal infections of the joint, as opposed to bacterial ones, are rare. As of 1988 only eight cases of such were reported in the literature, but they were serious. Fungal infections usually require removal of the artificial joint.[28]

Loosening of the knee prostheses is much less of a problem than with total hip replacements. The rarity of loosening allows the surgeon to select either a cemented or cementless approach, depending on the quality of the patient's bone. In the cementless approach, bone grows into and bonds to the textured surface of the metal prosthesis, eventually giving support to the knee as strong as that of the original bone.[29] Especially critical is proper placement of the artificial knee components relative to the remaining bone. One study found that thinning of bone, which if it progresses too far can lead to knee replacement failure, was related both to misaligned components and to placement of components that raised the knee joint higher than the original position of the knee.[30] In a 1990 series of patients on which doctors had used cementless components with bone-growth-encouraging surfaces, there was no loosening in any case and evidence of bone thickening in all.[31] Animal studies suggest that the degree of bone growth that is stimulated (or permitted) by the prosthesis depends greatly on the design of the surfaces.[32]

Late complications appear to be related to failure to duplicate the position of the original knee components relative to the rest of the leg.[33]

A review of the Sheehan total knee arthroplasty, one of the many possible variations of knee replacement surgery, found only 48.3% of knees totally free from pain, even though all had improvements in range of motion, and 8.3% of knees required reoperation. There were three cases of deep infection (5%). The authors concluded that other knee designs are superior.[34]

Failure of the soft tissues surrounding the knee to heal, as a result of infection, steroid use, and other causes has been successfully treated with flaps of muscle and **fascia**.[35]

Damage to the peroneal nerve, which wraps around the knee joint in a way that exposes it to injury, occurs in 0.87% of knee replacement procedures. Three-year follow-ups indicated complete recovery of function in less than one-third of patients. The most common consequence of damage of peroneal nerve is foot drop, which causes the toe of the dropped foot to hit the ground when it is brought forward for walking. This can be corrected with a brace.[36]

Most surgical instruments and many knee replacement components are made of alloys containing nickel. High blood levels of nickel and excretion of nickel in the urine have been reported following artificial joint surgery. This may reflect either contamination of the surgical site with tiny metal fragments, a response triggered by the nickel in the prosthetic surfaces, or both.[37] The long-term significance, if any, is uncertain.

As with any procedure in which anesthesia is used, death from reaction to the anesthetic drugs, error on the part of the anesthetist, or machine failure is a remote possibility. (See Glossary, p. 309)

? IS THIS THE MOST APPROPRIATE PROCEDURE FOR THE CONDITION?

If a knee is damaged beyond repair, say in a car accident or a bad fall, the only choices are replacement, permanent stiffening of the joint, or amputation. For most people, the artificial knee will be preferable to arthrodesis or amputation, and it is surely the best procedure in the vast majority of cases. For arthritis, it can relieve pain and restore sufficient function for all but the most strenuous athletics. The only instances in which it is inappropriate are those in which a trial of medical treatment of arthritis, with appropriately high dosages of appropriate anti-inflammatory drugs, has not been attempted.

? ARE THERE ALTERNATIVES TO THIS PROCEDURE?

If the damage caused by arthritis or other conditions is limited to the lower (tibial) component of the knee, it is possible to replace only the lower part of the knee joint. This procedure is referred to as a single-component replacement. Although this technique is controversial, a follow-up of single-component replacements after four years found good to excellent results in 76.3% of cases. All failures were associated with the use of thin rather than thick tibial components; if the tibial component is made thick enough, it never fails.[38]

If there is complete failure of the knee and the remaining bone is too thin or damaged to permit insertion of another artificial knee, a procedure called arthrodesis can be performed (see description above). Obviously, the results are much less satisfactory than a functioning knee joint, but the procedure avoids further deterioration of the leg and preserves some function.[39]

❓ WHAT IS CONTROVERSIAL ABOUT THE PROCEDURE?

A significant debate concerns the use of cementless versus cemented prostheses. Cement eventually wears, it generates heat as it sets, and the application of cement causes brief circulatory and respiratory reactions in many patients. Cementless versions avoid these problems, but do not adhere as tightly to bone as the cemented ones do, at least in the initial months of wear.

Most surgeons base their choice of prosthesis upon the patient's age and lifestyle, the amount of damage to the bone that has resulted from arthritis or trauma, and how good a fit they achieve with the artificial components after trimming the bones. Undoubtedly, doctors are influenced by sellers of prosthetic parts, but there is a growing trend to try to fit the parts to the patient, rather than the other way around.

Replacement of a single (the tibial or the femoral) component of the knee joint with an artificial material is still controversial. Widely varying rates of success have been reported, and experience with replacement of single hip joint components has not been good. All of this tends to cast doubt on the long-term results of replacement of only one knee component rather than total knee replacement.[40, 41]

How and at what rate new component designs should be introduced, followed up, and evaluated is a matter of discussion among orthopedic surgeons. Attempts to duplicate natural wear of knee components in the laboratory have not been particularly successful. At least one investigator counsels "extreme caution" in the introduction of new designs, and suggests that a five- to seven-year follow-up with no indication of progressive loosening and 10-year follow-ups of a significant number of patients be required before a design is put into general use.[42]

Transurethral Destruction of Bladder Lesion (15)

MORTALITY	MORBIDITY	CONTROVERSY
+	+	o

Examination of the inside of the bladder through a **cystoscope** or **resectoscope** inserted through the **urethra**, and destruction of abnormal tissue by cutting, **electrocautery,** or laser beam[1]

❓ WHAT CONDITION DOES THE PROCEDURE TREAT?

This procedure treats a wide variety of **lesions**—damaged tissue or tissue that should not be growing where it is—in the bladder and is usually done through a cystoscope. (See "Cystoscopy," p. 61.) Treatment of lesions associated with chronic interstitial cystitis, which is a repeated or continuous bladder infection associated with sexual intercourse, is quite successful.[2]

❓ WHAT IS THE PROCEDURE?

In this procedure, which is performed on both men and women, the patient is asked to empty his or her bladder of urine and is then given a spinal anesthetic or an injectable general anesthetic. He or she is placed on a special table much like that used for gynecological exams. The scope is lubricated and inserted through the urethra (through the penis in men and through the vagina in women), and the residual urine in the bladder is sucked out and measured. (Residual urine is measured to determine how well the bladder is functioning; it is the relationship of bladder capacity to what remains after voiding. If, for instance, the bladder holds 20 cc and there are 5 cc remaining, the bladder is functioning at 75%.) Then the bladder is inflated with saline or other solutions and visually examined. If a lesion is found that can be treated through the scope, **catheters**, **Randall stone forceps**, **cautery probes**, and biopsy knives can be passed through the scope to do the necessary work.

? WHO PERFORMS THE PROCEDURE?

This procedure is performed by a urologist.

? WHERE IS THE PROCEDURE PERFORMED?

This procedure is done on either an inpatient or outpatient basis in a hospital, in an outpatient surgery center, or in a well-equipped doctor's office.

? WHAT ARE THE MORTALITY (DEATH) AND MORBIDITY (COMPLICATION) RATES?

The mortality rate for diagnostic cystoscopy is zero. Other mortality from this procedure arises from the type of bladder lesion present and the methods used to destroy it. For example, **cryosurgery** of the prostate carries a mortality rate of 0.3% to 2.0%.[3]

Injury to the urethra is described as extremely common.[4] Possible injuries are tearing and bruising of the urethra, usually as a result of rough handling. Further, **fibrosis** and scarring following injury may cause the penis to bend and become impossible to straighten, and may require reconstructive surgery.[5] **Iatrogenic** (doctor-caused) injuries to the penis, including narrowing

of the urethra, are increasing, but can be prevented by very careful handling.[6]

? WHAT ARE THE OTHER COMPLICATIONS AND POSSIBLE SIDE EFFECTS?

Failure to adequately sterilize all parts of the cystoscope and the instruments used through it has been associated with repeated outbreaks of infection.[7] Some types of bladder tumors harbor bacteria in a noninfectious state; these become infectious when the tumor is destroyed and fragments are scattered about the bladder—an almost unavoidable situation. The condition can be handled through appropriate antibiotic treatment.[8]

Reflux of urine out of the bladder and back into the kidneys can occur in up to 20.6% of patients who have had cystoscopic treatment of bladder tumors.[9] Presumably sterile catheters still can carry bacterial toxins that can cause fever—even if all bacteria have been killed.[10]

Explosions inside the bladder can occur when electrosurgery probes dissociate water into hydrogen and oxygen, an explosive combination that can be ignited by the heated probe. Careful evacuation of all gas from the bladder as it is formed can prevent this complication, which is rare but can be devastating if it occurs.[11] Not usually fatal, this complication may cause severe damage to abdominal organs.

As with any procedure in which anesthesia is used, death from reaction to the anesthetic drugs, error on the part of the anesthetist, or machine failure is a remote possibility. (See Glossary, p. 309)

? IS THIS THE MOST APPROPRIATE PROCEDURE FOR THE CONDITION?

Because transurethral treatment with a cystoscope or a resectoscope is used for a wide variety of conditions, the answer depends upon the condition. There is little, if any, need for cystoscopy simply to measure residual urine or to evaluate stress incontinence as a first step. All of the other alternatives to cystoscopy are more invasive and are probably not preferable to cystoscopy or resectoscopy, but it is becoming quite clear that this procedure is not as innocuous as it was once believed to be.

Pathological examination of removed tumor fragments may indicate that all the tumor was not removed or that it has spread further than it appeared to on cystoscopic examination, or that it is an aggressive type that requires removal of all or part of the bladder. Use of the cystoscope can avoid surgery if any of these conditions are not present, so cystoscopic destruction is usually worth trying first; it can always be followed by more extensive surgery later.[12–14]

? ARE THERE ALTERNATIVES TO THIS PROCEDURE?

Monthly testing of urine for cancer cells has been shown to be an effective substitute for repeated cystoscopies to check for recurrence in treated cancer patients.[15]

? WHAT IS CONTROVERSIAL ABOUT THE PROCEDURE?

Little is controversial except the mounting evidence that the procedure is treated too cavalierly by those who do it and that there needs to be more attention paid to avoiding complications, even though complications other than urethral damage are relatively rare.

Transurethral Removal of Ureter Obstruction (54)

MORTALITY	MORBIDITY	CONTROVERSY
+	+	o

Insertion of a thin tube into the **ureter** to remove an obstruction

? WHAT CONDITION DOES THE PROCEDURE TREAT?

This procedure is used to remove obstructions in the ureter, generally those that are in the lower third of the ureters, or just above the bladder. The placement of stones dictates what they are called: If a stone remains in the kidney, it's a kidney stone; if it moves into the ureter, it's a ureteral stone; and if it moves down to the bladder, it's a bladder stone.

Small ureteral stones (which usually originate in the kidney and may be comprised of uric acid, an amino acid, or any mineral salt) can be removed from below the site where they are lodged in the ureter.[1, 2] Ureteral **catheters** can be used to insert **stents** for ureters that are invaded by cancer.[3] (The stent is inserted into the ureter because it has about the same diameter as the ureter. It holds the ureter open and prevents it from collapsing, thus allowing the stone to pass through it.) Balloons attached to catheters can be used to open blocked ureters in the same way that they are used for coronary angioplasty (see "Percutaneous Transluminal Coronary Angioplasty," p. 194).[4]

In the medical literature there is wide variation in the terms used to discuss this procedure; this occasionally makes it difficult to determine exactly what operation is being written about. A 1982 study[5] found that up to 70% of urologists preferred the use of "splint" to "stent." To make matters more complicated, a catheter can be used to place a stent or itself be used as a temporary stent. In what follows, we shall use the term "indwelling stent" to mean a stent—not a catheter—that is left in place for some period of time, usually as a permanent placement. We shall use the term "indwelling catheter" to mean a catheter that is left in place for only a brief period of time after surgery. The catheter that is used for stone removal and balloon dilation of strictures is withdrawn completely as soon as the procedure is finished.

Placement of indwelling stents can be used to correct surgical damage to the ureters without opening the abdomen.[6, 7] (Between 80% and 99% of all surgical injuries to the ureters occur during total abdominal hysterectomies.[8]) Such stents can also be used to open up blockage of the ureters caused by benign tumors[9] or scarring.[10] The ureters can also be cleared of blockages with stiff wires.

Not just a passive tube, the ureter is actively involved in the transport of urine from the kidney to the bladder by downward-pointing waves of contractions (**peristalsis**). To determine if the patient has a problem with the transport of urine, very small catheters can be inserted into the ureters to measure internal pressure and the rate and force of contractions.

Stones composed of uric acid or the amino acid cystine can be dissolved by catheter irrigation with appropriate chemicals.[11]

In one series, 95% success in removal of ureteral stones via catheters and similar methods was reported. The other 5% of patients required open operations (involving a large incision) for removal of the stones.[12] Another series reported a 92% success rate.[13]

Placement of stents reduces the incidence of complications following **extracorporeal shock-wave lithotripsy (ESWL)**, which uses sound waves from outside the body to break stones, from 26% to 7%.[14] One study reported a 97% success rate in fracturing ureteral stones after attempts to push the stone out of the urethra and into the kidney pelvis (a large open space in the middle of the kidney) failed.[15]

? WHAT IS THE PROCEDURE?

A ureteral catheter can be placed from within the bladder through a **cystoscope**,[16, 17] which requires regional or general anesthesia. Another option is to place the catheter through small incisions above the kidney; this can be done without regional or general anesthesia.[18] The catheter can also be placed via a small incision made in the bladder, a procedure requiring regional anesthesia or a local anesthetic. What happens after the catheter is maneuvered up the ureter to the site of the problem depends upon what the problem is—stone, **stricture**, pressure from a tumor, a gunshot injury, or some other abnormal condition.

Laser lithotripsy to break apart ureteral stones can be done through a ureteral catheter—one that is inserted through the urinary opening. The laser alone was successful in 64% of the cases, and the laser combined with ESWL succeeded in 79% of the cases. Combined with other means of stone retrieval, these two methods succeeded in 90% of cases. There were no complications associated with the use of the laser in this study; however, further operations to get rid of stones were required in 0.9% of cases.[19]

Use of a stone brush seems to improve the results of both extracorporeal and laser lithotripsy, probably by brushing away soft parts of the stone that absorb the laser or shock wave energy.[20] The stone brush, which is small and cone-shaped, is inserted into the ureter by way of a catheter and moved around. It brushes away the stones so that the ureter can carry away the stone particles.

A small study comparing open repair of ureteral strictures and treatment by catheterization showed that 100% of the open procedures were successful, versus 64.3% of the catheter procedures. Because an open procedure can be done if the catheterization and **dilation** fail, it seems reasonable to try the catheterization first.[21]

Use of a catheter to maneuver a stone back into the pelvis in the kidney so that it no longer blocks the ureter significantly increases the success of ESWL.[22]

? WHO PERFORMS THE PROCEDURE?

This procedure should only be done by a board-certified urologist with significant experience in the use of catheters and stents.

? WHERE IS THE PROCEDURE PERFORMED?

Depending upon the patient's condition and the reason for the surgery, this procedure can be performed on an inpatient or outpatient basis in a hospital, in an outpatient clinic, in a radiology office, or in a well-equipped doctor's office.

? WHAT ARE THE MORTALITY (DEATH) AND MORBIDITY (COMPLICATION) RATES?

Operative mortality (during the actual procedure) of zero and operative morbidity (during the actual procedure) of 0.68%, with total morbidity of 0.8%, have been reported for a 17-year series of ureteral stone removal with catheter devices. Indwelling catheters and antibiotics were not used routinely in this series.[23] Another study reports a morbidity rate of 1%.[24] Morbidity is significantly increased by the use of indwelling stents. What this means is that sometimes there may be no other option than to insert an indwelling stent even though risk of infection increases. If the ureter has a tendency to collapse, this could create more significant complications such as blockage of urine from the kidney, and perhaps greater infection.

Complications are reported to occur in about 6% of cases during the early part of the physician's "learning curve"; the rate declines after her technique is perfected.[25]

One death from infection closely following placement of a stent has been reported.[26] A 1981 German study reported a complication rate of 54.3% in patients given ureteral stents for various causes of ureteral obstruction.[27]

? WHAT ARE THE OTHER COMPLICATIONS AND POSSIBLE SIDE EFFECTS?

Failure to save the kidney from kidney failure by placing a **percutaneous** (or through-the-skin) ureteral stent occurs in about 40% of cases, about the same as for open kidney operations.[28] Attempts to open a ureteral stricture with an **angioplasty** balloon can fail in about 17% of cases.[29] In these cases, the kidney must be removed or an **open procedure** must be done.

Damage to the juncture between the kidney and the ureter during the removal of a stent has been reported.[30] Catheter blockage can lead to the need for additional surgery.[31] Some catheters can break off in the ureter; if they cannot be retrieved by another catheterization or a percutaneous procedure, an open procedure may be needed to remove them.

Rarely, an indwelling stent can cause **fistulas** between the ureter and a vein or artery and part of the intestines and ureter or artery. Fewer than 15 cases of such fistulas are reported in the literature. A case has been reported in which the patient developed a fistula between one ureter and an artery and between the **colon** and the other artery. The patient had **septicemia** and **hematuria**.[32, 33] If a catheter penetrates an artery by accident, it may block blood flow, leading to severe hemorrhaging when it is removed.[34]

The rationale for both indwelling catheters and indwelling stents is that they hold the ureter open, force urine to drain only into the bladder in cases of ureteral damage, and keep the ureter from collapsing under pressure from benign or malignant tumors.[35]

However, even perfectly placed indwelling stents or indwelling catheters can be uncomfortable or painful. Typically, an indwelling catheter is placed so that one end is high in the ureter and the other is led out through the urethra so that its removal will not require a cystoscopy procedure. It can also be wrapped around a **Foley catheter**—a rubber tube to drain urine that has a balloon on one end to hold it in the bladder. Because the catheter has to be a bit stiff to stay open inside the abdomen, it can cause pain. Symptoms—which are unpleasant but not harmful in the long run—include a continuous need to void (if the catheter distends the neck of the bladder sufficiently), frequent night voiding, flank and pubic pain, pain on removal of the catheter, and pain on urination.[36] These same symptoms are reported for indwelling stents.

In a 1990 study, 44% of patients reported mild to intolerable pain that was relieved by removal of the stent; 42% reported visible blood in the urine; 20% reported fever and chills; and 38% reported bladder or flank pain.[37] Most problems resolved when the stent was removed. A 1988 review suggests that the universal use of stents before lithotripsy should be avoided because the cure is worse than the disease—many patients report more pain with the use of the stent to hold the ureter open for stone passage than from the passage of small stones or stone fragments.[38] One small 1985 Japanese study found the stent ". . . neither safe nor effective" for more than short-term use.[39] A 1987 French study was less pessimistic, but still cited a complication rate of 11%.[40] A 1990 Japanese study found a complication rate of 17.2% and suggested that stents be removed as early as possible.[41] One study of stenting in **renal** transplant patients revealed that 76% of stented patients developed postoperative infections versus 45% of those without stents.[42]

Stent-associated pain may be caused by movement of the stent; it is possible that better methods to hold the stent in place might reduce the discomfort.[43, 44]

Crusts made of chemicals in the urine may form on the catheter and jam it inside the ureter. An encrusted catheter has been successfully removed by using laser lithotripsy inside the catheter.[45]

If a short catheter is placed in the ureter and held in position with a pigtail-shaped (not straight) catheter placed in the kidney, it is possible for the two catheters to wander about in the ureter; the authors recommend the use of catheters that are long enough to reach from the kidney to the bladder.[46]

While not a complication per se, **false-positive diagnoses** can result from x-ray studies of the kidney or bladder performed with a catheter in place when the bladder is full; the authors of the study cited recommend that all patients with indwelling catheters urinate before x-ray studies.[47]

As with any procedure in which anesthesia is used, death from reaction to the anesthetic drugs, error on the part of the anesthetist, or machine failure is a remote possibility. (See Glossary, p. 309)

? IS THIS THE MOST APPROPRIATE PROCEDURE FOR THE CONDITION?

"Watchful waiting" to see if stones will pass is always possible, but stone pain is among the most severe pains observed, and most patients will lose tolerance for waiting after a few days at most. If a kidney stone is hard and rigid, something that can only be guessed at based on the chemistry of the urine and x-ray studies, use of a catheter to push it back into the pelvis of the kidney, followed by ESWL, has a very high success rate. If the stone is composed of uric acid or cystine, it can be dissolved with chemicals passed through a catheter. If it is not in a position to be reached with a catheter from below and ESWL has failed, then some of the more complicated catheter manipulations are appropriate.

Given the variety of techniques that have emerged and the range of success rates reported for them by various authorities, it seems that research is needed to develop rules for treatment.

One thing that seems clear from the literature is that the indwelling stents, because they remain in the body a long time or even permanently, have a high rate of complications and should be used only if there is no other choice—for instance, if the patient's remaining lifetime is short, dilation of the ureter with a balloon has failed, or part of the ureter has been destroyed by cancer.

? ARE THERE ALTERNATIVES TO THIS PROCEDURE?

ESWL is the chief alternative to removal of stones by catheter, but is often combined with the latter procedure. For strictures and obstructions of the ureter from sources other than stones (for example, cancer), open operations are the only alternatives, and they have a significantly higher mortality rate than catheter manipulations.

? WHAT IS CONTROVERSIAL ABOUT THE PROCEDURE?

The main sources of controversy concern what to do with stones that are not shattered by ESWL or laser lithotripsy, and the merits and safety of long-term use of indwelling stents for which there is wide divergence of opinion among doctors.

Transurethral Resection of the Prostate (6)

MORTALITY	MORBIDITY	CONTROVERSY
+	−	●

- **MORBIDITY** is in the range of 18%, with major postoperative complications of narrowing of the urethra, infection, and excessive bleeding.
- Some studies report a higher long-term **MORTALITY** rate for men undergoing transurethral resection rather than an open procedure. The controversy is that many believe that the patient's age and other, nonrelated conditions that develop later are the primary factors in the observed higher mortality rate.

LAY TITLE: TURP

Removal of a portion of the prostate gland by means of a **cystoscope**

? WHAT CONDITION DOES THE PROCEDURE TREAT?

This procedure treats partial or complete blockage of the **urethra,** which is the tube in the penis through which urine and semen flow, by benign hypertrophy of the prostate gland—that is, noncancerous enlargement of the prostate—or cancer of the prostate gland. The prostate gland, which sits at the neck of the bladder and surrounds the urethra, grows rapidly at puberty and more slowly in later life. As men get older, it is common for the prostate to enlarge and thus interfere with urination. By age 60, about 70% of men have developed benign prostatic hypertrophy, or BPH, and about 90% of that 70% (or about 60% of all men) will have noticeable lower urinary tract symptoms, mainly the need to urinate frequently, pain on urination, and inability to empty the bladder completely. About 15% of men with symptoms eventually have a prostate operation of one sort or another.[1] Present data suggest that 30% to 40% of men who live to be 80 will undergo TURP or another prostate operation.[2] The cause of BPH is unknown, but there is some evidence that a virus called cytomegalovirus (CMV) may be involved.[3]

Statistical analyses indicate that being Protestant, being from a small town, and being fertile, as opposed to infertile, may increase the risk of both BPH and prostate cancer.[4] There is clearly a hormonal factor involved, and the finding that BPH arises from the muscle-cell–like portions of the prostate indicates that both **androgens** and **estrogens** play some role.[5] A prostate-specific growth factor, differing from previously known growth factors and growth hormones, has been isolated.[6] One Japanese study identified higher education and income and an urban lifestyle as risk factors; complex interactions of foods even may be involved in increasing the risk.[7] An American study found rural lifestyle to be a risk factor.[8] Exposure to the metal cadmium also increases the risk.[9]

In short, studies of the risk factors for BPH give widely varying results. The one constant finding is that reduction in male hormone levels results in reduction of BPH.

? WHAT IS THE PROCEDURE?

The patient is placed on a table that looks very much like the gynecologist's table with stirrups. A general or spinal anesthetic is given. If necessary, a small plastic **catheter** is inserted through the penis and urethra and into the bladder to drain it. A **trochar** is inserted into the bladder to inject irrigation fluid. A cystoscope (see "Cystoscopy," p. 61) is inserted into the penis, and the inside of the bladder is examined for tumors and signs of infection. The portion of the urethra compressed by the prostate gland is located, and an **electrosurgical loop,** which cuts with radio-frequency currents at low amperage, is used to cut away the diseased or malignant portions of the gland that are obstructing the flow of urine. The scope and trochar are then removed. Depending upon the surgeon's preferences, an irrigation catheter, which has tubes for inserting and draining irrigation solution, is put into the bladder. This is removed when the irrigation fluid has been clear of blood clots and tissue fragments for a day or so.

? WHO PERFORMS THE PROCEDURE?

This procedure is done by a urologist.

? WHERE IS THE PROCEDURE PERFORMED?

This procedure is done in a hospital.

? WHAT ARE THE MORTALITY (DEATH) AND MORBIDITY (COMPLICATION) RATES?

In 1988 the mortality rate for this procedure at community hospitals in the U.S. was 0.7%.[10]

Other studies cite mortality rates of 1%,[11] 2% to 3%,[12] 1.4%,[13] 0.7%,[14] 0.2%,[15] and 0.5%.[16] Reported morbidity rates are in the range of 18%—a rate that rises with the time required for the operation, the total weight of tissue removed, advancing age, minority status, and alcoholism.[17, 18] Major postoperative complications include narrowing of the urethra, infection, and excessive bleeding. A 1989 study suggests that 3% of patients will develop urethral **strictures** following the operation and that 9% will require reoperation **within one year.**[19] Another study indicates that excessive bleeding will occur in 4.7% of the procedures, urethral stricture in 4.4%, and total incontinence of urine will occur in about 0.9%.[20]

? WHAT ARE THE OTHER COMPLICATIONS AND POSSIBLE SIDE EFFECTS?

An oft-noted **intraoperative** complication is puncture or laceration of the bladder by the cutting tip of the cystoscope. This occurs when the current of the electrosurgical loop or pressure from the urine activates the obturator nerve—the nerve that signals the bladder to contract and expel urine—and produces a sudden contraction of the adductor muscle of the thigh, pulling the thigh against the body and jarring the cystoscope. Thigh muscle contractions occurred in about 10% of patients in one study. In 76% of the patients studied, this muscle contraction was eliminated by moving the receiving electrode—one of the two electrodes, emitting and receiving, that are necessary to run an electrical current —from under the buttocks to under the thigh. A small shot of local anesthetic can be used to block the obturator nerve before the procedure is begun.[21, 22]

Impotence and sterility may follow TURP. In one study patients followed up three years after the surgery noted reduced erections or an inability to become erect; all attributed this to the operation.[23] In another study, 11% of patients became completely impotent and 51% noted a decrease in sexual functioning. Retrograde ejaculation, in which the semen is pushed back into the bladder rather than out the urethra by the ejaculatory muscles, can also occur, and this affects sterility.[24] Healthy men usually have several erections per night, so sleep studies involving automatic recordings of erections are important in determining whether impotence has a psychological source. If the waking patient has no erections, but has a normal erection pattern when asleep, there is good reason to suspect that the cause is not physical. One sleep study showed no change in the frequency of nocturnal erections after TURP, which indicates that the impotence may have a psychological component.[25] Another study, however, showed a complete loss of nocturnal erections after TURP in one

patient.[26] Apparently, whether or not TURP causes impotence depends on factors in both the patient and the surgeon—in the latter case, specifically how skilled the surgeon is at maneuvering the tip of the cystoscope and at destroying the **lesion**—and not all these factors are well understood.

The medical literature for the last six years records the recognition of a TURP syndrome. The full-blown syndrome, which is apparently related to absorption of the surgical irrigating fluid, consists of difficulty in breathing, nausea, a rise in both arterial and venous blood pressure, swelling of the brain, cardiovascular shock, and **renal** insufficiency, in which the kidneys do not function at 100% capacity. It occurs in about 0.2% to 1.5% of patients.[27, 28] Although it is almost universally attributed to the irrigation fluid, one study using radioactive compounds to track irrigation fluid through the body found no change in total blood volume. This finding suggests that the procedure may force bacteria in the bladder into the bloodstream, producing **septicemia**. The chance of occurrence of TURP syndrome can be lessened by the use of irrigation fluids containing the amino acid glycine, whose **osmolality** is close to that of the blood.

As with any procedure in which anesthesia is used, death from reaction to the anesthetic drugs, error on the part of the anesthetist, or machine failure is a remote possibility. (See Glossary, p. 309)

? IS THIS THE MOST APPROPRIATE PROCEDURE FOR THE CONDITION?

This is a matter under heavy debate. In theory, TURP appears to be simpler and less traumatic to the patient than the open operation, a more complicated procedure involving an incision in the lower abdomen and removal of the prostate. It also seems that it should involve less blood loss, result in less morbidity, and allow a quicker return to normal living. At one time, the mortality rates for TURP were well below those for the open operation. At present, mortality for the open procedure is low. A variation of the procedure, which preserves at least one of the two bundles of nerves and vessels involved in causing an erection, apparently causes no impotence. (Advanced cancer may require that the neurovascular bundles be removed along with the tumor, in which case potency is not preserved, even by this new **open procedure**.)

Follow-up studies within the last decade indicate that patients who have TURP experience a higher postsurgical long-term mortality rate than those patients undergoing the open procedure. The reasons for this are hard to pin down because the demographic profiles of those having TURP and those having the open operation are very different.

? ARE THERE ALTERNATIVES TO THIS PROCEDURE?

Because prostate growth is triggered and maintained in part by male hormones, chemical castration by use of female hormones or male-hormone-receptor antagonists (drugs that block the entry of male hormones into cells) and surgical castration have long been advocated. Most patients have found the side effects, such as growth of the nipples and the underlying tissues ("gynecomastia"), reduction in facial and body hair, impotence, and loss of libido intolerable.

A class of drugs, called **alpha blockers**, which block a certain kind of receptor on the cells of the smooth muscle surrounding the urethra, have proven useful for treating both **urinary retention** and obstruction.[29] Some other studies have shown both reduction in symptoms and shrinkage of the prostate, but results have not been good enough to dislodge surgery from its place as the primary therapy for BPH.

? WHAT IS CONTROVERSIAL ABOUT THE PROCEDURE?

The finding that TURP has a higher long-term mortality rate than the open procedure totally contradicts medical wisdom about which kinds of procedures are least traumatic and which are not. A good deal of research has been devoted to finding out if the difference is real or a consequence of something else, such as a decision to use TURP on older and sicker patients. A 1990 study using reviews of hospital charts found that the difference remained even after age and general health status were accounted for: The risk of death following TURP was 28% higher than the risk following the open procedure.[30] An eight-year follow-up of Canadian patients revealed that 16.8% of those who had TURP required reoperation within eight years after surgery, versus 7% of those who had had the open procedure.[31]

The authors of the study that established the higher death rate for TURP have recommended that controlled clinical trials with random assignment be used to establish the safety and effectiveness of TURP.[32] In such a study, every other man needing prostate surgery would undergo TURP, and the others would have the open procedure.

This finding, coming long after TURP was adopted as a standard procedure because of presumed low mortality and morbidity, illustrates the flaws in the "cut first, study later" method by which most surgical procedures have been developed. Safety and effectiveness are proven, if proven at all, only in series of patients who are generally not randomly selected, and reported results may be based solely on patient populations in which little can be expected to go wrong in any case. Controlled, prospective clinical trials may well establish that many more apparently solid items of medical wisdom are in fact insupportable.

Unilateral External Simple Mastectomy (25)

MORTALITY	MORBIDITY	CONTROVERSY
+	−	o

- **SWELLING** in the surgical area has been reported in 47.1% of cases. Infection rates can soar to 25% in cancer patients who had preoperative radiation therapy.

Removal of a single breast without removal of underlying muscle or lymph nodes

? WHAT CONDITION DOES THE PROCEDURE TREAT?

This procedure treats breast cancer, which can occur in men as well as women.[1-3] The classical simple mastectomy consists of removal of all of the breast tissue including the nipple, areola (dark skin surrounding the nipple), and most of the overlying skin. Considerable confusion exists between this term and the term total mastectomy, which is exactly the same procedure.[4] Adding to this confusion is the use by some physicians of the term "total mastectomy" as shorthand for the modified radical mastectomy, which in fact is another procedure.[5] Simple mastectomy is often combined with sampling of the lymph nodes of the armpit on the affected side, to determine whether the cancer has spread beyond the breast.

Simple/total mastectomy is an alternative to the Halsted, radical, and extended radical mastectomies, all variations on breast removal that are much more extensive and disfiguring than this procedure.

? WHAT IS THE PROCEDURE?

The patient is given a general anesthetic. The breast to be removed is scrubbed with soap and antiseptic, and the body is draped with a sterile sheet so that only the appropriate area is exposed. An incision is made all the way around the breast, from the skin to the **fascia** of the pectoral muscles. Sufficient skin to cover the surgical wound is preserved. Bleeding vessels are **ligated** or **cauterized** with an **electrocautery device**. The breast is peeled away from the underlying muscle and sent to the pathologist. The fascia overlying the chest muscles and the exposed lymph nodes are examined for spread of the cancer. The operation may or may not include sampling of the lymph nodes in the armpit.

Finally, a drain is placed in the wound, which is closed by stretching the remaining (or reserved) skin over it. The drain is held in place by **sutures**, **clips**, or staples. (Generally, surgeons wait one or two days after draining stops to remove the drain. Most drains are out within a week because most patients' wounds heal within that time.) The wound is covered with a bandage. The patient is taken to the recovery room, and then to her room.

? WHO PERFORMS THE PROCEDURE?

This procedure can be done by a general or oncologic surgeon. Breast reconstruction is best done by a plastic surgeon unless the general or oncologic surgeon does a large number of them and can produce photographic evidence of good cosmetic results. Some insurance plans insist that breast reconstruction following a mastectomy be done by a general or oncologic surgeon and will not pay for the services of a plastic surgeon. However, usually the company will pay if the surgeon who removed the breast states that she is not qualified to do the reconstruction.

Reconstruction can be, and usually is, done at the same time as the mastectomy, but if the surgeon believes that skin grafting will be needed or that fat must be transplanted to reconstruct the breast, or if the patient has not responded well to the anesthetic (has falling blood pressure, difficulty with tissue oxygenation, or irregular pulse), the surgeon may elect to wait and do the reconstruction at another time.

? WHERE IS THE PROCEDURE PERFORMED?

Even though very short hospital stays have been achieved with selected patients, this surgery should be done in the inpatient department of a hospital.

? WHAT ARE THE MORTALITY (DEATH) AND MORBIDITY (COMPLICATION) RATES?

Mortality for this procedure in community hospitals in the U.S. in 1988 was 0.1%. Operative mortality (occurring during the operation) for total mastectomy and partial axillary lymph node dissection, a more traumatic operation than simple mastectomy, has been reported to be zero.[6]

Swelling in the surgical area can be expected in up to 47.1% of patients; tissue death (death of all or most of the cells) at the edge of reconstruction flaps occurs in as many as 5.8% of patients.[7] This generally occurs as a result of loss of blood supply or because of bacterial toxins.

? WHAT ARE THE OTHER COMPLICATIONS AND POSSIBLE SIDE EFFECTS?

Postoperative infections can be expected in up to 8.5% of patients,[8] and patients who have had preoperative radiation therapy, which can compromise the immune system, have shown an infection rate of up to 25%.[9] On the positive side, some studies have found no complications in breast reconstructions done at the same time as the mastectomy.[10] Because recent studies have shown lower complication rates with combined mas-

tectomy and reconstruction, and because the psychological response of the patient is better if she wakes up to discover that she still has two breasts, it is now the norm to do combined mastectomy and reconstruction —if the patient's condition at the conclusion of the mastectomy permits (see above discussion).

There is a definite tendency for surgeons to miss some cancerous lymph nodes when lymph node examination is carried out as part of the procedure, an oversight which can lead to erroneous choices of radiation/chemotherapy regimens.[11] The surgeon can miss cancerous cells because: the cells can't be seen with the naked eye; sometimes the cell changes are so subtle that they can't be seen even through an electron microscope; the distribution of cancer cells is not uniform; and cancer cells can travel through the bloodstream and lymph channels to reach other parts of the body.

As with any procedure in which anesthesia is used, death from reaction to the anesthetic drugs, error on the part of the anesthetist, or machine failure is a remote possibility. (See Glossary, p. 309)

? IS THIS THE MOST APPROPRIATE PROCEDURE FOR THE CONDITION?

Five-year recurrence-free survival with the simple procedure and no radiation or chemotherapy for low-risk patients is 61.7%. (Patients are considered low risk if there is no family history of breast cancer, no sign of spread of the breast cancer to other parts of the body, no sign of cancer in the other breast, and cancer cells in the biopsy specimen were well-differentiated—that is, looked more like breast cells than anything else.) Five-year survival with or without disease recurrence is 75.4%.[12] Because of the wide variation in types of breast cancer, it is best regarded as an appropriate procedure if the patient does not have contraindications, such as extremely advanced disease and extensive lymph node involvement. There is little reason to do the traditional, but more extensive and disfiguring, radical mastectomy unless the pectoral muscles of the chest have been invaded by the cancer to the extent that the disease cannot be treated by removal of the cancerous portion of the muscle.

A 25-year follow-up study, which compared women who had had simple mastectomy followed by radiation therapy with women who had had an extended radical mastectomy, found no difference in survival or disease-free survival.[13] ("Survival" is defined as survival with or without recurrence of the cancer; "disease-free survival" is survival without recurrence.) This strongly suggests that the extended radical mastectomy is unnecessarily mutilating and that simple mastectomy is a better treatment for operable breast cancer. It is important for both patient and doctor to remember that the surgeon cannot always get every cancerous breast cell and that residual, unremoved cancer has been found by biopsy in up to 77% of patients after surgery.[14] On that fact alone, one would expect to find that surgery plus radiation and/or chemotherapy would be more effective than surgery alone. Indeed, this is exactly what research has shown. Surgery alone is curative in only a minority of patients,[15] and the patient, the patient's family physician, oncologist, and surgeon have to be responsible for formulating a complete treatment program.[16]

A study of two anticancer drugs, cyclophosphamide (Cytoxan, Neosar), which is given at the time of surgery, and tamoxifen (Nolvadex), which is given for a longer period, suggests that these drugs can prevent cancer recurrence after a simple mastectomy.[17] An ongoing trial of these two drugs in combination with radiation suggests that recurrence of cancer at four years after simple mastectomy can be limited to 5% to 7% of patients.[18] (This study combined simple mastectomy and sampling of lymph nodes in the armpit on the affected side.)

A number of other studies indicate that simple mastectomy plus chemotherapy, or chemotherapy plus radiation, is far superior to simple mastectomy alone in ensuring five-year survival, even in people with advanced disease.[19] Some,[20] but by no means all,[21-25] chemotherapy regimens improve survival and extend the interval that the patient is disease-free.

The treatment of breast cancer is a "hot" area for current research, and knowledge in the field grows almost daily. It is very important that women with breast cancer be treated at a cancer center, or by an oncology group that knows the latest recommended protocols (conventions governing treatment accepted by the medical profession) and how they relate to various types of breast cancer, as well as the extent to which the cancer has spread when treatment is started.

A very good question to ask your doctor is whether she has computerized access to the medical literature on breast cancer and how often she uses it. With computerized access to either the National Library of Medicine via the search programs Paperchase or Grateful Med, or access to essentially the same literature via Colleague, a doctor can check the latest research daily. The computerized literature tends to be at least two months ahead of the print literature, and automatic searches that zero in on the questions the doctor has about a particular patient are far more efficient than reading more than 4,000 journals, most of them weekly or monthly—a necessity in order to ferret out the same information. Your doctor can be expected to read five to six pages of computerized search information every week; she cannot be expected to scan 4,000 journals.

? ARE THERE ALTERNATIVES TO THIS PROCEDURE?

There are a number of possible variations. For example, preservation of the nipple, which simplifies reconstruction of the breast after mastectomy and looks more normal, does not appear to lead to cancer recurrence in patients who have a mastectomy and radiation therapy. Preservation can lead to recurrence of the disease, however, if no radiation therapy is given following surgery.[26]

The other major alternative is lumpectomy, the simple removal of the tumor with or without follow-up radiation therapy. In a limited follow-up study comparing simple mastectomy, lymph node sampling, and radiation versus lumpectomy, radiation therapy, and insertion of a radioactive iridium wire (which emits radiation that kills cancer cells) at the site of the removed tumor, no difference in survival between the two procedures was found.[27] A later, larger study found the same results—simple mastectomy, in patients with Stage I or II cancer (two early stages in which the cancer has spread minimally), was no more effective than lumpectomy.[28]

Yet another alternative is sector resection, which is removal of the "wedge" of breast containing the lump. More extensive than the lumpectomy and less extensive than the simple/total mastectomy, this procedure has given good results.[29]

Although, strictly speaking, breast reconstruction is not part of sector resection, many women elect to have breast reconstruction done at the same time as the procedure. Immediate reconstruction using gel breast implants is associated with a failure rate (loss of the implant, which can range from slippage of the implant to implant rupture to infection at the site to scarring of the breast around the implant; the surgeon generally removes and replaces—if possible—any implant that fails due to rupture, infection, or scarring) of 18%. Smoking up to the time of surgery, failure to completely cover the implant with muscle tissue, and use of implants containing more than 400 ml—or about a pint —of gel were factors strongly associated with implant failure in one study.[30] If a breast reconstruction is difficult or problematic for any reason, it is better to postpone the procedure, even if the patient desires the psychological benefits of immediate breast reconstruction and even if the surgeon firmly believes that ". . . with early-stage disease, no patient need leave the operating room without a breast," according to one researcher.[31]

Although there should be a clear understanding between patient and doctor before surgery of what is to be done during surgery, the surgeon must have some leeway to decide not to do an immediate breast reconstruction if she realizes it is going to be a disaster, even if she and the patient have agreed on it before the operation.[32–35]

One small consolation for women who are on the plump side is that large breasts and "sufficient" abdominal tissue make breast reconstruction easier for the general or plastic surgeon.[36]

Postoperative depression can follow any surgery, but is particularly common following disfiguring operations. Some studies have found that postoperative depression is not influenced by the procedure chosen;[37, 38] others have found that depression is less frequent and less severe after lumpectomy.[39]

❓ WHAT IS CONTROVERSIAL ABOUT THE PROCEDURE?

There is little controversy about this procedure now, but, as noted above, new research results are coming thick and fast and it is essential that your doctor be reliably informed of the latest results.

Unilateral Salpingo-Oophorectomy or Salpingo-Ovariectomy (60)

MORTALITY	MORBIDITY	CONTROVERSY
+	+	o

Removal of a single ovary and **fallopian tube**

? WHAT CONDITION DOES THE PROCEDURE TREAT?

This procedure is done primarily to treat cancer of the ovary; cancer of the fallopian tube;[1,2] hormone-dependent breast cancer (cancer that is affected by the level of hormones, estrogen or progestogen, in the blood);[3-6] and infection of the ovary that does not respond to antibiotics.

A completely unresolved issue is whether unilateral (one-sided) or bilateral (two-sided) salpingo-oophorectomies should be done for conditions (such as a benign tumor of the ovary) that do not require suppression of female hormone production, a consequence of the removal of both ovaries. A recent article[7] states that "there are no generally accepted criteria." Leaving a normal ovary in the body has the theoretical advantage of promoting a normal hormonal flux even if supplemental estrogen is used.

? WHAT IS THE PROCEDURE?

An ovary and tube can be removed either via a **laparoscope** or with an **open procedure** involving an abdominal incision. In either case, the woman is given a general anesthetic. If the open procedure is used, the abdomen is shaved and scrubbed with soap and antiseptic, and an incision is made in the lower abdomen. The ovary and tube are located and removed. The surgeon should be careful to remove all of the ovary, to avoid the **ovarian remnant syndrome**. Once the ovary has been completely removed, the abdomen is closed in layers. The patient is taken to the recovery room and then to her room.

If this procedure is to be done with a laparoscope, the woman is prepared in exactly the same way as in the open procedure. A small incision is made in or just below the navel. Bleeding vessels are **cauterized** with an **electrocautery device**. The laparoscope is inserted through the navel incision, and the abdominal cavity is inflated with carbon dioxide to separate the organs. This also gives the surgeon the necessary room to maneuver the laparoscope and carry out the procedure. A **trochar** is then positioned over the ovary and tube to be removed and the abdomen is punctured.

The surgeon looks through the scope (or at a TV monitor connected to a TV camera in the scope) and locates the ovaries and tubes. Using the channels in the scope, the surgeon is able to pass small surgical instruments to where they are needed and the ovary and tube are removed. The abdomen is then deflated, and the scope and instruments are removed. The incisions are bandaged and the patient is taken to the recovery room and then to her room.

? WHO PERFORMS THE PROCEDURE?

This procedure is performed by a general surgeon or a gynecologist.

? WHERE IS THE PROCEDURE PERFORMED?

If the open procedure is done, it is performed in a hospital. The laparoscopic procedure can be done in the inpatient or outpatient department of a hospital or in an outpatient surgery facility.

? WHAT ARE THE MORTALITY (DEATH) AND MORBIDITY (COMPLICATION) RATES?

Mortality is essentially zero, with most deaths relating to anesthesia rather than to the procedure itself. As with any procedure in which anesthesia is used, death from reaction to the anesthetic drugs, error on the part of the anesthetist, or machine failure is a remote possibility. (See Glossary, p. 309)

? WHAT ARE THE OTHER COMPLICATIONS AND POSSIBLE SIDE EFFECTS?

The chief side effects of removal of both ovaries in premenopausal women include all those attributed to menopause—flushing, hot flashes, increased risk of cardiovascular disease,[8] and depression. However, these side effects are absent or diminished when a functioning ovary is left in place. Hormone replacement therapy for premenopausal women who have had both ovaries removed is controversial, but opinion seems to be leaning increasingly towards using estrogen supplements.[9] Much of the controversy and confusion result from studies that are contradictory or hard to interpret, especially those concerning the role of hormone replacement therapy in preventing heart disease or breast cancer. Many questions remain about the benefits and risks of long-term use of hormone replacement therapy.

Failure to remove all of the ovary can commonly lead to the **ovarian remnant syndrome**, which is difficult to treat,[10] and occasionally leads to blockage of the **ureters**.[11]

? IS THIS THE MOST APPROPRIATE PROCEDURE FOR THE CONDITION?

The answer depends upon whether we are talking about one or both ovaries. Clear standards and guidelines regarding bilateral and unilateral oophorectomies have simply not been developed in the medical profession. Given what we now know about the role of estrogen (which is secreted by the ovaries) in preventing osteoporosis and heart disease, it seems logical to leave at least one functioning ovary whenever possible.

There is usually no compelling reason to remove both ovaries, unless both are afflicted with infections that cannot be eradicated with antibiotics, or both are injured so severely that repair is impossible. A study of 1,000 hysterectomies with and without removal of the ovaries showed that the rate of undiagnosed cancer in the removed ovaries was zero. This lends support to the idea of leaving the ovaries in place if they appear normal during a hysterectomy.[12] The logic of the current studies, though not always reflected in the practices of surgeons, would suggest that it is safe to leave a normal ovary in when the other one is removed.

Neither a single ovary nor both ovaries should be removed for vague indications such as mild premenstrual syndrome or for painful menstruation, both of which usually can be treated with drugs.

? ARE THERE ALTERNATIVES TO THIS PROCEDURE?

Essentially, no. If there are clear reasons—such as malignancy, injury, or uncontrollable infection—for removal of the single ovary, the only question is whether the laparoscopic or the open procedure should be used.

? WHAT IS CONTROVERSIAL ABOUT THE PROCEDURE?

Other than the absence of standards and guidelines, there is little that is controversial about this procedure. Most of the controversy surrounds the removal of both ovaries and whether, and how, to treat the side effects that arise from the total loss of estrogen produced by the ovaries.

Because of the tendency of bowel cancer in women to spread to the ovaries, some researchers recommend removal of the ovaries in postmenopausal women who have cancer of the large intestine. The recommendation is considered controversial.[13]

Unilateral Thyroid Lobectomy (88)

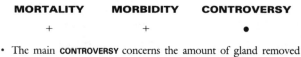

MORTALITY	MORBIDITY	CONTROVERSY
+	+	●

- The main **CONTROVERSY** concerns the amount of gland removed during the procedure. The decision is made by the surgeon based on the type, original location, and spread (if any) of the cancer.

Removal of one of the two lobes of the thyroid gland

? WHAT CONDITION DOES THE PROCEDURE TREAT?

This procedure is done almost exclusively for the treatment of cancer of the thyroid gland. (Located at the base of the neck, the thyroid gland consists of two lobes, one lobe on either side of the **trachea**, or windpipe.) This procedure can also be used in cases of hyperthyroidism (Graves' Disease) that do not respond to medical treatment. Radical dissection of the head and neck—involving an extensive Y-shaped incision, or actually series of incisions—was once done for thyroid cancer, but has since been totally replaced by surgery limited to the thyroid gland when the cancer has not spread beyond it. There have been very rare cases of a foreign body embedded in the thyroid, necessitating removal of a lobe.[1]

? WHAT IS THE PROCEDURE?

The front of the neck is shaved if necessary and scrubbed with soap and antiseptic. With the patient under general anesthesia, the surgeon makes an incision in the neck, following skinfold lines. Bleeding vessels are **ligated** or **cauterized** with an **electrocautery device**. The thyroid gland is exposed and the necessary portion is removed,

with care taken not to damage the nerves controlling the vocal cords if at all possible. The skin is closed with sutures or staples. The patient is taken to the recovery room and then to her room. Thyroid hormone activity should be carefully monitored after surgery.

? WHO PERFORMS THE PROCEDURE?

This operation is not technically difficult, but requires careful medical preparation and pre- and post-operative monitoring. To avoid the rare complication of thyroid storm—a state of increased thyroid secretion that leads to a syndrome of high fever, racing heartbeat, and delirium—it is important that the patient be treated medically (nonsurgically) and that thyroid function be rendered as close to normal as possible prior to surgery. A thoroughly experienced thyroid surgeon, or close cooperation between the surgeon and an endocrinologist, is required.

? WHERE IS THE PROCEDURE PERFORMED?

This surgery should be performed only in the inpatient department of a hospital.

? WHAT ARE THE MORTALITY (DEATH) AND MORBIDITY (COMPLICATION) RATES?

The mortality rate for the procedure itself is essentially zero. The mortality rate for thyroid storm, which is a rare complication, is high.

The main complication is damage to the nerves controlling the vocal cords. A surgical technique that reduces the incidence of this complication to between zero and 1% has been described.[2] If thyroid cancer is extensive, it may not always be possible to preserve the nerves, which can lead to hoarseness or loss of the voice in the worst cases.

? WHAT ARE THE OTHER COMPLICATIONS AND POSSIBLE SIDE EFFECTS?

The only other significant complication is infection.

As with any procedure in which anesthesia is used, death from reaction to the anesthetic drugs, error on the part of the anesthetist, or machine failure is a remote possibility. (See Glossary, p. 309)

? IS THIS THE MOST APPROPRIATE PROCEDURE FOR THE CONDITION?

For cancer of the thyroid diagnosed by examination of tissue samples, removal is the best alternative. For Graves' Disease and other varieties of hyperthyroidism, a "cocktail" of radioactive Iodine-131, which concentrates in the thyroid and destroys all or part of the gland, is preferable.

? ARE THERE ALTERNATIVES TO THIS PROCEDURE?

For thyroid cancer, no. For various forms of hyperthyroidism, see above.

? WHAT IS CONTROVERSIAL ABOUT THE PROCEDURE?

There is some controversy about the extent of tissue removal needed to effectively treat cancer. A prognostic scale developed at the Mayo Clinic can help in isolating some subgroups of patients who have better survival with total thyroid removal, as opposed to lobectomy.[3] The majority of patients with thyroid cancer can be treated with removal of only one lobe.[4] The extent of surgery has to be determined individually, based on the type, original location, and spread (if any) of the cancer.

Ureteral Catheterization (100)

MORTALITY	MORBIDITY	CONTROVERSY
+	+	o

Insertion of a thin tube into one or both of the **ureters**

Ureteral catheterization is the all-encompassing name for any procedure that consists of inserting a **catheter** through the urethra, into the bladder, and into one or both of the ureters.

? WHAT CONDITION DOES THE PROCEDURE TREAT?

Ureteral catheterization is a technique that has a wide (and often bewildering) variety of applications, and more are now under investigation. Among the most common uses are the following:

- Small ureteral stones, which usually originate in the kidney, can be removed from above[1] and below the site where they are lodged in the ureter.[2, 3]
- For cancerous ureters, ureteral catheters can be used to insert **shunts,** or tubes to support the natural channel of the ureter and hold it open. A **stent** may be placed in a damaged or weakened ureter.[4]
- Balloons attached to catheters can be used to open blocked ureters in the same way that they are used for coronary angioplasty (see "Percutaneous Transluminal Coronary Angioplasty, p. 194).[5]

The procedure goes by many names in the medical literature, so it is sometimes difficult to determine exactly what operation is being discussed. Terminology for equipment also varies. A 1982 study found that up to 70% of urologists preferred the use of "splint" to "stent."[6] To make matters more complicated, a catheter can be used to place a stent or used as a temporary stent.

Below, we use the term "indwelling stent" to mean a stent, not a catheter, that is usually permanently left in place, and "indwelling catheter" to mean a catheter that is briefly left in place after surgery. The catheter that is used for stone removal and balloon **dilation** of **strictures** is withdrawn completely as soon as the procedure is finished.

Placement of indwelling stents can correct surgical damage to the ureters without opening the abdomen.[7, 8] (Between 80% and 99% of all surgical injuries to the ureters occur during total abdominal hysterectomies.[9]) They can also be used to open up blockages of the ureters caused by benign tumors[10] or scarring.[11] Blockages in the ureters can also be cleared with stiff wires.

Not merely a passive tube, the ureter is actively involved in transport of urine from the kidney to the bladder by downward-pointing waves of contractions called **peristalsis**. To determine if the patient has a problem with the transport of urine, very small catheters can be inserted into the ureters to measure internal pressure and the rate and force of contractions.

Stones composed of uric acid or the amino acid cystine can be dissolved by catheter irrigation with appropriate chemicals.[12]

In one series, 95% success in removal of ureteral stones via catheters and similar methods was reported. The other 5% of patients required open operations for removal of the stones.[13] Another series reported a 92% success rate.[14]

Placement of stents reduces the incidence of complications following **extracorporeal shock-wave lithotripsy (ESWL)**, which uses sound waves from outside the body to break stones, from 26% to 7%.[15] One study reported a 97% success rate in fracturing ureteral stones after attempts to push the stone out of the urethra and into the kidney pelvis failed.[16]

? WHAT IS THE PROCEDURE?

A ureteral catheter can be placed from within the bladder through a **cystoscope**,[17, 18] which requires regional or general anesthesia. The catheter also can be placed through small incisions above the kidney; this can be done without regional or general anesthesia.[19] The catheter can also be placed via a small incision made in the bladder, a procedure requiring regional anesthesia or a local anesthetic. What happens after the catheter is maneuvered up the ureter to the site of the problem depends upon what the problem is—stones, stricture, pressure from a tumor, a gunshot injury, or whatever.

Laser lithotripsy to break apart ureteral stones can be done through a ureteral catheter—one that is inserted through the urinary opening. The laser alone was successful in 64% of the cases, and the laser combined with ESWL succeeded in 79% of the cases. Combined with other means of stone retrieval, these two methods succeeded in 90% of cases. There were no complications associated with the use of the laser in this study; however, further operations to deal with stones were required in 0.9% of cases.[20]

Use of a stone brush seems to improve the results of both extracorporeal and laser lithotripsy, probably by brushing away soft parts of the stone that absorb the laser or shock wave energy.[21] The stone brush, which is small and cone-shaped, is inserted into the ureter by way of a catheter and moved around, brushing away the stones so that the ureter can carry away the stone particles.

A small study comparing open repair of ureteral strictures and treatment by catheterization showed that 100% of the **open procedures** were successful, versus 64.3% of the catheter procedures. Because an open procedure can be done if the catheterization and dilation fails, it seems reasonable to try the catheterization first.[22]

Use of a catheter to maneuver a stone back into the pelvis, or large open space, in the kidney so that it no longer blocks the ureter significantly increases the success of ESWL.[23]

Balloon dilation of the ureter via a catheter can result in painless passage of kidney stones as large as 0.236 inches (6 mm).[24]

? WHO PERFORMS THE PROCEDURE?

This procedure should be done only by a board-certified urologist with significant experience in use of catheters and stents. Those procedures that are part of interventional radiology for kidney problems may be performed by a board-certified radiologist with additional training in interventional radiology—which is the use of catheters, needles, and scopes to drain abscesses and growths that can only be done under direct visualization techniques, such as x ray and **ultrasound**.

? WHERE IS THE PROCEDURE PERFORMED?

Depending on the patient's condition and the reason for the surgery, this procedure can be performed in the inpatient or outpatient department of a hospital, an outpatient clinic, a radiology office, or a well-equipped doctor's office.

? WHAT ARE THE MORTALITY (DEATH) AND MORBIDITY (COMPLICATION) RATES?

Operative mortality of zero and operative morbidity of 0.68%, with total morbidity of 0.8%, have been reported for a 17-year series of ureteral stone removal with catheter devices. Indwelling catheters and antibiotics were not used routinely in this series.[25] Another study reports a morbidity rate of 1%.[26] Morbidity is significantly increased by the use of indwelling stents.

Complications are reported to occur in about 6% of cases during the early part of the physician's "learning curve"; the rate declines after her technique is perfected.[27]

One death from infection closely following placement of a stent has been reported.[28] A 1981 German study reported a complication rate of 54.3% in patients given ureteral stents for various causes of ureteral obstruction.[29]

? WHAT ARE THE OTHER COMPLICATIONS AND POSSIBLE SIDE EFFECTS?

Failure to save the kidney from kidney failure by placing a **percutaneous** ureteral stent occurs in about 40% of cases, about the same as for open kidney operations.[30] Attempts to open a ureteral stricture with an **angioplasty** balloon fail in about 17% of cases.[31]

Damage to the juncture between the kidney and the ureter during the removal of a stent has been reported.[32] Catheter blockage can lead to the need for additional surgery.[33] Some catheters break off in the ureter; if they cannot be retrieved by another catheterization or a percutaneous procedure, an open procedure (which involves a large incision) may be needed to remove them.

Rarely, an indwelling stent can cause **fistulas** between the ureter and a vein or artery and part of the intestines and ureter or artery. Fewer than 15 cases are reported in the literature. A case has been reported in which the patient developed a fistula between one ureter and an artery and between the **colon** and the other artery. The patient had a bacterial infection of the bloodstream and bloody urine.[34, 35] If a catheter penetrates an artery by accident, it may block blood flow, leading to severe hemorrhaging when it is removed.[36]

The rationale for both indwelling catheters and indwelling stents is that they hold the ureter open, force urine to drain only into the bladder in cases of ureteral damage, and keep the ureter from collapsing under pressure from benign or malignant tumors.[37]

However, even indwelling stents or indwelling catheters placed with perfect technique can be uncomfortable or painful. Typically, an indwelling catheter is placed so that one end is high in the ureter and the other is led out through the urethra so that its removal will not require a cystoscopy procedure (see "Cystoscopy," p. 61). It can also be wrapped around a **Foley catheter**. Because the catheter has to be a bit stiff to stay open inside the abdomen, it can cause pain. Symptoms—which are unpleasant but not harmful in the long run—include a continuous need to void (if the catheter distends the neck of the bladder sufficiently), frequent night voiding, flank and pubic pain, pain on removal of the catheter, and pain on urination.[38] These symptoms are also reported for indwelling stents.

In a 1990 study, 44% of patients reported mild to intolerable pain that was relieved by removal of the stent, 42% reported visible blood in the urine, 20% reported fever and chills, and 38% reported bladder or flank pain.[39] Most problems resolved when the stent was removed. A 1988 review suggests that the universal use of stents before lithotripsy should be avoided because the cure is worse than the disease—many patients report more pain with the use of the stent to hold the ureter open for stone passage than from the passage of small stones or stone fragments.[40] One small 1985 Japanese study found the stent ". . . neither safe nor effective" for more than short-term use.[41] A 1987 French study was less pessimistic, but still cited a complication rate of 11%.[42] A 1990 Japanese study found a complication rate of 17.2% and suggested that stents be removed as early as possible.[43] One study of stenting in **renal** transplant patients revealed that 76% of stented patients developed postoperative infections versus 45% of those without stents.[44]

Stent-associated pain may be caused by movement of the stent; it is possible that better methods to hold the stent in place might reduce the discomfort.[45, 46]

Crusts composed of chemicals in the urine may form on the catheter and jam it inside the ureter. An encrusted catheter has been successfully removed by using laser lithotripsy inside the catheter.[47]

If a short catheter is placed in the ureter and held in position with a pigtail-shaped (not straight) catheter placed in the kidney, it is possible for the two catheters to move about in the ureter; the authors recommend the use of catheters long enough to reach from the kidney to the bladder.[48]

Although not a complication per se, **false positive diagnoses** can result from x-ray studies of the kidney or bladder performed with a catheter in place when the bladder is full; the authors of the study cited recommend that all patients with indwelling catheters urinate before x-ray studies.[49]

As with any procedure in which anesthesia is used, death from reaction to the anesthetic drugs, error on the part of the anesthetist, or machine failure is a remote possibility. (See Glossary, p. 309)

? IS THIS THE MOST APPROPRIATE PROCEDURE FOR THE CONDITION?

"Watchful waiting" to see if stones will pass is always possible, but stone pain is among the most severe pains observed, and most patients will lose tolerance for waiting after a few days at most. If a kidney stone is hard and rigid, something that can only be guessed at based on the chemistry of the urine and x-ray studies, use of a catheter to push it back into the pelvis of the kidney, followed by ESWL, has a very high success rate. If the stone is composed of uric acid or cystine, it can be dissolved with chemicals passed through a catheter. If it is not in a position to be reached with a catheter from below and EWSL has failed, then some of the more complicated catheter manipulations are appropriate.

Given the variety of techniques that have emerged and the range of success rates reported for them by various authorities, it seems that research is needed to develop rules for treatment.

One thing that seems clear from the literature is that the long-term use of stents has a high rate of complications and should be used only if no other choice presents itself—for instance, the patient's remaining lifetime is short, dilation of the ureter with a balloon has failed, or part of the ureter has been destroyed by cancer.

? ARE THERE ALTERNATIVES TO THIS PROCEDURE?

ESWL is the chief alternative to removal of stones by catheter, but is often combined with it. For strictures and obstructions of the ureter from sources other than stones (cancer, for example), open operations are the only alternatives, and they have a significantly higher mortality rate than catheter manipulations.

? WHAT IS CONTROVERSIAL ABOUT THE PROCEDURE?

The main sources of controversy concern what to do with stones that are not shattered by ESWL or laser lithotripsy, and the merits and long-term safety of indwelling stents, about which there is wide divergence of opinion among doctors.

Uterine Lesion Destruction (93)

MORTALITY	MORBIDITY	CONTROVERSY
+	+	o

Destruction of a **lesion** in or on the uterus by various means

? WHAT CONDITION DOES THE PROCEDURE TREAT?

Similar to the other female reproductive organs, the uterus is subject to a variety of lesions and tumors, both malignant and nonmalignant. The general recommendation for uterine cancer is removal of the uterus, but a premenopausal woman who wishes to retain her uterus in order to have children or to avoid the possible side effects of a hysterectomy can have conization of the **cervix** (removal of a cone of tissue from the cervical opening to eliminate a lesion) for cervical cancer, with careful follow-up at six-month intervals. This is possible only if the lesion is located in a position where it can be completely removed by a conization small enough to leave a functioning cervix.

One study has shown that when certain anatomic and microscopic criteria for the location of cervical cancer are met, it is highly unlikely that there is any cancer in the uterus itself.[1]

A laser may also be used to treat lesions in or on the cervix and preserve a woman's childbearing capability. A carbon dioxide laser can be aimed precisely at the lesion and causes less damage to adjacent tissue than other types of lasers. The laser may be used to treat lesions on the vaginal portion of the cervix and inside the neck of the uterus.

The other uterine lesion of major concern is nonmalignant: It is called a fibromyoma—or myoma, for short—and is a benign tumor of the uterine muscle. Depending upon the size, a myoma can be removed with a scalpel, **electrocautery device,** or laser, thus avoiding the loss of the uterus.

? WHAT IS THE PROCEDURE?

For hot (electrosurgical) or cold (scalpel) conization of the cervix, the patient is given a general anesthetic. The vagina is held open with a **speculum**, and a cone of the tissue surrounding the opening of the cervix is cut out, removed, and sent for study to determine the extent of any malignancy that may be present. In the cold procedure, the electrocautery may be used to control bleeding.

Removal of small fibromyomas[2] and other local lesions can be achieved with the resectoscope, a form of cystoscope that has recently come into use for uterine conditions.[3] During a resectoscope procedure, the patient is given a spinal anesthetic and positioned on a gynecologic examination table. The cervix is widened enough to insert the scope, and an **electrocautery probe** is guided through the scope to remove the tumor or other diseased tissue.

In laser removal of lesions, the surgeon inserts a **speculum** into the vagina and, through the use of a specialized gynecologic scope called a **colposcope**, directs the laser beam. Tissue may be vaporized or cut and removed for laboratory analysis.

? WHO PERFORMS THE PROCEDURE?

This procedure is performed by an obstetrician-gynecologist.

? WHERE IS THE SURGERY PERFORMED?

This procedure can be done on an inpatient or outpatient basis in a hospital, in an outpatient surgery facility, or in a well-equipped doctor's office.

? WHAT ARE THE MORTALITY (DEATH) AND MORBIDITY (COMPLICATION) RATES?

The death rate is essentially zero. Most complications result from anesthesia, not the procedure. As with any procedure in which anesthesia is used, death from re-

action to the anesthetic drugs, error on the part of the anesthetist, or machine failure is a remote possibility. (See Glossary, p. 309)

? WHAT ARE THE OTHER COMPLICATIONS AND POSSIBLE SIDE EFFECTS?

Other than rare **perforation** of the uterus, there are no major complications or side effects.

? IS THIS THE MOST APPROPRIATE PROCEDURE FOR THE CONDITION?

Yes, because this is a conservative procedure that can always be followed by hysterectomy if it fails. Use of LHRH antagonists (drugs that control and suppress part of the female hormonal cycle) can shrink myomas to the point at which surgery may not be needed, but these drugs cannot be taken on a long-term basis.

? ARE THERE ALTERNATIVES TO THIS PROCEDURE?

See above.

? WHAT IS CONTROVERSIAL ABOUT THE PROCEDURE?

There are few controversies about this procedure, because it is a conservative alternative to the more radical alternatives such as removal of the uterus.

Vacuum Extraction Delivery with Episiotomy (19)

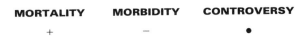

MORTALITY	MORBIDITY	CONTROVERSY
+	−	●

- Soft tissue **DAMAGE** is reported in 21.6% of vacuum deliveries. Damage in the form of vaginal and cervical laceration occurs in 18% of vacuum deliveries.

- The major **CONTROVERSY** is the further medicalization of birth through the active intervention of the physician. Studies have shown very little improvement in maternal and infant mortality and morbidity as a result of vacuum extraction delivery.

Use of a suction instrument to deliver a baby stuck low in the vagina, after making a surgical incision to enlarge the vaginal opening

? WHAT CONDITION DOES THE PROCEDURE TREAT?

This procedure is used when a baby's head is already deep into the vagina during birth and labor stops completely, the mother is in danger or exhausted, or the infant develops indications of sudden distress requiring immediate delivery. A vacuum extractor (description follows) can also be used to rotate the baby from a face-up to a face-down position if necessary and to manipulate the infant if there is an indication that its shoulders are in a position to become wedged in the birth canal. This latter use is rare.

Most childbirths go well, but the size of a baby's head is approximately the maximum that the female anatomy will permit, and it is not surprising that complete or partial tears of the **perineum** occur occasionally during delivery. A surgical cut in the perineum, called an **episiotomy**—which is done to (theoretically) prevent a large tear—seems to prevent some kinds of tears and increase the chance of others. (We have more to say about episiotomy below.)

? WHAT IS THE PROCEDURE?

This procedure lacks elegance. It is a variation on **forceps** delivery (see "Low-Forceps Delivery with Episiotomy," p. 177), a rather old practice that obstetricians believe has stood the test of time. An instrument that looks like the furniture duster attachment to a household vacuum cleaner with a suction cup at the end is slid into the vagina until it touches the baby's head. The doctor starts pulling, also rotating the baby if it is not in the face-down position.

Since the use of vacuum extraction has the potential to tear the vaginal opening, an episiotomy is done. An episiotomy is simply an incision, made with a pair of surgical scissors, from the vaginal opening into the tissue of the pelvic floor, called the perineum, to avoid a natural tear. The cut may be made directly down towards the anus or off to one side.

With the top of the infant's head securely in the suction cup, the baby is pulled out of the vagina, the vacuum is turned off, and delivery is finished normally.

? WHO PERFORMS THE PROCEDURE?

This procedure is performed by an obstetrician-gynecologist or family or general practitioner who delivers babies. Because studies indicate that junior hospital staff cause much more maternal pelvic trauma than do senior hospital staff,[1] you should discuss with the doctor—well before the delivery date—her philosophy of vacuum use, as well as how many vacuum deliveries she has done and with what results. To ensure that there is a written record of the discussion, it may be useful to write a letter to the doctor about agreements made, prior to labor and delivery, regarding the birth process and your preferences in medical interventions. (The doctor may or may not note the agreements in your chart.) Also make sure that any agreements with the doctor about vacuum use are in writing.

? WHERE IS THE PROCEDURE PERFORMED?

This procedure can be performed anywhere it is needed and where the doctor has the vacuum device. Usually, it is performed in a hospital or birthing center.

? WHAT ARE THE MORTALITY (DEATH) AND MORBIDITY (COMPLICATION) RATES?

Without detailed autopsy studies, it is hard to distinguish the mortality rate associated with any particular manipulation late in delivery with the mortality rate of delivery per se. The mortality rate for all vacuum deliveries with episiotomies for community hospitals in the U.S. in 1988 was less than 0.1%.[2] The chief complication of vacuum deliveries for the mother is damage to the vagina, the vaginal opening, and the tissues of the pelvic floor. A good deal of the medical literature on assisted deliveries consists of studies comparing forceps deliveries with vacuum deliveries. Looking at the figures for forceps deliveries and vacuum deliveries side by side can serve as a useful review of how harmful forceps deliveries can be. As one might expect, third- and fourth-degree perineal lacerations and vaginal and cervical lacerations were found to be fewer with vacuum extractions as opposed to forceps deliveries.[3] (The most serious kind, a fourth-degree tear, runs all the way through the perineum and causes complete separation of all tissue layers.) For further information on degrees of lacerations, see "Repair of Obstetric Laceration," p. 208.

Low-forceps deliveries are done when the baby's presenting part is firmly lodged in the woman's pelvis and clearly visible in the birth canal—this condition is called **engagement;** anything else is mid- or high-forceps, depending upon the position of the head in the canal.[4] "Significant" maternal soft tissue trauma was found in 48.9% of mothers delivered by the low-forceps method versus 21.6% of those delivered with the Mityvac vacuum system in one study.[5] Maternal fever occurred in 48% of cesarean-section births but in only 6% of vacuum extraction births. The same study found that vaginal and cervical lacerations occurred in 48% of forceps deliveries but in only 18% of vacuum deliveries, and maternal anemia occurred in 30% of mothers who had cesarean section versus 4% of those who had delivery with the vacuum extractor.[6]

? WHAT ARE THE OTHER COMPLICATIONS AND POSSIBLE SIDE EFFECTS?

What about the baby? A Viennese study found the infant death rate associated with the use of forceps to be 2.8% and the death rate associated with vacuum extraction to be 0.95%.[7] A study of Norwegian military recruits found that males delivered by forceps had significantly higher IQs at age 18 than those who were delivered by a vacuum extractor,[8] but this finding may be an **artifact**.

The incidence of skull fractures in newborns was found to be essentially identical for spontaneous vaginal and vacuum delivery births.[9]

A study of forceps versus the Kobayashi vacuum extractor (a variation, named after the doctor who invented it) found that infants delivered with the vacuum extractor had a higher risk of **cephalhematoma** and neonatal jaundice. There was no difference in major morbidity between the forceps and vacuum extraction groups.[10] Forceps deliveries cause hematomas of the scalp in 5.1% to 6% of deliveries done with them, versus 22.9% with vacuum extraction.[11, 12] Another study found the incidence of neurological injuries to the infant to be essentially the same for vacuum extraction and forceps deliveries.[13] A 1987 comparison of vacuum and mid-forceps deliveries found that cephalhematoma was more common with the use of forceps than with vacuum extraction.[14]

The use of Kielland's forceps (yet another variation

on forceps, named after the doctor who invented them) was associated with an infant mortality rate of 3.49%, a 23.3% rate of **transient neurological deficits** and abnormal behavior that resolved quickly, and a 15.1% incidence of birth trauma. Found following both instrument deliveries and natural births, **subgaleal hematomas**—which form between the brain and a band of fibrous tissue that forms the cap of the skull in newborns—result in a mortality rate of 22.8%. Fifty-two percent of the cases of subgaleal hematomas reported in a 1980 review of the literature were associated with vacuum deliveries, 11% occurred after mid-forceps deliveries, 28% occurred following normal vaginal deliveries, and 8.9% occurred following cesarean section.[15]

Normal births produce stress on the infant too, a fact that should not be forgotten in thinking about various modes of delivery. A study of the incidence of retinal hemorrhage (bleeding of the membrane at the back of the eye) found that infants born by cesarean section had a 2.6% incidence, those delivered by forceps had a 25% incidence, and those born without intervention had an incidence of 38%.[16] Broken bones have been reported following delivery of the infant by forceps, vacuum extraction, and cesarean section.[17] The incidence of broken collarbones in spontaneous vaginal deliveries is around 1.25%.[18]

? IS THIS THE MOST APPROPRIATE PROCEDURE FOR THE CONDITION?

Forceps deliveries, vacuum extractions, and cesarean sections compete for usage among doctors. Examination of the studies from 1975 to the present indicates that both forceps deliveries and vacuum extractions are becoming safer, and the mortality rate from cesarean sections is "only" six times that of vaginal deliveries now. Because both infant and maternal mortality, as opposed to morbidity, are quite low, the question of what

method to use turns on weighing the amount of damage that it is likely to inflict on the mother and baby against the risk of not performing that procedure. Yet who decides? Many, if not most, women no longer regard childbirth as open season for scalpel and scissors, regardless of what the doctor thinks.

We believe that the sum of the evidence indicates that just about anything that can be done with a forceps can be done with a vacuum extractor. Vacuum extractors produce less trauma to the mother, do not require the stretching of the vaginal canal that forceps do, and allow the infant to rotate to the easiest position for delivery. They do produce scalp trauma, but this is serious in only a few cases. Infant mortality of 0.6% and no maternal mortality have been reported.[19] The risk of scalp trauma can be lessened by the use of plastic rather than metal suction cups.[20]

? ARE THERE ALTERNATIVES TO THIS PROCEDURE?

Keep in mind that there is a question about the overall benefit of obstetrical manipulations, and the suggestion that they may do more harm than good in the aggregate (see below).

Cesarean section is an alternative if the infant is not mostly out of the womb. In cases in which the infant is low in the birth canal, a forceps or vacuum delivery is almost always possible. In addition, the maternal mortality rate for cesarean section is six to 20 times higher than the vaginal delivery rate, with the better ratios coming in later years.[21]

Of course, unassisted birth is an option. The present climate of litigation rewards the doctor who cuts, not the doctor who waits, but it is certainly reasonable for parents to insist that the doctor wait until there is clear evidence of continuing fetal distress before using any surgical means to remove the infant. A 1983 study of low-forceps versus spontaneous vaginal deliveries of low-birthweight infants found that the use of forceps did not improve survival,[22] so the benefit is questionable in any case.

? WHAT IS CONTROVERSIAL ABOUT THE PROCEDURE?

The biggest question is whether the "medicalization" of birth—transforming it from a natural, albeit uncomfortable, process, into a disease—and the further "gadgetization" of the process have contributed to the decline in maternal mortality that has been observed in this century. A comparison of Holland, where home births are the norm, and Denmark, where hospitals are the usual location, found essentially identical infant mortality rates.[23] In one study, investigators concluded that obstetrical medical intervention (as distinct from medical measures to improve maternal health prior to birth, and general public health measures) has nothing whatsoever to do with the improvements in maternal and infant mortality and morbidity that have been seen.[24] They further concluded that maternal and infant morbidity would have declined even more without obstetrical intervention. If these conclusions are true in the aggregate, then it must follow that obstetrical manipulations, in the aggregate, impose wholly unnecessary mortality, morbidity, and expense.

Even if we accept the legitimacy of continued intervention in the case of clear doubts about the aggregate benefits of the procedures, an associated question is the scientific foundation of the practices that are used. A study of European countries found that operative delivery rates (rates of cesarean sections, forceps deliveries, and vacuum extractions combined) varied from 6% to 24%, and the rate of artificial induction of labor ranged from 12% to 36%. No obvious health benefit other than a very slight reduction in infant mortality rates was found, with most of the variation in infant mortality rates being accounted for by other factors.[25] Further, use of fetal monitoring seems to increase the rate of all sorts of obstetrical surgery and medical intervention, but the extent to which problematic readings on the monitor indicate real fetal problems is much debated.

If conducted, a **meta-analysis** would probably indicate that the one group to clearly benefit from increased obstetrical intervention is high-risk infants. Overall, it would seem best to let nature take its course and only use the vacuum extractor if it becomes quite clear that labor will not proceed normally. More invasive approaches should be used only when both a trial of labor and attempted vacuum extraction have failed.

Vaginal Hysterectomy (21)

MORTALITY	MORBIDITY	CONTROVERSY
+	−	●

- The reported **MORBIDITY** rate for abdominal and vaginal hysterectomies is 24.2%. However, some studies have reported rates between 6.6% and 41%.

- The **CONTROVERSY** concerning this procedure is one of appropriateness, because less radical surgical and medical treatments are available.

Removal of the uterus through the vaginal opening without an abdominal incision

? WHAT CONDITION DOES THE PROCEDURE TREAT?

See "Total Abdominal Hysterectomy," p. 243.

The medical literature recommends that vaginal hysterectomies not be used as means of sterilization because several other procedures (**ligation** of the **fallopian tubes** via **laparoscope**, for example) have lower morbidity and mortality.[1] For conditions that are valid **indications** for hysterectomy, the vaginal hysterectomy, which does not require an abdominal incision, is the procedure of choice.[2]

In operations for cancer, the radical vaginal hysterectomy, a variation on the standard operation, produced five-year survival rates of 76% to 91%, depending upon the stage and size of the cancer when it was initially diagnosed.[3] Another study found a 97.6% five-year survival rate.[4]

WHAT IS THE PROCEDURE?

When the patient is under general or spinal anesthesia, she is placed in the **lithotomy position**. The vaginal lips, which have usually been shaved the night before, are washed with an antiseptic. The patient's legs and abdomen are draped so that only the vaginal opening is exposed and a **speculum** is inserted. The **cervix** is grasped with **forceps** and cut away from the upper part of the vagina, and the skin, **tendons**, muscles, and **ligaments** connecting the uterus to the upper part of the vaginal pouch are cut away. "Bleeders"—small veins and arteries that ooze blood—are cauterized; larger vessels are ligated, **clipped**, or clamped.

When the sides of the uterus are sufficiently exposed, the ligaments holding it from the top and the arteries and veins supplying blood are identified, ligated, and cut one by one. Because damage to the bladder and **ureters** can occur at this stage, the surgeon should take care to determine the identity of the structures being exposed so there is no accidental damage to the urinary tract. One or more ligaments are left intact to provide support for the upper part of the vagina; others are trimmed back.

When the uterus is completely free of its various supports and connections, it is pulled out through the vagina unless it is abnormally large, in which case it is cut into sections and removed piece by piece. The supporting ligaments are stitched to the top of the vaginal "cuff" that remains, and the roof of the cuff is sewn shut. If needed, any repairs to the muscles supporting the bladder and rectum are made at this time, in a procedure called **colporrhaphy**. A **catheter** is placed in the bladder, either through the **urethra** or by an incision below the pubic bone, and the patient is taken to the recovery room.

If the procedure is undertaken for cancer that has spread to the vagina, a new vagina can be constructed from **peritoneal** tissue, which is accessible through the incision without opening the abdominal cavity through a skin incision.

A modification of the usual procedure—which removes almost as much tissue as the total abdominal hysterectomy but is done through the vagina and requires no abdominal incision—has been developed and proposed as an operation for early, microinvasive (not grossly apparent) cancer of the cervix.[5] Another variation, which preserves normal anatomic relationships of the structures by leaving the **fascia** intact, has been developed for the treatment of noncancerous conditions only.[6] Yet another modification that does not involve ligation of as many ligaments as the standard procedure is associated with a low complication rate.[7]

WHO PERFORMS THE PROCEDURE?

This procedure should be performed by a general surgeon or a gynecologist who has had special training for it.

WHERE IS THE PROCEDURE PERFORMED?

This is major surgery that should always be performed as an inpatient procedure in a hospital.

WHAT ARE THE MORTALITY (DEATH) AND MORBIDITY (COMPLICATION) RATES?

In community hospitals in the U.S. in 1988, the mortality rate for vaginal hysterectomies was less than 0.1%. Mortality rates quoted in the medical literature since

1975 range from 0.82% (in a series of women with preexisting medical problems)[8] to 0.07% (less than one per 1000) in a recent German study.[9] In a nationwide study from 1979 to 1980 using data from hospitals participating in the Commission on Professional and Hospital Activities, the mortality rate for vaginal hysterectomies was 0.038%. The mortality for total abdominal hysterectomies was 0.15%—almost four times as high. Mortality rates rose with age and were twice as high for black women.[10] (In general, black women have less access to adequate medical care, and so may have other complicating illnesses.) A 1981 study of vaginal hysterectomies in women over the age of 65 found a mortality rate of zero and no complications resulting in extra days of hospital stay.[11] A 1976 study of Greek women found a mortality rate of 0.60% for vaginal hysterectomy and 0.645% for abdominal hysterectomy, with 2.966% for hysterectomies for cancer and 0.20% for noncancerous conditions.

Morbidity rates for the vaginal and abdominal groups were similar (24.21%), with a 48% rate of complications in patients operated on for cancer.[12] Other studies report morbidity rates as low as 6.6%[13] and as high as 41.07%.[14]

In a German study conducted between 1968 and 1973, the complication rate for the abdominal hysterectomy was almost twice as high as for vaginal hysterectomy (19.1% versus 9.6%), and total mortality for the abdominal procedure was five times as high as the vaginal procedure (1.7% versus 0.37%).[15]

Infection is a very common complication of this procedure, related both to the normal microbial population of the area and the use of bladder catheters following surgery. In one study, 49.1% of the women who had no preoperative antibiotics of any kind had fever, compared with patients who had had preventive antibiotics for 10 days (10.1% of whom had fever), those who had had three injections of antibiotics before surgery (8.6% of whom had fever), and those who had had a **cauterization** of cervical tissue (called a hot conization of the cervix) and an iodine scrub of the cervix (4.3% of whom had fever).[16] Another study, which cultured swabs of the cut edge of the vaginal cuff, found a high incidence of bacterial contamination and recommended preoperative antibiotics.[17] Many studies suggest that postoperative infections can be almost totally eliminated with preoperative antibiotics.[18–30]

One study found that the use of antibiotics cut three days off the average length of hospital stay.[31] A few other studies using various antibiotics have not found as large a reduction in infection rates, but have found that use of preoperative antibiotics reduced the postoperative infection rate by more than 80%. Without antibiotics, almost three-quarters of the women in some studies,[32] and nearly half[33–35] of the women operated on in others, had postoperative infections.[36–43] A review of studies published in the English language found that 96.7% of them reported a lower incidence of infection with preoperative antibiotics.[44] There is a higher rate of infection, even with these antibiotics, in women who have anemia or diabetes.[45]

Leaving the ovaries and tubes in place after either a vaginal or abdominal hysterectomy is associated with a low rate of complications. In a study of 2,132 women who had had hysterectomies, 0.66% required further gynecological surgery; there were two deaths (0.09%), both from cancer.[46] If the tubes and ovaries are left intact, ectopic pregnancy (implantation of fertilized egg outside the womb) following vaginal hysterectomy rarely occurs.

Catheters in the bladder are routinely used after gynecologic surgery (remaining in place anywhere from one to two days or even a week) to ensure proper urinary drainage. Either a **Foley catheter** (inserted through the urethra) or a suprapubic catheter, inserted into the bladder through the skin between the pubic bone and the top of the vaginal lips, may be used. Both are associated with high rates of infection, blockage, and bleeding from the bladder. Many patients find the suprapubic catheter more acceptable than the Foley catheter, despite the need for the skin puncture. The reason is that, if its diameter is large enough to stretch the bladder sphincter,[47] the Foley catheter can induce a sensation of constantly having to void. Infection rates with the Foley catheter can be as high as 67.1%, versus 20.9% for the suprapubic catheter.[48]

A change in sexual responsiveness and ability to enjoy intercourse following hysterectomy is frequently reported by women, and until quite recently has been dismissed by many in the medical profession as simply the product of an inflamed female imagination. The official position of the American College of Obstetricians and Gynecologists was that "neither the production of hormones nor a woman's ability to have satisfying sexual relations is affected. . . ."[49] Concerning this potential complication, one needs to distinguish carefully between hysterectomy that includes removal of the ovaries—which clearly causes dramatic hormonal changes—and hysterectomy that leaves the ovaries in place, a procedure that preserves the normal female hormonal balance but may alter pelvic and vaginal sensations, which play a large role in women's sexual responsiveness.

In a 1983 German study that focused on sexual responsiveness and female self-image, 56% of women under age 45 and 69% of women over age 45 reported no changes in their sex lives as a result of hysterectomy. These women did report significant changes in their self-image, however. Clearly, for about 44% of women under age 45 and one-third of women over age 45, the procedure does produce a perceived alteration in sexual response.[50] Another German study, reported in 1989, found significant changes in sexual behavior and responsiveness even if the ovaries were left in place, and recommended hormone therapy for changes in sexual responsiveness—even for women with intact ovaries.[51] Because sexual response has a very large mental component, both alterations in subjective perception and objective physical changes can produce objective changes in sexual response; neither of them are under the control of the patient to any significant degree. Surgery anywhere on the body frequently leads to diminished sensation, at least for a period following surgery, because most of the nerves that are cut are not individually reconnected.

❓ WHAT ARE THE OTHER COMPLICATIONS AND POSSIBLE SIDE EFFECTS?

The urge to void frequently is a complication associated more often with vaginal hysterectomies than with abdominal ones, according to one study.[52] For women who prior to surgery had complaints of a sensation of residual urine in the bladder after voiding, vaginal hysterectomy produced better results than total abdominal hysterectomy.[53]

A study of complications of vaginal and abdominal hysterectomy between 1978 and 1981 showed that women having vaginal hysterectomies had fewer infections, less bleeding, less fever, and shorter hospital stays than women who had the abdominal operation.[54] However, vaginal hysterectomies were associated with additional major surgical procedures to correct problems following the hysterectomy. The investigators strongly recommended the use of the vaginal hysterectomy with preoperative antibiotics to prevent infection for women in whom it was technically possible and clinically indicated. (It is technically impossible to perform vaginal hysterectomy (1) when the woman has a long narrow vagina in which no speculum can fit; and (2) when a woman has scar tissue in the vaginal vault and all attempts to **dilate** the vagina tear the tissue. In the final analysis, however, sometimes the issue is more a function of the surgeon's capabilities than with the actual anatomical position of the uterus.)

A **prospective study** of transfusion needs of women having vaginal hysterectomies found that two units of blood should be set aside when vaginal hysterectomy included pelvic floor repair.[55]

Complications following vaginal and abdominal hysterectomy can include **enterocele** (a **herniation** of the vagina into the pelvic cavity) and complete and incomplete **prolapse** of the vaginal vault. These complications can be treated with low operative morbidity (other than fever) by sewing the residual vaginal cuff to the sacrospinous ligament (between the base of the pelvis and the bottom of the spine), a procedure that can be done through the vagina and does not require an abdominal incision. This produced complete resolution of the prolapse in 90% of the patients treated. Slightly more than 14% (14.1%) had laxity of the vaginal walls without symptoms, 12.67% had vaginal **stenosis** or stress incontinence (inability to hold urine while coughing or laughing), 5.63% developed herniations of the bladder into the vaginal vault (called **cystocele**), and 4.22% had recurrent vaginal prolapse. (Numbers total more than 100% because some patients fell into multiple categories.)[56] A further modification of the surgical technique apparently can completely prevent prolapse.[57]

A procedure that essentially closes off the vagina has been recommended for the avoidance of vaginal prolapse and stress incontinence in elderly, nonsexually active women who have stress incontinence.[58] Completely aside from the fact that vaginal prolapse appears to be associated with ineffective operative technique in the first place, the same result can be achieved with the purchase of a box of adult diapers.

If a woman has previously been sterilized by clamping of the fallopian tubes with Hulka-Clemens spring-loaded clips, these may be dislodged during a vaginal hysterectomy. The clips were spontaneously squeezed out of the vaginal vault in two cases reported.[59]

As a late consequence of hysterectomy, **fistulas** between the **colon** and the vagina have been observed. The authors of the study note that the eruptions of pus when the cul-de-sac was opened were "volcanic" and propose naming the disease the "Io Syndrome" after the most eruptive body in the solar system. (The cul-de-sac is a blind pouch between the vagina and the neck of the cervix, which is reduced to a single, open pouch via most hysterectomy techniques.) The illness is life-threatening, but can be treated with surgery and antibiotics.[60]

The first, and only, case of an enormous pararenal **hematoma** (in the region of the kidney), which stretched from the vaginal stump to the kidney, was reported in 1987. The portion of the hematoma near the vaginal stump was seen by an **ultrasound**, but only a **CT scan** revealed the full extent. Such hematomas can be treated with surgery, but can be devastating if they become a focus of infection.[61]

There are three cases in the literature of herniation of the **small intestine** into the bladder through a defect caused in the course of a vaginal hysterectomy. These are hard to diagnose via bowel x ray if the **contrast medium** does not flow into the bladder. The second and third cases were reported in 1987.[62]

Pulmonary embolism is a potentially fatal complication of any surgery in the lower body. The rate of embolism in vaginal hysterectomies is about one-fifth that of abdominal hysterectomies (0.3% versus 1.7%).[63] Abdominoplastic surgery (cosmetic operations on the abdomen, such as "tummy tucks") performed at the same time as a number of different gynecological operations, including vaginal hysterectomy, were associated with significantly greater blood loss and increased incidence of pulmonary embolism. This is an important finding, because embolisms can be fatal.[64] The combining of procedures can reduce morbidity and mortality in some situations, but this is apparently not one of them.

Urinary retention can follow almost any surgery, but is especially common after operations on the abdomen and pelvis. In a highly detailed 1987 study from Germany, the frequency of urinary tract problems following vaginal hysterectomy was between one-half to one-fifth of that following abdominal hysterectomy, with the sole exception of retention of urine in an amount greater than 10% of maximum bladder capacity, for which the rate was 24.2% after vaginal surgery and 13.2% after abdominal hysterectomies.[65] Injection through a catheter of a solution of **prostaglandin** F2, a chemical produced naturally by the body, into the bladder was significantly more effective than salt water in overcoming urinary retention.[66] A similar result was found with the related compound prostaglandin E2.[67] Prostaglandins were first identified in the prostate gland of men. One of their functions is to stimulate smooth muscle tissue, such as that found in the bladder, to contract.

Accidental damage to the **ureters** sometimes occurs in the process of a hysterectomy: The ureters lie close to the paracervical ligaments that support the uterus in the region of the cervix. Some surgeons believe that the paracervical ligaments must be **ligated**, or tied off, before they are cut in order to prevent excess bleeding. This is a part of both the standard vaginal and standard open abdominal procedures, but of course is more difficult to perform vaginally. In both procedures, ligation and division of the paracervical ligaments may result in accidental ligation and cutting of the ureter. Relatively delicate corrective surgery is required to repair damaged ureters. Apparently, however, the paracervical ligaments are not as prone to bleeding as had been thought, and it appears that hysterectomies may be performed without tying them off. A surgical variation that does not involve ligation of the paracervical ligaments was found to reduce ureteral damage to 0.03% and reduced the need for further surgery to control bleeding to 0.02%.[68]

Damage to the peripheral **femoral** nerves can occur as a result of prolonged use of stirrup and operating table positions that are designed to give the surgeon room to work but force the legs to rotate outward at the hip joint when they are already extended as far to the side as they can go. Such a position crushes the femoral nerve beneath the inguinal ligament and produces a complication that usually clears within two months. This complication can be avoided by thigh supports that limit how far towards the patient's head the thighs can be pushed when the hip joint is rotated.[69]

A very large uterus—some have been found that are almost triple the average weight—may require the uterus to be dissected into pieces, a process called morcellation, before it is removed through the vagina. Morcellation is accompanied by no excess mortality or morbidity when used as part of a vaginal hysterectomy.[70]

Tumors of the retained ovaries appear less frequently after vaginal than after abdominal hysterectomies. The reasons for this are not at all clear, and the finding may represent an **artifact**.[71]

One case of spontaneous rupture of a normal spleen, considered a rare complication, has been reported following vaginal hysterectomy since 1975.[72]

As with any procedure in which anesthesia is used, death from reaction to the anesthetic drugs, error on the part of the anesthetist, or machine failure is a remote possibility. (See Glossary, p. 309)

? IS THIS THE MOST APPROPRIATE PROCEDURE FOR THE CONDITION?

As already noted, the only conditions for which clear medical consensus for hysterectomy exists are cancer and obstetrical emergencies. Few decision-support models (devices for making better medical decisions based on accumulated outcome data) appear in the literature, but a cost-benefit analysis[73] suggests that cancer prevention is a faulty rationale for hysterectomy. "Quality of life" considerations often play a role in the decision to use this procedure, but the medical profession has clearly failed to inform women adequately about possible effects of hysterectomy on mood and sexual enjoyment, and about lasting postoperative discomfort. As with virtually all procedures for nonmalignant conditions, nothing is lost by trying more conservative therapies first and operating only if they fail. The operation is always available if conservative therapies do not work.

? ARE THERE ALTERNATIVES TO THIS PROCEDURE?

There are three categories of alternatives: variations on the vaginal operation; the total abdominal hysterectomy; and medical treatment.

A variation on the standard technique appears to reduce the incidence of some problems.[74] This variation aligns the vaginal canal with the long axis of the body to avoid pressure from the abdominal organs. Using ligaments left over from the removal of the womb, the surgeon reinforces the point on the remaining vaginal cuff where fistulas to the bladder typically form.

Another surgical variation, which leaves the vaginal cuff open rather than closing it at the top, was found to result in more morbidity than the standard technique of stitching the vaginal cuff closed.[75]

Elective cesarean hysterectomy at the time of delivery of a baby is one alternative for women with cervical cancer.[76]

Beyond these variations on the standard technique, the abdominal **open procedure** is an option, but it seems to be indicated only for women with anatomical variations that make the vaginal procedure impossible or cancer that has spread so widely that the greater exposure afforded by the open, abdominal hysterectomy is needed to remove it all. There are less radical surgical alternatives now for almost every other indication for hysterectomy, although there is widespread disagreement about the merits of some of these, compared with a vaginal or abdominal hysterectomy.

What we are learning about the role of estrogen in preserving health in the older woman, even after menopause, argues for leaving the ovaries in place unless their removal is absolutely necessary for some reason, such as cancer. Studies of postmenopausal women show that the loss of estrogen accompanying the shut-down of the ovaries can lead to bone loss and osteoporosis.

? WHAT IS CONTROVERSIAL ABOUT THE PROCEDURE?

The short answer is "almost everything." As we have noted, all the indications for this procedure other than cancer and obstetrical emergencies are controversial; beyond these, there is only general agreement that it should not be used for sterilization. In general, if the indication is not cancer or obstetrical emergency, medical treatment and less radical surgical treatment (such as excision of fibroid tumors from the uterus, rather than removal of the uterus itself) should be tried first. A hysterectomy should be performed only if symptoms are intolerable and the operative risks and potential disruption of sexual response are worth it—and those decisions are best left to the patient.

Vascular Shunt and Bypass (31)

MORTALITY	MORBIDITY	CONTROVERSY
–	–	o

- The reported **MORTALITY** rate for this procedure ranges from 10% to 25%, and is more a function of a person's health than of the procedure itself.
- **INFECTION** is the primary complication in 21% of all cases. In cases of infection, the shunt must be removed.

Rerouting of a blood or fluid flow within the body to relieve circulatory problems, accumulation of fluid, etc. Virtually any circulatory system disorder, whether **congenital** or acquired, can be corrected by surgically rerouting the vessels causing the problem.

? WHAT CONDITION DOES THE PROCEDURE TREAT?

The term vascular shunt and bypass actually covers a wide variety of procedures, the most common of which is the **LeVeen peritoneovenous shunt**—used to treat **ascites** that cannot be successfully treated with other therapy. Ascites occurs when the rate of conversion of blood plasma to peritoneal fluid exceeds the rate of conversion of peritoneal fluid back to plasma, and causes death from kidney failure. To prevent death, the excess fluid is returned to the circulation, by the use of the shunt.

Ascites is caused by severe damage to the liver, called **cirrhosis,** which almost always arises from long-term alcoholism, but in rare cases can result from viral and parasitic infections. Individuals for whom vascular shunt and bypass surgery is considered are generally quite ill. The use of the shunt can dramatically improve the health of people with **alcoholic cirrhosis**, provided they stop drinking alcohol.

The procedure is also used to treat accumulation of fluid in the chest cavity caused by lung cancer that has spread to the **pleura**.[1] It is also effective in diminishing fluid accumulation in the chest cavity resulting from alcoholic cirrhosis.[2]

Vascular shunts and bypasses are also constructed temporarily during surgery. Their function is to keep blood flowing to and from major organs and parts of the body when damage to the regular route of blood supply requires that the route be cut off for extended periods for surgical repair. If, for example, a major portion of the **vena cava** must be repaired, a shunt can be constructed to route blood from below the site of the operation directly into the **atrium** of the heart. The vena cava is then clamped above the shunt, and repair of the vessel is begun. This allows the surgeon to work without haste, and keeps blood flowing to and from the lower body. Depending upon the success of the surgery, the shunt may be removed when repair is complete, or it may be left in place.[3]

A shunt running from beneath the membrane that covers the brain (the dura) and into the peritoneal cavity can relieve pressure on the brain in children who suffer from subdural effusion, a condition in which there is excess fluid below the membrane. The shunt is removed when the condition clears itself.[4] Similar shunts can be used to control fluid accumulation in the ventricles of the brain and can be left in place permanently. (The ventricles are structures in the center of the brain that are filled with cerebrospinal fluid. They help to cushion the brain and maintain its shape. If the fluid does not drain properly, the condition is called hydrocephalus. Left untreated, hydrocephalus can damage and eventually destroy brain tissue.)

? WHAT IS THE PROCEDURE?

For the insertion of a LeVeen peritonoeovenous shunt, the patient is usually given a general anesthetic,[5] but a local anesthetic can also be used.[6] The abdomen is shaved and scrubbed with soap and antiseptic, and draped so that only the incision site is exposed. The skin, fat, **fascia**, muscle, and **peritoneum** are cut; bleeding vessels are tied off and **cauterized**. Ascitic fluid is drained from the peritoneum by suction. The LeVeen shunt, with its multitube collecting system, one-way valve, and long upper **catheter**, is put into the abdomen and sutured in place. The upper catheter is run under the skin of the chest to one of the jugular veins (located on each side of the neck) or to the subclavian vein (located under the collarbone), threaded through a puncture in the vein, and pushed down into the **superior vena cava** at the point above the heart where blood from the upper body returns to it. The functioning of the shunt is checked by the injection of dye or tiny radioactive beads. If the shunt is working properly, the abdomen is closed in layers and bandaged. The patient is taken to the recovery room. Because of the high rate of early complications, the patient is usually kept in the intensive care unit for a few days after a shunt is placed.[7]

Other vascular shunts are done in much the same way, but are technically simpler than the LeVeen shunt (and so require a shorter operative time and result in less anesthesia stress on the patient). For example, in the procedure to treat excess fluid in the ventricles of the brain, surgeons open the skull and puncture the brain by making a small incision that allows a catheter to be threaded into the ventricles. When a good flow of fluid from the ventricles is obtained, the surgeons suture the shunt to the membranes covering the brain and tunnel it under the skin of the neck and chest down into the abdominal cavity. Because conditions that call for the use of a shunt are generally permanent, shunts are rarely removed unless they or the structures surrounding them become infected. In this event, they are generally replaced as soon as the infection is cured.

WHO PERFORMS THE PROCEDURE?

This procedure is performed by a general surgeon, vascular surgeon, or neurosurgeon.

WHERE IS THE PROCEDURE PERFORMED?

Because of the potential for complications, these procedures are always performed in a hospital.

WHAT ARE THE MORTALITY (DEATH) AND MORBIDITY (COMPLICATION) RATES?

When a peritoneovenous shunt, which routes fluid from the abdominal cavity into the venous circulation for disposal by the kidneys, is inserted, operative mortality ranges from 10% to 25%, depending upon how sick the patient is when the operation begins. Drainage of the ascitic fluid before the shunt is opened, so that the venous circulation is not hit with a massive amount of ascitic fluid, lessens the mortality. Around 81% of patients survive the first year with the shunt in place.

Bleeding from **esophageal varices** occurs in 7.9% of patients, as does late infection after placement of the shunt. Of the patients studied, 30.5% had a recurrence of ascites; most were attributable to obstructions of the shunt.[8] Dr. LeVeen, who invented the shunt, achieved a mortality rate of under 1% in patients who were not jaundiced and did not have fluid accumulation in the chest cavity.[9]

In patients in whom the cause of the accumulation of ascitic fluid is cancer, the major complication rate is 4% and the rate of **embolization of tumor** through the shunt is 5%. The outcome of tumor embolization can range from no symptoms to death, depending upon the size of the tumor **emboli** and the veins or arteries that are ultimately blocked by them.[10]

Other studies indicate that infection occurs in up to 21% of cases and usually requires removal of the shunt to clear up the infection.[11] The shunt can be an occasional source of a fatal **air embolism**[12, 13]; the surgeon can avoid this during repair procedures by clamping off the shunt before opening the peritoneum.

LeVeen shunts can also trigger a fatal condition called adult respiratory distress syndrome (ARDS),[14] which is an inability to adequately oxygenate the blood through breathing. ARDS can result from a wide variety of conditions that affect the way the alveoli (the small sacs in the lungs) exchange air with the blood. It is unknown precisely why LeVeen shunts can trigger this condition, but they probably cause a disturbance in the circulation of blood in the lungs. For the shunt to function effectively, the venous end must lie within the superior vena cava. Shunts can occasionally move out of position; this can be detected on x rays if the shunt has a **radiopaque** line on it.[15] (A radiopaque line on a shunt allows detection of the otherwise invisible shunt on an x ray.)

WHAT ARE THE OTHER COMPLICATIONS AND POSSIBLE SIDE EFFECTS?

For LeVeen shunts, subclinical disorders of blood clotting develop in about 75% of patients (subclinical disorders are those that are detectable on lab tests but do not produce symptoms). Few develop clotting problems or bleeding, although both have been noted.[16]

Blockage of a LeVeen shunt occurs in about 12% of cases. It must be treated with some delicacy, usually by detection of the blocked portion followed by surgical replacement, because flushing obstructions out of the tube into the venous circulation under pressure can be fatal.[17] Even if the LeVeen shunt controls the ascites, patients can die at a later time of the underlying liver disease (infectious and alcoholic cirrhosis, mainly) that causes the ascites.[18] Patients should be aware that placement of the shunt can be fatal if system-wide clotting occurs when the ascitic fluid enters the bloodstream.[19]

Some patients develop fluid in the lungs as a result of circulatory changes induced by the placement of the shunt; most respond to **diuretics**, but in a few, removal of the shunt may be required to avoid fluid accumulation in the lungs.[20]

A LeVeen shunt may occasionally cause **perforation** of the **colon** if the abdominal end migrates out of position.[21]

As with any procedure in which anesthesia is used, death from reaction to the anesthetic drugs, error on the part of the anesthetist, or machine failure is a remote possibility. (See Glossary, p. 309)

? IS THIS THE MOST APPROPRIATE PROCEDURE FOR THE CONDITION?

Yes, provided that everything else that might work is tried first, a precaution that most surgeons who implant shunts would endorse.

? ARE THERE ALTERNATIVES TO THIS PROCEDURE?

Yes—a "bedside" version of the LeVeen shunt is available. The shunt is placed by penetrating the abdomen with a **trochar** and routing the fluid collected into the

venous circulation through an IV set. The bedside system can serve as a temporary shunt and also can predict which patients will respond well to a permanent shunt.[22]

The general recommendation in the surgical literature is that use of the bedside version of the LeVeen shunt be used only after less radical treatment, such as **paracentesis**, diuretics, and operations to correct malignant and inflammatory conditions have failed. All of these alternatives should be tried first.

Although the bedside system works well in children, there is so little pediatric experience with it so far that it should be a "last-chance" procedure.

? WHAT IS CONTROVERSIAL ABOUT THE PROCEDURE?

Some studies show bleeding or disseminated blood clotting the veins and arteries in virtually every patient treated with a LeVeen shunt; others show it in no patients. The concentration of various substances in the ascitic fluid that is introduced into the bloodstream may have something to do with this complication, as sicker patients (with the presumably more concentrated fluid) seem to have more problems with clotting. The common practice now is to remove the fluid from the abdomen when the shunt is placed so that the immediate burden on the circulation is kept low. In addition, heparin, a clot-retarding drug, is used to slow clotting.

Wound Debridement and Excision (20)

MORTALITY	MORBIDITY	CONTROVERSY
+	+	o

Removal of dead tissue and restructuring of wounds to allow closure, reduce scarring, and lessen the chance of infection

? WHAT CONDITION DOES THE PROCEDURE TREAT?

This procedure is used to treat any condition in which a wound needs to be cleaned of debris, dead tissue, foreign particles (such as bullet fragments, glass, gravel, and dirt); it is also done to restructure the wound so that it can be closed, thus restoring as nearly as possible the normal structure of the tissues. Because the body does not deal well with most foreign materials and because dead tissue interferes with wound healing, wound excision and debridement are necessary to restructure wounds to allow closure, to produce a smaller scar, and to avoid infection.

The removal of dead tissue is particularly important, because it is an ideal growth medium for bacteria and inhibits the bacteria-killing action of white blood cells.[1] The long-standing surgical doctrine that all wounds have to be considered contaminated until successfully closed is periodically supported by repeated studies of bacteria in wounds.[2]

Most wounds resulting from injuries are not nice, neat, surgically precise cuts that can simply be closed with **sutures**. Often, extensive surgery is needed to produce a wound that will allow skin closure with minimal scarring.

Many wound debridement and excision techniques aim, directly or indirectly, to reduce the amount of bacteria present in the wound. Wounds heal well if there are fewer than 100,000 bacteria present per gram of exposed tissue, or about three million bacteria per ounce of tissue. Techniques for reducing bacterial count include pressure jet cleaning (a variation on the Water Pik used for cleaning teeth),[3] **ligating** or **cauterizing** all bleeding vessels, removal of all old blood and prompt removal of fresh blood in the wound, and antibiotics.[4] **Ultrasonic** debridement of hand wounds has recently been shown to produce no tissue damage and to be as effective as water-jet irrigation.[5]

? WHAT IS THE PROCEDURE?

The exact method used varies with the type of wound and the extent of the damage. The general procedure is to administer a local or general anesthetic depending upon the extent of the wound and the procedures planned; clean out debris; remove all dead tissue; close the various tissue layers with appropriate sutures or staples; and deal with the skin defect, if any, that results from skin grafting (transplanting skin from another part of the body) or coverage with skin substitutes.

There are numerous variations. It has been shown, for example, that closure of gunshot wounds with synthetic skin substitutes, and debridement every 48 hours, followed by definitive closure and skin grafting if needed, can reduce the rate of infection, which is often a problem with gunshot wounds.[6] The surgical doctrine that all gunshot wounds should be considered contaminated is periodically reconfirmed through experimental studies.[7]

Chronically infected open wounds have been treated by extensive removal of dead tissue and coverage with a transplanted piece of muscle, with a success rate of 93% to 100%.[8, 9] Either the muscles of the chest or the abdomen may be transplanted for this purpose.[10, 11]

An interesting new technique for treating orthopedic surgical wounds is to place a few small antibiotic-impregnated plastic beads in the wound before it is closed. This produces local concentrations of antibiotics in the wound that are higher than those attained with intravenous antibiotics; the beads do not have to be removed.[12]

? WHO PERFORMS THE PROCEDURE?

This procedure is performed by a general surgeon or trauma surgeon. Repair of scars, and procedures to avoid extensive scarring, are best done by a plastic or reconstructive surgeon.

? WHERE IS THE PROCEDURE PERFORMED?

Depending upon the extent of the wound, the planned procedure, and the patient's other conditions, the procedure can be done in a hospital (on an inpatient or outpatient basis), outpatient surgery facility, or well-equipped doctor's office.

? WHAT ARE THE MORTALITY (DEATH) AND MORBIDITY (COMPLICATION) RATES?

Mortality from successful wound excision and debridement is zero; mortality and complications arise when the procedure fails. For instance, massive fungal infection of burn wounds has a mortality rate of 93.5%.[13] Generalized abdominal wall infections—a potentially devastating complication in which infections affect all or most of the layers of the muscular wall of the abdomen—have a mortality rate of 19%.[14] **Muscle flap transplant coverage** of chronically infected wounds has a failure rate of about 7%.[15]

Postoperative peritonitis and infection of abdominal surgical incisions has a mortality rate of 24.6%, a complication rate of 20.3%, and an incisional hernia rate of 19.2% (see "Incisional Hernia Repair," p. 154), even with wound repair techniques that are considered successful.[16] **Muscle flap transplant closures** of infected perineal wounds can have a complication rate as high as 31%.[17]

Deep sternal wound infection occurs in about 1.2% of open-heart surgeries. The mortality rate from infection varies from zero to 35%, depending upon the method of treatment.[18]

The mortality rate from burn wound infection in children can be as high as 14%.[19]

? WHAT ARE THE OTHER COMPLICATIONS AND POSSIBLE SIDE EFFECTS?

Patients who have operations involving extensive perineal surgery—incisions in the floor of the pelvis such as for removal of the rectum for cancer—should be prepared for a stormy postoperative period. Failure of perineal surgical wounds to heal is quite common. No technique for management of perineal surgical wounds is completely satisfactory. There does seem to be a major difference in the infection rate for various techniques of perineal wound management; for example, infections are more common in patients in whom the anus is closed before the rectum is removed. Failure of the surgical incision can be expected in up to 50% of patients[20] and healing time can be as long as six months.[21] Some studies report that **topical** antibiotics applied during the operation help; other studies do not. Adequate drainage of the wound for an extended period seems to be critical.[22–24]

Irrigation of wounds with iodine solutions can cause **systemic** absorption of iodine and result in fatal iodine poisoning.[25]

As with any procedure in which anesthesia is used, death from reaction to the anesthetic drugs, error on the part of the anesthetist, or machine failure is a remote possibility. (See Glossary, p. 309)

? IS THIS THE MOST APPROPRIATE PROCEDURE FOR THE CONDITION?

There is ample evidence, going back centuries, that removal of foreign material and dead tissue from wounds reduces the chance of infection and speeds healing. It's also obvious that if possible, the wound margins should be trimmed surgically to produce a better-looking scar or avoid scarring, because scar tissue can cause limitations of function later on. The issue is generally not whether a wound should be debrided, but how. There seems to be extensive controversy among doctors, a general lack of completely satisfactory techniques for treating some types of wounds such as gunshot wounds, burns, and abrasions, and major problems of infection with abdominal and perineal wounds.

In the unfortunate case that a reader suffers one of these wounds, it is advisable to discuss beforehand the surgeon's plans for avoiding and managing infections. This seems to be one of the areas in which antibiotics cannot be overused, and it seems far better to give a sufficient dose before surgery than to take a "too little, too late" approach later once the infection develops.

? ARE THERE ALTERNATIVES TO THIS PROCEDURE?

As noted in the section above, the issue is not whether the procedure should be done, but which variation should be used.

? WHAT IS CONTROVERSIAL ABOUT THE PROCEDURE?

Although the nutrition of patients with severe wounds is not a point of controversy, it is good to see the medical profession finally recognizing, after much debate, that proper nutrition—in particular, adequate levels of vitamin A—is essential for wound healing.[26] While there seems to be general recognition of the need for adequate protein intake for healing of burn wounds, little attention is given to the value of dietary protein in the healing of other types of wounds.[27]

Many techniques in current use for treating non-military gunshot wounds are identical to those used in military medicine, although bullets from civilian weapons tend to have a lower velocity than bullets from military weapons and do not produce as much tissue damage.[28] A 1990 trial of less extensive treatment for civilian gunshot wounds showed that the infection rate was lower when the military techniques were not used.[29] There is some controversy regarding whether the clas-sical military technique of complete removal of all tissue along the path of the bullet is needed in uncomplicated wounds.[30] On the other hand, complex bullet wounds from military-type weapons (machine guns and assault rifles) should probably be treated with the military techniques.[31–33]

Maggots secrete both protein-dissolving and antibacterial substances and can have a role in debriding certain wounds (such as gunshot wounds and abrasions in delicate tissue) that cannot be healed with conventional therapy.[34]

In children with burns, a single-procedure treatment (as opposed to treatment in multiple stages) involving removal of the burned tissue and closure with skin grafts can be done with low mortality and low blood loss, and is as effective as multistage procedures, even when the burned area is extensive.[35]

Application of direct current at 200 to 800 microamps seems to accelerate wound healing and reduce infection and pain, for reasons that are not well understood. A partial explanation is that the body is believed to use weak electric currents to "guide" cells to their proper location. Increased currents, then, could be expected to result in faster cell movement into wounds and faster healing. This technique is not widely used[36]—one reason may be that the study of the effects of low-dose electromagnetic radiation on the body is in its infancy.

Excision of burn wounds down to the fascia did not enhance survival in a group of military patients, indicating that less radical procedures are acceptable.[37] Some military surgeons speculate that the high success rate of radical excision of burn wounds may be a statistical fluke, arising from the fact that only patients who are strong enough to withstand the operation undergo it.[38]

Anecdotal reports that honey has the power to sterilize infected wounds, destroy dead tissue, enhance skin coverage, and reduce swelling have appeared repeatedly. One of the latest of these reported a 98.3% success rate in a group of patients who were treated with honey after conventional treatment failed.[39]

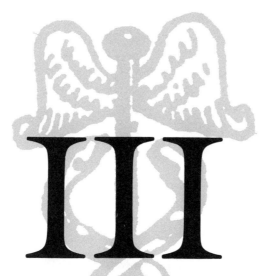

III

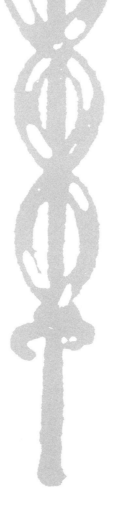

Additional Resources

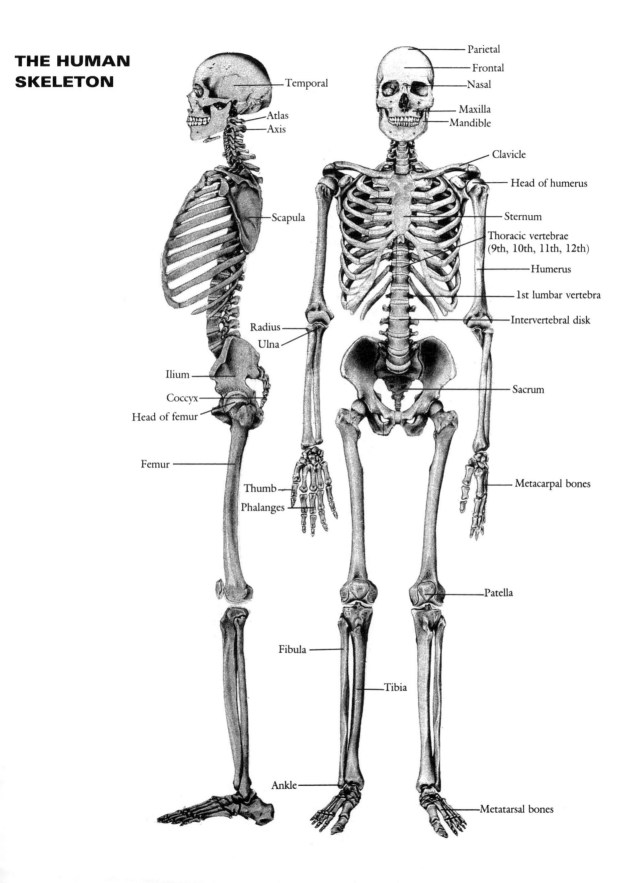

THE HUMAN SKELETON

Temporal

Atlas
Axis

Scapula

Radius
Ulna

Ilium

Coccyx

Head of femur

Femur

Thumb
Phalanges

Fibula

Ankle

Parietal
Frontal
Nasal
Maxilla
Mandible

Clavicle

Head of humerus

Sternum

Thoracic vertebrae
(9th, 10th, 11th, 12th)

Humerus

1st lumbar vertebra

Intervertebral disk

Sacrum

Metacarpal bones

Patella

Tibia

Metatarsal bones

THE VASCULAR SYSTEM

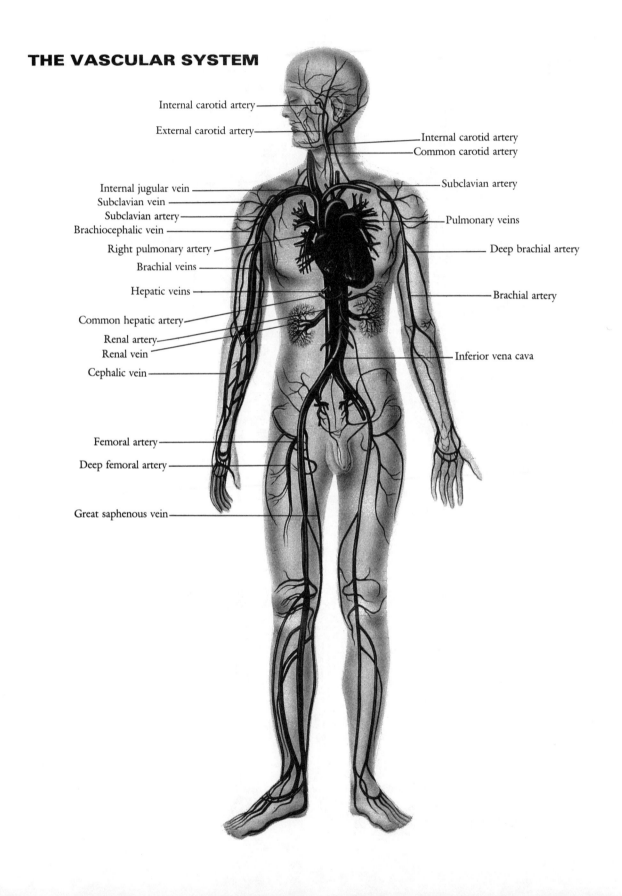

Internal carotid artery

External carotid artery

Internal carotid artery
Common carotid artery

Subclavian artery

Internal jugular vein
Subclavian vein
Subclavian artery
Brachiocephalic vein
Right pulmonary artery
Brachial veins

Pulmonary veins

Deep brachial artery

Hepatic veins

Brachial artery

Common hepatic artery
Renal artery
Renal vein

Cephalic vein

Inferior vena cava

Femoral artery

Deep femoral artery

Great saphenous vein

THE HUMAN HEART

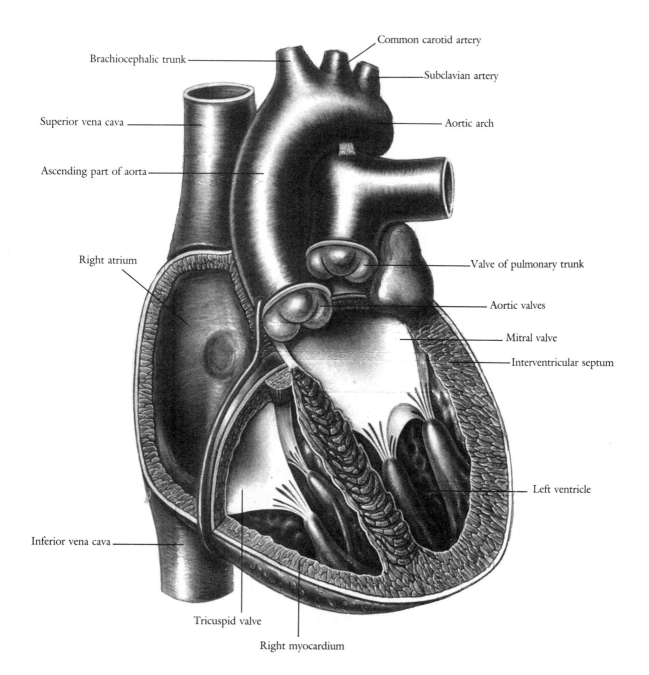

Brachiocephalic trunk

Common carotid artery

Subclavian artery

Aortic arch

Superior vena cava

Ascending part of aorta

Right atrium

Valve of pulmonary trunk

Aortic valves

Mitral valve

Interventricular septum

Left ventricle

Inferior vena cava

Tricuspid valve

Right myocardium

THE DIGESTIVE SYSTEM

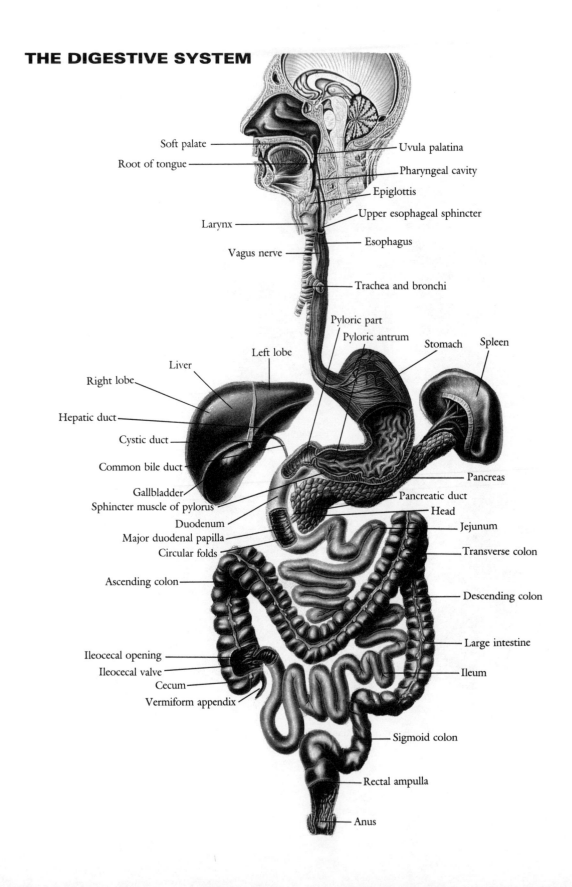

Soft palate

Root of tongue

Uvula palatina

Pharyngeal cavity

Epiglottis

Upper esophageal sphincter

Larynx

Esophagus

Vagus nerve

Trachea and bronchi

Pyloric part

Pyloric antrum

Left lobe

Stomach

Spleen

Liver

Right lobe

Hepatic duct

Cystic duct

Common bile duct

Gallbladder

Pancreas

Pancreatic duct

Sphincter muscle of pylorus

Head

Duodenum

Jejunum

Major duodenal papilla

Transverse colon

Circular folds

Ascending colon

Descending colon

Large intestine

Ileocecal opening

Ileocecal valve

Ileum

Cecum

Vermiform appendix

Sigmoid colon

Rectal ampulla

Anus

THE HUMAN SPINE

C 1 Atlas

C 2 Axis

C 3

C 4

C 5

C 6

C 7

Cervical vertebrae

Th 1

Th 2

Th 3

Th 4

Th 5

Th 6

Th 7

Th 8

Th 9

Th 10

Th 11

Th 12

Thoracic vertebrae

L 1

L 2

L 3

L 4

L 5

Lumbar vertebrae

Intervertebral disk

Sacrum (lateral view)

Coccyx

FEMALE GENITAL ORGANS

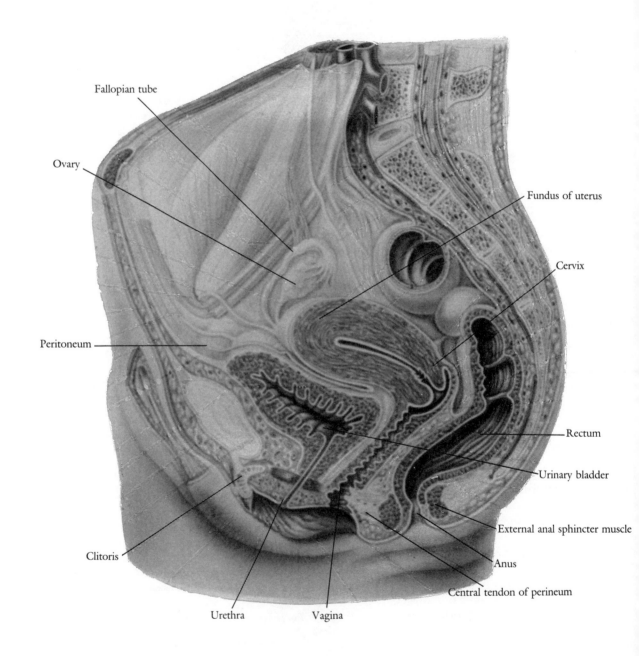

Fallopian tube

Ovary

Fundus of uterus

Cervix

Peritoneum

Rectum

Urinary bladder

External anal sphincter muscle

Clitoris

Anus

Central tendon of perineum

Urethra

Vagina

Glossary

Medical Terms

ABSCESS: A collection of pus which forms as the result of infection.

ACTINIC KERATOSES: Overgrowths of the horny outer layer of the skin caused by sun exposure; a benign skin disorder.

ACUTE: Characterized by sharpness or severity; having a sudden onset.

ADHESION: A band of scar tissue that forms between cut surfaces of organs; an abnormal union of body surfaces caused by fibrous scars.

ADRENAL GLANDS: Two important glands that perch on top of the kidneys and produce, among other chemicals, steroids such as sex hormones and hormones concerned especially with metabolism.

ADULT RESPIRATORY DISTRESS SYNDROME (ARDS): A condition in which the lungs suddenly fill with fluids making breathing very difficult. It is usually brought on by trauma.

AIR EMBOLISM: Air within the circulatory system, blocking the flow of blood.

ALCOHOLIC CIRRHOSIS: See *cirrhosis*.

ALIMENTARY CANAL: The digestive tract leading from the mouth through the intestines to the anus.

ALPHA-BLOCKERS: Drugs used to treat prostate conditions. They work by relaxing the muscles around the urethra and prostate.

AMBLYOPIA: A condition in which one eye dominates over the other; also known as "lazy eye."

AMENORRHEA: The failure to menstruate.

AMNIOCENTESIS: Extraction of a small amount of amniotic fluid in order to test for genetic and other disorders in the fetus.

ANAPHYLACTIC SHOCK: A severe allergic reaction that can include shock, breathing difficulty, itching and hives, convulsions, and coma.

ANASTOMOSIS: The joint formed by the sewing together of small and large intestines.

ANDROGEN: A male hormone.

ANESTHESIA RISK: The mortality rate from all types of anesthesia was estimated to be between 0.001% and 0.004% in the 1970s and early 1980s.[1] The most recent figures available from several Western nations suggest a death rate in the range of 0.004% to 0.007%, roughly a tenfold reduction. This is further supported by a close study of concluded malpractice cases in Massachusetts.[2] If an anesthesia complication is serious enough to warrant admission to an intensive care unit, the mortality is about 17%.[3]

ANEURYSM: A bulging and ballooning of the wall of an artery due to the pressure of blood flowing through a weakened area.

ANGINA PECTORIS: A crushing, squeezing chest pain that results from the heart muscle not receiving enough blood (and therefore not receiving enough oxygen).

ANGIOGRAM: An x ray of the blood vessels.

[1] E. C. Pierce, Jr., "The Patient's Safety in Anesthesia," *Resident and Staff Physician* 35 (Feb. 1989): 51–52, 54.
[2] G. L. Zeitlin, "Possible Decrease in Mortality Associated with Anaesthesia," *Anaesthesia* 44 (May 1989): 432–33.
[3] A. L. Cooper, J. M. Leigh, and I. C. Tring, "Admissions to the Intensive Care Unit After Complications of Anesthetic Techniques over 10 Years," *Anesthesia* 44 (Dec. 1989): 953–58.

ANGIOPLASTY: A technique used to treat severely blocked or narrowed coronary arteries, as well as arteries diseased with atherosclerotic plaque in other parts of the body. See *balloon angioplasty* and *laser angioplasty*.

ANTECUBITAL FOSSA: The shallow depression on the inside of the forearm, just below the elbow joint.

ANTICOAGULANT DRUG: A drug that hinders the clotting of blood.

ANTI-INFLAMMATORY MEDICATIONS: Medications that reduce inflammation or swelling.

AORTA: The body's primary artery that receives blood from the heart's left ventricle and distributes it to the body.

AORTIC VALVE: The valve between the left ventricle and the aorta.

APLASTIC ANEMIA: A blood defect in which the bone marrow can no longer make blood cells.

ARRHYTHMIA: An abnormal heart rhythm.

ARTERIOSCLEROSIS: A condition characterized by the thickening and loss of elasticity of the arteries; sometimes referred to as "hardening of the arteries."

ARTHRODESIS: Stiffening of a joint.

ARTHROPATHY: Joint disease.

ARTIFACT: An incidental finding that results from a faulty methodology or study design and does not represent a naturally occurring phenomenon; for example, a study that predicts adverse drug reactions in women over 35, when in fact the incidence of adverse drug reaction is no greater or is less than in the general population.

ASCENDING AORTA: The main vessel carrying blood from the heart to the rest of the body.

ASCITES: An accumulation of fluid in the abdomen.

ASTIGMATISM: A condition marked by an irregularly shaped cornea, which misdirects some of the light rays and thereby blurs some of what the person sees.

ATHEROEMBOLI: Clots composed of plaque.

ATHEROSCLEROSIS: An accumulation of mineral and fatty deposits on the inner lining of the walls of arteries.

ATHEROSCLEROTIC PLAQUE: A combination of blood platelets and fatty deposits that accumulate on the inside walls of arteries, usually at a spot where the arterial wall has been damaged.

ATRIAL FIBRILLATION: A heart rhythm disturbance marked by rapid, unsystematic contractions of the upper heart chambers.

ATRIUM: Either of the chambers of the heart that receive blood from the veins and force it into the ventricle or ventricles.

AURICLE: A term formerly used to designate an atrium of the heart.

AUTOLOGOUS TRANSPLANTS: Surgical movement of tissue from one place on the body to another.

AVASCULAR NECROSIS: The death of cells associated with deficient blood supply.

AZATHIOPRINE: An immunosuppressant drug (brand name: Imuran).

BALLOON ANGIOPLASTY: A method of opening a clogged or narrowed blood vessel with a balloon inserted into the vessel by means of a catheter and then inflated.

BACTEREMIA: Presence of bacteria in the bloodstream.

BARIUM ENEMA: A diagnostic x ray in which the colon is filled with a solution of barium that blocks x rays and outlines the colon.

BARIUM IMPACTION: Blockage of the intestines that results when barium hardens while in the colon.

BENIGN PROSTATIC HYPERTROPHY (BPH): A noncancerous enlargement of the prostate gland.

BETA-BLOCKERS: Drugs that prevent stimulation of the heart and vessels by blocking reception of chemical signals.

BILE PERITONITIS: Inflammation and irritation in which the infection comes from bile (bitter fluid secreted by the liver to aid in digestion) dripping into the peritoneal cavity.

BLOOD ELECTROLYTES: Charge-carrying molecular fragments that control muscle contraction to some extent.

BLUNT TRAUMA: Trauma from something other than a sharp instrument; a nonpenetrating injury.

BONE GRAFTING: Process of implanting a piece of bone to take the place of a removed bone or bony defect.

BOWEL INFARCTION: Loss of blood supply to the bowel resulting from atherosclerosis in the arteries supplying it.

BRACHIAL ARTERY: The major artery in the arm.

BRANCHED-CHAIN AMINO ACIDS: Building blocks of protein that have "Y" shapes in their molecular structure.

BROAD-SPECTRUM ANTIBIOTICS: A class of drugs that are effective against a wide range of bacteria.

BRONCHI: Tubes, composed of fibrous, elastic rings that run off the windpipe and divide in two, with one running to each lung, just above the top of the heart.

BYPASS SURGERY: Open-heart surgery to relieve a blocked heart artery.

CADAVER: A human body preserved for anatomical study or organ harvesting.

CALCULI: Hard, stonelike formations of mineral salts which may be found in the gallbladder, kidneys, or ureters.

CANCER IN SITU: Cancer that has not spread beyond the original site.

CANNULA: A tube that is inserted into a duct or body cavity, for example for the purpose of running a continuous flow of liquid into and out of an organ.

CARBON-FILAMENT GRAFT: A graft woven of carbon fibers called filaments; may be twisted or woven into thin sheet and may be used to replace vessels or tendons.

CARDIAC TAMPONADE: Compression of the heart caused by an accumulation of fluid or blood in the sac around the heart.

CAROTID ARTERY: Any of the four principal arteries of the neck and head.

CAROTID ARTERY STENOSIS: A narrowing of the main artery of the neck due to a buildup of mineral and fatty deposits.

CAROTID BRUITS: Sounds in the carotid arteries attributable to narrowing of the arteries.

CARPAL TUNNEL SYNDROME: A painful condition that results when the median nerve in the wrist is compressed, resulting in tingling and burning sensations in the hands and fingers.

CARTILAGE: Tissue that connects and supports.

CATHETER: A thin, flexible plastic tube that can be placed inside some part of the body, for example a Foley catheter which is used to drain urine from the bladder.

CAUTERIZE: To burn or sear tissue with a hot instrument such as a cautery probe.

CAUTERY PROBE: An instrument used to destroy tissue.

CECUM: The end of the large intestine nearest the appendix.

CENTRAL VENOUS SYSTEM: Large veins of the trunk of the body (thorax and abdomen).

CEPHALHEMATOMA: A collection of blood under the skin at the top of the skull.

CEREBRAL: Pertaining to the brain.

CEREBRAL ANGIOGRAPHY: X-ray pictures of the arteries of the brain.

CEREBRAL EDEMA: Retention of water in the tissues of the brain.

CEREBRAL EMBOLISM: The occlusion, or obstruction, of a blood vessel in the brain by a blood clot.

CERVICAL INCOMPETENCE: Abnormality of the cervix that prevents it from keeping the fetus securely within the womb.

CERVIX: Mouth of the uterus.

CHEMONUCLEOLYSIS: A procedure that involves the dissolution of intervertebral disk fragments with chemicals.

CHEMOTHERAPY: Generally, the treatment of any disease by drugs; usually applied to drug therapy for cancer.

CHOLANGIOGRAPHY: A procedure that enables the bile ducts to be seen on x-ray film after they have been filled with a contrast medium, which is opaque to x rays.

CHORIONIC VILLUS SAMPLING (CVS): Extraction and examination of a small fragment of the early placenta to detect genetic abnormalities in the fetus.

CIRCULATORY COLLAPSE: Cessation of effective blood circulation in the peripheral vessels of the body, the heart-lung system, or both.

CIRRHOSIS: The formation of fibrous scar tissue in place of healthy cells, obstructing the flow of blood through the liver. As a result, the various functions of the liver deteriorate.

CLAVICLE: Collarbone.

CLIPS: Pieces of metal or plastic with latching mechanism; used to stop blood flow, clip vein around lesion that is removed, and close a tube in the body.

CLOSED FRACTURE: A break or rupture of hard tissue, such as bone, that does not produce an open wound in the skin.

CLOSED PROCEDURE: One that does not involve cutting through the skin or an incision.

COAGULATE: To clot.

COLLAGEN: A main supportive protein of skin, tendon, bone, cartilage, and connective tissue.

COLLATERAL VESSELS: Vessels that parallel the veins in question and carry blood away from the same areas of the body.

COLON: The part of the large intestine that extends to the rectum.

COLOSTOMY: A surgical procedure that creates a new opening for the colon by leading the colon out through the abdominal wall.

COLPORRHAPHY: Repair of a rupture of the vagina by excision and suturing the edges of the tear.

COMMINUTED FRACTURE: That in which the bone is broken or crushed into several pieces.

COMMON BILE DUCT: The tube or duct running from the gallbladder and liver to the small intestine.

CONGENITAL: Present at birth.

CONTRAST MEDIUM: A solution of iodine compounds which block x rays; often called a dye or radiopaque dye.

CONTRAST PHLEBOGRAM: X ray of one or more veins of the leg using a contrast medium (a solution of iodine compounds which block x rays).

CORONARY: Pertaining to the heart, especially the two arteries that originate in the aorta and supply blood to the heart tissue.

CORONARY ARTERY: One of a pair of arteries that branch from the aorta, the main artery of the heart.

CORONARY ARTERY BYPASS GRAFTING (CABG): A procedure that uses arteries taken from another part of the body and attaches them to the aorta, the body's primary artery, in order to bypass clogged coronary arteries.

CORTICOSTEROID: Used principally as an anti-inflammatory drug.

CREMASTER MUSCLE: Muscle located in the groin that supports and holds in the pelvic organs.

CROHN'S DISEASE: Chronic inflammation of the intestines of unknown cause.

CRYOSURGERY: A process that utilizes extremely cold substances to destroy tissue.

CT SCAN: Also known as computerized axial tomography. CT is a noninvasive diagnostic procedure that takes a series of cross-sectional x rays, then uses a computer to construct highly detailed pictures of internal body parts, for example of the brain.

CULDOSCOPY: Examination of the union between the vagina and uterus at the top of the vagina, which offers a route into the abdomen.

CURETTE: A spoon-shaped instrument used for scraping or removing material from an organ or surface.

CYCLOPHOSPHAMIDE: An anticancer drug (brand names: Cytoxan, Neosar).

CYSTOCELE: Protrusion of the urinary bladder through the vaginal wall.

DEBRIDEMENT AND EXCISION: Removal of dead tissue and restructuring of wounds to allow closure, to reduce scarring, and to lessen the chance of infection.

DELTOID MUSCLE: Large muscle that covers the shoulder joint.

DIAPHRAGM: Muscle that separates the abdomen from the chest.

DIAGNOSTIC YIELD: Percentage of cases that have a definite diagnosis established by a diagnostic test or procedure.

DIGITAL SUBTRACTION ANGIOGRAPHY: A computer-directed x-ray system that reveals blood flow to the heart. This is accomplished by taking one x ray of the blood vessels of the heart and storing that image in a computer; a second x ray is taken of the heart after a contrast medium, or dye, has been injected into the vessels. The computer then compares the two pictures and removes (or subtracts) what is not needed, leaving a clear indication of where blood flow is restricted.

DILATION: Stretching or expanding of an organ or part of the body.

DISK: A plate-like structure, such as the cartilage cushion found between each vertebra.

DIURETIC: A drug that increases the output of urine and thus drains fluid from the body.

DIVERTICULITIS: Formation of small outpouchings from the colon, a condition more common in the aged and possibly due to a lack of fiber in the diet.

DOPPLER ULTRASONOGRAPHY: A diagnostic procedure that uses ultrasound to measure blood flow through major arteries and veins of the arms, legs, and neck.

DOUBLE-CONTRAST, OR AIR-CONTRAST, BARIUM ENEMA: A diagnostic procedure in which the colon is coated with a thin layer of barium and then filled with air. This method produces a more detailed view of the inner lining (mucosa) of the colon.

DUODENUM: First part of the small intestine just below the stomach.

ECHOCARDIOGRAPHY: An ultrasound study of the heart.

ECLAMPSIA: A condition affecting pregnant women that is a severe form of toxemia characterized by convulsions and coma.

ECTOPIC PREGNANCY: A pregnancy that occurs with the fetus outside, rather than inside, the womb. It frequently occurs in one of the fallopian tubes.

EDEMA: The swelling of body tissue.

EJECTION FRACTION: The amount of blood pumped out into the body by the left ventricle of the heart.

ELECTROCAUTERY: The use of electric current to seal blood vessels by heat and, thus, stop bleeding.

ELECTROCAUTERY DEVICE: An instrument with a wire, heated by an electrical current, that is used to cauterize tissue.

ELECTROCAUTERY LOOP: The portion of the electrocautery device that is heated and does the actual destroying or cauterizing of tissue.

ELECTROCOAGULATION: The application of an electric current to produce fusion of tissue.

ELECTROENCEPHALOGRAPHIC (EEG) CHANGES: Changes in the tracings of brain waves recorded on an EEG machine.

ELECTROLYTES: Mineral salts that are involved in nerve signal transmission and muscle contractions.

ELECTROMYOGRAPHY: A diagnostic procedure that uses very fine needles placed in the muscles to measure the speed and strength of signals carried in the nerves.

EMBOLECTOMY: The removal of an embolus, which is a solid particle, usually a fragment of clotted blood or a fatty deposit, carried along in the bloodstream.

EMBOLISM: The occlusion, or obstruction, of a blood vessel by a blood clot.

EMBOLIZATION OF FAT: The plugging of a blood vessel by a fragment of fat from the bone marrow.

EMBOLIZATION OF TUMOR: The plugging of a blood vessel due to tumor fragments, especially from stomach cancer.

EMBOLUS: A solid particle, usually a fragment of clotted blood or a fatty deposit, carried along in the bloodstream.

ENDOMETRIOSIS: A gynecological disease in which endometrial tissue, normally found in the uterus, grows outside of it.

ENDOMETRITIS: Inflammation of the lining of the uterus.

ENDOMETRIUM: Tissue lining the uterus that responds to hormone levels and is shed every month as menstrual flow.

ENDOSCOPIC: Relating to the use of a lighted device, called an endoscope, to look at the inside of a body cavity or organ.

ENDOTRACHEAL TUBE: A tube inserted in the trachea for anesthesia or breathing assistance.

ENGAGEMENT: Lodging of the baby's presenting part (the part of the fetus that is closest to the opening of the cervix during labor) firmly in the pelvis during childbirth; also called lightening or dropping.

ENTEROCELE: A herniation of the vagina into the pelvic cavity.

EPISIOTOMY: An incision, made with a surgical scissors, from the vaginal opening into the tissue of the pelvic floor, called the perineum, to avoid a natural tear during childbirth.

ESOPHAGEAL VARICES: Varicose veins of the esophagus, which have lost the support of the surrounding tissue, are bulging into the channel of the esophagus, and are irritated by the passage of food. They are almost always due to changes in the liver circulation caused by cirrhosis, which in turn is generally due to alcoholism. Although rare, a few cases are due to congenital weakness of the esophageal tissue.

ESOPHAGUS: The tube from the mouth to the stomach.

ESTROGENS: Female hormones.

ETIOLOGY: Cause or origin of disease or an abnormal condition.

EUSTACHIAN TUBES: Tubes leading from the ears and terminating in the upper portion of the throat.

EXTERNAL FIXATION: In repair of a broken bone, when the fixation device is attached to a limb without making a large incision in the limb; hole drilled in bone and metal tongs applied for the purpose of traction or to immobilize the limb.

EXTRACORPOREAL SHOCK-WAVE LITHOTRIPSY (ESWL): A process for shattering gallstones or kidney stones by using highly focused sound waves, which strike the stones and shatter them; positioning of the sound wave device is accomplished by x ray.

EXTRAVASATION: Leakage out of the vessels.

FALLOPIAN TUBES: Paired structures that carry eggs from the ovaries to the uterus.

FALSE-NEGATIVE DIAGNOSIS: Test results that appear normal even though a disease or condition is present, for example a negative pregnancy test when a woman is indeed pregnant.

FALSE-POSITIVE DIAGNOSIS: Test results that appear abnormal indicating the presence of a disease or condition when in fact no disease is present.

FASCIA: The sheet of tough, fibrous tissue that covers the body beneath the skin and encloses muscles and the separate layers of muscles.

FEMORAL ARTERY: The major artery in the thigh.

FEMORAL VEIN: The major vein in the thigh.

FEMUR: The thighbone.

FIBRIN: A protein in blood that is the major component of blood clots.

FIBROSIS: The formation of tough or sinewy (fibrous) tissue.

FIBULA: The smaller of the two bones of the lower leg.

FISSURE: A break or split in tissue.

FISTULA: A passage or tunnel formed in the body by disease, injury, congenital abnormalities, or, occasionally, surgery.

FLUOROSCOPY: An x-ray system that works like a television camera and produces "real-time" pictures of deep body structures. The images may be recorded on film or videotape for later study.

FOLEY CATHETER: A tube inserted through the urethra to drain the bladder.

FORCEPS: Surgical instrument like tongs, used to compress or grasp tissues.

GAMETE INTRAFALLOPIAN TRANSFER (GIFT): A method of conception that involves removing eggs from a woman's ovary, combining them with sperm, and placing the mixture directly in the fallopian tube for fertilization to occur.

GANGRENE: Death of tissue brought on by the loss of blood flow and bacterial infection.

GASTROESOPHAGEAL REFLUX: Occurs when acid enters the esophagus from the stomach through a weakly closing lower esophageal sphincter.

GLANS: The head of the penis.

GLAUCOMA: Disease of the eye in which increased pressure damages the retina and optic nerve.

GLENOID CAVITY: The depression on the front part of the shoulder blade; the arm socket.

GRAFT: Any tissue or organ for implantation or transplantation.

HEART DISEASE: Any condition that affects the vessels or chambers of the heart or interferes with the normal electrical activity of the cardiac muscle.

HEMATOLOGIST: A physician who specializes in the study of the blood and its diseases.

HEMATOMA: A collection of blood and clots usually in an organ, cavity, or tissue.

HEMATURIA: Bloody urine.

HEMODIALYSIS: The use of a machine to cleanse the blood in a patient whose kidneys have failed.

HEMOPERICARDIUM: An effusion of blood within the pericardium, the tissue that surrounds the heart.

HEPARIN: A drug that reduces the tendency of the blood to clot; commonly referred to as a "blood thinner."

HEPATIC VEIN: The main vein of the liver.

HERNIA: The protrusion of an organ or part of an organ through a muscular wall that usually supports it.

HERNIAL SAC: A pouch of the peritoneum containing a hernia.

HERNIATED, OR RUPTURED, DISK: A disk that abnormally protrudes from the vertebrae.

HERNIATION: The abnormal protrusion of an organ or other body part through a defect or natural opening in a membrane covering muscles or bone.

HETEROTROPHIC OSSIFICATION: Bone growing into the flesh surrounding a prosthesis.

HODGKIN'S DISEASE: A cancer of the lymph glands.

HUMERUS: The upper bone of the arm.

HYDRONEPHROSIS: A condition that results when the ureters are blocked and the pelvis fills with urine.

HYPERALIMENTATION: Feeding a complete protein/carbohydrate/fat/vitamin/mineral solution through a central venous catheter placed in the neck or the chest.

HYPERTENSION: A chronic increase in blood pressure above its normal range.

HYPERTHYROIDISM: Excessive functioning of the thyroid gland. Also known as Graves' disease.

HYPOTENSION: Low blood pressure.

HYSTEROSALPINGOGRAM: An x ray of the uterus and fallopian tubes.

IATROGENIC: Pertaining to a condition or illness that is caused by the doctor or is a result of medical care, such as a nosocomial infection.

ILEOCECAL VALVE: A sphincter that allows partially digested food to pass in only one direction; the joint between the large and small intestines.

ILEOSTOMY: An opening of the small bowel through the skin of the abdomen.

ILEUM: The lower portion of the small intestine.

IMMUNOLOGIST: A specialist in the study of the immune system of the body.

INDICATION: A reason to give a particular treatment.

INFARCTION: The development of an area of dead tissue as a result of interruption of blood supply to the area.

INFERIOR VENA CAVA: The large vein located in the lower portion of the abdomen and that serves the lower extremities and the pelvis.

INFLAMMATORY BOWEL DISEASE: A condition that is characterized by pain, heat, swelling, and loss of normal bowel function.

INFRASPINATUS MUSCLE: Muscle in the upper back that supports the spine and shoulder blades.

INFUNDIBULOPELVIC LIGAMENTS: The ligaments that support the ovaries.

INFUSION: The process of putting a fluid other than blood into a vein or body cavity.

INGUINAL CANAL: A canal containing two rings of fibrous tissue located in the groin in both men and women; in men, where the spermatic cord passes out of the abdomen into the scrotum, it supports the testicles, vas deferens (tubes that carry sperm from the testicles to the seminal vesicles), and blood vessels; in women, where the round ligament of the uterus leaves the abdomen to connect with the labium majus.

INHALATION THERAPY: Therapeutic use of respirators, aerosol-producing devices, oxygen, helium-oxygen, and carbon dioxide mixtures to assist breathing.

INTERLOBAR FISSURE: The line between the two largest lobes of the lung.

INTERMEDULLARY: Within the marrow.

INTERMITTENT AUSCULTATION: Act of listening with a stethoscope for sounds within the body to determine the condition of the lungs, heart, pleura, and other organs.

INTERMITTENT CLAUDICATION: A deficiency in the blood flow to a limb while walking, resulting in weakness or pain.

INTERNAL FIXATION: The use of plate, nails, screws, wires or some combination thereof in the repair of a broken bone.

INTERNAL JUGULAR VEIN: The branch of the jugular vein that lies deepest in the neck and carries blood to the brain.

INTRAABDOMINAL SEPSIS: Infection within the abdomen.

INTRAOPERATIVE: During surgery.

INTUBATE: To treat by intubation.

INTUBATION: The insertion of a tube into a hollow organ (such as the trachea), for the introduction of air.

INVASIVE CANCER: Cancer that has spread beyond the tissue layer in which it started.

INVASIVE PROCEDURE: One that involves an insertion of a probe or instrument through an incision or one of the natural orifices of the body.

IONIC: Related to or characterized by ions, which are positively and negatively charged molecules.

IONIC MEDIUM: A medium that separates into positively charged and negatively charged molecular fragments, or ions, when it is dissolved; a nonionic one does not.

ISCHEMIA: A localized deficiency of blood flow, due to an obstruction in the blood vessel.

ISCHEMIC BOWEL DISEASE: A condition that is characterized by a decreased flow of blood to the bowels.

JIG: A preformed plastic tray of molded nylon that keeps a bone aligned and prevents it from rotating while the surgeon is applying pressure to realign it into correct position.

LABIUM MAJUS: One of the two long lips of skin, one on each side of the vaginal opening, that form the outer genitals of a woman.

LABOR, TRIAL OF: Watching a laboring woman who has previously had a cesarean delivery to determine whether she can deliver vaginally.

LACERATION: A torn and ragged wound.

LAPAROTOMY: An open (involving a large incision) examination of the abdomen.

LASER ANGIOPLASTY: Use of a laser beam to treat severely blocked or narrowed arteries. The beam of light vaporizes the plaque.

LASER LITHOTRIPSY: A procedure that uses shock waves to shatter solid substances within the body such as kidney stones and gallstones.

LASER MICROSURGERY: Surgery done through a microscope, using a laser.

LEFT ATRIUM: A chamber on the left side of the heart; it receives blood from the pulmonary veins and delivers it to the left ventricle.

LEFT BUNDLE BRANCH BLOCK: A heart rhythm disturbance.

LEFT VENTRICLE: A chamber on the left side of the heart; it receives blood from the left atrium and pumps it into the aorta and then to the rest of the circulatory system.

LEPTOSPIROSIS: A bacterial infection caused by a microorganism, transmitted in the urine of infected animals, which may produce muscular pain, fever, chills, and jaundice.

LESION: An abnormal growth or localized condition, such as a tumor, wart, or cyst.

LEVEEN PERITONEOVENOUS SHUNT: A tube that routes fluid from the abdominal cavity into venous circulation for disposal by the kidneys.

LIGAMENT: Strong fibrous connective tissue that connects a bone to another bone.

LIGATE: To tie or bind with a loop of suture material.

LIGATION: The tying or binding of a blood vessel or duct with a loop of suture material.

LITHOTOMY POSITION: The conventional (supine) position for giving birth or for gynecologic examination. The woman lies flat on her back with her knees bent and legs spread wide apart with stirrups.

LITHOTRIPSY: See extracorporeal shock-wave lithotripsy (ESWL).

LOW SENSITIVITY TEST: A test that does not differentiate well between who is sick and who is not.

LOW SPECIFICITY TEST: A test that does not differentiate well between someone who is sick and has a specific condition and someone who does not have that condition.

LUMEN: The cavity or channel within a tube or tubular organ.

LYMPHOGRANULOMATOSIS: An inflammatory condition of the lymph glands.

LYMPHATIC SYSTEM: A vast network of capillaries, thin vessels, valves, ducts, nodes, and organs that helps to protect and maintain the fluid environment of the body.

MRI SCAN: Also known as magnetic resonance imaging. MRI employs a strong magnetic field (rather than x rays) and a computer to produce detailed pictures of the body's internal structures.

MACULAR DEGENERATION: A disease in which the surface of the macula (the part of the retina with the sharpest sight) degenerates enough to cause legal blindness.

MAJOR MORBIDITY: Any complication that extends the length of stay in the hospital beyond the expected discharge date.

MALIGNANT HYPERTHERMIA: An uncontrollable fever.

MEDULLARY CANAL: The canal in the center of bone. It contains the bone marrow.

MENISCUS: A fibrous cartilage within a joint, especially of the knee.

MESENTERY: The fold in the lining of the abdomen attaching the intestine to the back of the abdominal wall and containing the arteries and veins that supply the intestines.

META-ANALYSIS: A study that uses combined data from other studies.

METASTASES: Cancers that have spread beyond their original sites.

MICRO-EMBOLIZATION: Breaking off of small pieces of plaque or clots from the vessels that block small arteries, veins, and capillaries, causing organ damage.

MICROSURGERY: Surgical techniques performed on structures too small to see clearly with the naked eye, which require the surgeon to use an operating microscope and tiny versions of regular surgical instruments.

MORCELLATION: Dissection of solid tissue.

MUCOSA: Any tissue in the body that secretes mucus.

MUSCLE FLAP TRANSPLANT CLOSURE: Used when it is necessary to replace all layers of a body wall, as in the case of generalized abdominal infections. Usually, a section of the latissimus dorsi muscle of the back is taken and used to replace the abdominal wall or other major wall defect. Used interchangeably with muscle flap transplant coverage.

MUSCLE FLAP TRANSPLANT COVERAGE: Essentially the same as muscle flap transplant closure but implies that skin grafting may be needed later.

MUSCLE OVERLAP TECHNIQUE: A surgical technique for moving a section of skin and underlying tissue, including the blood supply, to an area where blood supply is poor and a skin graft would not be appropriate. Muscle overlaps can be used to cover areas that are burned or areas that require thick coverings, such as the hip.

MYELOGRAM: An x ray of the spinal cord.

MYOCARDIUM: The middle and thickest layer of the heart wall.

MYOMA: A benign tumor of the uterine muscle.

MYOPIA: Nearsightedness.

NASOGASTRIC TUBE: A tube that is inserted through the nose and runs down to the stomach.

NECROSIS: Death of living tissue.

NECROTIZING ENTEROCOLITIS: Infectious destruction of the bowel.

NECROTIZING FASCIITIS: A condition in which the fascia (the tough tissue containing the muscles) is destroyed, with destruction spreading to the overlying and underlying tissues.

NONSTEROIDAL ANTI-INFLAMMATORY DRUGS (NSAIDS): Analgesic agents, such as ibuprofen, that do not contain any synthetic derivatives of testosterone (steroids); drugs in the same class as aspirin.

NOSOCOMIAL INFECTION: An infection acquired while in a health care setting such as a hospital, outpatient center, or clinic.

OBSTRUCTIVE JAUNDICE: Collection of liver products in the blood, as a result of blockage of the liver ducts.

OCCLUSION: Blockage of any passage, canal, vessel, or opening in the body.

OMENTUM: A fatty "apron" that hangs down from the bottom of the stomach. It seems to have the role of plugging intestinal leaks and walling off abscesses.

ONCOLOGIST: A physician who specializes in the study and treatment of cancer.

OPEN FRACTURE: An open wound that reaches all the way down to the site of a break or rupture of hard tissue, such as bone, with at least part of the bone exposed through the skin.

OPEN PROCEDURE: A surgical procedure that involves cutting into the abdomen.

OPERATIVE MORTALITY: Death that occurs during a surgical procedure; depending upon other factors, could also include death that occurs in the process of recovery.

OSMOLALITY: Refers to the concentration of dissolved solids in the contrast media (a solution of an iodine compound used to make a body part or vein or artery visible on x rays); high-osmolality solutions have more dissolved solids than low-osmolality solutions.

OSMOSIS: Tendency for the concentration of solutions on either side of a semipermeable membrane (such as that used in a dialysis machine) to equalize over time.

OSTEOARTHRITIS: A noninflammatory degenerative joint disease that is characterized by pain and stiffness.

OVARIAN REMNANT SYNDROME: A condition that results when an ovarian fragment remains after the ovaries have been removed. It causes pelvic pain and can lead to ureteral obstruction.

PARACENTESIS: Tapping the abdomen with a large needle to remove fluid.

PATELLA: The kneecap.

PATENCY: The condition of being wide open.

PECTORALIS MAJOR: Large chest muscle that runs from the clavicle (collarbone) to just below the nipple.

PELVIC ADHESIONS: Bands of scar tissue that form between cut surfaces of organs inside the abdomen.

PERCUTANEOUS: Through the skin.

PERCUTANEOUS DISKECTOMY: Removal of all or part of an intervertebral disk with a mechanical device that fits into a needle and is inserted through the skin.

PERFORATION: Tearing or boring through a vessel, duct, intestine, or organ.

PERICARDIUM: The tissue that surrounds the heart; the heart sac.

PERINEUM: Pelvic area extending from the pubic bone and genitals in front to the coccyx (tailbone) and anus in the back; also includes part of the hipbone.

PERIOPERATIVE: The time period from admission to the hospital for surgery to discharge from the hospital.

PERIOPERATIVE MORTALITY: Death within 30 days of surgery or during the same hospital admission.

PERIPHERAL VENOUS SYSTEM: Veins of the limbs and head of the body.

PERISTALSIS: Wavelike actions of the alimentary canal, or digestive tract, that force the contents onward.

PERITONEAL: Relating to the peritoneum, the transparent covering of the organs that lies just behind the muscular wall of the abdomen.

PERITONEUM: The transparent covering of the organs that lies just behind the muscular wall of the abdomen.

PERITONITIS: An inflammation of the transparent membrane that covers most of the abdomen beneath the muscle layer.

PERITONSILLAR ABSCESS: Abscess associated with tonsillitis; occurs when one of the tonsils becomes infected and a collection of pus forms between the tonsil and the tissue around it.

PHLEBITIS: Inflammation of a vein, usually caused by infection or injury.

PLAQUE: A deposit of fatty buildup in the inner lining of the artery wall.

PLATELET-FIBRIN THROMBI: Blood clots composed mainly of fibrin, a blood protein.

PLEURA: The membrane surrounding the lungs.

PNEUMOPERITONEUM: Air in the peritoneal cavity.

PNEUMOTHORAX: Air in the chest cavity that can cause lung collapse.

POLYP: A protruding growth from any mucous membranes, especially those found in the nose, throat, uterus, and colon.

POLYPECTOMY: Removal of polyps.

POPLITEAL ARTERY: The portion of the femoral artery (in the thigh) that runs behind the knee and supplies virtually all the blood to the lower leg.

POSTOPERATIVE ANEMIA: A condition in which the blood is deficient in red blood cells, in hemoglobin, or in total volume. It results when there is any loss of red blood cells during surgery that lowers or reduces the concentration below what is considered normal.

PRE-ECLAMPSIA: A toxic condition of late pregnancy marked by very high blood pressure, swelling, and kidney malfunction.

PREPUCE: The foreskin of the penis.

PROLAPSE: The slippage of a body part from its normal position.

PROLAPSE OF THE RECTUM: Bulging outward of the rectum.

PROSTAGLANDINS: A group of hormonelike fatty acids found in many parts of the body. They affect many organs, and are responsible for stimulation of uterine contractions during labor and birth.

PROSTHESIS: An artificial body part.

PSEUDOANEURYSM: Dilation and twisting of a vessel, giving the appearance of an aneurysm.

PULMONARY: Pertaining to the lungs.

PULMONARY ARTERY: The main artery carrying blood from the heart to the lungs.

PULMONARY EMBOLISM: A blood clot that lodges in the pulmonary artery or in another vessel in a lung.

PULMONARY HYPERTENSION: High blood pressure limited to the vessels of the lungs.

QUADRICEPS: The large muscle of the front of the thigh.

RADIOISOTOPE STUDY: A diagnostic procedure that uses a radioactive isotope to view a body organ and examine its structure or function.

RADIOPAQUE: The property of a material (such as barium) that blocks x rays.

RADIUS: The smaller of the two bones in the lower arm.

RANDALL STONE FORCEPS: Forceps with curved slender blades and serrated jaws used to extract calculi (usually composed of mineral salts) from the renal pelvis.

RECTOCELE: Protrusion of part of the rectum into the vagina; also called a proctocele.

RENAL: Pertaining to the kidney.

RENAL PELVIS: The center of the kidney where various tubules enter into the ureters.

REOCCLUSION: Reclogging of a vessel.

RESPIRATORY DEPRESSION: Inability to fill the lungs, which results in suppressed or shallow breathing.

RESURFACING: Planing off any bone spurs or protrusions to create a very smooth surface for repair or replacement of joints.

RESUSCITATIVE THORACOTOMY: Opening the chest to restart and repair the heart.

RETRACT: To pull apart.

RETRACTORS: Surgical devices for holding back the edges of tissues or organs to keep tissues and organs exposed.

REVISION: A surgical alteration performed to correct or repair a previous surgery.

RHEUMATOID ARTHRITIS: A chronic systemic disease of the joints, characterized by inflammation and loss of bone.

RIGHT ATRIUM: Chamber on the right side of the heart; it receives blood from the superior and inferior vena cava and delivers it to the right ventricle.

RIGHT VENTRICLE: Chamber on the right side of the heart; it receives blood from the right atrium and pumps it into the pulmonary artery and then to the lungs.

ROTATOR CUFF: The muscles surrounding the shoulder that control the movement of the arm and enable it to move forward and backward.

ROTATOR CUFF ARTHROPATHY: Disease of the bones in the rotator cuff, which affects the attachments of the ligaments and tendons that make up the rotator cuff.

SAPHENOUS VEIN: The longest vein in the body, called the "great" saphenous vein, running from the pelvic region to the foot (each leg has one saphenous vein).

SARTORIUS MUSCLE: The muscle located in the groin/hip region.

SCLEROSIS: Hardening of tissue.

SCLEROTHERAPY: Injection of an irritating solution into a varicose vein, causing it to close.

SEPSIS: Presence of disease-causing microorganisms in the bloodstream.

SEPTIC ARTHRITIS: Triggering of additional arthritic responses by infection.

SEPTICEMIA: Generalized bacterial infection of the bloodstream; blood poisoning.

SEPTUM: Generally refers to a dividing wall or partition, such as the nasal septum, that separates the nasal cavities.

SHOULDER ARTHRODESIS: Freezing or fixing in place of the shoulder joint through surgery.

SHUNT: A tube, with or without a one-way valve, that carries some fluid from one place to another place; a passage between two natural channels, especially between blood vessels.

SIGMOID COLON: Lower portion of the large intestine just above the rectum; it looks something like an angular "S."

SILASTIC: Silicone-based elastic that should not react with tissue; can be used to cover a wound or replace certain tissues.

SINUSES: Air pockets that surround the nasal structures in the skull.

SKIN HOOKS: Instruments to hold skin in position, which look like knitting needles.

SLEEP APNEA: Momentary cessation of breathing during sleep, due to airway obstruction, that disrupts the normal sleep pattern.

SMALL INTESTINE: The part of the digestive tract concerned with the digestion of food and the absorption of food into the bloodstream.

SPECULUM: Device used to examine body canals, such as the vagina.

SPHENOID SINUS: The sinus, or cavity, that is lowest and farthest to the rear in the skull.

SPHINCTER: A ring of muscles found at the opening of an orifice such as the anus, bladder, or esophagus.

SPINAL TAP: A process in which a long, thin needle is used to remove cerebrospinal fluid from the spine.

SPINAL STENOSIS: A narrowing of the spinal canal.

SPINOUS PROCESSES: The backward-pointing extensions, or projections, of the bones of the spine.

SPLENIC FLEXURE: The right-angle bend in the colon right under the spleen.

STENOSIS: A narrowing or closing of a vessel or passageway in the body.

STENT: An appliance, such as a stiff tube, that is placed inside a vessel to prevent it from closing.

STERNUM: Breastbone.

STRESS INCONTINENCE: Inability to hold urine while coughing or laughing.

STRICTURE: A narrowing of a canal, duct, or other passage.

STRICTUREPLASTY: A procedure that removes only the portions of the bowel that are narrowed due to Crohn's disease.

SUBCAPSULARIS MUSCLE: The muscle under the shoulder capsule that is part of the supporting structure.

SUBCLAVIAN VEIN: Large vein that runs under the collarbone. It leads to the superior vena cava, which feeds into the right side of the heart.

SUBCLINICAL INFECTION: An infection with no detectable symptoms or signs (such as pain, fever, redness, or swelling) but which nonetheless destroys tissue or prevents healing after surgery.

SUBGALEAL HEMATOMA: A pool of blood that forms between the brain and the band of fibrous tissue at the cap of the skull.

It puts pressure on blood vessels, causes pain and possible brain damage, and causes alteration of neurons.

SUBMUCOSAL RESECTION: Excising of the tissue under the mucus membranes in the mouth, nose, intestines, or anywhere else there are such membranes.

SUPERIOR VENA CAVA: A major vein that drains blood from the head, neck, upper extremities, and chest and returns it to the right atrium of the heart.

SUPRASPINATUS MUSCLE: The diamond-shaped muscle that extends from the base of the skull to the shoulder blades.

SUTURE: To stitch together cut or torn edges of tissue with suture material, such as catgut, wire, or synthetic material.

SYSTEMIC: Affecting the body generally.

TAMOXIFEN: An anticancer drug (brand name: Nolvadex) used to relieve advanced breast cancer in premenopausal and postmenopausal women whose tumors are estrogen-dependent.

TELANGIECTASIA: A patch of dilated blood vessels visible on the skin.

TENDON: Cordlike tissue that connects muscles to bones.

TERES MINOR MUSCLE: A muscle in the shoulder that helps support the shoulder structure.

TERMINAL ILEUM: The portion of the small intestine that joins the large intestine and contains the ileocecal valve.

THORACIC AORTA: Part of the aorta that is in the chest above the diaphragm.

THORACOTOMY: Surgical incision of the chest wall.

THROMBOEMBOLECTOMY: Removal of a blood clot blocking a vein or artery.

THROMBOEMBOLISM: Blockage of a vessel or passage by a blood clot.

THROMBOSIS: Formation or development of a blood clot.

THROMBUS: A blood clot.

THYROID STORM: A state of increased thyroid secretion that leads to a syndrome of high fever, racing heartbeat, and delirium.

TIBIA: The large bone of the lower leg.

TOPICAL: Pertaining to a particular surface area.

TOTAL PARENTERAL NUTRITION (TPN): A type of extremely nutritious long-term intravenous feeding that bypasses the stomach and contains all of the necessary fats, proteins, and carbohydrates (and nutrients in general) that the body requires; usually used in a long coma, extensive burns, stomach and intestinal fistulas, and other conditions in which feeding by mouth cannot give adequate amounts of essential nutrients.

TOXEMIA: Bacterial toxins in the bloodstream.

TOXIC MEGACOLON: Massive swelling of the colon caused by bacterial toxins.

TOXIC SHOCK SYNDROME: An illness characterized by high fever, vomiting, diarrhea, and muscle tenderness; associated with the use of tampons.

TRACHEA: The tube that connects the throat to the bronchial tubes in the lungs; the windpipe.

TRACHEOSTOMY: A breathing hole cut into the throat below the larynx to bypass a breathing problem higher up in the body.

TRANSESOPHAGEAL ECHOCARDIOGRAPHY: An ultrasound procedure using an ultrasound source placed down the esophagus (the tube that leads from the mouth to the stomach) for the purpose of a graphic recording of internal structures of the heart.

TRANSLUMINAL: Pertaining to the inside of any tubular structure in the body; pertaining to anything done across or through the lumen.

TRANSIENT ELECTROCARDIOGRAPHIC CHANGES: Short-term, temporary changes that are observed in an electrocardiogram (EKG) and are present only during the procedure.

TRANSIENT ISCHEMIC ATTACK: Often called a "little stroke" because it interrupts the flow of blood to the brain; usually lasts only a minute or two.

TRANSIENT NEUROLOGICAL DEFICIT: A diagnosable brain or nerve problem that disappears quickly, and abnormal behavior that resolves quickly.

TRANSIENT VAGAL REACTION: Characterized by pallor, nausea, sweating, rapid fall in arterial blood pressure, and loss of consciousness; more properly called vasovagal attack.

TRANSVERSE COLON: The portion of the colon that runs across the middle of the abdomen.

TROCHAR: A sharp-pointed, hollow tube that is used to puncture the wall of a body cavity such as the abdomen.

TRUSS: An elastic, canvas, or padded metal appliance used to hold an abdominal hernia in place.

ULCERATIVE COLITIS: An inflammation of the colon and rectum in which ulcers in the digestive tract cause bloody stool.

ULNA: The larger of the two bones in the lower arm.

ULTRASONIC: Pertaining to ultrasound.

ULTRASOUND: Use of sound waves at very high frequency for diagnostic purposes. The resulting echoes are translated into pictures on a TV monitor; the image itself is called a sonogram.

UREMIA: Accumulation of waste products in the blood.

URETERS: Tubes that carry the urine from the kidneys to the bladder.

URETHRA: The tube through which urine is excreted from the bladder.

URINARY RETENTION: Inability to partially or completely empty the bladder.

UROGRAPHY: A kidney and bladder x ray using a contrast medium given by vein.

UTERINE MYOMA: A benign tumor of the muscular wall of the uterus; formerly called fibroid tumor.

UTERINE PROLAPSE: Bulging of the uterus into the vagina.

VACUUM EXTRACTOR: A medical device that is used during delivery; consists of a small suction cup, which is placed on the baby's head and is attached to a hose on a vacuum device; involves the creation of a vacuum to draw out the baby.

VAS DEFERENS: Tubes that carry sperm from the testicles to the seminal vesicles, the two glands that store sperm.

VASOCONSTRICTOR: A drug that causes the constricting of blood vessels.

VASODILATOR: A drug that causes the expanding of blood vessels.

VENA CAVA: The large vein in the center of the body.

VENOGRAPHY: An x ray of veins after the injection of a contrast medium (a solution of iodine compounds which block X rays).

VENTRICLE: One of the two lower chambers of the heart; or, any small cavity.

VENTRICULAR FIBRILLATION: Rapid, ineffective, very uneven beating of the two lower pumping chambers of the heart; blood pressure falls to zero, which results in unconsciousness. Condition may lead to death.

VERTEBRAE: Bones that comprise the spinal column.

VOLVULUS: An intestinal obstruction caused by the twisting and knotting of the bowel.

Research Terms

CONTROLLED CLINICAL TRIAL: A study in which the effects of chance are "controlled for" by using (at least) two groups. One group receives the treatment being researched, and the other group receives either a treatment known to be effective, a placebo (a sugar pill, which is presented as real medicine, or a sham treatment), or no treatment.

CROSSOVER STUDY: A controlled trial in which all patients receive all real or sham treatments at some time during the course of the trial.

DOUBLE BLIND CLINICAL TRIAL: A controlled trial in which neither the patients nor the doctors know which patients are receiving what treatment at what time during the study.

PROSPECTIVE STUDY: A study whose rules for data collection and evaluation are formulated before any data is collected on any patient, and which uses only data gathered after the study is formally begun; a study that "looks forward."

RETROSPECTIVE STUDY: A study that relies on data collected before the study rules for data collection and evaluation are formulated. It uses data gathered before the study is done; a study that "looks backward."

SERIES: A study that uses all the patients seen between a starting date and ending date who meet criteria for inclusion in the study; a study in which the patients are not randomly selected, and which uses all patients seen in a defined time interval.

STATISTICALLY SIGNIFICANT: Not likely to be due to chance alone; likely to be due to real effects, to an arbitrarily selected degree (usually 95% or 99%—meaning that the chance that the effects seen are due to chance alone is 5% or 1%, respectively). An alternative way to think about statistical significance is this: if a study that reports statistically significant findings at the 99% confidence level were repeated 100 times, 99 of the repeats would show an effect as large as, or larger than, the effect actually found.

Fiber-Optic Scopes

Technology has certainly changed the practice of medicine forever. Nowhere is this more apparent than in the use of endoscopes to examine interior parts of the body. Endoscopes are hollow tubes that contain a light source and a viewing lens. Some tubes are rigid for direct viewing, and others are flexible so that they can be "snaked" through various parts of the body. The newer flexible scopes owe their success in large part to the development and application of fiber-optic technology.

Fiber-optic devices are thin, flexible tubes containing bundles of glass filaments that can transmit light around bends and curves to illuminate the inside of the body. Scopes are viewing instruments that utilize a "light-at-the-end-of-the-tunnel" approach, but some offer more than just a look. Forceps, scissors, or other tiny instruments can be threaded through channels in some scopes, to facilitate surgical procedures. In addition, the pictures taken by the lens of the scope can be fed to TV monitor for better viewing.

Here are some of the more common endoscopes:

ARTHROSCOPE: A fiber-optic instrument used to examine the interior of a joint such as a knee or shoulder. The arthroscope is inserted through a small incision made above the joint.

BRONCHOSCOPE: An instrument inserted through the mouth to examine the lungs and bronchial tree. The rigid bronchoscope is a straight, hollow tube that permits direct viewing of the airway passages. The flexible bronchoscope uses a fiber-optic system that permits the doctor to inspect the full bronchial system.

COLONOSCOPE: A flexible fiber-optic instrument inserted through the anus to examine the large intestine from the anus to the cecum (the first part of the large intestine).

COLPOSCOPE: A thin, lighted instrument that is inserted into the vagina to permit examination of the cervix and to obtain tissue samples for biopsy.

CULDOSCOPE: A thin, lighted instrument that is inserted through an incision made in the vagina to view the uterus, fallopian tubes, and rectal wall.

CYSTOSCOPE: A rigid instrument with a viewing lens and light source that is used to view the urethra and bladder. Inserted through the urethra, the cystoscope may also be used to obtain urine and tissue samples.

GASTROSCOPE: A flexible fiber-optic instrument that is inserted through the mouth or the nose. It is used to examine the upper portion of the digestive tract—the esophagus, stomach, and duodenum.

HYSTEROSCOPE: A short, rigid instrument with a light source that is inserted through the vagina and cervix to examine the uterus.

LAPAROSCOPE: A thin, lighted instrument that is inserted through a small incision in the abdomen, usually near the navel. It is used to examine the liver, spleen, intestines, and in women the uterus, ovaries, and fallopian tubes.

LARYNGOSCOPE: A thin fiber-optic instrument that is inserted through a nostril in order to view the base of the tongue, epiglottis, larynx, and vocal cords.

PROCTOSCOPE: A short, rigid or flexible tube (about five or six inches long) that is inserted through the anus to examine the rectum.

SIGMOIDOSCOPE: A rigid or flexible tube inserted through the anus to examine the sigmoid colon (the "S"-shaped portion of the colon just above the rectum). The rigid sigmoidoscope is a lighted tube about 12 inches long and one inch in diameter. The flexible sigmoidoscope employs fiber-optics and is about two feet long.

Consumer Resources

The following organizations may be contacted when you need information about your condition or a surgical procedure. Some of these organizations have toll-free telephone numbers for your convenience. In order to give you the broadest range of information, we are including professional as well as consumer organizations.

Medical Specialty Boards: M.D.s

To verify the credentials of medical or osteopathic doctors, contact one of the following boards, or you may call the American Board of Medical Specialties toll-free at 800—776—CERT.

Allergy and Immunology, American Board of
University City Science Center
3624 Market Street
Philadelphia, PA 19104
215–349–9466

Anesthesiology, American Board of
100 Constitution Plaza, Room 1668
Hartford, CT 06103
302–522–9857

Colon and Rectal Surgery, American Board of
8750 Telegraph Road, Suite 410
Taylor, MI 48180
313–295–1740

Dermatology, American Board of
Henry Ford Hospital
Detroit, MI 48202
313–871–8739

Emergency Medicine, American Board of
200 Woodland Pass, Suite D
East Lansing, MI 48823
517–332–4800

Family Practice, American Board of
2228 Young Drive
Lexington, KY 40505
606–269–5626

Internal Medicine, American Board of
University City Science Center
3624 Market Street
Philadelphia, PA 19104
215–243–1500

Neurological Surgery, American Board of
Smith Tower
6550 Fannin Street, Suite 2139
Houston, TX 77030–2701
713–790–6015

Nuclear Medicine, American Board of
900 Veteran Avenue, Room 12–200
Los Angeles, CA 90024
213–825–6787

Obstetrics and Gynecology, American Board of
4225 Roosevelt Way, NE, Suite 305
Seattle, WA 98105
206–547–4884

Ophthalmology, American Board of
111 Presidential Boulevard, Suite 241
Bala Cynwyd, PA 19004
215–664–1175

Orthopedic Surgery, American Board of
737 North Michigan Avenue, Suite 1150
Chicago, IL 60611
312–664–9444

Otolaryngology, American Board of
5615 Kirby Drive, Suite 936
Houston, TX 77005
713–528–6200

Pathology, American Board of
5401 West Kennedy Boulevard, Suite 780
P.O. Box 25915
Tampa, FL 33622
813–286–2444

Pediatrics, American Board of
111 Silver Cedar Court
Chapel Hill, NC 27514
919–929–0461

Physical Medicine and Rehabilitation, American Board of
Northwest Center, Suite 674
21 First Street, SW
Rochester, MN 55902
507–282–1776

Plastic Surgery, American Board of
7 Penn Center
1635 Market Street
Philadelphia, PA 19103–2204
215–587–9322

Preventive Medicine, American Board of
Department of Community Medicine
Wright State University School of Medicine
P.O. Box 927
Dayton, OH 45401
513–278–6914

Psychiatry and Neurology, American Board of
500 Lake Cook Road, Suite 335
Deerfield, IL 60015
312–945–7900

Radiology, American Board of
300 Park, Suite 440
Birmingham, MI 48009
313–645–0600

Surgery, American Board of
1617 John F. Kennedy Boulevard, Suite 860
Philadelphia, PA 19103–1847
215–568–4000

Thoracic Surgery, American Board of
1 Rotary Center, Suite 803
Evanston, IL 60201
312–475–1520

Urology, American Board of
31700 Telegraph Road, Suite 150
Birmingham, MI 48010
313–646–9720

Medical Specialty Boards: D.O.s

Anesthesiology, American Osteopathic Board of
17201 East 40 Highway, Suite 204
Independence, MO 64055
816–373–4700

Dermatology, American Osteopathic Board of
25510 Plymouth Road
Detroit, MI 48239
313–937–1200

Emergency Medicine, American Osteopathic Board of
Philadelphia Osteopathic Medical Center
4190 City Avenue
Philadelphia, PA 19131
215–871–2811

General Practice, American Osteopathic Board of
2474 Dempster Street, Suite 217
Des Plaines, IL 60016
312–635–8477

Internal Medicine, American Osteopathic Board of
5200 South Ellis Avenue
Chicago, IL 60615
312–947–4880

Neurology and Psychiatry, American Osteopathic Board of
Department of Psychiatry
401 Haddon Avenue
Camden, NJ 08103–1505
609–757–7765

Nuclear Medicine, American Osteopathic Board of
5200 South Ellis Avenue
Chicago, IL 60615
312–947–4490

Obstetrics and Gynecology, American Osteopathic Board of
Ohio University College of Osteopathic Medicine
Grosvenor Hall, West 064
Athens, OH 45701
614–593–2239

Ophthalmology and Otorhinolaryngology, American Osteopathic Board of
405 Grand Avenue
Dayton, OH 45405
513–222–4213

Orthopedic Surgery, American Osteopathic Board of
5155 Raytown Road, Suite 103
Kansas City, MO 64133
816–353–6400

Pathology, American Osteopathic Board of
13355 East Ten Mile Road
Warren, MI 48089
313–759–7565

Pediatrics, American Osteopathic Board of
2700 River Road, Suite 407
Des Plaines, IL 60018
312–635–0201

Preventive Medicine, American Osteopathic Board of
12535 Lt. Nichols Road
Fairfax, VA 22033
703–648–3834

Proctology, American Osteopathic Board of
75 Skylark Road
Springfield, NJ 07081
201–687–2062

Radiology, American Osteopathic Board of
Route 2, Box 75
Milan, MO 63556
816–265–4991

Rehabilitation Medicine, American Osteopathic Board of
9058 West Church
Des Plaines, IL 60016
312–699–0048

Surgery, American Osteopathic Board of
405 Grand Avenue
Dayton, OH 45404
513–226–2656

Professional Academies, Colleges, and Societies

You may also obtain consumer information from professional academies, colleges, and societies. In addition to their consumer-oriented publications, some of these organizations operate referral services.

PROFESSIONAL ACADEMIES

Cosmetic Surgery, American Academy of
159 East Live Oak Avenue, Suite 204
Arcadia, CA 91006
800–221–9808
818–447–1579

Dermatology, American Academy of
1567 Maple Avenue
P.O. Box 3116
Evanston, IL 60201–3116
798–869–3954

Facial Plastic Reconstructive Surgery, American Academy of
1110 Vermont Avenue, NW
Washington, DC 20005
800–332-FACE
800–523-FACE (Canada)
202–842–4500

Orthopedic Surgeons, American Academy of
222 South Prospect Avenue
Park Ridge, IL 60068
708–823–7186

Otolaryngology (Head & Neck Surgery), American Academy of
1 Prince Street
Alexandria, VA 22314–3357
703–836–4444

PROFESSIONAL COLLEGES

Cardiology, American College of
9111 Old Georgetown Road
Bethesda, MD 20814
301–897–5400

Foot Surgeons (Podiatry), American College of
1601 Dolores Street
San Francisco, CA 94110
415–826–3200

Obstetricians and Gynecologists, American College of
409 12th Street, SW
Washington, DC 20024
202–638–5577

PROFESSIONAL SOCIETIES

Cataract and Refractive Surgery, American Society of
3702 Pender Drive, Suite 250
Fairfax, VA 22030
703–591–2220

Colon and Rectal Surgeons, American Society of
800 East Northwest Highway, Suite 1080
Palatine, IL 60067
708–359–9184

Dermatological Surgery, American Society of
1567 Maple Avenue
Evanston, IL 60201
800–441–2737
708–869–3959

Laser Medicine & Surgery, American Society for
2404 Stewart Square
Wausau, WI 54401
715–845–9283

Lipo-Suction Surgery, American Society of
159 East Live Oak Avenue, Suite 204
Arcadia, CA 91006
800–221–9808
818–447–1579

Plastic and Reconstructive Surgeons, American Society of
444 East Algonquin Road
Arlington Heights, IL 60005
800–635–0635
708–228–9900

Consumer and Government Organizations

There's a wealth of material available to consumers from national health organizations, consumer support groups, clearinghouses, and government agencies. This section lists toll-free hot lines, clearinghouses, national health organizations, and government agencies.

TOLL-FREE HOT LINES

ALZHEIMER'S DISEASE
Alzheimer's Disease Foundation
800–621–0379
800–572–6037 in IL

CANCER
AMC Cancer Information
American Medical Center Cancer Research Center
800–525–3777
303–233–6501 in CO

American Cancer Society
800–227–2345

Cancer Information Service
National Cancer Institute
800–4–CANCER

DIABETES
American Diabetes Association
800–232–3472

Diabetes Center, Inc.
800–848–2793

Juvenile Diabetes Foundation
800–223–1138
212–889–7575

ENDOMETRIOSIS
Endometriosis Association
800–922–ENDO

HEAD INJURY
National Head Injury Foundation
800–444–NHIF

HEALTH INFORMATION
American Trauma Society
800–556–7890

National Library of Medicine
800–272–4787

HEARING AND SPEECH
Deafness Research Foundation
800–535–3323

National Association for Hearing and Speech
800–638–8255
301–897–8682 in MD (call collect)

HEART DISEASE
Heartlife
800–241–6993
404–523–0826 in GA

HOSPITAL CARE
Shriners Hospital Referral Line
800–237–5055
800–282–9161 in FL

KIDNEY DISEASE
American Kidney Fund
800–638–8299

Kidney Stones
800–333–3032

LIVER DISEASE
American Liver Foundation
800–223–0179
201–857–2626 in NJ

LUNG DISEASE
Lung Line, National Asthma Center
800–222–5864
303–355–LUNG in Denver

LUPUS
Lupus Foundation of America
800–558–0121
202–328–4550 in Washington, DC

ORGANS
The Living Bank
800–528–2971
713–528–2971 in TX

Organ Donor Hot Line
800–24–DONOR
800–552–2138 in VA

PARKINSON'S DISEASE
American Parkinson's Disease Association
800–223–2732

National Parkinson's Foundation
800–327–4545
800–433–7022
305–547–6666 in Miami area

Parkinson's Education Program
800–344–7872
714–640–0218 in CA

RARE ILLNESSES
National Organization for Rare Diseases
800–999–NORD

PROSTATE
Prostate Information Hot Line
800–543–9632

SPINAL CORD INJURY
National Spinal Cord Injury Association
800–962–9629

Spinal Cord Injury Hot Line
800–526–3456

STROKE
Courage Stroke Network
800–553–6321

SURGERY SERVICES
American Society of Plastic and Reconstructive Surgeons
800–635–0635

Cosmetic Surgery Information Service
800–221–9808

Facial, Plastic and Reconstructive Surgery
800–332–FACE
800–532–FACE—Canada

International Craniofacial Foundation
800–535–3643

SELF-HELP CLEARINGHOUSES

California
California Self-Help Center UCLA
Los Angeles, CA
800–222–LINK—CA only
213–825–1799

Bay Area Self-Help Center
San Francisco, CA
415–921–4401

Central Region Self-Help Center
Merced, CA
209–385–6937

Northern Region Self-Help Center
Sacramento, CA
916–456–2070

Self-Help Clearinghouse of Yolo County
Davis, CA
916–756–8181

Southern Region Self-Help Center
San Diego, CA
619–298–3152

Connecticut
Connecticut Self-Help Mutual Support Network
203–789–7645

Illinois
Illinois Self-Help Center
Evanston, IL
800–322–MASH—IL only
708–328–0470

Champaign Self-Help Center
Champaign, IL
217–352–0092

Iowa
Iowa Self-Help Clearinghouse
Fort Dodge, IA
800–383–4777
515–576–5870

Kansas
Kansas Self-Help Network
Wichita, KS
800–445–0116—KS only
316–689–3170

Massachusetts
Massachusetts Clearinghouse of Mutual Help Groups
Amherst, MA
413–545–2313

Michigan
Michigan Self-Help Clearinghouse
Lansing, MI
800–752–5858—MI only
517–484–7373

Center for Self-Help
Benton Harbor, MI
800–336–0341—MI only
616–925–0594

Minnesota
Minnesota First Call For Help
St. Paul, MN
612–224–1133

Missouri
The Support Group Clearinghouse
Kansas City, MO
816–561–HELP

Nebraska
Nebraska Self-Help Information Services
Lincoln, NE
402–476–9668

New Jersey
New Jersey Self-Help Clearinghouse
Denville, NJ
800–367–6274—NJ only
201–625–9565
201–625–9053 TDD

New York
New York State Self-Help Clearinghouse
Albany, NY
518–442–5337

New York City Self-Help Clearinghouse
Brooklyn, NY
718–596–6000

Brooklyn Self-Help Clearinghouse
Brooklyn, NY
718–834–7341
718–834–7332

Westchester Self-Help Clearinghouse
Valhalla, NY
914–347–3620

Long Island Self-Help Clearinghouse
Central Islip, NY
516–348–3030

North Carolina
North Carolina Supportworks
Charlotte, NC
704–331–9500

Oregon
Northwest Regional Self-Help Clearinghouse
Portland, OR
503–222–5555

Pennsylvania
Self-Help Groups Network of the Pittsburgh Area
Pittsburgh, PA
412–261–5363

Self-Help Information & Networking Exchange
Scranton, PA
717–961–1234

Philadelphia Clearinghouse
Philadelphia, PA
215–482–4316

Rhode Island
The Support Group Helpline
Providence, RI
401–277–2231

South Carolina
Midland Area Support Group
West Columbia, SC
803–791–9227

Texas
Texas Self-Help Clearinghouse
Austin, TX
512–476–0611

Dallas Self-Help Clearinghouse
Dallas, TX
214–871–2420

Houston Area Self-Help Clearinghouse
Houston, TX
713–523–8963

San Antonio Self-Help Clearinghouse
San Antonio, TX
512–826–2288

Tarrant County Self-Help Clearinghouse
Ft. Worth, TX
817–335–5405

Tennessee
Support Group Clearinghouse
Knoxville, TN
615–584–6736

Vermont
Vermont Self-Help Clearinghouse
Waterbury, VT
800–442–5356—VT only
802–241–2249

Washington, DC
Self-Help Clearinghouse of Greater Washington
Falls Church, VA
703–536–4100

NATIONAL HEALTH ORGANIZATIONS

American Association of Kidney Patients
1 Davis Boulevard, Suite LL-1
Tampa, FL 33606
813–251–0725

American Cancer Society
1599 Clifton Road, NE
Atlanta, GA 30329
404–320–3333

American Diabetes Foundation
Two Park Avenue
New York, NY 10016
212–683–7444

American Digestive Disease Society
7720 Wisconsin Avenue, Suite 217
Bethesda, MD 20814
301–652–9293

American Heart Association
7320 Greenville Avenue
Dallas, TX 75231
214–373–6300

American Liver Foundation
998 Pompton Avenue
Cedar Grove, NJ 07009
201–857–2626

American Lung Association
1740 Broadway
New York, NY 10019
212–889–3370

Arthritis Foundation
1314 Spring Street, NW
Atlanta, GA 30309
404–872–7100

Asthma and Allergy Foundation of America
1717 Massachusetts Avenue, NW, Suite 305
Washington, DC 20036
202–265–0265

Crohn's Disease & Colitis Foundation of America
444 Park Avenue, South, 11th Floor
New York, NY 10016
212–685–3440

Cystic Fibrosis Foundation
3384 Peachtree Road, NE
Suite 558
Atlanta, GA 30326
404–233–2195

Leukemia Society of America
800 Second Avenue
New York, NY 10017
212–573–8484

Muscular Dystrophy Association of America
810 Seventh Avenue
New York, NY 10019
212–586–0808

National Foundation for Asthma
P.O. Box 30069
Tucson, AZ 85751
602–642–7481

National Health Information Clearinghouse
U.S. Office of Disease Prevention & Health Promotion
800–336–4797

National Kidney Foundation
80 East 33rd Street
New York, NY 10016
212–889–2210

National Multiple Sclerosis Society
205 East 42nd Street
New York, NY 10017
212–986–3240

National Stroke Association
1565 Clarkson Street
Denver, CO 80218
303–839–1992

National Women's Health Network
224 Seventh Street, NE
Washington, DC 20003
202–543–9222

GOVERNMENT CLEARINGHOUSES

High Blood Pressure Information Center
National Institutes of Health
Bethesda, MD 20892
301–496–1809

National Arthritis and Musculoskeletal and Skin Diseases Information Clearinghouse
P.O. Box AMS
Bethesda, MD 20892
301–468–3225

National Diabetes Information Clearinghouse
P.O. Box NDIC
Bethesda, MD 20892
301–468–2162

National Digestive Diseases Information Clearinghouse
P.O. Box NDDIC
Bethesda, MD 20892
301–468–6344

National Kidney and Urologic Disease Information Clearinghouse
P.O. Box NKU-DIC
Bethesda, MD 20892
301–468–6345

Notes

Arterial Catheterization

1. D. Elias, P. Lasser, and P. Rougier, "A simplified surgical technical procedure for intra-arterial chemotherapy in secondary liver cancer," *European Journal of Surgical Oncology* 13 (October 1987): 441–48.

2. K. Morimoto et al., "Combined transcatheter arterial embolization and regional chemotherapy for locally advanced carcinoma of the breast," *Acta Radiologica* 24 (May–June 1985): 241–45.

3. M. Markman, "Cytotoxic intracavitary chemotherapy," *American Journal of the Medical Sciences* 291 (March 1986): 175–79.

4. R. W. Carlson and B. I. Sikic, "Continuous infusion or bolus injection in cancer chemotherapy," *Annals of Internal Medicine* 99 (December 1983): 823–33.

5. H. J. Hartung and U. Lenk, "Intra- and postoperative complications in infrarenal abdominal aortic aneurysms," *Anaesthetist* 38 (March 1989): 128–35.

6. J. M. Daly et al., "Long-term hepatic arterial infusion chemotherapy: Anatomic considerations, operative technique, and treatment morbidity," *Archives of Surgery* 119 (August 1984): 936–41.

7. A. G. Bledin et al., "Technetium-99m-labeled macroaggregated albumin arteriography for detection of abnormally positioned arterial catheters during infusion chemotherapy," *Cancer* 53 (15 February 1984): 858–62.

8. P. W. de Graaf et al., "Complications of Tenckhoff catheter implantation in patients with multiple previous intraabdominal procedures for ovarian carcinoma," *Gynecologic Oncology* 29 (January 1988): 43–49.

9. N. M. Sheiner, J. Zeltzer, and E. MacIntosh, "Arterial embolectomy in the modern era," *Canadian Journal of Surgery* 25 (July 1982): 373–75.

10. E. G. Shifrin et al., "Practice and theory of 'delayed' embolectomy: A 22-year perspective," *Journal of Cardiovascular Surgery* 27 (September–October 1986): 553–56.

11. C. M. Purut et al., "Intraoperative management of severe endobronchial hemorrhage," *Annals of Thoracic Surgery* 51 (February 1991): 304–6.

12. A. G. Fleisher et al., "Management of massive hemoptysis secondary to catheter-induced perforation of the pulmonary artery during cardiopulmonary bypass," *Chest* 95 (June 1989): 1340–41.

13. W. C. Feng et al., "Swan-Ganz catheter-induced massive hemoptysis and pulmonary artery false aneurysm," *Annals of Thoracic Surgery* 50 (October 1990): 644–46.

14. C. Lazzam, T. A. Sanborn, and F. Christian, Jr., "Ventricular entrapment of a Swan-Ganz catheter: A technique for nonsurgical removal," *Journal of the American College of Cardiology* 13 (May 1989): 1422–24.

15. C. H. Pegelow et al., "Experience with a totally implantable venous device in children," *American Journal of Diseases of Children* 140 (January 1986): 69–71.

16. D. G. Maki et al., "Septic endarteritis due to intra-arterial catheters for cancer chemotherapy: Guidelines for prevention," *Cancer* 44 (October 1979): 1228–40.

17. M. L. Goldman et al., "Complications of in-dwelling chemotherapy catheters," *Cancer* 36 (December 1975): 1983–90.

18. J. P. Kapp, R. L. Ross, and E. M. Tucker, "Supraophthalmic carotid infusion for brain-tumor chemotherapy," *Journal of Neurosurgery* 58 (April 1983): 616–18.

19. R. J. Lutz et al., "Mixing studies during intracarotid ar-

tery infusions in an in vitro model," *Journal of Neurosurgery* 64 (February 1986): 277–83.

20. J. P. Kapp, J. L. Parker, and E. M. Tucker, "Supra-ophthalmic carotid infusion for brain chemotherapy: Experience with a new single-lumen catheter and maneuverable tip," *Journal of Neurosurgery* 62 (June 1985): 823–25.

21. K. T. Moran et al., "Long-term brachial artery catheterization: Ischemic complications," *Journal of Vascular Surgery* 8 (July 1988): 76–78.

22. S. Lifshitz, L. D. Railsback, and H. J. Buchsbaum, "Intraarterial pelvic infusion chemotherapy in advanced gynecologic cancer," *Obstetrics and Gynecology* 52 (October 1978): 476–80.

23. K. Minakuchi et al., "The availability of digital subtraction angiography using continuous intra-arterial infusion tubes," *Gan To Kagaku Ryoho* 14 (October 1987): 2900–2905. (Published in Japanese)

24. F. Christ and H. J. Straehler-Pohl, "Angiographic localization diagnosis via intra-arterial cytostasis catheters for the perfusion of orocavitary and pharyngeal tumours," *Rontgenblatter* 35 (July 1982): 270–74. (Published in German)

25. *Journal de Radiologie* 65 (December 1984): 833–38. (Published in French)

26. H. D. Piroth et al., "Regional transfemoral intra-arterial chemotherapy using selective catheter placement," *Strahlentherapie und Onkologie* 162 (February 1986): 115–22. (Published in German)

27. K. J. Tuman et al., "Effect of pulmonary artery catheterization on outcome in patients undergoing coronary artery surgery," *Anesthesiology* 70 (February 1989): 199–206.

28. W. C. Shoemaker et al., "The efficacy of central venous and pulmonary artery catheters and therapy based upon them in reducing mortality and morbidity," *Archives of Surgery* 125 (October 1990): 1332–37.

29. L. L. Schrader et al., "Is routine preoperative hemodynamic evaluation of nonagenarians necessary?" *Journal of the American Geriatrics Society* 39 (January 1991): 1–5.

30. M. A. Matthay and K. Chatterjee, "Bedside catheterization of the pulmonary artery: Risks compared with benefits," *Annals of Internal Medicine* 109 (November 1988): 826–34.

31. W. C. Shoemaker et al., "Prospective trial of supranormal values of survivors as therapeutic goals in high-risk surgical patients," *Chest* 94 (December 1988): 1176–86.

32. C. S. Hesdorffer et al., "The value of Swan-Ganz catheterization and volume loading in preventing renal failure in

patients undergoing abdominal aneurysmectomy," *Clinical Nephrology* 28 (December 1987): 272–76.

33. W. P. Joyce et al., "The role of central haemodynamic monitoring in abdominal aortic surgery," *European Journal of Vascular Surgery* 4 (December 1990): 633–36.

Aspiration and Curettage, Postdelivery

1. P. A. King et al., "Secondary postpartum haemorrhage," *Australian and New Zealand Journal of Obstetrics and Gynaecology* 29 (November 1989): 394–98.

2. M. S. Beksac et al., "Stress-induced release of cortisol and prolactin during dilatation and curettage under general and local anesthesia," *Neuropsychobiology* 11 (Number 4, 1984): 227–28.

3. C. M. Sledmere et al., "Psychological aspects of Vabra curettage in menopause clinics," *Maturitas* 3 (December 1981): 205–13.

4. M. E. Boyd, "Dilatation and curettage," *Canadian Journal of Surgery* 32 (January 1989): 9–13.

5. F. Hald et al., "Diagnostic accuracy of outpatient endocervical curettage using conventional and Vabra curettage of the cervix," *ACTA Obstetricia et Gynecologica Scandinavica* 67 (Number 1, 1988): 71–74.

6. S. Alberico et al., "Diagnostic validity of the Vabra curettage," *European Journal of Gynaecologic Oncology* 7 (Number 2, 1986): 135–8.

7. J. A. Lubbers, "Diagnostic suction curettage without anesthesia: An investigation into the practical usefulness of the Vabra aspirator," *ACTA Obstetricia et Gynecologica Scandinavica Supplement* (Number 62, 1977): 1–12.

8. Ibid.

9. N. C. Siddle et al., "A controlled trial of naproxen sodium for relief of pain associated with Vabra suction curettage," *British Journal of Obstetrics and Gynaecology* 90 (September 1983): 864–69.

10. T. J. Helmerhorst et al., "Endocervical curettage by Vabra aspiration as part of colposcopic evaluation," *Gynecologic Oncology* 36 (March 1990): 312–16.

11. A. M. Kaunitz et al., "Comparison of endometrial biopsy with the endometrial pipelle and Vabra aspirator," *Journal of Reproductive Medicine* 33 (May 1988): 427–31.

12. G. L. Goldberg, G. Tsalacopoulos, and D. A. Davey, "A

comparison of endometrial sampling with the Accurette and Vabra aspirator and uterine curettage," *South African Medical Journal* 61 (23 January 1982): 114–16.

13. S. Danero et al., "Critical review of dilatation and curettage in the diagnosis of malignant pathology of the endometrium," *European Journal of Gynaecologic Oncology* 7 (Number 3, 1986): 162–65.

14. R. J. Gimpelson and H. O. Rappold, "A comparative study between panoramic hysteroscopy with directed biopsies and dilatation and curettage," *American Journal of Obstetrics and Gynecology* 158 (March 1988): 489–92.

Bone Marrow Biopsy

1. W. D. James and R. B. Odom, "Graft-v-host disease," *Archives of Dermatology* 119 (August 1983): 683–89.

2. E. J. Kanfer, "Bone marrow transplantation: Current controversies," *Bone Marrow Transplant* 3 (September 1988): 501–8.

3. HealthCare Knowledge Resources/Commission on Professional and Hospital Activities, Ann Arbor, Mich. (*HealthWeek,* November 6, 1989).

4. B. M. Camitta et al., "Severe aplastic anemia: A prospective study of the effect of early marrow transplantation on acute mortality," *Blood* 48 (July 1976): 63–70.

5. E. D. Thomas, "Karnofsky Memorial Lecture: Marrow transplantation for malignant diseases," *Journal of Clinical Oncology* 1 (September 1983): 517–31.

6. H. L. Seewann, "Jamshidi biopsy in clinical hematology: Method, indications and results of over 1,000 completed biopsies with special reference to chronic myeloproliferative diseases," *Wiener Medizinische Wochenschrift Supplement* 100 (1986): 1–24. (Published in German)

7. W. E. Stamm et al., "Infection due to *Corynebacterium* species in marrow transplant patients," *Annals of Internal Medicine* 91 (August 1979): 167–73.

8. K. M. Sullivan, "Immunoglobulin therapy in bone marrow transplantation," *American Journal of Medicine* 83 (October 1987): 34–45.

9. T. Hays, P. A. Lane, Jr., and F. Shafer, "Transient erythroblastopenia of childhood. A review of 26 cases and reassessment of indications for bone marrow aspiration," *American Journal of Diseases of Children* 143 (May 1989): 605–7.

Combined Right and Left Cardiac Catheterization

1. V. Fuster et al., "Atherosclerotic plaque rupture and thrombosis: Evolving concepts," *Circulation* 82 (September 1990, Supplement): II47–59.

2. R. W. Wissler and D. Vesselinovitch, "An update on the pathogenesis of atherosclerosis: Principles of prevention, intervention, retardation, and regression," *Hawaiian Medical Journal* 49 (July 1990): 237–40, 261.

3. M. Marzilli et al., "Some clinical considerations regarding the relation of coronary vasospasm to coronary atherosclerosis: A hypothetical pathogenesis," *American Journal of Cardiology* 45 (April 1980): 882–86.

4. W. B. Kannel, W. P. Castelli, and T. Gordon, "Cholesterol in the prediction of atherosclerotic disease: New perspectives based on the Framingham study," *Annals of Internal Medicine* 90 (January 1979): 85–91.

5. D. Levy, "Left ventricular hypertrophy: Epidemiological insights from the Framingham Heart Study," *Drugs* 5 (1988, Supplement): 1–5.

6. R. E. Vlietstra et al., "Effect of cigarette smoking on survival of patients with angiographically documented coronary artery disease: Report from the CASS registry," *Journal of the American Medical Association* 255 (28 February 1986): 1023–27.

7. P. M. Cinciripini, "Cognitive stress and cardiovascular reactivity. II. Relationship to atherosclerosis, arrhythmias, and cognitive control," *American Heart Journal* 112 (November 1986): 1051–65.

8. P. D. Hirsh et al., "Prostaglandins and ischemic heart disease," *American Journal of Medicine* 71 (December 1981): 1009–26.

9. A. Rozanski, D. S. Krantz, and C. N. Bairey, "Ventricular responses to mental stress testing in patients with coronary artery disease: Pathophysiological implications," *Circulation* 83 (April 1991, Supplement): II137–44.

10. R. S. Eliot et al., "Influence of environmental stress on pathogenesis of sudden cardiac death," *Federation Proceedings* 36 (April 1977): 1719–24.

11. R. S. Eliot and J. C. Buell, "Role of emotions and stress in the genesis of sudden death," *Journal of the American College of Cardiology* 5 (June 1985, Supplement): 95B–98B.

12. B. Dorian and C. B. Taylor, "Stress factors in the devel-

opment of coronary artery disease," *Journal of Occupational Medicine* 26 (October 1984): 747–56.

13. A. P. Goldberg, "Aerobic and resistive exercise modify risk factors for coronary heart disease," *Medicine and Science in Sports and Exercise* 21 (December 1989): 669–74.

14. J. M. Morgan et al., "Left heart catheterization by direct ventricular puncture: Withstanding the test of time," *Catheterization and Cardiovascular Diagnosis* 15 (February 1989): 87–90.

15. J. V. Kelly and F. J. Hellinger, "Heart disease and hospital deaths: An empirical study," *Health Services Research* 22 (August 1987): 369–95.

16. D. F. Adams and H. L. Abrams, "Complications of coronary arteriography: A follow-up report," *Cardiovascular Radiology* 2 (27 April 1979): 89–96.

17. P. R. Mahrer and N. Eshoo, "Outpatient cardiac catheterization and coronary angiography," *Catheterization and Cardiovascular Diagnosis* 7 (Number 4, 1981): 355–60.

18. C. E. Hansing et al., "Cardiac catheterization experience in hospitals without cardiovascular surgery programs," *Catheterization and Cardiovascular Diagnosis* 3 (Number 3, 1977): 207–14.

19. M. N. Jackson, "Cardiac catheterization in a freestanding setting," *Health Technology Assessment Reports* (Number 6, 1989): 1–8.

20. J. W. Kennedy et al., "Mortality related to cardiac catheterization and angiography," *Catheterization and Cardiovascular Diagnosis* 8 (Number 4, 1982): 323–40.

21. C. H. Croft and K. Lipscomb, "Modified technique of transseptal left heart catheterization," *Journal of the American College of Cardiology* 5 (April 1985): 904–10.

22. E. C. Lozner et al., "Coronary arteriography 1984–1987: A report of the Registry of the Society for Cardiac Angiography and Interventions," *Catheterization and Cardiovascular Diagnosis* 17 (May 1989): 11–14.

23. B. C. Morton and D. S. Beanlands, "Complications of cardiac catheterization: One centre's experience," *Canadian Medical Association Journal* 131 (15 October 1984): 889–92.

24. Kennedy et al., "Mortality related to cardiac catheterization and angiography," *Catheterization and Cardiovascular Diagnosis* 1 (Number 3, 1975): 323–40.

25. A. Rashid et al., "Coronary arteriography: Prevention of thromboembolic complications using a pressure-drip flushing technique," *Catheterization and Cardiovascular Diagnosis* 1 (Number 3, 1975): 283–91.

26. C. E. Hansing, "The risk and cost of coronary angiography. II. The risk of coronary angiography in Washington State," *Journal of the American Medical Association* 242 (24 August 1979): 735–38.

27. E. D. Folland et al., "Complications of cardiac catheterization and angiography in patients with valvular heart disease," *Catheterization and Cardiovascular Diagnosis* 17 (May 1989): 15–21.

28. J. Gwost et al., "Analysis of the complications of cardiac catheterization over nine years," *Catheterization and Cardiovascular Diagnosis* 8 (Number 1, 1982): 13–21.

29. C. J. Porter et al., "Cardiac catheterization in the neonate: A comparison of three techniques," *Journal of Pediatrics* 93 (July 1978): 97–101.

30. A. Bernard et al., "Analysis of the complications of coronarography: Apropos of a series of 2,300 consecutive tests," *Journal de Radiologie* 68 (May 1987): 353–60. (Published in French)

31. L. W. Johnson et al., "Coronary arteriography 1984–1987: A report of the Registry of the Society for Cardiac Angiography and Interventions. I. Results and complications," *Catheterization and Cardiovascular Diagnosis* 17 (May 1989): 5–10.

32. H. E. Cohn et al., "Complications and mortality associated with cardiac catheterization in infants under one year: A prospective study," *Pediatric Cardiology* 6 (Number 3, 1985): 123–31.

33. D. G. Human, I. D. Hill, and C. B. Fraser, "Critical congenital heart disease," *South African Medical Journal* 65 (16 June 1984): 958–60.

34. W. Gross-Fengels et al., "Complications of intravenous digital subtraction angiography—results in 500 patients," *Rontgenblatter* 40 (September 1987): 281–85. (Published in German)

35. D. Pelz, A. J. Fox, and F. Vinuela, "Clinical trial of Iohexol vs. Conray 60 for cerebral angiography," *American Journal of Nuclear Radiology* 5 (September–October 1984): 565–68.

36. T. Khalikov, A. F. Tsyb, and T. V. Oliper, "Cerebral complications of cervical angiography," *Vopr Neirokhir* (January-February 1976): 47–52. (Published in Russian)

37. J. Jamie Caro, Evelinda Trindade, and Maurice McGregor, "The risks of death and of severe nonfatal reactions with high- and low-osmolality contrast media: A meta-analysis," *American Journal of Roentgenology, Radium Therapy and Nuclear* 156 (April 1991): 825–32.

38. S. A. Schroeder, K. I. Marton, and B. L. Strom, "Fre-

quency and morbidity of invasive procedures: Report of a pilot study from two teaching hospitals," *Archives of Internal Medicine* 138 (December 1978): 1809–11.

39. K. G. Oldroyd et al., "Cardiac catheterization by the Judkins technique as an outpatient procedure," *British Medical Journal* 298 (1 April 1989): 875–76.

40. Folland et al., "Complications of cardiac catheterization and angiography in patients with valvular heart disease," 15–21.

41. Hansing, "The risk and cost of coronary angiography. II. The risk of coronary angiography in Washington State," 735–38.

42. S. Pink, L. Fiutowski, and R. E. Gianelly, "Outpatient cardiac catheterizations: Analysis of patients requiring admission," *Clinical Cardiology* 12 (July 1989): 375–78.

43. Rashid et al., "Coronary arteriography: Prevention of thromboembolic complications using a pressure-drip flushing technique," 283–91.

44. J. T. Stewart et al., "Major complications of coronary arteriography: The place of cardiac surgery," *British Heart Journal* 63 (February 1990): 74–77.

45. Morton and Beanlands, "Complications of cardiac catheterization: One centre's experience," 889–92.

46. Ibid.

47. W. Gross-Fengels et al., "Complications of brachiocephalic catheter angiography using a non-ionic contrast medium," *Radiologe* 27 (February 1987): 83–88. (Published in German)

48. M. R. Nicholson et al., "Fatal atheromatous embolization during coronary angiography," *Cardiovascular Interventional Radiology* 5 (Number 3–4, 1982): 174–76.

49. V. M. Walley et al., "Death at cardiac catheterization: Coronary artery embolization of calcium debris from Ionescu-Shiley bioprosthesis," *Catheterization and Cardiovascular Diagnosis* 21 (October 1990): 92–94.

50. J. S. Ladowski and R. L. Hardesty, "Repair of an iatrogenic aortoatrial fistula," *Catheterization and Cardiovascular Diagnosis* 10 (Number 1, 1984): 43–46.

51. Croft and Lipscomb, "Modified technique of transseptal left heart catheterization," 904–10.

52. H. C. Redman, "The Budd-Chiari syndrome: Angiography and its complications," *Journal of the Canadian Association of Radiologists* 26 (December 1975): 271–8.

53. E. J. Andrews, Jr., "The vagus reaction as a possible cause of severe complications of radiological procedures," *Radiology* 121 (October 1976): 1–4.

54. C. L. Anthony et al., "A double-blind randomized clinical study of the safety, tolerability and efficacy of Hexabrix in pediatric angiocardiography," *Investigative Radiology* 19 (November–December 1984, Supplement): S335–43.

55. M. Sovak, C. A. Halkovich, and S. J. Foster, "Current contrast media and ioxilan. Comparative evaluation of vascular pain by aversion conditioning," *Investigative Radiology* 23 (September 1988, Supplement): S84–87.

56. B. Hagen et al., "Experimental evaluation of radiographic contrast media in perivascular pain receptors in the perfused isolated rabbit ear," *Fortschritte auf dem Gebiete der Rontgenstrahlen und der Nuklearmed Erganzungsband* 128 (1989): 46–53. (Published in German)

57. B. Hagen, "Systematic and local reactions during phlebography of the leg with special reference to postphlebographic complications. Randomized, prospective, intraindividual double-blind study of iopamidol and ioxithalamate (250 mg I/ml) using the 125I-fibrinogen test: II," *Radiologe* 25 (June 1985): 260–64. (Published in German)

58. R. L. Feldman et al., "Contrast media-related complications during cardiac catheterization using Hexabrix or Renografin in high-risk patients," *American Journal of Cardiology* 61 (1 June 1988): 1334–37.

59. G. H. Whitehouse and S. L. Snowdon, "An assessment of iopamidol, a nonionic contrast medium, in aorto-femoral angiography," *Clinical Radiology* 33 (March 1982): 231–34.

60. E. W. Gertz et al., "Clinical superiority of a new nonionic contrast agent (iopamidol) for cardiac angiography," *Journal of the American College of Cardiology* 5 (February 1985): 250–58.

61. Redman, "The Budd-Chiari syndrome: Angiography and its complications," 271–78.

62. S. R. Mills et al., "The incidence, etiologies, and avoidance of complications of pulmonary angiography in a large series," *Radiology* 136 (August 1980): 295–99.

63. J. L. Mills et al., "Minimizing mortality and morbidity from iatrogenic arterial injuries: The need for early recognition and prompt repair," *Journal of Vascular Surgery* 4 (July 1986): 22–27.

64. G. Zocholl et al., "Inadequate configurational stability of a DSA pigtail catheter as a cause of complications. Case report and study of the mechanism," *Rofo Fortschritte auf dem Gebiete der Rontgenstrahlen und der* 146 (January 1987): 62–65. (Published in German)

65. Pelz, Fox, and Vinuela, "Clinical trial of Iohexol vs. Conray 60 for cerebral angiography," 565–68.

66. P. M. Schofield, "Follow-up study of morbidity in patients with angina pectoris and normal coronary angiograms and the value of investigation for esophageal dysfunction," *Angiology* 41 (April 1990): 286–96.

67. M. A. Krupp and M. J. Chatton, eds., *Current Medical Diagnosis and Treatment* (Los Altos, Calif.: Lange Medical Publishers, 1984), 211.

68. G. D. Plotnick et al., "Clinical indicators of left main coronary artery disease in unstable angina," *Annals of Internal Medicine* 91 (August 1979): 149–53.

10. P. G. Dalldorf et al., "Traumatic rupture of the aorta. Indications for aortography," *American Surgeon* 56 (August 1990): 500–503.

11. D. G. Marsh and J. T. Sturm, "Traumatic aortic rupture: Roentgenographic indications for angiography," *Annals of Thoracic Surgery* 21 (April 1976): 337–40.

12. S. R. Gundry et al., "Indications for aortography in blunt thoracic trauma: A reassessment," *Journal of Trauma* 22 (August 1982): 664–71.

13. S. H. Skotnicki et al., "Traumatic rupture of the thoracic aorta," *ACTA Chirurgica Belgica* 82 (September–October 1982): 485–91.

Contrast Aortogram

1. R. Takolander et al., "Fatal thrombo-embolic complications at aorto-femoral angiography," *ACTA Radiologica: Diagnosis* 26 (January–February 1985): 15–19.

2. G. W. Hartman et al., "Mortality during excretory urography: Mayo Clinic experience," *American Journal of Roentgenology, Radium Therapy and Nuclear* 139 (November 1982): 919–22.

3. M. O. Perry, "Spinal cord injury following aortorenal bypass," *Journal of Cardiovascular Surgery* 20 (May–June 1979): 260–64.

4. R. E. Latchaw et al., "Iohexol vs. metrizamide: Study of efficacy and morbidity in cervical myelography," *American Journal of Nuclear Radiology* 6 (November–December 1985): 931–33.

5. D. J. Sahn, et al., "Real-time cross-sectional echocardiographic diagnosis of coarctation of the aorta: A prospective study of echocardiographic-angiographic correlations," *Circulation* 56 (November 1977): 762–69.

6. W. H. Chow et al., "Two-dimensional and pulsed Doppler echocardiographic diagnosis of an acquired aortic right ventricular fistula," *Clinical Cardiology* 12 (September 1989): 544–45.

7. P. Probst et al., "Postoperative evaluation of composite aortic grafts: Comparison of angiography and CT," *British Journal of Radiology* 56 (November 1983): 797–804.

8. P. J. Strouse et al., "Aortic dissection presenting as spinal cord ischemia with a false-negative aortogram," *Cardiovascular and Interventional Radiology* 13 (April–May 1990): 77–82.

9. W. Auffermann et al., "MR imaging of complications of aortic surgery," *Journal of Computer Assisted Tomography* 11 (November–December 1987): 982–89.

Contrast Cerebral Arteriogram

1. D. P. Swanson et al., "Product selection criteria for intravascular ionic contrast media," *Clinical Pharmacy* 4 (September–October 1985): 527–38.

2. M. Ramirez-Lassepas et al., "Cervical myelopathy complicating cerebral angiography. Report of a case and review of the literature," *Neurology* 27 (September 1977): 834–37.

3. H. Vogel, "Radiation risks and gonadal exposure in radiodiagnosis," *Munchener Medizinische Wochenschrift* 121 (13 July 1979): 943–46. (Published in German)

4. P. R. Cooper, K. Maravilla, and J. Cone, "Computerized tomographic scan and gunshot wounds of the head: Indications and radiographic findings," *Neurosurgery* 4 (May 1979): 373–80.

5. E. J. Angtuaco and E. F. Binet, "High-resolution computed tomography in intracranial aneurysms," *Critical Reviews in Diagnostic Imaging* 25 (Number 2, 1986): 113–58.

6. R. F. Carmody and J. F. Seeger, "Intracranial applications of digital subtraction angiography," *Critical Reviews in Diagnostic Imaging* 23 (Number 1, 1984): 1–40.

7. J. E. McKittrick, J. Henrikson, and G. W. Iwasiuk, "Indications for contralateral carotid endarterectomy: Role of the noninvasive laboratory," *American Journal of Surgery* 140 (August 1980): 206–8.

8. J. Rohr, C. Hillion, and G. Gauthier, "Ultrasonic studies and indications for angiography. Comparative study of 547 carotid arteries," *Schweizer Archiv fur Neurologie und Psychiatrie* 137 (Number 2, 1986): 45–62. (Published in French)

9. A. L. Day, "Indications for surgical intervention in middle

cerebral artery obstruction," *Journal of Neurosurgery* 60 (February 1984): 296–304.

Contrast Phlebogram of the Leg

1. S. A. Schroeder et al., *Current Medical Diagnosis and Treatment* (Norwalk, Conn.: Appleton & Lange, 1991), 330–31.
2. U. Albrechtsson, "Side-effects at phlebography with ionized and nonionized contrast medium," *Diagnostic Imaging* 48 (Number 4, 1979): 236–40.
3. K. Reinhardt, "Formation of a large blister with subsequent necrosis of the skin following paravenous contrast medium injection at the dorsum of the foot in a patient with edema and deep phlebothrombosis," *Rontgenblatter* 32 (May 1979): 277–79. (Published in German)
4. Schroeder et al., *Current Medical Diagnosis and Treatment*, 331.
5. Ibid., 330.
6. Ibid., 331.

Cystoscopy

1. W. G. Guerriero, "Operative injury to the lower urinary tract," *Urologic Clinics of North America* 12 (May 1985): 339–48.
2. Ibid.
3. A. Mosbah et al., "Iatrogenic urethral strictures of the male urethra," *Acta Urologica Belgica* 58 (Number 3, 1990): 87–93. (Published in French)
4. C. L. Strand et al., "Nosocomial *Pseudomonas aeruginosa* urinary tract infections," *Journal of the American Medical Association* 248 (1 October 1982): 1615–18.
5. J. V. Ricos Torrent et al., "Incidence of vesico-ureteral reflux after endoscopic surgery of superficial tumors of the bladder. A prospective study," *Archivos Espanoles de Urologia* 43 (March 1990): 136–9. (Published in Spanish)
6. J. F. Gephart, "Endotoxin contamination of Foley catheters associated with fevers following transurethral resection of the prostate," *Infection Control* 5 (May 1984): 231–34.
7. C. Viville, R. de Petriconi, and L. Bietho, "Intravesical explosion during endoscopic resection," *Journal of Urology (Paris)* 90 (Number 5, 1984): 361–63. (Published in French)

8. A. Orandi and M. Orandi, "Urine cytology in the detection of bladder tumor recurrence," *Journal of Urology* 116 (November 1976): 568–69.
9. Mosbah et al., "Iatrogenic urethral strictures of the male urethra," 87–93.

Diagnostic Laparoscopy

1. I. Vido et al., "Diagnostic value of cytological investigations in metastatic tumours of the liver: Comparison of laparoscopy, histology, and cytology," *Deutsche Medizinische Wochenschrift* 100 (19 December 1975): 2602–4. (Published in German)
2. E. U. Snowden, J. C. Jarrett, 2d, and M. Y. Dawood, "Comparison of diagnostic accuracy of laparoscopy, hysteroscopy, and hysterosalpingography in evaluation of female infertility," *Fertility and Sterility* 41 (May 1984): 709–13.
3. J. A. Fayez, G. Mutie, and P. J. Schneider, "The diagnostic value of hysterosalpingography and laparoscopy in infertility investigation," *International Journal of Fertility* 33 (March–April 1988): 98–101.
4. D. H. Barad et al., "Gamete intrafallopian tube transfer (GIFT): Making laparoscopy more than 'diagnostic,'" *Fertility and Sterility* 50 (December 1988): 928–30.
5. P. R. Gindoff et al., "Efficacy of assisted reproductive technology during diagnostic and operative infertility laparoscopy," *Obstetrics and Gynecology* 75 (February 1990): 299–301.
6. C. M. Whitworth et al., "Value of diagnostic laparoscopy in young women with possible appendicitis," *Surgery, Gynecology and Obstetrics* 167 (September 1988): 187–90.
7. A. Abi Aad et al., "The value of laparoscopy in the diagnostic evaluation of cryptorchism with non-palpable testicles," *Acta Urologica Belgica* 58 (Number 2, 1990): 69–78. (Published in French)
8. K. A. Dugan, "Diagnostic laparoscopy under local anesthesia for evaluation of infertility," *Journal of Obstetric, Gynecologic and Neonatal Nursing* 14 (September–October 1985): 363–66.
9. D. Fermelia and G. Berci, "Diagnostic and therapeutic laparoscopy. An entity often overlooked by the surgeon," *Surgical Endoscopy* 1 (Number 2, 1987): 73–77.
10. D. A. van Lith, K. J. van Schie, and W. Beekhuizen, "Diagnostic miniculdoscopy preceding laparoscopy when

bowel adhesions are suspected," *Journal of Reproductive Medicine* 23 (August 1979): 87–90.

11. E. Wildhirt, "The diagnostic value of laparoscopy—A perspective study," *Tokai Journal of Experimental and Clinical Medicine* 6 (July 1981): 223–27.

12. P. C. De Groen et al., "Diagnostic laparoscopy in gastroenterology. A 14-year experience," *Digestive Diseases and Sciences* 32 (July 1987): 677–81.

13. M. G. Kane and G. J. Krejs, "Complications of diagnostic laparoscopy in Dallas: A 7-year prospective study," *Gastrointestinal Endoscopy* 30 (August 1984): 237–40.

14. J. Rattan et al., "Diagnostic gastrointestinal laparoscopy: Experience and changing indications," *Israel Journal of Medical Sciences* 23 (November 1987): 1132–36.

15. M. F. El-Minawi et al., "Physiologic changes during CO_2 and N_2O pneumoperitoneum in diagnostic laparoscopy. A comparative study," *Journal of Reproductive Medicine* 26 (July 1981): 338–46.

16. R. S. Phillips et al., "Experience with diagnostic laparoscopy in a hepatology training program," *Gastrointestinal Endoscopy* 33 (December 1987): 417–20.

17. Kane and Krejs, "Complications of diagnostic laparoscopy in Dallas: A 7-year prospective study," 237–40.

18. M. Sauer and J. C. Jarrett, 2d, "Small bowel obstruction following diagnostic laparoscopy," *Fertility and Sterility* 42 (October 1984): 653–54.

19. G. Sotrel, E. Hirsch, and K. C. Edelin, "Necrotizing fasciitis following diagnostic laparoscopy," *Obstetrics and Gynecology* 62 (September 1983, Supplement): 67s–69s.

20. U. M. Irsigler and J. V. van der Merwe, "Diagnostic laparoscopy v. combined screening laparoscopy and timed follicle aspiration for in vitro fertilization," *South African Medical Journal* 10 (January 1987): 20–22.

21. O. Ferret Maldonado, R. Bueno Bruzon, and R. Arendt, "Diagnostic reliability of emergency laparoscopy," *Deutsche Zeitschrift fur Verdauungs-Und Stoffwechselkrankheiten* 40 (Number 3–4, 1980): 119–25. (Published in German)

22. H. K. Ho, L. N. Sim, and L. K. Ho, "The diagnostic value of laparoscopy in women with pelvic pain," *Singapore Medical Journal* 30 (October 1989): 453–56.

Dilation and Curettage

1. R. J. Gimpelson and H. O. Rappold, "A comparative study between panoramic hysteroscopy with directed biopsies and dilatation and curettage. A review of 276 cases," *American Journal of Obstetrics and Gynecology* 158 (March 1988): 489–92.

2. M. E. Boyd, "Dilatation and curettage," *Canadian Journal of Surgery* 32 (January 1989): 9–13.

3. A. A. Hodari et al., "Dilatation and curettage for second-trimester abortions," *American Journal of Obstetrics and Gynecology* 127 (15 April 1977): 850–54.

4. I. Z. MacKenzie and J. G. Bibby, "Critical assessment of dilatation and curettage in 1029 women," *Lancet* 2 (9 September 1978): 566–68.

5. P. G. Brooks and S. P. Serden, "Hysteroscopic findings after unsuccessful dilatation and curettage for abnormal uterine bleeding," *American Journal of Obstetrics and Gynecology* 158 (June 1988): 1354–57.

6. J. R. Dingfelder et al., "Reduction of cervical resistance by prostaglandin suppositories prior to dilatation for induced abortion," *American Journal of Obstetrics and Gynecology* 122 (May 1975): 25–30.

7. W. Grunberger and P. Riss, "Cervical incompetence after previous cervical dilatation and curettage," *Wiener Medizinische Wochenschrift* 129 (15 July 1979): 390–92. (Published in German)

8. G. R. Struthers, D. L. Scott, and M. Farr, "Septic arthritis and thigh abscess after dilatation and curettage," *Clinical Rheumatology* 3 (March 1984): 71–73.

9. M. S. Beksac et al., "Stress-induced release of cortisol and prolactin during dilatation and curettage under general and local anesthesia," *Neuropsychobiology* 11 (Number 4, 1984): 227–28.

10. C. M. Sledmere et al., "Psychological aspects of Vabra curettage in menopause clinics," *Maturitas* 3 (December 1981): 205–13.

11. J. J. Smith and H. Schulman, "Current dilatation and curettage practice: A need for revision," *Obstetrics and Gynecology* 65 (April 1985): 516–18.

12. S. Danero et al., "Critical review of dilatation and curettage in the diagnosis of malignant pathology of the endometrium," *European Journal of Obstetrics, Gynecology, and Reproductive Biology* 7 (Number 3, 1986): 162–65.

13. Gimpelson and Rappold, "A comparative study between panoramic hysteroscopy with directed biopsies and dilatation and curettage," 489–92.

14. M. E. Boyd, "Dilatation and curettage," 9–13.

15. F. Hald et al., "Diagnostic accuracy of outpatient endocervical curettage using conventional and Vabra curettage of the cervix," *ACTA Obstetricia et Gynecologica Scandinavica* 67 (Number 1, 1988): 71–74.

16. S. Alberico et al., "Diagnostic validity of the Vabra Curettage. Compared study on 172 patients who underwent Vabra Curettage and the fractional curettage of the uterine cavity," *European Journal of Gynaecological Oncology* 7 (Number 2, 1986): 135–38.

17. J. A. Lubbers, "Diagnostic suction curettage without anesthesia. An investigation into the practical usefulness of the Vabra aspirator," *ACTA Obstetricia et Gynecologia Scandinavica* (1977 Supplement): 1–12.

18. Ibid.

19. N. C. Siddle et al., "A controlled trial of naproxen sodium for relief of pain associated with Vabra suction curettage," *British Journal of Obstetrics and Gynaecology* 90 (September 1983): 864–69.

20. T. J. Helmerhorst et al., "Endocervical curettage by Vabra aspiration as part of colposcopic evaluation," *Gynecologic Oncology* 36 (March 1990): 312–16.

21. A. M. Kaunitz et al., "Comparison of endometrial biopsy with the endometrial Pipelle and Vabra aspirator," *Journal of Reproductive Medicine* 33 (May 1988): 427–31.

22. G. L. Goldberg, G. Tsalacopoulos, and D. A. Davey, "A comparison of endometrial sampling with the Accurette and Vabra aspirator and uterine curettage," *South African Medical Journal* 61 (23 January 1982): 114–16.

Endoscopic Biopsy of the Bronchus

1. L. Hernandez Blasco et al., "Safety of the transbronchial biopsy in outpatients," *Chest* 99 (March 1991): 562–65.

Endoscopic Large Bowel Examination

1. N. W. Agrawal, K. Akdamar, and M. S. Litwin, "Postoperative adhesions causing colon obstruction," *American Surgeon* 50 (September 1984): 479–81.

2. P. Rutgeerts et al., "Natural history of recurrent Crohn's disease at the ileocolonic anastomosis after curative surgery," *Gut* 25 (June 1984): 665–72.

3. A. Montori et al., "Therapeutic colonoscopy," *Endoscopy* 8 (May 1977): 81–84.

4. A. Kappas et al., "Diagnosis of pseudomembranous colitis," *British Medical Journal* 1 (18 March 1978): 675–78.

5. A. Sugawara et al., "Clinical study of pseudomembranous colitis: A neurosurgical viewpoint," *No Shinkei Geka* 18 (September 1990): 807–12. (Published in Japanese)

6. D. C. Brewster et al., "Intestinal ischemia complicating abdominal aortic surgery," *Surgery* 109 (April 1991): 447–54.

7. F. Gabrielli, U. Ginanneschi, and F. M. Fazio, "Emergency situations in pathology of the left colon: Validity of fibrosigmoidoscopy in differential diagnosis," *Chirurgia Italiana* 35 (October 1983): 733–41. (Published in Italian)

8. N. O. Aston, W. J. Owen, and J. D. Irving, "Endoscopic balloon dilatation of colonic anastomotic strictures," *British Journal of Surgery* 76 (August 1989): 780–82.

9. V. Pietropaolo et al., "Endoscopic dilation of colonic postoperative strictures," *Surgical Endoscopy* 4 (Number 1, 1990): 26–30.

10. S. Eidt and M. Stolte, "Gastric glandular cysts—investigations into their genesis and relationship to colorectal epithelial tumors," *Zeitschrift fur Gastroenterologie* 27 (April 1989): 212–17.

11. R. Ottenjann and B. Wormann, "Multiple colorectal polyps and risk of cancer," *Deutsche Medizinische Wochenschrift* 110 (6 December 1985): 1879–82. (Published in German)

12. "Future requirements for colonoscopy in Britain. Report by the Endoscopy Section Committee of the British Society of Gastroenterology," *Gut* 28 (June 1987): 772–75.

13. W. Matek et al., "Initial experience with the new electronic endoscope," *Endoscopy* 16 (January 1984): 20–21.

14. R. G. Norfleet, "Colonoscopy and polypectomy in nonhospitalized patients," *Gastrointestinal Endoscopy* 28 (February 1982): 15–16.

15. R. C. Haggitt et al., "Prognostic factors in colorectal carcinomas arising in adenomas: Implications for lesions removed by endoscopic polypectomy," *Gastroenterology* 89 (August 1985): 328–36.

16. J. Nevoral et al., "Endoscopic colorectal polypectomy in children and adolescents," *Ceskoslovenska Pediatrie* 45 (June 1990): 347–49. (Published in Czech)

17. R. Hesterberg et al., "Endoscopic resection of colorectal polyps," *Deutsche Medizinische Wochenschrift* 112 (6 February 1987): 210–13. (Published in German)

18. F. A. Macrae, K. G. Tan, and C. B. Williams, "Towards safer colonoscopy: A report on the complications of 5,000 diagnostic or therapeutic colonoscopies," *Gut* 24 (May 1983): 376–83.

19. P. Fruhmorgen and L. Demling, "Complications of diagnostic and therapeutic colonoscopy in the Federal Republic of Germany. Results of an inquiry," *Endoscopy* 11 (May 1979): 146–50.

20. F. J. Theuerkauf, Jr., "Colonoscopy and polypectomy," *American Surgeon* 42 (January 1976): 33–43.

21. L. E. Smith, "Fiberoptic colonoscopy: Complications of colonoscopy and polypectomy," *Diseases of the Colon and Rectum* 19 (July–August 1976): 407–12.

22. S. E. Silvis et al., "Endoscopic complications. Results of the 1974 American Society for Gastrointestinal Endoscopy Survey," *Journal of the American Medical Association* 235 (1 March 1976): 928–30.

23. B. Ostyn et al., "Retroperitoneal abscess complicating colonoscopy polypectomy," *Diseases of the Colon and Rectum* 30 (March 1987): 201–3.

24. S. Nivatvongs, "Complications in colonoscopic polypectomy. An experience with 1,555 polypectomies," *Diseases of the Colon and Rectum* 29 (December 1986): 825–30.

25. P. Fric et al., "Therapeutic methods of digestive endoscopy in persons of advanced age," *Czechoslovak Medicine* 13 (Number 2–3, 1990): 45–51.

26. W. H. Isbister, "Colorectal polyps: An endoscopic experience," *Australian and New Zealand Journal of Surgery* 56 (September 1986): 717–22.

27. W. E. Strodel et al., "Therapeutic and diagnostic colonoscopy in nonobstructive colonic dilatation," *Annals of Surgery* 197 (April 1983): 416–21.

28. Hesterberg et al., "Endoscopic resection of colorectal polyps," 210–13.

29. G. Jimenez Mesa et al., "Endoscopic polypectomy of the colon in children," *Acta Gastroenterologica Latinoamericana* 15 (Number 4, 1985): 221–24. (Published in Spanish)

30. R. Holtzman et al., "Repeat colonoscopy after endoscopic polypectomy," *Diseases of the Colon and Rectum* 30 (March 1987): 185–88.

31. Hesterberg et al., "Endoscopic resection of colorectal polyps," 210–13.

32. K. Nagasako, "Endoscopic diagnosis of early colon cancer," *Gan No Rinsho* 34 (August 1988): 1326–32. (Published in Japanese)

33. T. Muto et al., "Endoscopic diagnosis and management of colonic polyps," *Gan To Kagaku Ryoho* 13 (July 1986): 2273–81. (Published in Japanese)

34. G. Hoff and M. Vatn, "Epidemiology of polyps in the rectum and sigmoid colon. Endoscopic evaluation of size and localization of polyps," *Scandinavian Journal of Gastroenterology* 20 (April 1985): 356–60.

35. D. E. Low et al., "Prospective assessment of risk of bacteremia with colonoscopy and polypectomy," *Digestive Diseases and Sciences* 32 (November 1987): 1239–43.

36. C. I. Bartram and M. A. Hall-Craggs, "Interventional colorectal endoscopic procedures: Residual lesions on follow-up double-contrast barium enema study," *Radiology* 162 (March 1987): 835–38.

37. D. D. Wadas and R. A. Sanowski, "Complications of the hot biopsy forceps technique," *Gastrointestinal Endoscopy* 34 (January–February 1988): 32–37.

38. J. P. Christie, "Malignant colon polyps—cure by colonoscopy or colectomy?" *American Journal of Gastroenterology* 79 (July 1984): 543–47.

39. E. J. Gyorffy et al., "Large colorectal polyps: Colonoscopy, pathology, and management," *American Journal of Gastroenterology* 84 (August 1989): 898–905.

40. I. K. Woolfson et al., "Usefulness of performing colonoscopy one year after endoscopic polypectomy," *Diseases of the Colon and Rectum* 33 (May 1990): 389–93.

41. P. Barillari et al., "Effect of preoperative colonoscopy on the incidence of synchronous and metachronous neoplasms," *ACTA Chirurgica Scandinavica* 156 (February 1990): 163–66.

42. Hesterberg et al., "Endoscopic resection of colorectal polyps," 210–13.

43. C. B. Williams, J. E. Whiteway, and J. R. Jass, "Practical aspects of endoscopic management of malignant polyps," *Endoscopy* 19 (November 1987, Supplement): 31–37.

44. A. Gaugg, "Limits of endoscopic polypectomy," *Wiener Medizinische Wochenschrift* 138 (15 July 1988): 331–32. (Published in German)

45. Haggitt et al., "Prognostic factors in colorectal carcinomas arising in adenomas," 328–36.

46. A. R. Rosseland, A. Bakka, and O. Reiertsen, "Endoscopic treatment of colorectal carcinoma," *Scandinavian Journal of Gastroenterology Supplement* 149 (1988): 102–5.

47. C. Fucini, B. G. Wolff, and R. J. Spencer, "An appraisal of endoscopic removal of malignant colonic polyps," *Mayo Clinic Proceedings* 61 (February 1986): 123–26.

48. V. D. Fedorov et al., "Results of the removal of malignant colonic polyps," *Endoscopy* 18 (July 1986): 138–41.

49. M. Jung et al., Endoscopic and surgical therapy of malignant colorectal polyps," *Zeitschrift fur Gastroenterologie* 26 (March 1988): 179–84. (Published in German)

50. T. Van Wymersch et al., "Risk of recurrence of colorectal polyps following endoscopic resection," *Acta Gastroenterologica Belgica* 51 (July–October 1989): 391–96. (Published in French)

51. V. P. Strekalovskii and G. N. Emukhvari, "Long-term results of endoscopic polypectomy of the colon," *Khirurgiia (Mosk)* (February 1989): 59–62. (Published in Russian)

52. C. Barthelemy et al., "Endoscopic excision of malignant colorectal polyps. Study of a series of 82 cases," *Annales de Gastroenterologie et D Hepatologie (Paris)* 22 (January–February 1986): 5–8. (Published in French)

53. A. Rasinski et al., "Fiber-optic endoscopy of the lower gastrointestinal tract in children," *Pediatria Polska* 64 (May 1989): 281–87. (Published in Polish)

Endoscopic Lung Biopsy

1. A. Overlack et al., "Bronchography during flexible bronchoscopy. Indications and results in bronchiectasis," *Deutsche Medizinische Wochenschrift* 112 (10 July 1987): 1126–29. (Published in German)

2. A. Jover et al., "Bronchial fibroscopy. Indications and results," *Poumon et le Coeur* 34 (Number 4, 1978): 283–90. (Published in French)

3. P. A. Willcox and S. R. Benatar, "Use of the flexible fibre-optic bronchoscope in the diagnosis of lung carcinoma," *South African Medical Journal* 21 (21 May 1983): 799–801.

4. A. M. Barr and F. L. Kurer, "General anaesthesia for transbronchial lung biopsy," *Anaesthesia* 39 (August 1984): 822–25.

5. J. E. Duckett et al., "General anaesthesia for Nd:YAG laser resection of obstructing endobronchial tumours using the rigid bronchoscope," *Canadian Anaesthetists Society Journal* 32 (January 1985): 67–72.

6. H. Hildmann, "Removal of foreign bodies from the trachea. Indications for tracheobronchoscopy with a rigid instrument," *HNO* 38 (October 1990): 382–84. (Published in German)

7. R. G. Vanderschueren and C. J. Westermann, "Complications of endobronchial neodymium-Yag (Nd:Yag) laser application," *Lung* 168 (Supplement, 1990): 1089–94.

8. R. F. Ward, J. E. Arnold, and G. B. Healy, "Flexible minibronchoscopy in children," *Annals of Otology, Rhinology and Laryngology* 96 (November–December 1987): 645–49.

9. B. Strauss et al., "Complications in endoscopic and endoscopic biopsy studies—analysis of a one-year patient sample," *Zeitschrift fur Erkrankungen der Atmungsorgane* 170 (Number 2, 1988): 140–47. (Published in German)

10. P. M. Suratt, J. F. Smiddy, and B. Gruber, "Deaths and complications associated with fiberoptic bronchoscopy," *Chest* 69 (June 1976): 747–51.

11. D. B. Groff, H. S. Nagaraj, and J. S. Janik, "Bronchoscopy in childhood," *Journal of Pediatric Surgery* 16 (August 1981, Supplement): 627–30.

12. A. M. Barr and F. L. Kurer, "General anaesthesia for trans-bronchial lung biopsy," *Anaesthesia* 39 (August 1984): 822–25.

13. I. D. Conacher, M. L. Paes, and G. N. Morritt, "Carbon dioxide laser bronchoscopy. A review of problems and complications," *Anaesthesia* 42 (May 1987): 511–18.

14. F. Konrad et al., "Monitoring of bronchoscopy in artificially ventilated patients using peripheral pulse oximetry—a useful monitoring method?" *Anasthesie, Intensivtherapie, Notfallmedizin* 23 (August 1988): 205–8. (Published in German)

15. G. Kessler, A. Rauchfuss, and C. Werner, "Pulse oximetry in surgery of the bronchial system," *HNO* 37 (May 1989): 216–19. (Published in German)

16. L. L. Schulman et al., "Utility of airway endoscopy in the diagnosis of respiratory complications of cardiac transplantation," *Chest* 93 (May 1988): 960–67.

17. D. Weiland et al., "Aspergillosis in 25 renal transplant patients. Epidemiology, clinical presentation, diagnosis, and

management," *Annals of Surgery* 198 (November 1983): 622–29.

18. F. R. Cockerill, 3d, et al., "Open lung biopsy in immunocompromised patients," *Archives of Internal Medicine* 145 (August 1985): 1398–1404.

19. C. L. Snyder et al., "Diagnostic open-lung biopsy after bone marrow transplantation," *Journal of Pediatric Surgery* 25 (August 1990): 871–76.

20. C. Personne et al., "Indications and technique for endoscopic laser resections in bronchology. A critical analysis based upon 2,284 resections," *Journal of Thoracic and Cardiovascular Surgery* 91 (May 1986): 710–15.

Esophagogastroduodenoscopy

1. D. A. Lieberman, C. K. Wuerker, and R. M. Katon, "Cardiopulmonary risk of esophagogastroduodenoscopy. Role of endoscope diameter and systemic sedation," *Gastroenterology* 88 (February 1985): 468–72.

2. F. Cosentino et al., "Alizapride versus placebo in premedication for esophagogastroduodenoscopy. Double-blind clinical study. Experimental research in vitro," *Minerva Dietologica E Gastroenterologica* 35 (January–March 1989): 35–37. (Published in Italian)

3. W. M. Rodney et al., "Esophagogastroduodenoscopy by family physicians," *Journal of the American Board of Family Practice* 3 (April–June 1990): 73–79.

4. Ibid.

5. J. Libor, G. Pocsai, and J. Ivanyi, "ECG studies during esophagogastroduodenoscopy," *Zeitschrift fur Gastroenterologie* 15 (May 1977): 293–99. (Published in German)

6. F. Cosentino et al., "Holter's ECG monitoring in esophagogastroduodenoscopy. Premedication with tiropramide," *Minerva Dietologica E. Gastroenterologica* 35 (January–March 1989): 31–34. (Published in Italian)

7. M. L. Beck, "Diagnostic tests: Preparing your patient psychologically for an esophagogastroduodenoscopy," *Nursing* 11 (January 1981): 28–30.

8. A. Sagripanti et al., "Platelet activation in outpatients undergoing esophagogastroduodenoscopy," *Journal of Nuclear Medicine and Allied Sciences* 33 (January–March 1989): 22–25.

9. M. J. Gordon, "Transient submandibular swelling following esophagogastroduodenoscopy," *American Journal of Digestive Diseases* 21 (June 1976): 507–8.

10. G. C. Secchi et al., "Predictability of the anamnesis in pathology of the upper tract of the digestive system. Computerized analysis concerning 1000 subjects submitted to esophagogastroduodenoscopy," *Annali Italiani Di Medicina Interna* 4 (January–March 1989): 16–22. (Published in Italian)

11. R. McHenry et al., "The yield of routine duodenal aspiration for *Giardia lamblia* during esophagogastroduodenoscopy," *Gastrointestinal Endoscopy* 33 (December 1987): 425–26.

12. J. E. Geenen, "New diagnostic and treatment modalities involving endoscopic retrograde cholangiopancreatography and esophagogastroduodenoscopy," *Scandinavian Journal of Gastroenterology, Supplement* 77 (1982): 93–106.

13. R. A. Erickson and M. E. Glick, "Why have controlled trials failed to demonstrate a benefit of esophagogastroduodenoscopy in acute upper gastrointestinal bleeding? A probability model analysis," *Digestive Diseases and Sciences* 31 (July 1986): 760–68.

14. G. C. Vitale et al., "A computerized 24-hour ambulatory esophageal pH monitoring and esophagogastroduodenoscopy in the reflux patient. A comparative study," *Annals of Surgery* 200 (December 1984): 724–28.

Exploratory Laparotomy

1. D. D. Coker et al., "Restaging laparotomy for Hodgkin's disease," *Annals of Surgery* 197 (January 1983): 79–83.

2. B. Neidhardt et al., "Exploratory laparotomy and splenectomy in lymphogranulomatosis," *Deutsche Medizinische Wochenschrift* 100 (11 July 1975): 1487–92. (Published in German)

3. H. Tera and C. Aberg, "Mortality after laparotomy. A 10-year series," *ACTA Chirurgica Scandinavica* 142 (Number 1, 1976): 67–72.

4. S. E. Ross and P. D. Morehouse, "Urgent and emergent re-laparotomy in trauma. A preventable cause of increased mortality?" *American Surgeon* 52 (June 1986): 308–11.

5. T. J. Bunt, "Non-directed relaparotomy for intraabdominal sepsis. A futile procedure," *American Surgeon* 52 (June 1986): 294–98.

6. D. V. Feliciano et al., "Abdominal gunshot wounds. An

urban trauma center's experience with 300 consecutive patients," *Annals of Surgery* 208 (September 1988): 362–70.

7. P. J. Harbrecht, R. N. Garrison, and D. E. Fry, "Role of infection in increased mortality associated with age in laparotomy," *American Surgeon* 49 (April 1983): 173–78.

8. J. A. Butler, J. Huang, and S. E. Wilson, "Repeated laparotomy for postoperative intra-abdominal sepsis. An analysis of outcome predictors," *Archives of Surgery* 122 (June 1987): 702–6.

9. C. J. Rutherford et al., "The decision to perform staging laparotomy in symptomatic Hodgkin's disease," *British Journal of Haematology* 44 (March 1980): 347–58.

10. Neidhardt et al., "Exploratory laparotomy and splenectomy in lymphogranulomatosis," 1487–92.

11. M. H. Torosian and A. D. Turnbull, "Emergency laparotomy for spontaneous intestinal and colonic perforations in cancer patients receiving corticosteroids and chemotherapy," *Journal of Clinical Oncology* 6 (February 1988): 291–96.

12. P. Powell-Jackson, B. Greenway, and R. Williams, "Adverse effects of exploratory laparotomy in patients with unsuspected liver disease," *British Journal of Surgery* 69 (August 1982): 449–51.

13. H. Tera and C. Aberg, "Relaparotomy. A ten-year series," *ACTA Chirurgica Scandinavica* 141 (Number 7, 1975): 637–44.

14. J. P. Cederna et al., "Necrotizing fasciitis of the total abdominal wall after sterilization by partial salpingectomy. Case report and review of literature," *American Journal of Obstetrics and Gynecology* 163 (July 1990): 138–39.

15. Neidhardt et al., "Exploratory laparotomy and splenectomy in lymphogranulomatosis," 1487–92.

16. F. R. Sutherland et al., "Predicting the outcome of exploratory laparotomy in ICU patients with sepsis or organ failure," *Journal of Trauma* 29 (February 1989): 152–57.

Fetal Electrocardiogram (EKG)

1. C. Tchobroutsky, "Obstetric management and delivery in diabetics," *Diabete et Metabolisme* 16 (Number 2, 1990): 125–30. (Published in French)

2. J. A. Crowhurst, R. W. Burgess, and R. J. Derham, "Monitoring epidural analgesia in the parturient," *Anaethesia and Intensive Care* 18 (August 1990): 308–13.

3. J. Y. Col, "Fetal bradycardia caused by arrhythmia. Apropos of a case of blocked staggered atrial extrasystole," *Journal de Gynecologie, Obstetrique et Biologie Reproduction (Paris)* 18 (Number 6, 1989): 777–84. (Published in French)

4. W. Stoll, "Indications for cesarean section," *Schweizerische Medizinische Wochenschrift* 128 (24 February 1990): 255–59. (Published in German)

5. J. Heinrich and D. Radmann, "Diagnosis of biophysical status in pregnancy," *Zentralblatt Fur Gynakologie* 110 (Number 24, 1988): 1537–45. (Published in German)

6. G. H. Visser, D. J. Bekedam, and L. S. Ribbert, "Changes in antepartum heart rate patterns with progressive deterioration of the fetal condition," *International Journal of Biomedical Computing* 25 (May 1990): 239–46.

7. L. D. Devoe, "The nonstress test," *Obstetrics and Gynecology Clinics of North America* 17 (March 1990): 111–28.

8. V. K. Iyer, Y. Ploysongsang, and P. A. Ramamoorthy, "Adaptive filtering in biological signal processing," *Critical Reviews in Biomedical Engineering* 17 (Number 6, 1990): 531–84.

9. *Stedman's Medical Dictionary,* 25th ed. (Baltimore: Williams and Wilkins, 1990), 154.

10. H. F. Sandmire, "Whither electronic fetal monitoring?" *Obstetrics and Gynecology* 76 (December 1990): 1130–34.

11. J. M. Grant, "The fetal heart rate trace is normal, isn't it? Observer agreement of categorical assessments," *Lancet* 337 (26 January 1991): 215–18.

12. R. Gagnon, "Acoustic stimulation: Effect on heart rate and other biophysical variables," *Clinics in Perinatology* 16 (September 1989): 643–60.

Fetal Monitoring

1. C. Tchobroutsky, "Obstetric management and delivery in diabetics," *Diabete et Metabolisme* 16 (Number 2, 1990): 125–30. (Published in French)

2. J. A. Low, "The current status of maternal and fetal blood flow velocimetry," *American Journal of Obstetrics and Gynecology* 164 (April 1991): 1049–63.

3. P. Jouppila, "Doppler findings in the fetal and uteroplacental circulation: A promising guide to clinical decisions," *Annals of Medicine* 22 (April 1990): 109–13.

4. J. A. Crowhurst, R. W. Burgess, and R. J. Derham, "Monitoring epidural analgesia in the parturient," *Anaesthesia and Intensive Care* 18 (August 1990): 308–13.

5. G. P. Becks and G. N. Burrow, "Thyroid disease and pregnancy," *Medical Clinics of North America* 75 (January 1991): 121–50.

6. D. A. Fyfe and C. H. Kline, "Fetal echocardiographic diagnosis of congenital heart disease," *Pediatric Clinics of North America* 37 (February 1990): 45–67.

7. J. D. Schulman, "Treatment of the embryo and the fetus in the first trimester: current status and future prospects," *American Journal of Medical Genetics* 35 (February 1990): 197–200.

8. Y. Tannirandorn and C. H. Rodeck, "New approaches in the treatment of haemolytic disease of the fetus," *Baillieres Clinical Haematology* 3 (April 1990): 289–320.

9. H. J. Finberg et al., "The biophysical profile. A literature review and reassessments of its usefulness in the evaluation of fetal well-being," *Journal of Ultrasound in Medicine* 9 (October 1990): 583–91.

10. W. F. Rayburn, "Fetal body movement monitoring," *Obstetrics and Gynecology Clinics of North America* 17 (March 1990): 95–110.

11. F. Szanto and L. Kovacs, "Significance in unilateral intermittent breast stimulation in prenatal diagnosis," *Orvosi Hetilap* 132 (24 February 1991): 417–19. (Published in Hungarian)

12. R. Romero et al., "Sonographically monitored amniocentesis to decrease intraoperative complications," *Obstetrics and Gynecology* 65 (March 1985): 426–30.

13. T. H. Hasaart and G. G. Essed, "Amniotic fluid embolism after transabdominal amniocentesis," *European Journal of Obstetrics, Gynecology, and Reproductive Biology* 16 (September 1983): 25–30.

Fiber-Optic Bronchoscopy

1. R. S. Snell, *Clinical Anatomy for Medical Students,* 3rd ed., (Boston: Little, Brown, and Company, 1986), 136.

2. S. B. Fitzpatrick et al., "Indications for flexible fiberoptic bronchoscopy in pediatric patients," *American Journal of Diseases of Children* 137 (June 1983): 595–97.

3. R. Kurzrock et al., "Mycobacterial pulmonary infections after allogeneic bone marrow transplantation," *American Journal of Medicine* 77 (July 1984): 35–40.

4. D. Emanuel et al., "Rapid immunodiagnosis of cytomegalovirus pneumonia by bronchoalveolar lavage using human and murine monoclonal antibodies," *Annals of Internal Medicine* 104 (April 1986): 476–81.

5. T. K. Choi et al., "Bronchoscopy and carcinoma of the esophagus. II. Carcinoma of the esophagus with tracheobronchial involvement," *American Journal of Surgery* 147 (June 1984): 760–62.

6. T. L. Gueldner and G. H. Lawrence, "Prognostic implications of bronchogenic carcinoma proven by bronchoscopic biopsy," *American Surgeon* 42 (July 1976): 503–6.

7. C. H. Van Meter, Jr., et al., "Tracheoplasty for congenital long-segment intrathoracic tracheal stenosis," *American Surgeon* 57 (March 1991): 157–60.

8. "Lung lobe torsion following lobectomy," *American Surgeon* 56 (October 1990): 639–42.

9. C. Mallios et al., "One lung high frequency ventilation for peroral sealing of bronchial stump fistulae," *Anaesthesia* 43 (May 1988): 409–10.

10. J. S. Reilly et al., "Liver transplants in children: Importance for the otolaryngologist," *Annals of Otology, Rhinology and Laryngology* 93 (September–October 1984): 494–97.

11. G. R. Kerby, G. Pierce, and W. E. Ruth, "Clinical experience with pleuroscopy utilizing the bronchofiberscope," *Annals of Otology, Rhinology, and Laryngology* 84 (September–October 1975): 602–6.

12. A. A. Garzon and A. Gourin, "Surgical management of massive hemoptysis. A ten-year experience," *Annals of Surgery* 187 (March 1978): 267–71.

13. V. Tsang and P. Goldstraw, "Endobronchial stenting for anastomotic stenosis after sleeve resection," *Annals of Thoracic Surgery* 48 (October 1989): 568–71.

14. A. Overlack et al., "Bronchography during flexible bronchoscopy. Indications and results in bronchiectasis," *Deutsche Medizinische Wochenschrift* 112 (10 July 1987): 1126–29. (Published in German)

15. A. Jover et al., "Bronchial fibroscopy. Indications and results," *Poumon et le Coeur* 34 (Number 4, 1978): 283–90. (Published in French)

16. P. A. Willcox and S. R. Benatar, "Use of the flexible fibreoptic bronchoscope in the diagnosis of lung carcinoma," *South African Medical Journal* 63 (21 May 1983): 799–801.

17. A. M. Barr and F. L. Kurer, "General anaesthesia for trans-bronchial lung biopsy," *Anaesthesia* 39 (August 1984): 822–25.

18. J. E. Duckett et al., "General anaesthesia for Nd:YAG laser resection of obstructing endobronchial tumours using

the rigid bronchoscope," *Canadian Anaesthetists Society Journal* 32 (January 1985): 67–72.

19. H. Hildmann, "Removal of foreign bodies from the trachea. Indications for tracheobronchoscopy with a rigid instrument," *HNO* 38 (October 1990): 382—84. (Published in German)

20. R. G. Vanderschueren and C. J. Westermann, "Complications of endobronchial neodymium-Yag (Nd:Yag) laser application," *Lung* 168 (Supplement, 1990): 1089–94.

21. R. F. Ward, J. E. Arnold, and G. B. Healy, "Flexible minibronchoscopy in children," *Annals of Otology, Rhinology, and Laryngology* 96 (November–December 1987): 645–49.

22. L. R. Joyner, Jr., et al., "Neodymium-YAG laser treatment of intrabronchial lesions. A new mapping technique via the flexible fiberoptic bronchoscope," *Chest* 87 (April 1985): 418–27.

23. G. G. De Vane, "Laser initiated endotracheal tube explosion," *Journal of the American Association of Nurse Anesthetists* 58 (June 1990): 188–92.

24. T. Peachey et al., "Systemic air embolism during laser bronchoscopy," *Anaesthesia* 43 (October 1988): 872–75.

25. J. F. Dumon et al., "Principles for safety in application of neodymium-YAG laser in bronchology," *Chest* 86 (August 1984): 163–68.

26. P. M. Suratt, J. F. Smiddy, and B. Gruber, "Deaths and complications associated with fiberoptic bronchoscopy," *Chest* 69 (June 1976): 747–51.

27. D. B. Groff, H. S. Nagaraj, and J. S. Janik, "Bronchoscopy in childhood," *Journal of Pediatric Surgery* 16 (August 1981, Supplement): 627–30.

28. R. B. McElvein and G. L. Zorn, Jr., "Indications, results, and complications of bronchoscopic carbon dioxide laser therapy," *Annals of Surgery* 199 (May 1984): 522–25.

29. A. Arabian and S. V. Spagnolo, "Laser therapy in patients with primary lung cancer," *Chest* 86 (October 1984): 519–23.

30. Fitzpatrick et al., "Indications for flexible fiberoptic bronchoscopy in pediatric patients," 595–97.

31. B. Fischer et al., "HIV-associated infections: Indications and importance of fiberoptic bronchoscopy," *Pneumologie* 44 (Supplement, 1990): 316–17. (Published in German)

32. Barr and Kurer, "General anaesthesia for trans-bronchial lung biopsy," 822–25.

33. I. D. Conacher, M. L. Paes, and G. N. Morritt, "Carbon dioxide laser bronchoscopy. A review of problems and complications," *Anaesthesia* 42 (May 1987): 511–18.

34. F. Konrad et al., "Monitoring of bronchoscopy in artificially ventilated patients using peripheral pulse oximetry—a useful monitoring method?" *Anasthesie, Intensivtherapie, Notfallmedizin* 23 (August 1988): 205–8. (Published in German)

35. G. Kessler, A. Rauchfuss, and C. Werner, "Pulse oximetry in surgery of the bronchial system," *HNO* 37 (May 1989): 216–19. (Published in German)

36. L. L. Schulman et al., "Utility of airway endoscopy in the diagnosis of respiratory complications of cardiac transplantation," *Chest* 93 (May 1988): 960–67.

37. G. G. De Vane, "Laser initiated endotracheal tube explosion," 188–92.

38. S. Krawtz et al., "Nd-YAG laser-induced endobronchial burn. Management and long-term follow-up," *Chest* 95 (April 1989): 916–18.

39. R. G. Hooper and F. N. Jackson, "Endobronchial electrocautery," *Chest* 87 (June 1985): 712–14.

40. D. Weiland et al., "Aspergillosis in 25 renal transplant patients. Epidemiology, clinical presentation, diagnosis, and management," *Annals of Surgery* 198 (November 1983): 622–29.

41. F. R. Cockerill, 3d, et al., "Open lung biopsy in immunocompromised patients," *Archives of Internal Medicine* 145 (August 1985): 1398–1404.

42. C. L. Snyder et al., "Diagnostic open-lung biopsy after bone marrow transplantation," *Journal of Pediatric Surgery* 25 (August 1990): 871–76.

43. C. Personne et al., "Indications and technique for endoscopic laser resections in bronchology. A critical analysis based upon 2,284 resections," *Journal of Thoracic and Cardiovascular Surgery* 91 (May 1986): 710–15.

Left Cardiac Catheterization

1. J. M. Morgan et al., "Left heart catheterization by direct ventricular puncture: Withstanding the test of time," *Catheterization and Cardiovascular Diagnosis* 16 (February 1989): 87–90.

Myelogram with Contrast Enhancement

1. F. Postacchini and M. Massobrio, "Outpatient lumbar myelography. Analysis of complications after myelography comparing outpatients with inpatients," *Spine* 10 (July–August 1985): 567–70.

2. *National Inpatient Profile, Diagnosis Volume 1989* (Ann Arbor, Mich.: HealthCare Knowledge Resources, 1990).

3. F. Postacchini and M. Massobrio, "Outpatient lumbar myelography," 567–70.

4. L. Carfagna et al., "Gaseous myelography. Accidents and complications. Case reports," *Minerva Anestesiologica* 45 (December 1979): 901–6. (Published in Italian)

5. F. Postacchini and M. Massobrio, "Outpatient lumbar myelography," 567–70.

6. K. Tallroth, "Metrizamide myelography in patients with iodine allergy or previous adverse reactions to iodinated contrast media," *Spine* 12 (July–August 1987): 574–76.

7. D. G. Potts, D. G. Gomez, and G. F. Abbott, "Possible causes of complications of myelography with water-soluble contrast medium," *Acta Radiologica Supplementum* 355 (1977): 390–402.

8. H. J. Robertson and R. D. Smith, "Cervical myelography: Survey of modes of practice and major complications," *Radiology* 174 (January 1990): 79–83.

9. I. O. Skalpe and P. Amundsen, "Lumbar radiculography with metrizamide. A nonionic water-soluble contrast medium," *Radiology* 115 (April 1975): 91–95.

10. J. C. Holder et al., "Iohexol lumbar myelography: Clinical study," *American Journal of Neuroradiology* 5 (July–August 1984): 399–402.

11. T. Hindmarsh et al., "Lumbar myelography with iohexol and metrizamide. A double-blind clinical trial," *ACTA Radiologica: Diagnosis* 25 (Number 5, 1984): 365–68.

12. J. Bohutova et al., "Some unusual complications of myelography and lumbosacral radiculography," *Diagnostic Imaging* 48 (Number 6, 1979): 320–25.

13. D. D. Shaw, T. Bach-Gansmo, and K. Dahlstrom, "Iohexol: Summary of North American and European clinical trials in adult lumbar, thoracic, and cervical myelography with a new nonionic contrast medium," *Investigative Radiology* 20 (January–February 1985, Supplement):S44–50.

14. A. Kuhner et al., "Lesions of the cauda equina after dimer-X myelography," *Neurochirurgia* 20 (November 1977): 216–21. (Published in German)

15. R. Bonneau and J. M. Morris, "Complications of water-soluble contrast lumbar myelography. Review of the literature and case report," *Spine* 3 (December 1978): 343–45.

16. P. Salenius and L. E. Laurent, "Results of operative treatment of lumbar disc herniation. A survey of 886 patients," *Acta Orthopaedica Scandinavica* 48 (Number 6, 1977): 630–34.

17. O. Troisier and D. Cypel, "Discography: An element of decision. Surgery versus chemonucleolysis," *Clinical Orthopedics and Related Research* (May 1986): 70–78.

18. T. J. Masaryk et al., "High-resolution MR imaging of sequestered lumbar intervertebral disks," *American Journal of Roentgenology* (May 1988).

Percutaneous Liver Biopsy

1. M. Mayer et al., "Is liver biopsy in gallbladder operations still indicated?" *Chirurg* 61 (August 1990): 592–94. (Published in German)

2. E. Moller and E. Wildhirt, "An unusual case of a fatal delayed hemorrhage following liver biopsy," *Acta Hepatosplenologica* 16 (July–August 1969): 265–68. (Published in German)

3. L. Greiner and F. H. Franken, "Sonographically assisted liver biopsy—replacement for blind needle biopsy?" *Deutsche Medizinische Wochenschrift* 108 (11 March 1983): 368–72. (Published in German)

Spinal Canal Exploration

1. L. H. Perling, J. P. Laurent, and W. R. Cheek, "Epidural hibernoma as a complication of corticosteroid treatment," *Journal of Neurosurgery* 69 (October 1988): 613–16.

2. J. P. Nguyen, M. Djindjian, and S. Badiane, "Vertebral hemangioma with neurologic signs. Clinical presentation, results of a survey by the French Society of Neurosurgery," *Neurochirurgie* 35 (Number 5, 1989): 270–74, 305–8. (Published in French)

3. B. S. Epstein, J. A. Epstein, and M. D. Jones, "Cervical

spinal stenosis," *Radiologic Clinics of North America* 15 (August 1977): 215–26.

4. A. Sances, Jr., et al., "The biomechanics of spinal injuries," *Critical Reviews in Biomedical Engineering* 11 (Number 1, 1984): 1–76.

5. M. Ericsson, G. Algers, and S. E. Schliamser, "Spinal epidural abscesses in adults: Review and report of iatrogenic cases," *Scandinavian Journal of Infectious Diseases* 22 (Number 3, 1990): 249–57.

6. P. K. Toshniwal and R. P. Glick, "Spinal epidural lipomatosis: Report of a case secondary to hypothyroidism and review of literature," *Journal of Neurology* 234 (April 1987): 172–76.

7. H. Verbiest, "Results of surgical treatment of idiopathic developmental stenosis of the lumbar vertebral canal. A review of twenty-seven years' experience," *Journal of Bone and Joint Surgery (British Volume)* 59 (May 1977): 181–88.

8. Ericsson, G. Algers, and Schliamser, "Spinal epidural abscesses in adults," 249–57.

9. R. Gershater and E. L. St. Louis, "Lumbar epidural venography. Review of 1,200 cases," *Radiology* 131 (May 1979): 409–21.

10. F. P. Gargano, "Transverse axial tomography of the spine," *CRC Critical Reviews in Clinical Radiology and Nuclear Medicine* 8 (December 1976): 279–328.

11. J. F. Cusick, "Pathophysiology and treatment of cervical spondylotic myelopathy," *Clinical Neurosurgery* 37 (1991): 661–81.

12. W. D. Tobler and S. Weil, "Epidural lipomatosis and renal transplantation," *Surgical Neurology* 29 (February 1988): 141–44.

Abdominal Aorta Resection and Replacement

1. R. P. Leather et al., "Comparative analysis of retroperitoneal and transperitoneal aortic replacement for aneurysm," *Surgery, Gynecology and Obstetrics* 168 (May 1989): 387–93.

2. T. Dueyama et al., "Clinical experience with PTFE graft replacement in the descending thoracic aorta," *International Angiology* 6 (July–September 1987): 243–46.

3. R. Waneck and P. Polterauer, "Sonographic studies of the aorta after prosthetic replacement," *Wiener Klinische Wochenschrift* 97 (15 March 1985): 274–82. (Published in German)

4. M. C. Oz et al., "Replacement of the abdominal aorta with a sutureless intraluminal ringed prosthesis," *American Journal of Surgery* 158 (August 1989): 121–26.

5. M. C. Oz et al., "Twelve-year experience with intraluminal sutureless ringed graft replacement of the descending thoracic and thoracoabdominal aorta," *Journal of Vascular Surgery* 11 (February 1990): 331–38.

6. J. Lavee et al., "Tube graft replacement of abdominal aortic aneurysm: Is concomitant iliac disease a contraindication?" *Journal of Cardiovascular Surgery* 29 (July–August 1988): 449–52.

7. J. Ennker et al., "Replacement of the infrarenal aorta in advanced age," *Langenbecks Archiv fur Chirurgie* 369 (1986): 345–48. (Published in German)

8. W. E. Walker et al., "The management of aortoduodenal fistula by in situ replacement of the infected abdominal aortic graft," *Annals of Surgery* 205 (June 1987): 727–32.

9. M. J. Jacobs et al., "In-situ replacement and extra-anatomic bypass for the treatment of infected abdominal aortic grafts," *European Journal of Vascular Surgery* 5 (February 1991): 83–86.

10. P. M. Spagna et al., "Rigid intraluminal prosthesis for replacement of thoracic and abdominal aorta," *Annals of Thoracic Surgery* 39 (January 1985): 47–52.

11. W. E. Evans and J. P. Hayes, "Tube graft replacement of abdominal aortic aneurysm," *American Journal of Surgery* 156 (August 1988): 119–21.

12. J. M. Thomas, N. J. Mortensen, and C. R. Bayliss, "Ureteric obstruction after Dacron vascular replacement," *Annals of the Royal College of Surgeons* 65 (November 1983): 385–88.

13. E. S. Crawford et al., "Aortic arch aneurysm. A sentinel of extensive aortic disease requiring subtotal and total aortic replacement," *Annals of Surgery* 199 (June 1984): 742–52.

14. E. S. Crawford et al., "Diffuse aneurysmal disease (chronic aortic dissection, Marfan, and mega aorta syndromes) and multiple aneurysm. Treatment by subtotal and total aortic replacement emphasizing the elephant trunk operation," *Annals of Surgery* 211 (May 1990): 521–37.

15. T. Yamada et al., "Reconstruction of radicular arteries in the total replacement of thoracoabdominal aorta," *Kyobu Geka* 43 (November 1990): 942–48. (Published in Japanese)

16. T. Kazui et al., "Total graft replacement of the thora-

coabdominal aorta with reconstruction of visceral branches, intercostal and lumbar arteries in expanding chronic dissecting aneurysms of the thoracoabdominal aorta," *Nippon Kyobu Geka Gakkai Zasshi* 37 (July 1989): 1436–40. (Published in Japanese)

Above-the-Knee Amputation

1. G. Kolde et al., "Kaposi-like acroangiodermatitis in an above-knee amputation stump," *British Journal of Dermatology* 120 (April 1989): 575–80.

2. E. L. Marin, S. S. Bifulco, and A. Fast, "Obesity. A risk factor for knee dislocation," *American Journal of Physical Medicine and Rehabilitation* 69 (June 1990): 132–34.

3. E. Markgraf, G. Clausner, and W. Lungershausen, "Traumatic vascular lesions of the knee joint," *Beitrage Zur Orthopadie und Traumatologie* 36 (September 1989): 401–11. (Published in German)

4. H. B. Kram, P. L. Appel, and W. C. Shoemaker, "Prediction of below-knee amputation wound healing using noninvasive laser Doppler velocimetry," *American Journal of Surgery* 158 (July 1989): 29–31.

5. D. D. Thomas, R. F. Wilson, and R. G. Wiencek, "Vascular injury about the knee," *American Surgeon* 55 (June 1989): 370–77.

6. C. C. Huston et al., "Morbid implications of above-knee amputations. Report of a series and review of the literature," *Archives of Surgery* 115 (February 1980): 165–67.

7. J. K. Prasad et al., "Rehabilitation of burned patients with bilateral above-knee amputations," *Burns* 16 (August 1990): 297–301.

8. N. Ellitsgaard et al., "Outcome in 282 lower extremity amputations. Knee salvage and survival," *ACTA Orthopaedica Scandinavica* 61 (April 1990): 140–42.

9. S. G. Friedman and K. V. Krishnasastry, "The possibility of distal embolization from a femoral-popliteal prosthesis above the knee. A consideration against its routine use in this position," *Archives of Surgery* 125 (May 1990): 668–70.

10. J. A. Michaels, "Choice of material for above-knee femoropopliteal bypass graft," *British Journal of Surgery* 76 (January 1989): 7–14.

11. F. Laurendeau and J. Lassonde, "Above-knee femoropopliteal reconstruction with polytetrafluoroethylene: A good alternative to saphenous vein bypass," *Canadian Journal of Surgery* 32 (January 1989): 48–50.

12. J. Matsubara et al., "Clinical results of femoropopliteal bypass using externally supported (EXS) Dacron grafts: With a comparison of above- and below-knee anastomosis," *Journal of Cardiovascular Surgery (Torino)* 31 (November–December 1990): 731–34.

13. J. F. Vollmar et al., "Aortic aneurysms as late sequelae of above-knee amputation," *Lancet* 2 (7 October 1989): 834–35.

14. S. F. Crouse et al., "Oxygen consumption and cardiac response of short-leg and long-leg prosthetic ambulation in a patient with bilateral above-knee amputation: Comparisons with able-bodied men," *Archives of Physical Medicine and Rehabilitation* 71 (April 1990): 313–17.

15. F. Flandry et al., "The effect of the CAT-CAM above-knee prosthesis on functional rehabilitation," *Clinical Orthopaedics and Related Research* (February 1989): 249–62.

16. C. A. Mitchell and T. L. Versluis, "Management of an above-knee amputee with complex medical problems using the CAT-CAM prosthesis," *Physical Therapy* 70 (June 1990): 389–93.

17. D. J. DiAngelo et al., "Performance assessment of the Terry Fox jogging prosthesis for above-knee amputees," *Journal of Biomechanics* 22 (Number 6–7, 1989): 543–58.

18. R. Torres-Moreno et al., "Computer-aided design and manufacture of an above-knee amputee socket," *Journal of Biomedical Engineering* 13 (January 1991): 3–9.

19. R. Torres-Moreno et al., "A reference shape library for computer-aided socket design in above-knee prostheses," *Prosthetics and Orthotics International* 13 (December 1989): 130–39.

20. L. Peeraer et al., "Development of EMG-based mode and intent recognition algorithms for a computer-controlled above-knee prosthesis," *Journal of Biomedical Engineering* 12 (May 1990): 178–82.

21. K. J. Sandin and B. S. Smith, "Above-knee amputation with insidious pulmonary embolism and hypercoagulability secondary to protein C deficiency," *Archives of Physical Medicine and Rehabilitation* 70 (September 1989): 699–701.

22. S. Bengston, K. Knutson, and L. Lidgren, "Treatment of infected knee arthroplasty," *Clinical Orthopaedics and Related Research* (August 1989): 173–78.

23. F. M. Ivey et al., "Treatment options for infected knee arthroplasties," *Reviews of Infectious Diseases* 12 (May–June 1990): 468–78.

24. N. A. Purry and M. A. Hannon, "How successful is below-knee amputation for injury?" *Injury* 20 (January 1989): 32–36.

25. T. J. Bunt et al., "Iatrogenic tibial pseudoaneurysm following below-knee amputation," *American Surgeon* 56 (September 1990): 546–47.

26. Kolde et al., "Kaposi-like acroangiodermatitis in an above-knee amputation stump," 575–80.

27. B. J. Moran et al., "Through-knee amputation in high-risk patients with vascular disease: Indications, complications and rehabilitation," *British Journal of Surgery* 77 (October 1990): 1118–20.

28. A. Houghton et al., "Rehabilitation after lower limb amputation: A comparative study of above-knee, through-knee and Gritti-Stokes amputations," *British Journal of Surgery* 76 (June 1989): 622–24.

29. R. R. Lexier, I. J. Harrington, and J. M. Woods, "Lower extremity amputations: A 5-year review and comparative study," *Canadian Journal of Surgery* 30 (September 1987): 374–76.

30. D. Rosenthal et al., "Prosthetic above-knee femoropopliteal bypass for intermittent claudication," *Journal of Cardiovascular Surgery (Torino)* 31 (July-August 1990): 462–68.

31. E. J. Prendiville et al., "Long-term results with the above-knee popliteal expanded polytetrafluoroethylene graft," *Journal of Vascular Surgery* 11 (April 1990): 517–24.

32. R. B. Patterson et al., "Preferential use of EPTFE for above-knee femoropopliteal bypass grafts," *Annals of Vascular Surgery* 4 (July 1990): 338–43.

33. D. W. Gray and R. L. Ng, "Anatomical aspects of the blood supply to the skin of the posterior calf: Technique of below-knee amputation," *British Journal of Surgery* 77 (June 1990): 662–64.

34. C. W. Jamieson and D. Hill, "Amputation for vascular disease," *British Journal of Surgery* 63 (September 1976): 683–90.

Aortocoronary Bypass

1. K. Ennabli and L. C. Pelletier, "Morbidity and mortality of coronary artery surgery after the age of 70 years," *Annals of Thoracic Surgery* 42 (August 1986): 197–200.

2. M. Sunamori et al., "The characteristics of coronary artery revascularization in aged patients," *Japanese Journal of Surgery* 20 (March 1990): 163–69.

3. F. H. Edwards et al., "True emergency coronary artery bypass surgery," *Annals of Thoracic Surgery* 49 (April 1990): 603–10.

4. F. D. Loop et al., "J. Maxwell Chamberlain memorial paper. Sternal wound complications after isolated coronary artery bypass grafting: Early and late mortality, morbidity, and cost of care," *Annals of Thoracic Surgery* 49 (February 1990): 179–86.

5. K. Ennabli and L. C. Pelletier, "Morbidity and mortality of coronary artery surgery after the age of 70 years," 197–200.

6. D. M. Rose et al., "Analysis of morbidity and mortality in patients 70 years of age and over undergoing isolated coronary artery bypass surgery," *American Heart Journal* 110 (August 1985): 341–46.

7. W. K. Summers, "Psychiatric sequelae to cardiotomy," *Journal of Cardiovascular Surgery (Torino)* 20 (September–October 1979): 471–76.

8. C. J. Rabiner and A. E. Willner, "Psychopathology observed on follow-up after coronary bypass surgery," *Journal of Nervous and Mental Disease* 163 (November 1976): 295–301.

9. Sunamori et al., "The characteristics of coronary artery revascularization in aged patients," 163–69.

10. P. C. Ferry, "Neurologic sequelae of cardiac surgery in children," *American Journal of Diseases of Children* 141 (March 1987): 309–12.

11. E. Vasquez and W. R. Chitwood, Jr., "Postcardiotomy delirium: An overview," *International Journal of Psychiatry in Medicine* 6 (Number 3, 1975): 373–83.

12. H. Speidel et al., "Problems in the classification of psychopathological disorders following cardiac surgery with extracorporeal circulation," *Psychiatria Clinica (Basel)* 12 (Number 2, 1979): 57–79. (Published in German)

13. B. D. Townes et al., "Neurobehavioral outcomes in cardiac operations. A prospective controlled study," *Journal of Cardiovascular Surgery* 98 (November 1989): 774–82.

14. D. G. Folks et al., "Coronary artery bypass surgery in older patients: Psychiatric morbidity," *Southern Medical Journal* 79 (March 1986): 303–6.

15. "Die extrakorporale Zirkulation als Risikofaktor der Herzchirurgie," *Zeitschrift fur Kardiologie* 79 (1990 Supplement): 87–93. (Published in German)

16. T. J. Gardner et al., "Stroke following coronary artery bypass grafting: A 10-year study," *Annals of Thoracic Surgery* 40 (December 1985): 574–81.

17. J. Landercasper et al., "Perioperative stroke risk in 173 consecutive patients with a past history of stroke," *Archives of Surgery* 125 (August 1990): 986–89.

18. B. J. Brener et al., "The risk of stroke in patients with asymptomatic carotid stenosis undergoing cardiac surgery: A follow-up study," *Journal of Vascular Surgery* 5 (February 1987): 269–79.

19. T. J. Gardner et al., "Major stroke after coronary artery bypass surgery: Changing magnitude of the problem," *Journal of Vascular Surgery* 3 (April 1986): 684–87.

20. G. L. Reed, 3d et al., "Stroke following coronary-artery bypass surgery. A case-control estimate of the risk from carotid bruits," *New England Journal of Medicine* 319 (10 November 1988): 1246–50.

21. G. S. Weinstein and B. Levin, "The Coronary Artery Surgery Study (CASS). A critical appraisal," *Journal of Thoracic and Cardiovascular Surgery* 90 (October 1985): 541–48.

22. B. R. Chaitman et al., "Effect of coronary bypass surgery on survival patterns in subsets of patients with left main coronary artery disease. Report of the Collaborative Study in Coronary Artery Surgery (CASS)," *American Journal of Cardiology* 48 (October 1981): 765–77.

23. W. J. Rogers et al., "Ten-year follow-up of quality of life in patients randomized to receive medical therapy or coronary artery bypass graft surgery. The Coronary Artery Surgery Study (CASS)," *Circulation* 82 (November 1990): 1647–58.

24. J. B. Wong et al., "Myocardial revascularization for chronic stable angina. Analysis of the role of percutaneous transluminal coronary angioplasty based on data available in 1989," *Annals of Internal Medicine* 113 (1 December 1990): 852–71.

25. C. J. Glueck, "Role of risk factor management in progression and regression of coronary and femoral artery atherosclerosis," *American Journal of Cardiology* 57 (30 May 1986): 35G-41G.

26. D. H. Blankenhorn, "Regression of atherosclerosis: What does it mean?" *American Journal of Medicine* 90 (21 February 1991): 42S-47S.

27. D. Roth and W. J. Kostuk, "Noninvasive and invasive demonstration of spontaneous regression of coronary artery disease," *Circulation* 62 (October 1980): 888–96.

28. V. Hombach et al., "Regression of coronary sclerosis in familial hypercholesterolemia IIa by specific LDL apheresis," *Deutsche Medizinische Wochenschrift* 111 (7 November 1986): 1709–15. (Published in German)

29. D. H. Blankenhorn, "Regression of atherosclerosis: Dietary and pharmacologic approach," *Canadian Journal of Cardiology* 5 (May 1989): 206–10.

30. G. Weber, L. Resi, and P. Tanganelli, "Regression of atherosclerosis lesions," *Wiener Klinische Wochenschrift* 101 (27 October 1989): 698–702. (Published in German)

31. J. P. Kane et al., "Regression of coronary atherosclerosis during treatment of familial hypercholesterolemia with combined drug regimens," *Journal of the American Medical Association* 264 (19 December 1990): 3007–12.

32. G. Brown et al., "Regression of coronary artery disease as a result of intensive lipid-lowering therapy in men with high levels of apolipoprotein B," *New England Journal of Medicine* 323 (8 November 1990): 1289–98.

33. M. R. Malinow, "Experimental models of atherosclerosis regression," *Atherosclerosis* 48 (August 1983): 105–18.

34. M. G. Bourassa et al., "Long-term fate of bypass grafts: The Coronary Artery Surgery Study (CASS) and Montreal Heart Institute experiences," *Circulation* 72 (December 1985): V71–78.

35. T. Killip, E. Passamani, and K. Davis, "Coronary artery surgery study (CASS): A randomized trial of coronary bypass surgery. Eight years follow-up and survival in patients with reduced ejection fraction," *Circulation* 72 (December 1985): V102–9.

36. B. R. Chaitman et al., "Coronary Artery Surgery Study (CASS): Comparability of 10-year survival in randomized and randomizable patients," *Journal of the American College of Cardiology* 16 (November 1990): 1071–78.

37. "Coronary artery surgery study (CASS): A randomized trial of coronary bypass surgery. Survival data," *Circulation* 68 (November 1983): 939–50.

Appendectomy

1. M. A. Krupp and M. J. Chatton, *Current Medical Diagnosis and Treatment* (Los Altos, Calif.: Lange Medical Publications, 1984) 385 pp.

2. P. Monod-Broca, "Mortality in emergency abdominal surgery: Apropos of 304 cases. An argument for clinical medicine," *Bulletin de L'Academie Nationale de Medecine* 173 (November 1989): 1059–63. (Published in French)

3. R. Andersson, K. G. Tranberg, and S. Bengmark, "Bile peritonitis in acute cholecystitis," *HPB Surgery* 2 (March 1990): 7–12.

4. J. F. Renier et al., "Surgical treatment of perforated diverticular sigmoiditis. A retrospective study apropos of 45 cases," *Journal de Chirurgie (Paris)* 126 (November 1989): 567–74. (Published in French)

5. M. F. Mazurik et al., "Causes of fatal outcome in acute appendicitis," *Klinicheskaia Khirurgiia* (Number 4, 1990): 18–19. (Published in Russian)

6. HealthCare Knowledge Resources/Commission on Professional and Hospital Activities, *HealthWeek* (6 November 1989).

7. Mazurik et al., "Causes of fatal outcome in acute appendicitis," 18–19.

8. A. Dirksen and E. Kjoller, "Cardiac predictors of death after non-cardiac surgery evaluated by intention to treat," *British Medical Journal* 297 (22 October 1988): 1011–13.

9. E. N. Elechi, "Acute appendicitis: A clinical pattern in Port Harcourt Nigeria," *East African Medical Journal* 66 (May 1989): 328–32.

10. H. Tera and C. Aberg, "Mortality after laparotomy. A 10-year series," *ACTA Chirurgica Scandinavica* 142 (Number 1, 1976): 67–72.

11. R. Luckmann, "Incidence and case fatality rates for acute appendicitis in California. A population-based study of the effects of age," *American Journal of Epidemiology* 129 (May 1990): 905–18.

12. C. E. Vorhes, "Appendicitis in the elderly: The case for better diagnosis," *Geriatrics* 42 (March 1987): 89–92.

13. A. P. Ukhanov, "Causes of postoperative mortality in acute appendicitis," *Khirurgiia (Mosk)* (February 1989): 17–21. (Published in Russian)

14. M. Schein et al., "Peritoneal lavage in abdominal sepsis. A controlled clinical study," *Archives of Surgery* 125 (September 1990): 1132–35.

15. T. Calandra et al., "Clinical significance of *Candida* isolated from peritoneum in surgical patients," *Lancet* 2 (16 December 1989): 1437–40.

16. R. A. Mustard et al., "Pneumonia complicating abdominal sepsis. An independent risk factor for mortality," *Archives of Surgery* 126 (February 1991): 170–75.

17. V. I. Bondarev et al., "Analysis of mortality in acute diffuse peritonitis," *Klinicheskaia Khirurgiia* (Number 1, 1990): 21–23. (Published in Russian)

18. P. J. Blind and S. T. Dahlgren, "The continuing challenge of the negative appendix," *ACTA Chirurgica Scandinavica* 152 (October 1986): 623–27.

19. D. V. Young, "Results of urgent appendectomy for right lower quadrant tenderness," *American Journal of Surgery* 157 (April 1989): 428–30.

20. J. R. Izbicki et al., "Retro- and prospective studies on the value of clinical and laboratory chemical data in acute appendicitis," *Chirurg* 61 (December 1990): 887–93. (Published in German)

21. M. F. Mazurik et al., "Means of reducing mortality in acute appendicitis," *Khirurgiia (Mosk)* (February 1989): 13–17. (Published in Russian)

22. Y. Heloury et al., "Complications of appendicitis and appendectomies. Apropos of 106 cases," *Journal de Chirurgie (Paris)* 120 (November 1983): 615–22. (Published in French)

23. G. Sava et al., "Mortality in appendectomy. About an homogeneous series of 5 348 cases," *Semaine des Hospitaux de Paris* 57 (8 November 1981): 1713–18. (Published in French)

24. N. V. Karaman, IuG Kudinskii, and L. B. Alekseeva, "Causes of mortality in acute appendicitis," *Vestnik Khirurgii Imeni I. I. Grekova* 125 (December 1980): 66–69. (Published in Russian)

25. I. R. Gough et al., "Consequences of removal of a 'normal' appendix," *Medical Journal of Australia* 1 (16 April 1983): 370–72.

26. E. G. Waters, "Elective appendectomy with abdominal and pelvic surgery," *Obstetrics and Gynecology* 50 (November 1977): 511–17.

27. O. P. Ofili, "Simultaneous appendectomy and inguinal herniorrhaphy could be beneficial," *Ethiopian Medical Journal* 29 (January 1991): 37–38.

28. Gough et al., "Consequences of removal of a 'normal' appendix," 370–72.

29. A. Lansade et al., "Single preoperative intravenous dose of metronidazole for appendectomy in children," *Annales de Pediatrie (Paris)* 37 (January 1990): 62–64. (Published in French)

Below-the-Knee Amputation

1. F. M. Ivey et al., "Treatment options for infected knee arthroplasties," *Reviews of Infectious Diseases* 12 (May–June 1990): 468–78.

2. D. D. Thomas, R. F. Wilson, and R. G. Wiencek, "Vas-

cular injury about the knee. Improved outcome," *American Surgeon* 55 (June 1989): 370–77.

3. E. Markgraf, G. Clausner, and W. Lungershausen, "Traumatic vascular lesions of the knee joint," *Beitrage Zur Orthopadie und Traumatologie* 36 (September 1989): 401–11. (Published in German)

4. J. J. Peck et al., "Popliteal vascular trauma. A community experience," *Archives of Surgery* 125 (October 1990): 1339–43.

5. W. K. Brodzka et al., "Long-term function of persons with atherosclerotic bilateral below-knee amputation living in the inner city," *Archives of Physical Medicine and Rehabilitation* 71 (October 1990): 895–900.

6. R. R. Lexier, I. J. Harrington, and J. M. Woods, "Lower extremity amputations: A 5-year review and comparative study," *Canadian Journal of Surgery* 30 (September 1987): 374–76.

7. H. B. Kram, P. L. Appel, and W. C. Shoemaker, "Prediction of below-knee amputation wound healing using non-invasive laser Doppler velocimetry," *American Journal of Surgery* 158 (July 1989): 29–31.

8. C. B. Kernek and W. B. Rozzi, "Simplified two-stage below-knee amputation for unsalvageable diabetic foot infections," *Clinical Orthopaedics and Related Research* (December 1990): 251–56.

9. S. Torii et al., "Reverse flow saphenous island flap in the patient with below-knee amputation," *British Journal of Plastic Surgery* 42 (September 1989): 517–20.

10. M. S. Pinzur et al., "A safe, pre-fabricated, immediate postoperative prosthetic limb system for rehabilitation of below-knee amputations," *Orthopedics* 12 (October 1989): 1343–45.

11. I. J. Harrington et al., "A plaster-pylon technique for below-knee amputation," *Journal of Bone and Joint Surgery, British Volume* 73 (January 1991): 76–78.

12. N. A. Purry and M. A. Hannon, "How successful is below-knee amputation for injury?" *Injury* 20 (January 1989): 32–36.

13. H. A. Latimer, L. E. Dahners, and D. K. Bynum, "Lengthening of below-the-knee amputation stumps using the Ilizarov technique," *Journal of Orthopaedic Trauma* 4 (Number 4, 1990): 411–14.

14. C. V. Ruckley, P. A. Stonebridge, and R. J. Prescott, "Skewflap versus long posterior flap in below-knee amputations," *Journal of Vascular Surgery* 13 (March 1991): 423–27.

15. C. Aligne et al., "Primary closure of below-knee amputation stumps: A prospective study of 62 cases," *Annals of Vascular Surgery* 4 (March 1990): 143–46.

16. K. K. Au, "Sagittal flaps in below-knee amputations in Chinese patients," *Journal of Bone and Joint Surgery, British Volume* 71 (August 1989): 597–98.

17. Purry and Hannon, "How successful is below-knee amputation for injury?" 32–36.

18. C. H. Boniske, "Joint Replacement Surgery," letter, *New England Journal of Medicine* 324 (1991): 1367.

19. T. J. Bunt, J. M. Malone, and R. R. Karpman, "Iatrogenic tibial pseudoaneurysm following below-knee amputation," *American Surgeon* 56 (September 1990): 546–47.

20. R. O. Gregg, "Bypass or amputation? Concomitant review of bypass arterial grafting and major amputations," *American Journal of Surgery* 149 (March 1985): 397–402.

21. D. Rosenthal et al., "Prosthetic above-knee femoropopliteal bypass for intermittent claudication," *Journal of Cardiovascular Surgery (Torino)* 31 (July–August 1990): 462–68.

22. B. J. Moran et al., "Through-knee amputation in high-risk patients with vascular disease: Indications, complications and rehabilitation," *British Journal of Surgery* 77 (October 1990): 1118–20.

23. G. Dorros et al., "Below-the-knee angioplasty: Tibioperoneal vessels, the acute outcome," *Catheterization and Cardiovascular Diagnosis* 19 (March 1990): 170–78.

24. T. A. Sanborn et al., "Infrapopliteal and below-knee popliteal lesions: Treatment with sole laser thermal angioplasty. Work in progress," *Radiology* 172 (July 1989): 89–93.

25. D. W. Gray and R. L. Ng, "Anatomical aspects of the blood supply to the skin of the posterior calf: Technique of below-knee amputation," *British Journal of Surgery* 77 (June 1990): 662–64.

26. C. W. Jamieson and D. Hill, "Amputation for vascular disease," *British Journal of Surgery* 63 (September 1976): 683–90.

Bilateral Salpingo-Oophorectomy

1. W. W. Liang, Y. N. Lin, and Y. N. Lee, "Malignant mixed mullerian tumor of fallopian tube," *Chung-Hua Fu Chan Ko Tsa Chih* 45 (April 1990): 272–75.

2. H. G. Muntz et al., "Primary adenocarcinoma of the fal-

lopian tube," *European Journal of Gynaecological Oncology* 10 (Number 4, 1989): 239–49.

3. L. Bohr and C. F. Thomsen, "Low-grade stromal sarcoma: A benign-appearing malignant uterine tumour; a review of current literature. Differential diagnostic problems illustrated by four cases," *European Journal of Obstetrics, Gynecology, and Reproductive Biology* 39 (March 1991): 63–69.

4. W. H. Wolberg, "Adjunctive chemotherapy as an alternative to ovarian ablation in premenopausal women with carcinoma of the breast," *Surgery, Gynecology and Obstetrics* 165 (December 1987): 563–66.

5. M. Izuo, "Breast cancer and hormone therapy," *Gan To Kagaku Ryoho* 14 (October 1987): 2830–36. (Published in Japanese)

6. K. I. Pritchard and D. J. Sutherland, "The use of endocrine therapy," *Hematology/Oncology Clinics of North America* 3 (December 1989): 765–805.

7. W. R. Miller, "Fundamental research leading to improved endocrine therapy for breast cancer," *Journal of Steroid Biochemistry* 27 (Number 1–3, 1987): 477–85.

8. E. T. de Jonge and P. F. Venter, "Hysterectomy for septic abortion—is bilateral salpingo-oophorectomy necessary?" *South African Medical Journal* 74 (17 September 1988): 291–92.

9. M. Hernandez Avila, A. M. Walker, and H. Jick, "Use of replacement estrogens and the risk of myocardial infarction," *Epidemiology* 1 (March 1990): 128–33.

10. L. Weinstein, "Hormonal therapy in the patient with surgical menopause," *Obstetrics and Gynecology* 75 (April 1990, Supplement): 47S-50S.

11. F. V. Price, R. Edwards, and H. J. Buchsbaum, "Ovarian remnant syndrome: Difficulties in diagnosis and management," *Obstetrical and Gynecological Survey* 45 (March 1990): 151–56.

12. M. M. Zaitoon, "Ureteral obstruction secondary to retained ovarian remnants: A case report and review of the literature," *Journal of Urology* 137 (May 1987): 973–74.

13. P. Loizzi et al., "Removal or preservation of ovaries during hysterectomy: A six-year review," *International Journal of Gynaecology and Obstetrics* 31 (March 1990): 257–61.

14. H. K. Genant, D. J. Baylink, and J. C. Gallagher, "Estrogens in the prevention of osteoporosis in postmenopausal women," *American Journal of Obsterics and Gynecology* 161 (December 1989): 1842–46.

15. T. Matsumoto et al., "Effect of vitamin D metabolites on bone metabolism in a rat model of postmenopausal osteo-porosis," *Journal of Nutritional Science and Vitaminology (Tokyo)* 31 (December 1985, Supplement): S61–65.

16. A. Birnkrant, J. Sampson, and P. H. Sugarbaker, "Ovarian metastasis from colorectal cancer," *Diseases of the Colon and Rectum* 29 (November 1986): 767–71.

17. H. J. Chihal, "Indications for drug therapy in premenstrual syndrome patients," *Journal of Reproductive Medicine* 32 (June 1987): 449–52.

18. W. R. Keye, Jr., "Medical treatment of premenstrual syndrome," *Canadian Journal of Psychiatry* 30 (November 1985): 483–88.

19. I. Jacobs and D. Oram, "Prophylactic oophorectomy," *British Journal of Hospital Medicine* 38 (November 1987): 440–44, 448–49.

Bilateral Tubal Destruction

1. A. Nisanian, "Outpatient minilaparotomy sterilization with local anesthesia," *Journal of Reproductive Medicine* 35 (April 1990): 380–83.

2. P. V. Mehta, "Laparoscopic sterilization with the Falope ring: Experience with 10,100 women in rural camps," *Obstetrics and Gynecology* 57 (March 1981): 345–50.

3. H. B. Peterson et al., "Deaths attributable to tubal sterilization in the United States, 1977 to 1981," *American Journal of Obstetrics and Gynecology* 146 (15 May 1983): 131–36.

4. H. B. Peterson et al., "Mortality risk associated with tubal sterilization in United States hospitals," *American Journal of Obstetrics and Gynecology* 143 (15 May 1982): 125–29.

5. L. G. Escobedo et al., "Case-fatality rates for tubal sterilization in U.S. hospitals, 1979 to 1980," *American Journal of Obstetrics and Gynecology* 160 (January 1989): 147–50.

6. R. W. Rochat et al., "Mortality associated with sterilization: Preliminary results of an international collaborative observational study," *International Journal of Gynaecology and Obstetrics* 24 (August 1986): 275–84.

7. J. D. Keeping, A. Chang, and J. Morrison, "Sterilization: A comparative review," *Australian and New Zealand Journal of Obstetrics and Gynaecology* 19 (November 1979): 193–202.

8. F. Destefano et al., "Complications of interval laparoscopic tubal sterilization," *Obstetrics and Gynecology* 61 (February 1983): 153–58.

9. J. M. Aubert, I. Lubell, and M. Schima, "Mortality risk associated with female sterilization," *International Journal of*

Gynaecology and Obstetrics 18 (Number 6, 1980): 406–10.

10. E. Schneller et al., "Operative complications of laparoscopic tubal sterilization with Bleier clips," *Geburtshilfe und Frauenheilkunde* 42 (May 1982): 379–84. (Published in German)

11. A. L. Franks, J. S. Kendrick, and H. B. Peterson, "Unintended laparotomy associated with laparoscopic tubal sterilization," *American Journal of Obstetrics and Gynecology* 157 (November 1987): 1102–5.

12. C. Aranda et al., "A comparative clinical trial of the tubal ring versus the Rocket clip for female sterilization," *American Journal Obstetrics and Gynecology* 153 (1 December 1985): 755–59.

13. "Immediate sequelae following tubal sterilization. A multicentre study of the ICMR Task Force on Female Sterilization," *Contraception* 28 (October 1983): 369–84.

14. H. H. Riedel et al., "The frequency distribution of various pelviscopic (laparoscopic) operations, including complications rates—statistics of the Federal Republic of Germany in the years 1983–1985," *Zentralblatt fur Gynakologie* 111 (Number 2, 1989): 78–91.

15. M. M. Green et al., "Acute pelvic inflammatory disease after surgical sterilization," *Annals of Emergency Medicine* 20 (April 1991): 344–47.

16. "Open laparoscopy for tubal occlusion in the female," *Advances in Contraception* 1 (June 1985): 181–89.

17. H. B. Peterson et al., "Deaths associated with laparoscopic sterilization by unipolar electrocoagulating devices, 1978 and 1979," *American Journal of Obstetrics and Gynecology* 149 (15 January 1981): 141–43.

18. J. J. Kjer and L. B. Knudsen, "Ectopic pregnancy subsequent to laparoscopic sterilization," *American Journal of Obstetrics and Gynecology* 160 (May 1989): 1202–4.

19. J. C. Brantley, 3d, and P. M. Riley, "Cardiovascular collapse during laparoscopy: A report of two cases," *American Journal of Obstetrics and Gynecology* 159 (September 1988): 735–37.

20. P. L. Ostman et al., "Circulatory collapse during laparoscopy," *Journal of Clinical Anesthesia* 2 (March–April 1990): 129–32.

21. J. M. Cooper et al., "Incidence, significance and remission of tubal spasm during attempted hysteroscopic tubal sterilization," *Journal of Reproductive Medicine* 30 (January 1985): 39–42.

22. D. E. Gunatilake, "Case report: Fatal intraperitoneal explosion during electrocoagulation via laparoscopy," *International Journal of Gynaecology and Obstetrics* 15 (Number 4, 1978): 353–57.

23. G. L. Smith, G. P. Taylor, and K. F. Smith, "Comparative risks and costs of male and female sterilization," *American Journal of Public Health* 75 (April 1985): 370–74.

24. "Tubal sterilization with Filshie Clip. A multicentre study of the ICMR task force on female sterilization," *Contraception* 30 (October 1984): 339–53.

25. H. B. Peterson et al., "The safety and efficacy of tubal sterilization: An international overview," *International Journal of Gynecaeology and Obstetrics* 21 (April 1983): 139–44.

26. K. Limpaphayom et al., "Laparoscopic tubal electrocoagulation for sterilization: 5000 cases," *International Journal of Gynaecology and Obstetrics* 18 (Number 6, 1980): 411–13.

Bilateral Tubal Division

1. G. L. Smith, G. P. Taylor, and K. F. Smith, "Comparative risks and costs of male and female sterilization," *American Journal of Public Health* 75 (April 1985): 370–74.

2. "Tubal sterilization with Filshie Clip. A multicentre study of the ICMR task force on female sterilization," *Contraception* 30 (October 1984): 339–53.

3. H. B. Peterson et al., "The safety and efficacy of tubal sterilization: An international overview," *International Journal of Gynaecology and Obstetrics* 21 (April 1983): 139–44.

4. K. Limpaphayom et al., "Laparoscopic tubal electrocoagulation for sterilization: 5000 cases," *International Journal of Gynaecology and Obstetrics* 18 (Number 6, 1980): 411–13.

Cataract Removal with Intraocular Lens Implant

1. A. Donn, "The Eyes" in *The Columbia University College of Physicians and Surgeons Complete Home Medical Guide* (New York: Crown, 1989): 690–710.

2. *Dorland's Illustrated Medical Dictionary,* 26th ed. (Philadelphia: W. B. Saunders, 1981): 229.

3. D. E. Larsen et al., "The Eyes" in *Mayo Clinic Family Health Book* (New York: William Morrow, 1990): 735–80.

4. B. T. Hutchinson, "Cataracts," *Harvard Medical School Health Letter* (April 1988): 6–8.

5. Donn, "The Eyes," 690–710.

6. B. Thomas Hutchinson, "Cataracts," 6–8.

7. Donn, "The Eyes," 690–710.

8. Ibid.

9. Larsen et al., "The Eyes," 735–80.

10. P. S. Koch, H. Bradley, and N. Swenson, "Visual acuity recovery rates following cataract surgery and implantation of soft intraocular lenses," *Journal of Cataract and Refractive Surgery* 17 (March 1991): 143–47.

11. O. Nishi and K. Nishi, "Intercapsular cataract surgery with lens epithelial cell removal. Part III: Long-term follow-up of posterior capsular opacification," *Journal of Cataract and Refractive Surgery* 17 (March 1991): 218–20.

12. M. Yanoff and E. G. Redovan, "Anterior eyewall perforation during subconjunctival cataract block," *Ophthalmic Surgery* 21 (May 1990): 362–63.

13. S. E. Brady, E. J. Cohen, and D. H. Fischer, "Diagnosis and treatment of chronic postoperative bacterial endophthalmitis," *Journal of Ophthalmic Nursing and Technology* 9 (January–February 1990): 22–26.

14. B. Jansen, C. Hartman, and F. Schumacher-Perdreau et al., "Late onset endophthalmitis associated with intraocular lens: A case of molecularly proved *S. epidermidis* aetiology," *British Journal of Ophthalmology* 75 (July 1991): 440–41.

15. R. F. Steinert, S. F. Brint, and S. M. White et al., "Astigmatism after small incision cataract surgery. A prospective randomized, multicenter comparison of 4- and 6.5-mm incisions," *Ophthalmology* 98 (April 1991): 415–16.

16. S. M. Bloom, R. E. Wysaynski, and A. J. Brucker, "Scleral fixation suture for dislocated posterior chamber intraocular lens," *Ophthalmic Surgery* (December 1990): 851–54.

17. M. Blumenthal, E. Assia, and Y. Schochot, "Lens anatomical principles and their technical implications in cataract surgery. Part I: The lens capsule," *Journal of Cataract and Refractive Surgery* 17 (March 1991): 205–10.

18. M. Blumenthal, E. Assia, and D. Neuman, "Lens anatomical principles and their technical implications in cataract surgery. Part II: The lens nucleus," *Journal of Cataract and Refractive Surgery* 17 (March 1991): 211–17.

Cervical Cesarean Section

1. D. N. Danforth, "Cesarean section," *Journal of the American Medical Association* 253 (8 February 1985): 811–18.

2. G. Burkett et al., "Evaluation of surgical staples in cesarean section," *American Journal of Obstetrics and Gynecology* 161 (September 1989): 540–45.

3. P. Duff, "Pathophysiology and management of post-cesarean endomyometritis," *Obstetrics and Gynecology* 67 (February 1986): 269–76.

4. F. J. Spielman and B. C. Corke, "Advantages and disadvantages of regional anesthesia for cesarean section. A review," *Journal of Reproductive Medicine* 30 (November 1985): 832–40.

5. N. Cirau-Vigneron et al., "Evolution of the indications for caesareans. Comparison of 1971–1976 and 1976–1979 at the Maternity Center of the Louis-Mourier Hospital," *Journal de Gynecologie, Obstetrique et Biologie de la Reproduction (Paris)* 14 (Number 3, 1985): 375–84.

6. P. Bingham and R. J. Lilford, "Management of the selected term breech presentation: Assessment of the risks of selected vaginal delivery versus cesarean section for all cases," *Obstetrics and Gynecology* 69 (June 1987): 965–78.

7. R. S. Stafford, "The impact of nonclinical factors on repeat cesarean section," *Journal of the American Medical Association* 265 (2 January 1991): 59–63.

8. J. T. Parer, "The current role of intrapartum fetal blood sampling," *Clinical Obstetrics and Gynecology* 23 (June 1980): 565–82.

9. T. M. Coltart, J. A. Davies, and M. Katesmark, "Outcome of a second pregnancy after a previous elective caesarean section," *British Journal of Obstetrics and Gynaecology* 97 (December 1990): 1140–43.

10. M. G. Rosen, J. C. Dickinson, and C. L. Westhof, "Vaginal birth after cesarean: A meta-analysis of morbidity and mortality," *Obstetrics and Gynecology* 77 (March 1991): 465–70.

11. G. Pridjian, J. U. Hibbard, and A. H. Moawad, "Cesarean: Changing the trends," *Obstetrics and Gynecology* 77 (February 1991): 195–200.

12. B. L. Flamm et al., "Vaginal birth after cesarean delivery: Results of a five-year multicenter collaborative study," *Obstetrics and Gynecology* 76 (November 1990): 750–54.

13. Bingham and Lilford, "Management of the selected term breech presentation," 965–78.

14. J. P. McKenna, B. R. Guerdan, and J. C. Wright, "Vaginal birth after cesarean section. A safe option in carefully selected patients," *Postgraduate Medicine* 84 (1 November 1988): 211–15.

15. A. Katsulov et al., "Vaginal delivery after two and more

cesarean sections," *Akusherstvo I Ginekologiia (Sofiia)* 29 (Number 4, 1990): 16–19. (Published in Bulgarian)

16. P. Audra and G. Putet, "Do any indications remain for vaginal delivery in breech presentation?" *Revue Francaise de Gynecologie et D'Obstetrique* 85 (October 1990): 545–48. (Published in French)

Circumcision

1. H. V. Kunz, "Circumcision and meatotomy," *Primary Care* 13 (September 1986): 513–25.

2. T. E. Wiswell, "Routine neonatal circumcision: A reappraisal," *American Family Physician* 41 (March 1990): 817.

3. D. H. Spach, A. E. Stapleton, and W. E. Stamm, "Lack of circumcision increases the risk of urinary tract infection in young men," *Journal of the American Medical Association* 267 (5 February 1992): 679–81.

4. T. L. Stull and J. J. LiPuma, "Epidemiology and natural history of urinary tract infections in children," *Medical Clinics of North America* 75 (March 1991): 287–97.

5. Wiswell, "Routine Neonatal Circumcision," 859–63.

6. T. Shealey, "Should Your Baby Boy Be Circumcised?" *Children* 2 (February 1988): 77–79.

7. S. Moses, J. E. Bradley, N. J. Nagelkerke, et al., "Geographical patterns of male circumcision practices in Africa: association with seroprevalence," *International Journal of Epidemiology* 19 (September 1990): 693–7.

8. Kunz, "Circumcision and meatotomy," 513–25.

9. Ibid.

10. A. V. Myron and D. P. Maguire, "Pain perception in the neonate: Implications for circumcision," *Journal of Professional Nursing* 7 (May–June 1991): 188–93.

11. A. L. Masciello, "Anesthesia for neonatal circumcision: Local is better than dorsal penile nerve block," *Obstetrics and Gynecology* 75 (May 1991): 834–38.

12. P. Fontaine and W. L. Toffler, "Dorsal penile nerve block for newborn circumcision," *American Family Physician* 43 (April 1991): 1327–33.

13. T. J. Metcalf, L. M. Osborn, and M. Mariani, "Circumcision: A study of current pediatrics," *Clinical Pediatrics* 22 (1983): 575–79.

14. American Academy of Pediatrics, "Report of the Task Force on Circumcision," *Pediatrics* 84 (1989): 388–91.

15. H. Speert, "Circumcision of the newborn: An appraisal of its present state," *Obstetrics and Gynecology* 2 (1953): 164–72.

16. Ibid.

17. W. F. Gee and J. S. Ansell, "Neonatal circumcision, a 10-year overview: With comparison of the Gomco clamp and the Plastibell device," *Pediatrics* 58 (1976): 824–27.

18. W. E. Schmidt, "A circumcision method draws new concern," *The New York Times* (8 October 1985): C1.

19. E. F. Crain and J. C. Gershel, "Urinary tract infections in febrile infants younger than eight weeks of age," *Pediatrics* 86 (September 1990): 363–67.

20. Myron and Maguire, "Pain perception in the neonate," 188–93.

21. L. Marchette, R. Main, and E. Redick et al., "Pain reduction interventions during neonatal circumcision," *Nursing Research* 40 (July–August 1991): 241–44.

Closed Fracture Reduction of the Radius and Ulna

1. T. S. Axelrod and R. Y. McMurtry, "Open reduction and internal fixation of comminuted, intraarticular fractures of the distal radius," *Journal of Hand Surgery, American Volume* 15 (January 1990): 1–11.

Closed Fracture Reduction of the Tibia and Fibula

1. W. G. Cimino, M. L. Corbett, and R. E. Leach, "The role of closed reduction in tibial shaft fractures," *Orthopaedic Review* 19 (March 1990): 233–40.

2. F. H. Savoie et al., "Tibial plateau fractures. A review of operative treatment using AO technique," *Orthopedics* 10 (May 1987): 745–50.

3. H. Griffith Winter, *Complete Guide to Symptoms, Illness, and Surgery,* 2nd ed. (Los Angeles: The Body Press, 1989), 754–55.

4. A. J. Sarokhan et al., "Total knee arthroplasty in juvenile rheumatoid arthritis," *Journal of Bone and Joint Surgery, American Volume* 65 (October 1983): 1071–80.

5. HealthCare Knowledge Resources/Commission on Profes-

sional and Hospital Activities, *HealthWeek* (6 November 1989).

6. G. J. Clancey and S. T. Hansen, Jr., "Open fractures of the tibia: A review of 102 cases," *Journal of Bone and Joint Surgery, American Volume* 60 (January 1978): 118–22.

7. P. Rommens et al., "The operative treatment of tibial shaft fractures: A review of 277 cases," *ACTA Chirurgica Belgica* 85 (July–August 1985): 268–73.

8. R. M. Simin et al., "Fractures of the neck of the talus and the Blair fusion: A review of the literature and case report," *Clinics in Podiatric Medicine and Surgery* 5 (April 1988): 393–420.

9. G. Donald and D. Seligson, "Treatment of tibial shaft fractures by percutaneous Kuntscher nailing. Technical difficulties and a review of 50 consecutive cases," *Clinical Orthopaedics and Related Research* (September 1983): 64–73.

10. W. D. Fisher and D. L. Hamblen, "Problems and pitfalls of compression fixation of long bone fractures: A review of results and complications," *Injury* 10 (November 1978): 99–107.

11. Donald and Seligson, "Treatment of tibial shaft fractures by percutaneous Kuntscher nailing," 64–73.

12. G. J. Clancey and S. T. Hansen, Jr., "Open fractures of the tibia: A review of 102 cases," *Journal of Bone and Joint Surgery, American Volume* 60 (January 1978): 118–22.

13. Donald and Seligson, "Treatment of tibial shaft fractures by percutaneous Kuntscher nailing," 64–73.

Closed Reduction and Internal Fixation of Fracture of the Femur

1. L. B. Bone et al., "Early versus delayed stabilization of femoral fractures," *Journal of Bone and Joint Surgery, American Volume* 71 (March 1989): 336–40.

2. J. H. Schafer et al., "Histological and biochemical changes in the lung in relation to survival time following femoral fracture in the dog," *Langenbecks Archiv Fur Chirurgie* (1975, Supplement): 221–24. (Published in German)

3. J. Kroupa, "Indications of primary osteosynthesis in patients with fractures of long bones of extremities with special regard to multiple and associated fractures of femur diaphysis," *Czechoslovak Medicine* 9 (Number 4, 1986): 218–32.

4. L. J. Harris, "Closed retrograde intramedullary nailing of peritrochanteric fractures of the femur with a new nail," *Journal of Bone and Joint Surgery, American Volume* 62 (October 1980): 1185–93.

5. P. Skinner et al., "Displaced subcapital fractures of the femur: A prospective randomized comparison of internal fixation hemiarthroplasty and total hip replacement," *Injury* 20 (September 1989): 291–93.

6. G. M. White et al., "The treatment of fractures of the femoral shaft with the Brooker-Wills distal locking intramedullary nail," *Journal of Bone and Joint Surgery* 68 (July 1986): 865–76.

7. M. Delmi et al., "Dietary supplementation in elderly patients with fractured neck of the femur," *Lancet* 335 (28 April 1990): 1013–16.

Cruciate Ligament Repair

1. P. Lass et al., "Muscle coordination following rupture of the anterior cruciate ligament. Electromyographic studies of 14 patients," *ACTA Orthopaedica Scandinavica* 62 (February 1991): 9–14.

2. R. S. Snell, *Clinical Anatomy for Medical Students*, 3rd ed. (Boston: Little, Brown, and Company, 1986), 690.

3. G. A. Hanks et al., "Meniscus repair in the anterior cruciate deficient knee," *American Journal of Sports Medicine* 18 (November–December 1990): 606–11.

4. K. D. Shelbourne, A. Mollabashy, and M. De Carlo, "Acute anterior cruciate ligament injury," *Indiana Medicine* 83 (December 1990): 896–900.

5. D. Saragaglia et al., "Rehabilitation of the knee movement after ligamentoplasty using MacIntosh's procedure augmented by Kennedy-Lad: A comparison between recent and old rupture of the anterior cruciate ligament," *Revue de Chirurgie Orthopedique et Reparatrice de L'Appareil Moteur* 76 (Number 5, 1990): 317–20. (Published in French)

6. A. Mitsou et al., "Acute rupture of anterior cruciate ligament: Histological study of 15 cases," *Archives D'Anatomie et De Cytologie Pathologiques* 38 (Number 5–6, 1990): 212–14.

7. D. A. McGuire and G. L. Grinstead, "Advances in anterior cruciate ligament surgery," *Alaska Medicine* 32 (July–September 1990): 101–5.

8. B. Gutin et al., "Does tourniquet use during anterior cruciate ligament surgery interfere with postsurgical recovery of function?" *Arthroscopy* 7 (Number 1, 1991): 52–56.

9. D. Daluga et al., "Primary bone grafting following graft

procurement for anterior cruciate ligament insufficiency," *Arthroscopy* 6 (Number 3, 1990): 205–8.

10. D. W. Jackson and R. K. Schaefer, "Cyclops syndrome: Loss of extension following intra-articular anterior cruciate ligament reconstruction," *Arthroscopy* 6 (Number 3, 1990): 171–8.

11. J. J. Bonamo, C. Fay, and T. Firestone, "The conservative treatment of the anterior cruciate deficient knee," *American Journal of Sports Medicine* 18 (November–December 1990): 618–23.

12. R. L. Barrack et al., "The outcome of nonoperatively treated complete tears of the anterior cruciate ligament in active young adults," *Clinical Orthopaedics and Related Research* (October 1990): 192–99.

13. F. L. Hefti et al., "Healing of the transected anterior cruciate ligament in the rabbit," *Journal of Bone and Joint Surgery, American Volume* 73 (March 1991): 373–83.

14. A. Finsterbush et al., "Secondary damage to the knee after isolated injury of the anterior cruciate ligament," *American Journal of Sports Medicine* 18 (September–October 1990): 475–79.

15. M. Salvi et al., "Ultrastructure of periprosthetic Dacron knee ligament tissue. Two cases of ruptured anterior cruciate ligament reconstruction," *ACTA Orthopaedica Scandinavica* 62 (April 1991): 174–77.

16. G. A. Woods, P. A. Indelicato, and T. J. Prevot, "The Gore-Tex anterior cruciate ligament prosthesis. Two- versus three-year results," *American Journal of Sports Medicine* 19 (January–February 1991): 48–55.

17. T. S. Roberts et al., "Anterior cruciate ligament reconstruction using freeze-dried, ethylene oxide-sterilized, bone-patellar tendon-bone allografts. Two-year results in thirty-six patients," *American Journal of Sports Medicine* 19 (January–February 1991): 35–41.

18. K. D. Shelbourne et al., "Anterior cruciate ligament injury: Evaluation of intraarticular reconstruction of acute tears without repair. Two- to seven-year follow-up of 155 athletes," *American Journal of Sports Medicine* 18 (September–October 1990): 484–88.

19. D. W. Jackson et al., "The effects of in situ freezing on the anterior cruciate ligament. An experimental study in goats," *Journal of Bone and Joint Surgery, American Volume* 73 (February 1991): 201–13.

20. M. J. Gibbons et al., "Effects of gamma irradiation on the initial mechanical and material properties of goat bone-patellar tendon-bone allografts," *Journal of Orthopaedic Research* 9 (March 1991): 209–18.

21. S. J. O'Brien et al., "The iliotibial band lateral sling procedure and its effect on the results of anterior cruciate ligament reconstruction," *American Journal of Sports Medicine* 19 (January–February 1991): 21–24.

22. K. Shino et al., "Reconstruction of the anterior cruciate ligament using allogeneic tendon," *American Journal of Sports Medicine* 18 (September–October 1990): 457–65.

23. C. Andersson, M. Odensten, and J. Gillquist, "Knee function after surgical or nonsurgical treatment of acute rupture of the anterior cruciate ligament: A randomized study with a long-term follow-up period," *Clinical Orthopaedics and Related Research* (March 1991): 255–63.

24. A. L. Doerr, Jr., et al., "A complication of interference screw fixation in anterior cruciate ligament reconstruction," *Orthopaedic Review* 19 (November 1990): 997–1000.

25. R. R. Wroble and R. A. Brand, "Paradoxes in the history of the anterior cruciate ligament," *Clinical Orthopaedics and Related Research* (October 1990): 183–91.

Dialysis Arteriovenostomy

1. C. R. Baker, Jr., "Complications and management of methods of dialysis access for renal failure," *American Surgeon* 42 (November 1976): 859–62.

2. R. B. Shack et al., "Expanded polytetrafluoroethylene as dialysis access grafts: Serial study of histology and fibrinolytic activity," *American Surgeon* 43 (December 1977): 817–25.

3. S. R. Mandel et al., "Vascular access in a University transplant and dialysis program. Results, costs, and manpower implications," *Archives of Surgery* 112 (November 1977): 1375–80.

4. R. Vanholder, N. Hoenich, and S. Ringoir, "Adequacy studies of fistula single-needle dialysis," *American Journal of Kidney Diseases* 10 (December 1987): 417–26.

5. A. P. Morgan et al., "Femoral triangle sepsis in dialysis patients: Frequency, management, and outcome," *Annals of Surgery* 191 (April 1980): 460–64.

6. A. R. Nissenson et al., "No-needle dialysis (NND): Experience with the new carbon transcutaneous hemodialysis (HD) access device (CTAD)," *Clinical Nephrology* 15 (June 1981): 302–8.

7. O. Ringden et al., "Subcutaneous arteriovenous fistulas for dialysis with special emphasis on vascular insufficiency," *Scandinavian Journal of Urology and Nephrology* 10 (Number 1, 1976): 73–79.

8. E. Cada et al., "Percutaneous transluminal angioplasty of failing arteriovenous dialysis fistulae," *Nephrology, Dialysis, Transplantation* 4 (Number 1, 1989): 57–61.

9. E. Minar and J. Zazgornik, "Local hirudin application— an aid in preventing occlusion of an arteriovenous fistula in dialysis patients?" *Klinische Wochenschrift* 63 (15 February 1985): 190–91.

10. Morgan et al., "Femoral triangle sepsis in dialysis patients," 460–64.

11. H. Bergrem, A. Flatmark, and S. Simonsen, "Dialysis fistulas and cardiac failure," *ACTA Medica Scandinavica* 204 (Number 3, 1978): 191–93.

12. C. B. Anderson et al., "Cardiac failure and upper extremity arteriovenous dialysis fistulas. Case reports and a review of the literature," *Archives of Internal Medicine* 136 (March 1976): 292–97.

13. H. von Bibra et al., "The effects of arteriovenous shunts on cardiac function in renal dialysis patients—an echocardiographic evaluation," *Clinical Nephrology* 9 (May 1978): 205–9.

14. C. B. Anderson and M. A. Groce, "Banding of arteriovenous dialysis fistulas to correct high-output cardiac failure," *Surgery* 78 (November 1975): 552–54.

15. R. K. Pearl et al., "The use of a moldable plastic splint to minimize early postoperative thrombosis of an internal arteriovenous fistula in the high-risk renal dialysis patient," *American Surgeon* 46 (June 1980): 333–34.

16. M. Rodriguez Moran et al., "Hand exercise effect in maturation and blood flow of dialysis arteriovenous fistulas ultrasound study," *Angiology* 35 (October 1984): 641–44.

17. S. K. Halter et al., "Carpal tunnel syndrome in chronic renal dialysis patients," *Archives of Physical Medicine and Rehabilitation* 62 (May 1981): 197–201.

18. M. Naito, K. Ogata, and T. Goya, "Carpal tunnel syndrome in chronic renal dialysis patients: Clinical evaluation of 62 hands and results of operative treatment," *Journal of Hand Surgery, British Volume* 12 (October 1987): 366–74.

19. J. E. Kenzora, "Dialysis carpal tunnel syndrome," *Orthopedics* 1 (May–June 1978): 195–203.

20. V. Seifert et al., "Carpal tunnel syndrome following arteriovenous forearm shunt in chronic dialysis patients—a review of 24 surgically treated patients," *Zeitschrift fur Orthopadie und Ihre Grenzgebiete* 125 (January–February 1987): 85–90. (Published in German)

21. M. S. Rohr et al., "Arteriovenous fistulas for long-term dialysis. Factors that influence fistula survival," *Archives of Surgery* 113 (February 1978): 153–55.

22. D. W. Hunter and S. K. So, "Dialysis access: Radiographic evaluation and management," *Radiologic Clinics of North America* 25 (March 1987): 249–60.

23. A. H. Moss et al., "Use of a silicone catheter with a Dacron cuff for dialysis short-term vascular access," *American Journal of Kidney Diseases* 12 (December 1988): 492–98.

24. G. F. Fant, V. W. Dennis, and L. D. Quarles, "Late vascular complications of the subclavian dialysis catheter," *American Journal of Kidney Diseases* 7 (March 1986): 225–28.

25. Nissenson et al., "No-needle dialysis (NND)," 302–8.

Endoscopic Colon Polypectomy

1. S. Eidt and M. Stolte, "Gastric glandular cysts—investigations into their genesis and relationship to colorectal epithelial tumors," *Zeitschrift fur Gastroenterologie* 27 (April 1989): 212–17.

2. R. Ottenjann and B. Wormann, "Multiple colorectal polyps and risk of cancer," *Deutsche Medizinische Wochenschrift* 110 (6 December 1985): 1879–82. (Published in German)

3. W. Matek et al., "Initial experience with the new electronic endoscope," *Endoscopy* 16 (January 1984): 20–21.

4. K. Eitner et al., "Endoscopic laser treatment of neoplasm and tubulovillous adenoma of the rectosigmoid. Initial experiences and review of the literature," *Gastroenterologisches Journal* 50 (Number 1, 1990): 38–42. (Published in German)

5. S. Naveau and J. C. Chaput, "Laser in gastroenterologic endoscopic therapy," *Revue du Praticien* 41 (21 January 1991): 232–34. (Published in French)

6. A. I. Morris, N. Krasner, and P. Cracknell, "Advances in gastrointestinal endoscopy and laser therapy," *Scandinavian Journal of Gastroenterology, Supplement* 117 (1985): 55–61.

7. R. C. Haggitt et al., "Prognostic factors in colorectal carcinomas arising in adenomas: Implications for lesions removed by endoscopic polypectomy," *Gastroenterology* 89 (August 1985): 328–36.

8. J. Nevoral et al., "Endoscopic colorectal polypectomy in

children and adolescents," *Ceskoslovenska Pediatrie* 45 (June 1990): 347–49. (Published in Czech)

9. P. Fric et al., "Therapeutic methods of digestive endoscopy in persons of advanced age," *Czechoslovak Medicine* 13 (Number 2–3, 1990): 45–51.

10. W. H. Isbister, "Colorectal polyps: An endoscopic experience," *Australian and New Zealand Journal of Surgery* 56 (September 1986): 717–22.

11. R. Hesterberg et al., "Endoscopic resection of colorectal polyps," *Deutsche Medizinische Wochenschrift* 112 (6 February 1987): 210–13. (Published in German)

12. G. Jimenez Mesa et al., "Endoscopic polypectomy of the colon in children," *Acta Gastroenterologica Latinoamericana* 15 (Number 4, 1985): 221–24. (Published in Spanish)

13. R. Holtzman et al., "Repeat colonoscopy after endoscopic polypectomy," *Diseases of the Colon and Rectum* 30 (March 1987): 185–88.

14. Hesterberg et al., "Endoscopic resection of colorectal polyps," 210–13.

15. K. Nagasako, "Endoscopic diagnosis of early colon cancer," *Gan No Rinsho* 34 (August 1988): 1326–32. (Published in Japanese)

16. T. Muto et al., "Endoscopic diagnosis and management of colonic polyps," *Gan To Kagaku Ryoho* 13 (July 1986): 2273–81. (Published in Japanese)

17. G. Hoff and M. Vatn, "Epidemiology of polyps in the rectum and sigmoid colon. Endoscopic evaluation of size and localization of polyps," *Scandinavian Journal of Gastroenterology* 20 (April 1985): 356–60.

18. C. I. Bartram and M. A. Hall-Craggs, "Interventional colorectal endoscopic procedures: Residual lesions on follow-up double-contrast barium enema study," *Radiology* 162 (March 1987): 835–38.

19. I. K. Woolfson et al., "Usefulness of performing colonoscopy one year after endoscopic polypectomy," *Diseases of the Colon and Rectum* 33 (May 1990): 389–93.

20. Hesterberg et al., "Endoscopic resection of colorectal polyps," 210–13.

Free Skin Graft

1. Y. Iwahira and Y. Maruyama, "Expanded preauricular full-thickness free skin graft," *Plastic and Reconstructive Surgery* 87 (January 1991): 150–52.

2. Y. Nakayama and S. Soeda, "Nylon threads used as drains in free skin grafting," *Annals of Plastic Surgery* 24 (January 1990): 91–95.

3. Y. Nakayama, T. Iino, and S. Soeda, "A new method for the dressing of free skin grafts," *Plastic and Reconstructive Surgery* 86 (December 1990): 1216–19.

4. N. D. Manchon et al., "Incidence and severity of drug interactions in the elderly: A prospective study of 639 patients," *Revue de Medecine Interne* 10 (November–December 1989): 521–25. (Published in French)

5. G. G. Hallock, "Free-flap coverage of the exposed Achilles tendon," *Plastic and Reconstructive Surgery* 83 (April 1989): 710–16.

6. R. P. Muller, "Free skin transplants," *Zeitschrift fur Hautkrankheiten* 63 (Supplement 2, 1988): 35–40. (Published in German)

Head and Neck Endarterectomy

1. M. L. Dyken and R. Pokras, "The performance of endarterectomy for disease of the extracranial arteries of the head," *Stroke* 15 (November–December 1984): 948–50.

2. M. C. Donaldson et al., "Recent experience with the asymptomatic cervical bruit," *Archives of Surgery* 122 (August 1987): 893–96.

3. T. C. Dehn and G. W. Taylor, "Cranial and cervical nerve damage associated with carotid endarterectomy," *British Journal of Surgery* 70 (June 1983): 365–68.

4. M. I. Aldoori and R. N. Baird, "Local neurological complication during carotid endarterectomy," *Journal of Cardiovascular Surgery (Torino)* 29 (July–August 1988): 432–36.

5. B. Messert and J. A. Black, "Cluster headache, hemicrania, and other head pains: Morbidity of carotid endarterectomy," *Stroke* 9 (November–December 1978): 559–62.

6. R. E. Welling et al., "Cervical wound hematoma after carotid endarterectomy," *Annals of Vascular Surgery* 3 (July 1989): 229–31.

7. E. R. Gomez et al., "Wound hematomas after carotid endarterectomy," *American Surgeon* 51 (February 1985): 111–13.

8. D. G. Dwells et al., "A theoretical mechanism for massive supraglottic swelling following carotid endarterectomy," *Australian and New Zealand Journal of Surgery* 58 (December 1988): 979–81.

9. J. W. Francfort et al., "Airway compromise after carotid surgery in patients with cervical irradiation," *Journal of Cardiovascular Surgery (Torino)* 30 (November–December 1989): 877–81.

10. V. K. Stojanovic and I. Saradnici, "Reconstructive surgery in diseases of the blood vessels of the neck," *ACTA Chirurgica Iugoslavica* 24 (Number 2, 1977): 145–52. (Published in Serbo-Croatian, Roman)

11. R. Pokras and M. L. Dyken, "Dramatic changes in the performance of endarterectomy for diseases of the extracranial arteries of the head," *Stroke* 19 (October 1988): 1289–90.

12. B. R. Chambers and J. W. Norris, "The case against surgery for asymptomatic carotid stenosis," *Stroke* 15 (November–December 1984): 964–67.

Hemodialysis

1. F. Coronel et al., "Morbidity and mortality of diabetic patients on dialysis in a 10-year program: Value of combined treatment," *Medicina Clinica* 92 (14 January 1989): 10–14. (Published in Spanish)

2. S. R. Acchiardo, L. W. Moore, and L. Burk, "Morbidity and mortality in hemodialysis patients," *ASAIO Transactions* 36 (July–September 1990): M148–51.

3. A. J. Collins and C. M. Kjellstrand, "Shortening of the hemodialysis procedure and mortality in 'healthy' dialysis patients," *ASAIO Transactions* 36 (July–September 1990): M145–48.

4. C. M. Kjellstrand, B. Hylander, and A. C. Collins, "Mortality on dialysis—on the influence of early start, patient characteristics, and transplantation and acceptance rates," *American Journal of Kidney Diseases* 15 (May 1990): 483–90.

5. P. W. Eggers, "Mortality rates among dialysis patients in Medicare's End-Stage Renal Disease Program," *American Journal of Kidney Diseases* 15 (May 1990): 414–21.

6. A. R. Nissenson et al., "Morbidity and mortality of continuous ambulatory peritoneal dialysis: Regional experience and long-term prospects," *American Journal of Kidney Diseases* 7 (March 1986): 229–34.

7. E. D. Avner et al., "Mortality of chronic hemodialysis and renal transplantation in pediatric end-stage renal disease," *Pediatrics* 67 (March 1981): 412–16.

8. B. Borlase, J. S. Simon, and G. Hermann, "Abdominal surgery in patients undergoing chronic hemodialysis," *Surgery* 102 (July 1987): 15–18.

9. A. J. Collins et al., "Changing risk factor demographics in end-stage renal disease patients entering hemodialysis and the impact on long-term mortality," *American Journal of Kidney Diseases* 15 (May 1990): 422–32.

10. Eggers, "Mortality rates among dialysis patients in Medicare's End-Stage Renal Disease Program," 414–21.

11. N. G. Levinsky and R. A. Rettig, "The Medicare End-State Renal Disease Program—A Report from the Institute of Medicine," *New England Journal of Medicine* 324 (1991): 1143–48.

12. Ibid.

13. W. M. McClellan et al., "Functional status and quality of life: Predictors of early mortality among patients entering treatment for end stage renal disease," *Journal of Clinical Epidemiology* 44 (Number 1, 1991): 83–89.

14. A. Murisasco et al., "Sequential sodium therapy allows correction of sodium-volume balance and reduces morbidity," *Clinical Nephrology* 24 (October 1985): 201–8.

15. M. D. Jameson and T. B. Wiegmann, "Principles, uses, and complications of hemodialysis," *Medical Clinics of North America* 74 (July 1990): 945–60.

16. E. G. Lowrie et al., "Effect of the hemodialysis prescription of patient morbidity: Report from the National Cooperative Dialysis Study," *New England Journal of Medicine* 305 (12 November 1981): 1176–81.

17. P. Degoulet et al., "Mortality risk factors in patients treated by chronic hemodialysis. Report of the Diaphane collaborative study," *Nephron* 31 (Number 2, 1982): 103–10.

18. Acchiardo, Moore, and Burk, "Morbidity and mortality in hemodialysis patients," M148–51.

19. S. R. Acchiardo, L. W. Moore, and P. A. Latour, "Malnutrition as the main factor in morbidity and mortality of hemodialysis patients," *Kidney International Supplement* 16 (December 1983): S199–203.

20. Levinsky and Rettig, "The Medicare End-State Renal Disease Program," 1143–48.

21. P. J. Held et al., "Mortality and duration of hemodialysis treatment," *Journal of the American Medical Association* 265 (20 February 1991): 871–75.

22. Collins and Kjellstrand, "Shortening of the hemodialysis procedure and mortality in 'healthy' dialysis patients," M145–48.

23. J. P. Wauters et al., "Short hemodialysis: long-term mor-

tality and morbidity," *Artificial Organs* 10 (June 1986): 182–84.

24. P. Schmidt et al., "Morbidity during regular dialysis treatment and after renal transplantation," *Wiener Klinische Wochenschrift* 91 (16 March 1979): 193–97. (Published in German)

25. Degoulet et al., "Mortality risk factors in patients treated by chronic hemodialysis," 103–10.

26. F. Coronel et al., "Analysis of factors in the prognosis of diabetics on continuous ambulatory peritoneal dialysis (CAPD): long-term experience," *Peritoneal Dialysis International* 9 (Number 2, 1989): 121–25.

27. A. Davenport, P. N. Bramley, and J. I. Wyatt, "Morbidity and mortality due to cerebral edema complicating the treatment of severe leptospiral infection," *American Journal of Kidney Diseases* 16 (August 1990): 160–65.

28. J. A. Chazan, N. L. Lew, and E. G. Lowrie, "Increased serum aluminum. An independent risk factor for mortality in patients undergoing long-term hemodialysis," *Archives of Internal Medicine* 151 (February 1991): 319–22.

29. J. A. Chazan et al., "Increased body aluminum. An independent risk factor in patients undergoing long-term hemodialysis?" *Archives of Internal Medicine* 148 (August 1988): 1817–20.

30. A. J. Smith et al., "Aluminum-related bone disease in mild and advanced renal failure: Evidence for high prevalence and morbidity and studies on etiology and diagnosis," *American Journal of Nephrology* 6 (Number 4, 1986): 275–83.

31. Ibid.

32. A. Holm, E. A. Rutsky, and J. S. Aldrete, "Short- and long-term effectiveness, morbidity, and mortality of peritoneovenous shunt inserted to treat massive refractory ascites of nephrogenic origin analysis of 14 cases," *American Surgeon* 55 (November 1989): 645–52.

33. M. Bruguera et al., "Incidence and features of liver disease in patients on chronic hemodialysis," *Journal of Clinical Gastroenterology* 12 (June 1990): 298–302.

34. T. P. Kalman, P. G. Wilson, and C. M. Kalman, "Psychiatric morbidity in long-term renal transplant recipients and patients undergoing hemodialysis. A comparative study," *Journal of the American Medical Association* 250 (1 July 1983): 55–58.

35. T. Sensky, "Psychiatric morbidity in renal transplantation," *Psychotherapy and Psychosomatics* 52 (Number 1–3, 1989): 41–46.

36. I. M. Numan, K. S. Barklind, and B. Lubin, "Correlates of depression in chronic dialysis patients: Morbidity and mortality," *Research in Nursing and Health* 4 (September 1981): 295–97.

37. F. G. Foster and F. P. McKegney, "Small group dynamics and survival on chronic hemodialysis," *International Journal of Psychiatry in Medicine* 8 (Number 2, 1977–78): 105–16.

38. Levinsky and Rettig, "The Medicare End-State Renal Disease Program," 1143–48.

39. V. E. Pollak et al., "Repeated use of dialyzers is safe: Long-term observations on morbidity and mortality in patients with end-stage renal disease," *Nephron* 42 (Number 3, 1986): 217–23.

40. A. J. Wing et al., "Mortality and morbidity of reusing dialysers. A report by the registration committee of the European Dialysis and Transplant Association," *British Medical Journal* 2 (23 September 1978): 853–55.

41. Levinsky and Rettig, "The Medicare End-State Renal Disease Program," 1143–48.

Hemorrhoidectomy

1. J. L. Masson, "Outpatient hemorrhoidectomy using the CO_2 laser," *Journal de Chirurgie (Paris)* 127 (April 1990): 227–29. (Published in French)

2. J. Bartizal and P. A. Slosberg, "An alternative to hemorrhoidectomy," *Archives of Surgery* 112 (April 1977): 534–36.

3. V. Wienert, "Ambulatory hemorrhoidectomy through rubber band ligation," *Fortschritte der Medizin* 95 (7 July 1977): 1619–22. (Published in German)

4. R. G. Saleeby, Jr., et al., "Hemorrhoidectomy during pregnancy: Risk or relief?" *Diseases of the Colon and Rectum* 34 (March 1991): 260–61.

5. J. Y. Wang et al., "The role of lasers in hemorrhoidectomy," *Diseases of the Colon and Rectum* 34 (January 1991): 78–82.

6. S. K. Asfar, T. H. Juma, and T. Ala-Edeen, "Hemorrhoidectomy and sphincterotomy. A prospective study comparing the effectiveness of anal stretch and sphincterotomy in reducing pain after hemorrhoidectomy," *Diseases of the Colon and Rectum* 31 (March 1988): 181–85.

7. P. E. Mortensen et al., "A randomized study on hemorrhoidectomy combined with anal dilatation," *Diseases of the Colon and Rectum* 30 (October 1987): 755–57.

8. C. D. Johnson, J. Budd, and A. J. Ward, "Laxatives after

hemorrhoidectomy," *Diseases of the Colon and Rectum* 30 (October 1987): 780–81.

9. L. E. Smith, J. J. Goodreau, and W. J. Fouty, "Operative hemorrhoidectomy versus cryodestruction," *Diseases of the Colon and Rectum* 22 (January–February 1979): 10–16.

10. V. Berta, M. Perelli-Ercolini, and G. Beani, "Criteria for choice of cryosurgical hemorrhoidectomy," *Chirurgia Italiana* 31 (February 1979): 78–82. (Published in Italian)

11. Y. Yamamoto and K. Sano, "Cryosurgical hemorrhoidectomy: How to prevent the postoperative swelling and prolapse," *Cryobiology* 19 (June 1982): 289–91.

12. P. M. Nieves, J. Perez, and J. A. Suarez, "Hemorrhoidectomy—how I do it: Experience with the St. Mark's Hospital technique for emergency hemorrhoidectomy," *Diseases of the Colon and Rectum* 20 (April 1977): 197–201.

13. J. C. McConnell and I. T. Khubchandani, "Long-term follow-up of closed hemorrhoidectomy," *Diseases of the Colon and Rectum* 26 (December 1983): 797–99.

14. Z. Cohen, "Symposium on outpatient anorectal procedures. Alternatives to surgical hemorrhoidectomy," *Canadian Journal of Surgery* 28 (May 1985): 230–31.

15. Ibid.

16. J. P. Thomson, "Hemorrhoidectomy—how I do it: Current views in Britain," *Diseases of the Colon and Rectum* 20 (April 1977): 173–76.

17. B. G. Wolff and C. E. Culp, "The Whitehead hemorrhoidectomy. An unjustly maligned procedure," *Diseases of the Colon and Rectum* 31 (August 1988): 587–90.

18. J. C. Bonello, "Who's afraid of the dentate line? The Whitehead hemorrhoidectomy," *American Journal of Surgery* 156 (September 1988): 182–86.

19. C. V. Devien and J. P. Pujol, "Total circular hemorrhoidectomy," *International Surgery* 74 (July–September 1989): 154–57.

Incisional Hernia Repair

1. J. O. DeLancey, R. A. Starr, and T. E. Elkins, "Incisional hernia of the vaginal apex following vaginal hysterectomy in a premenopausal, sexually inactive woman," *Obstetrics and Gynecology* 73 (May 1989): 880–81.

2. J. A. Fantl, H. B. Krebs, and L. J. Dunn, "Incisional bladder hernia and urinary incontinence: Report of three cases," *Obstetrics and Gynecology* 65 (March 1985, Supplement): 74S–77S.

3. C. S. Ubhi and D. L. Morris, "Fracture and herniation of bowel at bone graft donor site in the iliac crest," *Injury* 16 (November 1984): 202–3.

4. N. Gammelgaard and J. Jensen, "Wound complications after closure of abdominal incisions with Dexon or Vicryl. A randomized double-blind study," *ACTA Chirurgica Scandinavica* 149 (Number 5, 1983): 505–8.

5. T. E. Bucknall, "Factors influencing wound complications: A clinical and experimental study," *Annals of the Royal College of Surgeons of England* 65 (March 1983): 71–77.

6. C. D. George and H. Ellis, "The results of incisional hernia repair: A 12-year review," *Annals of the Royal College of Surgeons of England* 68 (July 1986): 185–87.

7. S. Langer and J. Christiansen, "Long-term results after incisional hernia repair," *ACTA Chirurgica Scandinavica* 151 (Number 3, 1985): 217–19.

8. J. D. McCarthy and M. W. Twiest, "Intraperitoneal polypropylene mesh support of incisional herniorraphy," *American Journal of Surgery* 142 (December 1981): 707–11.

9. G. M. Larson and H. W. Harrower, "Plastic mesh repair of incisional hernias," *American Journal of Surgery* 135 (April 1978): 559–63.

10. M. P. Elliott and G. L. Juler, "Comparison of Marlex mesh and microporous teflon sheets when used for hernia repair in the experimental animal," *American Journal of Surgery* 137 (March 1979): 342–44.

11. E. J. Cerise et al., "The use of Mersilene mesh in repair of abdominal wall hernias: A clinical and experimental study," *Annals of Surgery* 181 (May 1975): 728–34.

12. R. G. Molloy et al., "Massive incisional hernia: Abdominal wall replacement with Marlex mesh," *British Journal of Surgery* 78 (February 1991): 242–44.

13. S. F. Sener et al., "Technique and complications of reconstruction of the pelvic floor with polyglactin mesh," *Surgery, Gynecology, and Obstetrics* 168 (June 1989): 475–80.

14. J. R. Ausobsky, M. Evans, and A. V. Pollock, "Does mass closure of midline laparotomies stand the test of time? A random control clinical trial," *Annals of the Royal College of Surgeons of England* 67 (May 1985): 159–61.

15. J. R. Andersen et al., "Polyglycolic acid, silk, and topical ampicillin. Their use in hernia repair and cholecystectomy," *Archives of Surgery* 115 (March 1980): 293–95.

16. P. M. McNeil and H. J. Sugerman, "Continuous absorbable vs interrupted nonabsorbable fascial closure. A pro-

spective, randomized comparison," *Archives of Surgery* 121 (July 1986): 821–23.

17. J. C. Goligher et al., "A controlled clinical trial of three methods of closure of laparotomy wounds," *British Journal of Surgery* 62 (October 1975): 823–29.

18. C. P. Armstrong et al., "Wound healing in obstructive jaundice," *British Journal of Surgery* 71 (April 1984): 267–70.

19. T. T. Irvin et al., "Abdominal wound healing in jaundiced patients," *British Journal of Surgery* 65 (July 1978): 521–22.

20. T. T. Irvin, C. G. Koffman, and H. L. Duthie, "Layer closure of laparotomy wounds with absorbable and nonabsorbable suture materials," *British Journal of Surgery* 63 (October 1976): 793–96.

21. P. M. Lamont and H. Ellis, "Incisional hernia in reopened abdominal incisions: An overlooked risk factor," *British Journal of Surgery* 75 (April 1988): 374–76.

22. E. Hoffman, "Prophylactic antibiotic usage in clean surgical procedures," *American Surgeon* 50 (March 1984): 161–64.

23. Langer and Christiansen, "Long-term results after incisional hernia repair," 217–19.

24. Armstrong et al., "Wound healing in obstructive jaundice," 267–70.

25. Irvin et al., "Abdominal wound healing in jaundiced patients," 521–22.

26. F. W. Gierhake et al., "Immunologic aspects to the prevention of infection cardiac surgery," *Thoraxchirurgie Vaskulare Chirurgie* 23 (August 1975): 417–22. (Published in German)

Insertion of Intercostal Catheter

1. T. T. Huang, D. H. Parks, and S. R. Lewis, "Outpatient breast surgery under intercostal block anesthesia," *Plastic and Reconstructive Surgery* 63 (March 1979): 299–303.

2. D. J. Krauss, F. Khonsari, and O. M. Lilien, "Incapacitating flank pain of questionable renal origin," *Urology* 9 (January 1977): 61–67.

3. E. C. Ashby, "Abdominal pain of spinal origin. Value of intercostal block," *Annals of the Royal College of Surgeons of England* 59 (May 1977): 242–46.

4. P. P. Gerasimenko, "Thoracophrenotomy as an approach to the adrenal glands," *Vestnik Khirurgii Imeni I. I. Grekova* 117 (November 1976): 64–70. (Published in Russian)

5. J. Aubert, K. Koumare, and A. Dufrenot, "Anatomical study of the twelfth intercostal nerve and oblique lumbotomies," *Journal of Urology (Paris)* 87 (Number 5, 1981): 283–89. (Published in French)

6. A. T. Young et al., "Percutaneous extraction of urinary calculi: Use of the intercostal approach," *Radiology* 154 (March 1985): 633–38.

7. D. F. Murphy, "Continuous intercostal nerve blockade for pain relief following cholecystectomy," *British Journal of Anaethesia* 55 (June 1983): 521–24.

8. G. Engberg and L. Wiklund, "Pulmonary complications after upper abdominal surgery: Their prevention with intercostal blocks," *ACTA Anaesthesiologica Scandinavica* 32 (January 1988): 1–9.

9. L. H. Toledo-Pereyra and T. R. DeMeester, "Prospective randomized evaluation of intrathoracic intercostal nerve block with bupivacaine on postoperative ventilatory function," *Annals of Thoracic Surgery* 27 (March 1979): 203–5.

10. Ibid.

11. R. J. Faust and L. A. Nauss, "Post-thoracotomy intercostal block: Comparison of its effects on pulmonary function with those of intramuscular meperidine," *Anesthesia and Analgesia* 55 (July–August 1976): 542–46.

12. Toledo-Pereyra and DeMeester, "Prospective randomized evaluation of intrathoracic intercostal nerve block with bupivacaine on postoperative ventilatory function," 203–5.

13. A. D. Baxter et al., "Continuous intercostal blockade after cardiac surgery," *British Journal of Anaesthesia* 59 (February 1987): 162–66.

14. D. W. Noller et al., "Intercostal nerve block with flank incision," *Journal of Urology* 117 (June 1977): 759–61.

15. R. D. Miller, R. R. Johnston, and Y. Hosobuchi, "Treatment of intercostal neuralgia with 10 percent ammonium sulfate," *Journal of Thoracic and Cardiovascular Surgery* 69 (March 1975): 476–78.

16. W. B. Ross et al., "Intercostal blockade and pulmonary function after cholecystectomy," *Surgery* 105 (February 1989): 166–69.

17. J. E. Galway, P. K. Caves, and J. W. Dundee, "Effect of intercostal nerve blockade during operation on lung function and the relief of pain following thoracotomy," *British Journal of Anaesthesia* 47 (June 1975): 730–35.

18. Engberg and Wiklund, "Pulmonary complications after upper abdominal surgery," 1–9.

19. R. G. Berrisford et al., "Pulmonary complications after lung resection: The effect of continuous extrapleural intercostal nerve block," *European Journal of Cardiothoracic Surgery* 4 (Number 8, 1990): 407–10.

20. E. D. Crawford and D. G. Skinner, "Intercostal nerve block with thoracoabdominal and flank incisions," *Urology* 19 (January 1982): 25–28.

21. E. D. Crawford, D. G. Skinner, and D. B. Capparell, "Intercostal nerve block with thoracoabdominal incision," *Journal of Urology* 121 (March 1979): 290–91.

22. G. Engberg, "Respiratory performance after upper abdominal surgery. A comparison of pain relief with intercostal blocks and centrally acting analgesics," *ACTA Anaesthesiologica Scandinavica* 29 (May 1985): 427–33.

23. V. M. Pedersen et al., "Air-flow meter assessment of the effect of intercostal nerve blockade on respiratory function in rib fractures," *ACTA Chirurgica Scandinavica* 149 (Number 2, 1983): 119–20.

24. P. Bunting and J. F. McGeachie, "Intercostal nerve blockade producing analgesia after appendectomy," *British Journal of Anaesthesia* 61 (August 1988): 169–72.

25. E. Ishizuka et al., "Continuous intercostal nerve block for pain relief after lumbar incision," *Journal of Urology* 122 (October 1979): 506–7.

26. H. Vaghadia and L. C. Jenkins, "Use of a Doppler ultrasound stethoscope for intercostal nerve block," *Canadian Journal of Anaesthesia* 35 (January 1988): 86–89.

27. P. G. Atanassoff et al., "Intercostal nerve block for minor breast surgery," *Regional Anaesthesie* 16 (January–February 1991): 23–27.

28. Young et al., "Percutaneous extraction of urinary calculi," 633–38.

29. Berrisford et al., "Pulmonary complications after lung resection," 407–10.

30. Young et al., "Percutaneous extraction of urinary calculi," 633–38.

31. Huang, Parks, and Lewis, "Outpatient breast surgery under intercostal block anesthesia," 299–303.

32. S. Sabanathan et al., "Continuous intercostal nerve block for pain relief after thoracotomy," *Annals of Thoracic Surgery* 46 (October 1988): 425–26.

33. J. F. Nunn and G. Slavin, "Posterior intercostal nerve block for pain relief after cholecystectomy. Anatomical basis and efficacy," *British Journal of Anaesthesia* 52 (March 1980): 253–60.

34. D. C. Moore, "Intercostal nerve block for postoperative somatic pain following surgery of thorax and upper abdomen," *British Journal of Anaesthesia* 47 (February 1975, Supplement): 284–86.

35. K. D. Cronin and M. J. Davies, "Intercostal block for post operative pain relief," *Anaesthesia and Intensive Care* 4 (August 1976): 259–61.

36. M. P. Shelly and G. R. Park, "Intercostal nerve blockade for children," *Anaesthesia* 42 (May 1987): 541–44.

37. D. W. Blake, G. Donnan, and J. Novella, "Interpleural administration of bupivacaine after cholecystectomy: A comparison with intercostal nerve block," *Anaesthesia and Intensive Care* 17 (August 1989): 269–74.

38. J. A. Gallo, Jr., et al., "Complications of intercostal nerve blocks performed under direct vision during thoracotomy: A report of two cases," *Journal of Thoracic and Cardiovascular Surgery* 86 (October 1983): 628–30.

39. W. Scholl and H. V. Makowski, "High spinal anaesthesia following intrathoracic intercostal nerve block," *Anaesthesist* 26 (March 1977): 151–52. (Published in German)

40. C. W. Otto and C. L. Wall, "Total spinal anesthesia: A rare complication of intrathoracic intercostal nerve block," *Annals of Thoracic Surgery* 22 (September 1976): 289–92.

41. A. Mowbray, K. K. Wong, and J. M. Murray, "Intercostal catheterization. An alternative approach to the paravertebral space," *Anaesthesia* 42 (September 1987): 958–61.

42. D. C. Moore, W. H. Bush, and J. E. Scurlock, "Intercostal nerve block: A roentgenographic anatomic study of technique and absorption in humans," *Anesthesia and Analgesia* 59 (November 1980): 815–25.

43. D. C. Moore, "Anatomy of the intercostal nerve: Its importance during thoracic surgery," *American Journal of Surgery* 144 (September 1982): 371–73.

44. W. F. Casey, "Respiratory failure following intercostal nerve blockade," *Anaesthesia* 39 (April 1984): 351–54.

45. J. Ponten et al., "Bupivacaine for intercostal nerve blockade in patients on long-term beta-receptor blocking therapy," *ACTA Anaesthesiologica Scandinavica,* Supplement 76 (1982): 70–77.

46. Baxter et al., "Continuous intercostal blockade after cardiac surgery," 162–66.

47. Gallo et al., "Complications of intercostal nerve blocks performed under direct vision during thoracotomy," 628–30.

48. Ross et al., "Intercostal blockade and pulmonary function after cholecystectomy," 166–69.

49. N. Rawal et al., "Epidural morphine for postoperative pain relief: A comparative study with intramuscular narcotic and intercostal nerve block," *Anesthesia and Analgesia* 61 (February 1982): 93–98.

50. H. Shafei et al., "Intrapleural bupivacaine for early post-thoracotomy analgesia—comparison with bupivacaine intercostal block and cryofreezing," *Thoracic and Cardiovascular Surgery* 38 (February 1990): 38–41.

51. M. J. Jones and K. R. Murrin, "Intercostal block with cryotherapy," *Annals of the Royal College of Surgeons of England* 69 (November 1987): 261–62.

52. S. Sabanathan et al., "Efficacy of continuous extrapleural intercostal nerve block on post-thoracotomy pain and pulmonary mechanics," *British Journal of Surgery* 77 (February 1990): 221–25.

53. G. C. Roviaro et al., "Intrathoracic intercostal nerve block with phenol in open chest surgery. A randomized study with statistical evaluation of respiratory parameters," *Chest* 90 (July 1986): 64–67.

54. W. H. Fleming and L. B. Sarafian, "Kindness pays dividends: The medical benefits of intercostal nerve block following thoracotomy," *Journal of Thoracic and Cardiovascular Surgery* 74 (August 1977): 273–74.

Intervertebral Disk Excision

1. L. L. Wiltse, "Surgery for intervertebral disk disease of the lumbar spine," *Clinical Orthopaedics and Related Research* (November–December 1977): 22–45.

2. C. L. Branch and C. L. Branch, Jr., "Posterior lumbar interbody fusion with the keystone graft: Technique and results," *Surgical Neurology* 27 (May 1987): 449–54.

3. H. Bertalanffy and H. R. Eggert, "Complications of anterior cervical discectomy without fusion in 450 consecutive patients," *ACTA Neurochirurgica (Wien)* 99 (Number 1–2, 1989): 41–50.

4. Ibid.

5. Ibid.

6. M. E. Brooks et al., "Urologic complications after surgery on lumbosacral spine," *Urology* 26 (August 1985): 202–4.

7. N. Nakano, "Lower lumbar anterior discectomy without fusion: A several year follow-up indicating usefulness of this technique in surgery of the lower lumbar spine," *Nippon Seikeigeka Gakkai Zasshi* 57 (March 1983): 321–28.

8. J. A. Freischlag et al., "Vascular complications associated with orthopedic procedures," *Surgery, Gynecology, and Obstetrics* 169 (August 1989): 147–52.

9. J. L. Pinkowski and M. C. Leeson, "Anaphylactic shock associated with chymopapin skin test. A case report and review of the literature," *Clinical Orthopaedics and Related Research* (November 1990): 186–90.

10. S. Roukoz et al., "Critical study of 200 surgically treated lumbar disk hernias," *Annales de Chirurgie* 44 (Number 1, 1990): 44–48. (Published in French)

11. M. E. Taylor, "Return to work following back surgery: A review," *American Journal of Industrial Medicine* 16 (Number 1, 1989): 79–88.

12. G. Onik and C. A. Helms, "Automated percutaneous lumbar diskectomy." *American Journal of Roentgenology, Radium Therapy, and Nuclear* 156 (March 1991): 531–38.

13. P. Kambin and J. L. Schaffer, "Percutaneous lumbar discectomy. Review of 100 patients and current practice," *Clinical Orthopaedics and Related Research* (January 1989): 24–34.

14. "Diagnostic and therapeutic technology assessment. Chemonucleolysis for herniated lumbar disk," *Journal of the American Medical Association* 262 (18 August 1989): 953–56.

15. G. R. Cybulski, J. L. Stone, and R. Kant, "Outcome of laminectomy for civilian gunshot injuries of the terminal spinal cord and cauda equina: Review of 88 cases," *Neurosurgery* 24 (March 1989): 392–97.

16. G. Opitz et al., "Surgical therapy of backache," *Fortschritte der Medizin* 107 (20 June 1989): 69–70, 73–74. (Published in German)

Joint Replacement Revision

1. HealthCare Knowledge Resources/Commission on Professional and Hospital Activities, *HealthWeek* (25 February 1991).

2. J. A. Roberts, D. F. Finlayson, and P. A. Freeman, "The long-term results of the Howse total hip arthroplasty. With particular reference to those requiring revision," *Journal of Bone and Joint Surgery, British Volume* 69 (August 1987): 545–50.

3. D. J. Schurman et al., "Conventional cemented total hip arthroplasty. Assessment of clinical factors associated with re-

vision for mechanical failure," *Clinical Orthopaedics and Related Research* (March 1989): 173–80.

4. Y. Dohmae et al., "Reduction in cement-bone interface shear strength between primary and revision arthroplasty," *Clinical Orthopaedics and Related Research* (November 1988: 214–20.

5. D. S. Hungerford and L. C. Jones, "The rationale of cementless revision of cemented arthroplasty failures," *Clinical Orthopaedics and Related Research* (October 1988): 12–24.

6. N. S. Broughton and N. Rushton, "Revision hip arthroplasty. A retrospective survey," *ACTA Orthopaedica Scandinavica* 53 (December 1982): 923–28.

7. S. Esses, D. Hastings, and J. Schatzker, "Revision of total hip arthroplasty," *Canadian Journal of Surgery* 26 (July 1983): 345–47.

8. J. B. Retpen et al., "Clinical results after revision and primary total hip arthroplasty," *Journal of Arthroplasty* 4 (December 1989): 297–302.

9. E. T. James, G. A. Hunter, and H. U. Cameron, "Total hip revision arthroplasty: Does sepsis influence the results?" *Clinical Orthopaedics and Related Research* (October 1982): 88–94.

10. G. B. Miley et al., "Medical and surgical treatment of the septic hip with one-stage revision arthroplasty," *Clinical Orthopaedics and Related Research* (October 1982): 76–82.

11. W. R. Murray, "Acetabular salvage in revision total hip arthroplasty using the bipolar prosthesis," *Clinical Orthopaedics and Related Research* (February 1990): 92–99.

12. L. Sanzen et al., "Revision operations on infected total hip arthroplasties. Two- to nine-year follow-up study," *Clinical Orthopaedics and Related Research* (April 1988): 165–72.

13. A. K. Hedley et al., "Revision of failed total hip arthroplasties with uncemented porous-coated anatomic components," *Clinical Orthopaedics and Related Research* (October 1988): 75–90.

14. H. U. Cameron et al., "Revision of total knee replacement," *Canadian Journal of Surgery* 24 (July 1981): 418–20.

15. S. Bengtson, K. Knutson, and L. Lidgren, "Revision of infected knee arthroplasty," *ACTA Orthpaedica Scandinavica* 57 (December 1986): 489–94.

16. W. H. Harris, "Revision surgery for failed, nonseptic total hip arthroplasty: The femoral side," *Clinical Orthopaedics and Related Research* (October 1982): 8–20.

17. R. J. Friedman et al., "Results of revision total knee arthroplasty performed for aseptic loosening," *Clinical Orthopaedics and Related Research* (June 1990): 235–41.

18. B. F. Morrey and R. S. Bryan, "Revision total elbow arthroplasty," *Journal of Bone and Joint Surgery, American Volume* 69 (April 1987): 523–32.

19. M. P. Murray et al., "Function after revision of failed total hip arthroplasty," *ACTA Orthpaedica Scandinavica* 55 (February 1984): 59–62.

20. C. M. Christensen, B. M. Seger, and R. B. Schultz, "Management of intraoperative femur fractures associated with revision hip arthroplasty," *Clinical Orthopaedics and Related Research* (November 1989): 177–80.

21. O. A. Nercessian, E. G. Gonzalez, and F. E. Stinchfield, "The use of somatosensory-evoked potential during revision or reoperation for total hip arthroplasty," *Clinical Orthopaedics and Related Research* (June 1989): 138–42.

22. K. Steinbrink, "The case for revision arthroplasty using antibiotic-loaded acrylic cement," *Clinical Orthopaedics and Related Research* (December 1990): 19–22.

23. R. Soto-Hall et al., "Tobramycin in bone cement. An indepth analysis of wound, serum, and urine concentrations in patients undergoing total hip revision arthroplasty," *Clinical Orthopaedics and Related Research* (May 1983): 60–64.

24. B. M. Wroblewski, "One-stage revision of infected cemented total hip arthroplasty," *Clinical Orthopaedics and Related Research* (October 1986): 103–7.

25. R. A. Mollan and C. J. McClelland, "Instrumentation for the revision of total hip arthroplasty," *Clinical Orthopaedics and Related Research* (June 1984): 16–22.

26. R. D. Scott, "Revision total knee arthroplasty," *Clinical Orthopaedics and Related Research* (January 1988): 65–77.

27. R. H. Emerson, Jr., et al., "Noncemented acetabular revision arthroplasty using allograft bone," *Clinical Orthopaedics and Related Research* (December 1989): 30–43.

28. L. A. Whiteside, "Cementless reconstruction of massive tibial bone loss in revision total knee arthroplasty," *Clinical Orthopaedics and Related Research* (November 1989): 80–86.

Left Hemicolectomy

1. P. M. Griffin et al., "Adenocarcinomas of the colon and rectum in persons under 40 years old. A population-based study," *Gastroenterology* 100 (April 1991): 1033–40.

2. L. Rosenberg et al., "A hypothesis: Nonsteroidal anti-inflammatory drugs reduce the incidence of large-bowel cancer,"

Journal of the National Cancer Institute 83 (6 March 1991): 355–58.

3. J. M. Carstensen, L. O. Bygren, and T. Hatschek, "Cancer incidence among Swedish brewery workers," *International Journal of Cancer* 45 (15 March 1990): 393–96.

4. R. S. Snell, *Clinical Anatomy for Medical Students,* 3rd ed. (Boston: Little, Brown, and Company, 1986), 281–83.

5. R. W. Busuttil, R. P. Foglia, and W. P. Longmire, Jr., "Treatment of carcinoma of the sigmoid colon and upper rectum. A comparison of local segmental resection and left hemicolectomy," *Archives of Surgery* 112 (August 1977): 920–23.

6. W. J. Hoskins et al., "Right hemicolectomy and ileal resection with primary reanastomosis for irradiation injury of the terminal ileum," *Gynecologic Oncology* 26 (February 1987): 215–24.

7. B. A. Mizock, "Branched-chain amino acids in sepsis and hepatic failure," *Archives of Internal Medicine* 145 (July 1985): 1284–88.

8. F. Rouffet et al., "Surgical treatment of cancer of the left colon. True left hemicolectomy or segmental colectomy?" *Journal de Chirurgie (Paris)* 125 (December 1988): 712–16. (Published in French)

9. Busuttil, Foglia, and Longmire, "Treatment of carcinoma of the sigmoid colon and upper rectum," 920–23.

10. W. P. Morgan et al., "Management of obstructing carcinoma of the left colon by extended right hemicolectomy," *American Journal of Surgery* 149 (March 1985): 327–29.

11. Ibid.

12. N. Bouasakao et al., "Colo-duodenal fistula caused by cancer of the right colonic flexure treated by right extended hemicolectomy associated with a mucosal patch using a terminal ileal pedicled graft. Apropos of a case," *Journal de Chirurgie* 121 (December 1984): 757–63. (Published in French)

Ligation and Stripping of Varicose Veins of the Legs

1. E. W. Taylor et al., "Long saphenous vein stripping under local anaesthesia," *Annals of the Royal College of Surgeons of England* 63 (May 1981): 206–7.

2. P. Conrad, "Sclerostripping—a new procedure for the treatment of varicose veins," *Medical Journal of Australia* 2 (12 July 1975): 42–44.

3. B. Almgren et al., "The posterior approach for subfascial ligation of perforating veins," *ACTA Chirurgica Scandinavica* 148 (Number 3, 1982): 243–45.

4. J. B. Holme, K. Skajaa, and K. Holme, "Incidence of lesions of the saphenous nerve after partial or complete stripping of the long saphenous vein," *ACTA Chirurgica Scandinavica* 156 (February 1990): 145–48.

5. S. S. Ramasastry, G. O. Dick, and J. W. Futrell, "Anatomy of the saphenous nerve: Relevance to saphenous vein stripping," *American Surgeon* 53 (May 1987): 274–77.

6. H. M. Becker, "A successful blood vessel reconstruction following inadvertent exeresis of arteries during varicose vein surgery," *Chirurg* 46 (August 1975): 367–70. (Published in German)

7. A. H. Boontje, "Iatrogenic arterial injuries," *Journal of Cardiovascular Surgery (Torino)* 19 (July–August 1978): 335–40.

8. J. E. Liddicoat et al., "Inadvertent femoral artery 'stripping': Surgical management," *Surgery* 77 (February 1975): 318–20.

9. E. P. Lofgren, H. L. Coates, and P. C. O'Brien, "Clinically suspect pulmonary embolism after vein stripping," *Mayo Clinic Proceedings* 51 (February 1976): 77–80.

10. R. A. Nabatoff, "Technique for operation upon recurrent varicose veins," *Surgery, Gynecology and Obstetrics* 143 (September 1976): 463–67.

11. D. Reinharez, "Impotence following stripping," *Phlebologie* 33 (July–September 1980): 427–36. (Published in French)

12. J. P. Henriet et al., "A new case of impotence after stripping," *Phlebologie* 38 (April–June 1985): 319–32. (Published in French)

13. K. A. Lofgren, "Surgical management of chronic venous insufficiency," *ACTA Chirurgica Scandinavica, Supplement* (1988) 544: 62–68.

14. F. M. Ameli, "Current concepts in the management of varicose veins," *Canadian Journal of Surgery* 29 (January 1986): 21–23.

15. J. Tremblay, E. W. Lewis, and P. T. Allen, "Selecting a treatment for primary varicose veins," *Canadian Medical Association Journal* 133 (1 July 1985): 20–25.

16. E. J. Orbach, "Controversies and realities of therapy for varicosis," *International Surgery* 62 (March 1977): 149–51.

17. K. Koyano and S. Sakaguchi, "Selective stripping operation based on Doppler ultrasonic findings for primary varicose veins of the lower extremities," *Surgery* 103 (June 1988): 615–19.

Lobectomy of Lung

1. A. R. Gribetz et al., "Rhizopus lung abscess in renal transplant patient successfully treated by lobectomy," *Chest* 77 (January 1980): 102–4.

2. A. Schattenberg et al., "Allogeneic bone marrow transplantation after partial lobectomy for aspergillosis of the lung," *Bone Marrow Transplant* 3 (September 1988): 509–12.

3. F. J. Rescorla et al., "Pulmonary hypertension in neonatal cystic lung disease: Survival following lobectomy and ECMO in two cases," *Journal of Pediatric Surgery* 25 (October 1990): 1054–56.

4. D. K. Porter, M. J. Van Every, and J. W. Mack, Jr., "Emergency lobectomy for massive hemoptysis in cystic fibrosis," *Journal of Thoracic and Cardiovascular Surgery* 86 (September 1983): 409–11.

5. B. Frenckner and U. Freyschuss, "Pulmonary function after lobectomy for congenital lobar emphysema and congenital cystic adenomatoid malformation," *Scandinavian Journal of Thoracic and Cardiovascular Surgery* 16 (Number 3, 1982): 293–98.

6. E. B. Diethrich et al., "Postoperative complications necessitating right lower lobectomy in a heart-lung transplant recipient with previous sternotomy," *Journal of Thoracic and Cardiovascular Surgery* 94 (September 1987): 389–92.

7. J. A. Fleetham, H. Clarke, and N. R. Anthonisen, "Regional lung function in erect humans after lobectomy," *Journal of Applied Physiology* 54 (April 1983): 1018–24.

8. J. A. Barker, W. Z. Yahr, and B. P. Krieger, "Right upper lobectomy 20 years after left pneumonectomy. Preoperative evaluation and follow-up," *Chest* 97 (January 1990): 248–50.

9. R. K. Firmin et al., "Sleeve lobectomy (lobectomy and bronchoplasty) for bronchial carcinoma," *Annals of Thoracic Surgery* 35 (April 1983): 442–49.

10. J. M. Van Den Bosch et al., "Lobectomy with sleeve resection in the treatment of tumors of the bronchus," *Chest* 80 (August 1981): 154–57.

11. R. D. Weisel et al., "Sleeve lobectomy for carcinoma of the lung," *Journal of Thoracic and Cardiovascular Surgery* 78 (December 1979): 839–49.

12. V. V. Rodionov, A. G. Kunitsin, and N. G. Artem'eva, "Our 15 years' experience using lobectomy with resection and plastic surgery of the bronchi in lung cancer," *Vestnik Khirurgii Imeni I. I. Grekova* 132 (January 1984): 17–21. (Published in Russian)

13. J. Deslauriers et al., "Long-term clinical and functional results of sleeve lobectomy for primary lung cancer," *Journal of Thoracic and Cardiovascular Surgery* 92 (November 1986): 871–79.

14. R. T. Shipley and M. C. Mahoney, "Right middle lobe collapse following right upper lobectomy," *Radiology* 166 (March 1988): 725–28.

15. T. Ishihara et al., "Does pleural bronchial wrapping improve wound healing in right sleeve lobectomy?" *Journal of Thoracic and Cardiovascular Surgery* 89 (May 1985): 665–72.

16. M. L. Pinstein et al., "Middle lobe torsion following right upper lobectomy," *Radiology* 155 (June 1985): 580.

17. L. E. Quint, G. M. Glazer, and M. B. Orringer, "Central lung masses: Prediction with CT of need for pneumonectomy versus lobectomy," *Radiology* 165 (December 1987): 735–38.

18. M. Valente et al., "Lobectomy with bronchoplastic procedures for lung cancer," *Tumori* 65 (31 October 1979): 643–48.

19. T. H. Hoffmann and H. T. Ransdell, "Comparison of lobectomy and wedge resection for carcinoma of the lung," *Journal of Thoracic and Cardiovascular Surgery* 79 (February 1980): 211–17.

20. J. G. Llaurado et al., "Radioisotopic pulmonary lobectomy: Feasibility study in dogs," *Journal of Nuclear Medicine* 31 (May 1990): 594–600.

21. Deslauriers et al., "Long-term clinical and functional results of sleeve lobectomy for primary lung cancer," 871–79.

22. L. P. Faber, "Results of surgical treatment of stage III lung carcinoma with carinal proximity. The role of sleeve lobectomy versus pneumonectomy and the role of sleeve pneumonectomy," *Surgical Clinics of North America* 67 (October 1987): 1001–14.

23. W. Van Mieghem and M. Demedts, "Cardiopulmonary function after lobectomy or pneumonectomy for pulmonary neoplasm," *Respiratory Medicine* 83 (May 1989): 199–206.

24. N. Berend, A. J. Woolcock, and G. E. Marlin, "Effects of lobectomy on lung function," *Thorax* 35 (February 1980): 145–50.

25. A. Nonoyama et al., "Pulmonary function after lobectomy in children under ten years of age," *Japanese Journal of Surgery* 16 (November 1986): 425–34.

26. Firmin et al., "Sleeve lobectomy (lobectomy and bronchoplasty) for bronchial carcinoma," 442–49.

Local Destruction of Ovarian Lesion

1. H. Griffith Winter, *Complete Guide to Symptoms, Illness, and Surgery,* 2nd ed. (Los Angeles: The Body Press, 1989), 858–59.
2. S. A. Schroeder et al., *Current Medical Diagnosis and Treatment* (Norwalk, Conn.: Appleton & Lange, 1991), 518–20.

Local Destruction of Skin Lesion

1. T. Breza, R. Taylor, and W. H. Eaglstein, "Noninflammatory destruction of actinic keratoses by fluorouracil," *Archives of Dermatology* 112 (September 1976): 1256–58.
2. G. D. Lyons, R. E. Owens, and D. F. Mouney, "Argon laser destruction of cutaneous telangiectatic lesions," *Laryngoscope* 91 (August 1981): 1322–25.
3. S. A. Schroeder et al., *Current Medical Diagnosis and Treatment* (Norwalk, Conn.: Appleton & Lange, 1991), 95.
4. J. Menon and R. H. Gelberman, "Interphalangeal joint destruction: A complication of cryotherapy," *Journal of Hand Surgery, American Volume* 5 (November 1980): 600–1.

Low-Forceps Delivery with Episiotomy

1. A. S. Hagadorn-Freathy, E. R. Yeomans, and G. D. Hankins, "Validation of the 1988 ACOG forceps classification system," *Obstetrics and Gynecology* 77 (March 1977): 356–60.
2. *Stedman's Medical Dictionary,* 25th ed. (Baltimore: Williams and Wilkins, 1990), 409.
3. D. L. Healy, M. A. Quinn, and R. J. Pepperell, "Rotational delivery of the fetus: Kielland's forceps and two other methods compared," *British Journal of Obstetrics and Gynaecology* 89 (July 1982): 501–6.
4. HealthCare Knowledge Resources/Commission on Professional and Hospital Activities, *HealthWeek* (30 May 1989).
5. G. J. Ratten, "Changes in obstetric practice in our time," *Australian and New Zealand Journal of Obstetrics and Gynaecology* 25 (November 1985): 241–44.
6. D. A. Richardson, M. I. Evans, and L. A. Cibils, "Midforceps delivery: A critical review," *American Journal of Obstetrics and Gynecology* 145 (1 March 1983): 621–32.
7. L. Meyer et al., "Maternal and neonatal morbidity in instrumental deliveries with the Kobayashi vacuum extractor and low forceps," *ACTA Obstetricia et Gynecologica Scandinavica* 66 (Number 7, 1987): 643–47.
8. R. A. Bashore, W. H. Phillips, Jr., and C. R. Brinkman, 3d, "A comparison of the morbidity of midforceps and cesarean delivery," *American Journal of Obstetrics and Gynecology* 162 (June 1990): 1428–34.
9. D. L. Dell, S. E. Sightler, and W. C. Plauche, "Soft cup vacuum extraction: A comparison of outlet delivery," *Obstetrics and Gynecology* 66 (November 1985): 624–28.
10. J. B. Greis, J. Bieniarz, and A. Scommegna, "Comparison of maternal and fetal effects of vacuum extraction with forceps or cesarean deliveries," *Obstetrics and Gynecology* 57 (May 1981): 571–77.
11. H. Amirikia, B. Zarewych, and T. N. Evans, "Caesarean section: A 15-year review of changing incidence, indications, and risks," *American Journal of Obstetrics and Gynecology* 140 (1 May 1981): 81–90.
12. Healy, Quinn, and Pepperell, "Rotational delivery of the fetus," 501–6.
13. S. T. Nilsen, "Boys born by forceps and vacuum extraction examined at 18 years of age," *ACTA Obstetricia et Gynecologica Scandinavica* 63 (Number 6, 1984): 549–54.
14. P. Adelstein et al., "Obstetric practice and infant morbidity," *British Journal of Obstetrics and Gynaecology* 84 (October 1977): 721–25.
15. L. J. Dierker, Jr., et al., "Midforceps deliveries: Longterm outcome of infants," *American Journal of Obstetrics and Gynecology* 154 (April 1986): 764–68.
16. L. J. Dierker, Jr., et al., "The midforceps: Maternal and neonatal outcomes," *American Journal of Obstetrics and Gynecology* 152 (15 May 1985): 176–83.
17. P. A. Robertson, R. K. Laros, Jr., and R. L. Zhao, "Neonatal and maternal outcome in low-pelvic and midpelvic operative deliveries," *American Journal of Obstetrics and Gynecology* 162 (June 1990): 1436–42.
18. E. L. Silbar, "Factors related to the increasing cesarean section rates for cephalopelvic disproportion," *American Journal of Obstetrics and Gynecology* 154 (May 1986): 1095–98.

19. P. Altmann et al., "About the choice of extraction instrument for vaginal operative termination in vertex presentation," *Geburtshilfe und Frauenheilkunde* 35 (December 1975): 949–55. (Published in German)

20. J. Endl, G. Wolf, and A. Schaller, "Problems and results of skull X-ray following vacuum extraction," *Geburtshilfe und Frauenheilkunde* 35 (December 1975): 943–48. (Published in German)

21. Meyer et al., "Maternal and neonatal morbidity in instrumental deliveries with the Kobayashi vacuum extractor and low forceps," 643–47.

22. K. E. Thacker, T. Lim, and J. H. Drew, "Cephalhaematoma: A 10-year review," *Australian and New Zealand Journal of Obstetrics and Gynaecology* 27 (August 1987): 210–12.

23. G. M. Maryniak and J. B. Frank, "Clinical assessment of the Kobayashi vacuum extractor," *Obstetrics and Gynecology* 64 (September 1984): 431–35.

24. W. C. Plauche, "Fetal cranial injuries related to delivery with the Malmstrom vacuum extractor," *Obstetrics and Gynecology* 53 (June 1979): 750–57.

25. F. F. Broekhuizen et al., "Vacuum extraction versus forceps delivery: Indications and complications, 1979 to 1984," *Obstetrics and Gynecology* 69 (March 1987): 338–42.

26. W. C. Plauche, "Subgaleal hematoma. A complication of instrumental delivery," *Journal of the American Medical Association* 244 (3 October 1980): 1597–98.

27. R. Besio et al., "Neonatal retinal hemorrhages and influence of perinatal factors," *American Journal of Ophthalmology* 87 (January 1979): 74–76.

28. F. A. Chervenak et al., "Is routine cesarean section necessary for vertex-breech and vertex-transverse twin gestations?" *American Journal of Obstetrics and Gynecology* 148 (1 January 1984): 1–5.

29. H. Schrocksnadel, K. Heim, and O. Dapunt, "The clavicular fracture—a questionable achievement in modern obstetrics," *Geburtshilfe und Frauenheilkunde* 49 (May 1989): 481–84. (Published in German)

30. L. K. Angell, R. M. Robb, and F. G. Berson, "Visual prognosis in patients with ruptures in Descemet's membrane due to forceps injuries," *Archives of Ophthalmology* 99 (December 1981): 2137–39.

31. W. Lisch et al., "Corneal lesion by vacuum extraction," *Klinische Monatsblatter fur Augenheilkunde* 169 (October 1976): 520–23. (Published in German)

32. W. Wiegand, "Anophthalmos. Sequela of an unusual birth injury," *Fortschritte der Ophthalmologie* 87 (Number 5, 1990): 540–41. (Published in German)

33. S. J. Gould and J. F. Smith, "Spinal cord transection, cerebral ischaemic and brain-stem injury in a baby following a Kielland's forceps rotation," *Neuropathology and Applied Neurobiology* 10 (March–April 1984): 151–58.

34. M. C. Maheshwari, "Forceps delivery as a risk factor in epilepsy: A comparative prospective cohort survey," *Acta Neurologica Scandinavica* 81 (June 1990): 522–23.

35. N. Germane and L. Rubenstein, "The effects of forceps delivery on facial growth," *Pediatric Dentistry* 11 (September 1989): 193–97.

36. M. Camus, G. Lefebvre, and Y. Darbois, "Facial paralysis of obstetrical origin," *Revue Francaise de Gynecologie et D'Obstetrique* 81 (March 1986): 145–47. (Published in French)

37. H. Y. Ngan, G. W. Tang, and H. K. Ma, "Vacuum extractor: A safe instrument?" *Australian and New Zealand Journal of Obstetrics and Gynecology* 26 (August 1986): 177–81.

38. Maryniak and Frank, "Clinical assessment of the Kobayashi vacuum extractor," 431–35.

39. H. A. Krone and H. Heidegger, "Maternal mortality, its definition and assessment. Report of maternal mortality at the Bamberg Gynecologic Clinic 1963–1988," *Geburtshilfe und Frauenheilkunde* 49 (July 1989): 666–72. (Published in German)

40. D. B. Schwartz, M. Miodovnik, and J. P. Lavin, Jr., "Neonatal outcome among low birth weight infants delivered spontaneously or by low forceps," *Obstetrics and Gynecology* 62 (September 1983): 283–86.

41. B. J. Marshall and D. L. Healy, "Mid-cavity occipitoanterior forceps delivery—Laufe and Barnes forceps compared," *Australian and New Zealand Journal of Obstetrics and Gynecology* 27 (February 1987): 13–17.

42. S. Scherjon, "A comparison between the organization of obstetrics in Denmark and The Netherlands," *British Journal of Obstetrics and Gynaecology* 93 (July 1986): 684–89.

43. M. Tew, "Do obstetric intranatal interventions make birth safer?" *British Journal of Obstetrics and Gynecaeology* 93 (July 1986): 659–74.

44. P. Bergsjo, E. Schmidt, and D. Pusch, "Differences in the reported frequencies of some obstetrical interventions in Europe," *British Journal of Obstetrics and Gynaecology* 90 (July 1983): 628–32.

Medical Induction of Labor

1. "Eclampsie," *Presse Medicale* 19 (23 June 1990): 1188–90. (Published in French)
2. S. A. Schroeder et al., *Current Medical Diagnosis and Treatment* (Norwalk, Conn.: Appleton & Lange, 1991), 542–43.
3. W. Rath et al., "Principles of physiologic and drug-induced cervix ripening—recent morphologic and biochemical findings," *Geburtshilfe und Frauenheilkunde* 50 (September 1990): 657–64. (Published in German)
4. M. Porto, "The unfavorable cervix: Methods of cervical priming," *Clinical Obstetrics and Gynecology* 32 (June 1989): 262–68.
5. F. P. Meehan, G. Burke, and J. T. Kehoe, "Update on delivery following prior cesarean section: A 15-year review 1972–1987," *International Journal of Gynaecology and Obstetrics* 30 (November 1989): 205–12.
6. W. F. Rayburn, "Prostaglandin E2 gel for cervical ripening and induction of labor: A critical analysis," *American Journal of Obstetrics and Gynecology* 160 (March 1989): 529–34.
7. Porto, "The unfavorable cervix," 262–68.
8. Schroeder et al., *Current Medical Diagnosis and Treatment* 542.

Nephroureterectomy

1. T. Burghele, "Nephroureterectomy in urinary tuberculosis," *European Urology* 2 (Number 1, 1976): 1–3.
2. S. Pettersson et al., "Treatment of urothelial tumors of the upper urinary tract by nephroureterectomy, renal autotransplantation, and pyelocystostomy," *Cancer* 54 (1 August 1984): 379–86.

Open Reduction and Internal Fixation of Fracture of the Femur

1. HealthCare Knowledge Resources/Commission on Professional and Hospital Activities, *HealthWeek* (6 November 1989).

2. L. Tiret and F. Hatton, "Femoral neck fractures after age 65: Morbidity, mortality, lethality," *Revue D'Epidemiologie et De Sante Publique* 35 (Number 2, 1987): 157–63. (Published in French)
3. S. Holmberg et al., "Fixation of 220 femoral neck fractures. A prospective comparison of the Rydell nail and the LIH hook pins," *ACTA Orthopaedica Scandinavica* 61 (April 1990): 154–57.
4. J. S. Jensen and M. Michaelsen, "Trochanteric femoral fractures treated with McLaughlin osteosynthesis," *ACTA Orthopaedica Scandinavica* 46 (November 1975): 795–803.
5. R. N. Chan and J. Hoskinson, "Thompson prosthesis for fractured neck of femur. A comparison of surgical approaches," *Journal of Bone and Joint Surgery, British Volume* 57 (November 1975): 437–43.
6. H. Kuderna, N. Bohler, and D. J. Collon, "Treatment of intertrochanteric and subtrochanteric fractures of the hip by the Ender method," *Journal of Bone and Joint Surgery, American Volume* 58 (July 1976): 604–11.
7. O. Wihlborg, "Fixation of femoral neck fractures. A four-flanged nail versus threaded pins in 200 cases," *ACTA Orthopaedica Scandinavica* 61 (October 1990): 415–18.
8. R. A. Calandruccio, "Classification of femoral neck fractures in the elderly as pathologic fractures," *Hip* (1983): 9–33.
9. M. Delmi et al., "Dietary supplementation in elderly patients with fractured neck of the femur," *Lancet* 335 (28 April 1990): 1013–16.

Open Reduction and Internal Fixation of Fracture of the Radius and Ulna

1. T. S. Axelrod and R. Y. McMurtry, "Open reduction and internal fixation of comminuted, intraarticular fractures of the distal radius," *Journal of Hand Surgery, American Volume* 15 (January 1990): 1–11.
2. R. S. Smith et al., "Open reduction and internal fixation of volar lip fractures of the distal radius," *Journal of Orthopaedic Trauma* 2 (Number 3, 1988): 181–87.

Open Reduction and Internal Fixation of Fracture of the Tibia and Fibula

1. F. W. Rhinelander, "Minimal internal fixation of tibial fractures," *Clinical Orthopaedics and Related Research* (Number 107, 1975): 188–220.
2. Y. Masse, J. H. Aubriot, and N. Lamotte, "Fractures of the tibial shaft treated by blind intramedullary nailing. A review of 521 cases," *Revue de Chirurgie Orthopedique et Reparatrice de L Appareil Moteur* 63 (September 1977): 575–91. (Published in French)
3. A. J. Sarokhan et al., "Total knee arthroplasty in juvenile rheumatoid arthritis," *Journal of Bone and Joint Surgery, American Volume* 65 (October 1983): 1071–80.
4. R. M. Simin et al., "Fractures of the neck of the talus and the Blair fusion: A review of the literature and case report," *Clinics in Podiatric Medicine and Surgery* 5 (April 1988): 393–420.
5. G. Cierny, 3d, H. S. Byrd, and R. E. Jones, "Primary versus delayed soft tissue coverage for severe open tibial fractures. A comparison of results," *Clinical Orthopaedics and Related Research* (Number 178, 1983): 54–63.
6. K. Hasenhuttl, "The treatment of unstable fractures of the tibia and fibula with flexible medullary wires. A review of 235 fractures," *Journal of Bone and Joint Surgery, American Volume* 63 (July 1981): 921–31.
7. J. W. Mast, P. G. Spiege, and J. N. Pappas, "Fractures of the tibial pilon," *Clinical Orthopaedics and Related Research* (May 1988): 68–82.
8. R. W. Hood and E. J. Riseborough, "Lengthening of the lower extremity by the Wagner method. A review of the Boston Children's Hospital Experience," *Journal of Bone and Joint Surgery, American Volume* 63 (September 1981): 1122–31.

Partial Small Bowel Resection

1. D. M. Lutomski et al., "Warfarin absorption after massive small bowel resection," *American Journal of Gastroenterology* 80 (February 1985): 99–102.
2. M. D. Schuffler, S. H. Leon, and S. Krishnamurthy, "Intestinal pseudoobstruction caused by a new form of visceral neuropathy: Palliation by radical small bowel resection," *Gastroenterology* 89 (November 1985): 1152–56.
3. C. Partensky et al., "Resection of carcinoid tumors of the small intestine is still indicated in the presence of disseminated hepatic metastases," *Annales de Chirurgie de la Main* 44 (Number 1, 1990): 34–38. (Published in French)
4. A. Sitges-Serra et al., "Mesenteric infarction: An analysis of 83 patients with prognostic studies in 44 cases undergoing a massive small-bowel resection," *British Journal of Surgery* 75 (June 1988): 544–48.
5. E. J. Harju and T. T. Pessi, "Massive resection of the small bowel," *International Surgery* 72 (January–March 1987): 25–29.
6. Y. Ohsawa et al., "Surgical treatment and problem of massive small intestinal resection in children—assessment of background diseases and actual management," *Nippon Geka Gakkai Zasshi* 89 (September 1988): 1378–81. (Published in Japanese)
7. H. J. Freeman et al., "Sodium-dependent D-glucose transport after proximal small intestinal resection in rat," *American Journal of Physiology* 255 (September 1988): G292–97.
8. C. M. Vazquez, M. T. Molina, and A. Ilundain, "Role of rat large intestine in reducing diarrhea after 50% or 80% distal small bowel resection," *Digestive Diseases and Sciences* 34 (November 1989): 1713–19.
9. S. Miura et al., "Long-term outcome of massive small bowel resection," *American Journal of Gastroenterology* 86 (April 1991): 454–59.
10. V. S. Klimberg et al., "Intestinal glutamine metabolism after massive small bowel resection," *American Journal of Surgery* 159 (January 1990): 27–32.
11. D. Buttner, R. Pichlmayr, and H. Canzler, "Surgical and dietetic problems of subtotal resection of the small intestine in adults," *Munchener Medizinische Wochenschrift* 120 (10 November 1978): 1489–92. (Published in German)
12. Lutomski et al., "Warfarin absorption after massive small bowel resection," 99–102.
13. D. Darmaun et al., "Glutamine metabolism after small intestinal resection in humans," *Metabolism* 40 (January 1991): 42–44.
14. K. Hatakeyama et al., "Nutritional assessments in the long-term survivors following massive resection of the small intestine," *Nippon Geka Gakkai Zasshi* 89 (September 1988): 1414–17. (Published in Japanese)
15. A. A. Barros D'Sa, T. G. Parks, and A. D. Roy, "The problems of massive small bowel resection and difficulties en-

countered in management," *Postgraduate Medical Journal* 54 (May 1978): 323–27.

16. R. C. Chu, S. M. Barkowski, and J. Buhac, "Small bowel resection-associated urinary calcium loss in rats on long-term total parenteral nutrition," *Journal of Parenteral and Enteral Nutrition* 14 (January–February 1990): 64–67.

17. T. O. Nunan, J. E. Compston, and C. Tonge, "Intestinal calcium absorption in patients after jejuno-ileal bypass or small intestinal resection and the effect of vitamin D," *Digestion* 34 (Number 1, 1986): 9–14.

18. H. Uno et al., "Disorders of bone metabolism caused by small bowel resection in rats," *Gastroenterologica Japonica* 25 (December 1990): 693–99.

19. S. Hasegawa et al., "Problems and difficulties in adapting period in infants and children after massive intestinal resection," *Nippon Geka Gakkai Zasshi* 89 (September 1988): 1391–94. (Published in Japanese)

20. Y. Matsuo et al., "Long term prognosis after massive small bowel resection in children," *Nippon Geka Gakkai Zasshi* 89 (September 1988): 1406–9. (Published in Japanese)

21. S. Kamagata et al., "Endocrinological and metabolic disorders in the patients with massive bowel resection in the newborn period," *Nippon Geka Gakkai Zasshi* 89 (September 1988): 1399–1402. (Published in Japanese)

22. C. Ricour et al., "Extensive resection of the small intestine in children," *Archives Francaises de Pediatrie* 42 (April 1985): 285–90. (Published in French)

23. W. Rappaport and A. Guzauskas, "Tube enterostomy after small bowel resection," *American Journal of Surgery* 159 (February 1990): 256–57.

24. T. Myrhoj, K. Ladefoged, and S. Jarnum, "Chronic intestinal pseudo-obstruction in patients with extensive bowel resection for Crohn's disease," *Scandinavian Journal of Gastroenterology* 23 (April 1988): 380–84.

25. S. R. Hamilton et al., "The role of resection margin frozen section in the surgical management of Crohn's disease," *Surgery, Gynecology and Obstetrics* 160 (January 1985): 57–62.

26. J. Sayfan et al., "Recurrence after strictureplasty or resection for Crohn's disease," *British Journal of Surgery* 76 (April 1989): 335–38.

27. C. N. Ellis et al., "Small bowel obstruction after colon resection for benign and malignant diseases," *Diseases of the Colon and Rectum* 34 (May 1991): 367–71.

28. Barros D'Sa, Parks, and Roy, "The problems of massive small bowel resection and difficulties encountered in management," 323–27.

29. G. S. Sidhu et al., "Absorption studies after massive small bowel resection and antiperistaltic colon interposition in rhesus monkeys," *Digestive Diseases and Sciences* 30 (May 1985): 483–88.

30. P. Kinzel et al., "Disaccharidases and peptidases of intestinal mucosa after experimental subtotal small intestinal resection with and without retardation of the passage," *Zeitschrift fur Experimentelle Chirurgie, Transplantation, und Kunstliche Organe* 20 (Number 5, 1987): 280–89. (Published in German)

31. M. J. Koruda et al., "Effect of parenteral nutrition supplemented with short-chain fatty acids on adaptation to massive small bowel resection," *Gastroenterology* 95 (September 1988): 715–20.

32. A. S. Al-Jurf, M. K. Younoszai, and F. Chapman-Furr, "Effect of nutritional method on adaptation of the intestinal remnant after massive bowel resection," *Journal of Pediatric Gastroenterology and Nutrition* 4 (April 1985): 245–52.

Percutaneous Transluminal Coronary Angioplasty

1. S. G. Richardson et al., "Management of acute coronary occlusion during percutaneous transluminal coronary angioplasty: Experience of complications in a hospital without on-site facilities for cardiac surgery," *British Medical Journal* 300 (10 February 1990): 355–58.

2. H. Serota et al., "Predictors of cardiac survival after percutaneous transluminal coronary angioplasty in patients with severe left ventricular dysfunction," *American Journal of Cardiology* 67 (15 February 1991): 367–72.

3. G. Dorros et al., "In-hospital mortality rate in the National Heart, Lung and Blood Institute Percutaneous Transluminal Coronary Angioplasty Registry," *American Journal of Cardiology* 53 (15 June 1984): 17C–21C.

4. D. P. Faxon et al., "Role of percutaneous transluminal coronary angioplasty in the treatment of unstable angina. Report from the National Heart, Lung and Blood Institute Percutaneous Transluminal Coronary Angioplasty and Coronary Artery Surgery Study Registries," *American Journal of Cardiology* 53 (15 June 1984): 131C–135C.

5. G. Dorros et al., "Complex coronary angioplasty: Multiple coronary dilatations," *American Journal of Cardiology* 53 (15 June 1984): 126C–130C.

6. J. H. O'Keefe, Jr., et al., "Early and late results of coronary angioplasty without antecedent thrombolytic therapy for acute myocardial infarction," *American Journal of Cardiology* 64 (1 December 1989): 1221–30.

7. G. O. Hartzler et al., " 'High-risk' percutaneous transluminal coronary angioplasty," *American Journal of Cardiology* 61 (9 May 1988): 33G–37G.

8. J. R. Kramer et al., "Late follow-up of 781 patients undergoing percutaneous transluminal coronary angioplasty or coronary artery bypass grafting for an isolated obstruction in the left anterior descending coronary artery," *American Heart Journal* 118 (December 1989): 1144–53.

9. O'Keefe, et al., "Early and late results of coronary angioplasty without antecedent thrombolytic therapy for acute myocardial infarction," 1221–30.

10. Dorros et al., "Complex coronary angioplasty," 126C–130C.

11. F. Stammen et al., "Immediate and short-term results of a 1988–1989 coronary angioplasty registry," *American Journal of Cardiology* 67 (1 February 1991): 253–58.

12. M. Vandormael et al., "Predictors of long-term cardiac survival in patients with multivessel coronary artery disease undergoing percutaneous transluminal coronary angioplasty," *American Journal of Cardiology* 67 (1 January 1991): 1–6.

13. D. P. Faxon, "The risk of reperfusion strategies in the treatment of patients with acute myocardial infarction," *Journal of the American College of Cardiology* 12 (December 1988, Supplement A): 52A–57A.

14. M. J. Cowley et al., "Emergency coronary bypass surgery after coronary angioplasty: The National Heart, Lung and Blood Institute's Percutaneous Transluminal Coronary Angioplasty Registry experience," *American Journal of Cardiology* 53 (15 June 1984): 22C–26C.

15. R. A. Prayson and N. B. Ratliff, "An analysis of outcome following percutaneous transluminal coronary artery angioplasty. An autopsy series," *Archives of Pathology and Laboratory Medicine* 114 (December 1990): 1211–17.

16. Ibid.

17. R. G. McKay et al., "Combined percutaneous aortic valvuloplasty and transluminal coronary angioplasty in adult patients with calcific aortic stenosis and coronary artery disease," *Circulation* 76 (December 1987): 1298–1306.

18. B. S. George et al., "Brachial approach to emergency cardiac catheterization during thrombolytic therapy for acute myocardial infarction. TAMI Study Group," *Catheterization and Cardiovascular Diagnosis* 20 (August 1990): 221–26.

19. C. W. Akins et al., "Comparison of coronary artery bypass grafting and percutaneous transluminal coronary angioplasty as initial treatment strategies," *Annals of Thoracic Surgery* 47 (April 1989): 507–15.

Peritoneal Adhesiolysis

1. R. A. Bronson and E. E. Wallach, "Lysis of periadnexal adhesions for correction of infertility," *Fertility and Sterility* 28 (June 1977): 613–19.

2. C. M. March and R. Israel, "Gestational outcome following hysteroscopic lysis of adhesions," *Fertility and Sterility* 36 (October 1981): 455–59.

3. E. Diamond, "Lysis of postoperative pelvic adhesions in infertility," *Fertility and Sterility* 31 (March 1979): 287–95.

4. J. D. Barbot et al., "Use of the CO_2 laser in tubal microsurgery: Comparative study of the results of the lysis of adhesions by laparascopic control on the 8th day. Apropos of 172 cases," *Journal de Gynecologie, Obstetrique et Biologie de la Reproduction (Paris)* 14 (Number 6, 1985): 763–67. (Published in French)

5. March and Israel, "Gestational outcome following hysteroscopic lysis of adhesions," 455–59.

Placement of Central Venous Catheter

1. V. Vanholder, N. Hoenich, and S. Ringoir, "Morbidity and mortality of central venous catheter hemodialysis," *Nephron* 47 (Number 4, 1987): 274–79.

2. M. R. Kramer et al., "Pneumococcal bacteremia—no change in mortality in 30 years," *Israel Journal of Medical Sciences* 23 (March 1987): 174–80.

3. T. Eilard, "Isolation of fungi in blood cultures," *Scandinavian Journal of Infectious Diseases* 19 (Number 2, 1987): 145–56.

4. M. H. Armengaud et al., "Diaphragmatic paralysis after puncture of the internal jugular vein," *Annales Francaises d' Anestheste et de Reanimation* 10 (Number 1, 1991): 77–80.

5. W. C. Shoemaker et al., "The efficacy of central venous and pulmonary artery catheters and therapy based upon them

in reducing mortality and morbidity," *Archives of Surgery* 125 (October 1990): 1332–37, 1337–38.

Removal of Tube and Ectopic Pregnancy

1. F. Lubke, E. Focke, and E. H. Torabi-Tillig, "Changes in the diagnosis and therapy of extra-uterine pregnancy," *Geburtshilfe und Frauenheilkunde* 49 (February 1989): 172–78. (Published in German)

2. E. Coupet, "Ectopic pregnancy: The surgical epidemic," *Journal of the National Medical Association* 81 (May 1989): 567–72.

3. J. I. Makinen, R. U. Erkkola, and P. J. Laippala, "Causes of the increase in the incidence of ectopic pregnancy. A study on 1017 patients from 1966 to 1985 in Turku, Finland," *American Journal of Obstetrics and Gynecology* 160 (March 1989): 642–46.

4. M. A. Shafer and R. L. Sweet, "Pelvic inflammatory disease in adolescent females. Epidemiology, pathogenesis, diagnosis, treatment, and sequelae," *Pediatric Clinics of North America* 36 (June 1989): 513–32.

5. U. Banninger, J. Kunz, and W. E. Schreiner, "Laparoscopic sterilization with electrocautery: Complications and reliability," *Geburtshilfe und Frauenheilkunde* 39 (May 1979): 393–400. (Published in German)

6. T. al-Shawaf et al., "Gamete intra-fallopian transfer in non-endometriotic pelvic adhesions," *Human Reproduction* 5 (May 1990): 434–38.

7. G. Lavy et al., "Ectopic pregnancy: Its relationship to tubal reconstructive surgery," *Fertility and Sterility* 47 (April 1987): 543–56.

8. A. Rempen and P. Albert, "Diagnosis and therapy of a cesarean section scar implanted early pregnancy," *Zeitschrift fur Geburtshilfe und Perinatologie* 194 (January–February 1990): 46–48. (Published in German)

9. Steven A. Schroeder er al., *Current Medical Diagnosis and Treatment 1991* (Norwalk, Conn.: Appleton & Lange, 1991), 540.

10. M. A. Krupp and M. J. Chatton, *Current Medical Diagnosis and Treatment* (Los Altos, Calif.: Lange Medical Publications, 1984), 480.

11. J. F. Renier et al., "Surgical treatment of perforated diverticular sigmoiditis. A retrospective study apropos of 45 cases," *Journal de Chirurgie (Paris)* 126 (November 1989): 567–74. (Published in French)

12. Ibid.

13. M. Iuchtman and S. Grunstein, "Acute abdomen in ruptured interstitial pregnancy following unilateral salpingectomy," *European Journal of Obstetrics, Gynecology, and Reproductive Biology* 26 (October 1987): 165–68.

14. O. Zamir et al., "Peritonitis and empyema following the use of dextran in tubal operations," *International Journal of Gynaecology and Obstetrics* 29 (June 1989): 181–83.

15. R. E. Leach and S. J. Ory, "Management of ectopic pregnancy," *American Family Physician* 41 (April 1990): 1215–22.

16. P. A. Marchbanks et al., "Risk factors for ectopic pregnancy," *Journal of the American Medical Association* 259 (25 March 1988): 1823–27.

17. O. Lalos, "Risk factors for tubal infertility among infertile and fertile women," *European Journal of Obstetrics, Gynecology, and Reproductive Biology* 29 (October 1988): 129–36.

18. T. Tulandi, "Salpingo-ovariolysis: A comparison between laser surgery and electrosurgery," *Fertility and Sterility* 45 (April 1986): 489–91.

19. I. Stornes, K. R. Larsen, and J. Wiese, "Fertility after extrauterine pregnancy. A 16-year retrospective study," *Ugeskrift for Laeger* 152 (14 May 1990): 1439–41. (Published in Danish)

20. M. Gummerus and A. Saari-Kemppainen, "Ectopic pregnancy," *Zentralblatt fur Gynakologie* 108 (Number 2, 1986): 112–17. (Published in German)

21. J. B. Dubuisson et al., "Reproductive outcome after laparoscopic salpingectomy for tubal pregnancy," *Fertility and Sterility* 53 (June 1990): 1004–7.

22. G. Nakamura et al., "Vascular pedicle transposition of an ovary with subsequent intrauterine pregnancy," *Fertility and Sterility* 52 (October 1989): 688–90.

23. I. Timor-Tritsch and E. Paldi, "Tubal pregnancy treated by salpingectomy using operative culdoscopy," *ACTA Obstetricia et Gynecologica Scandinavica* 54 (Number 3, 1975): 285–86.

24. Krupp and Chatton, *Current Medical Diagnosis and Treatment*, 480.

25. J. B. Dubuisson, F. X. Aubriot, and V. Cardone, "Laparoscopic salpingectomy for tubal pregnancy," *Fertility and Sterility* 47 (February 1987): 225–28.

26. S. G. McNeeley and T. E. Elkins, "Gynecologic surgery and surgical morbidity in mentally handicapped women," *Obstetrics and Gynecology* 74 (August 1989): 155–58.

27. G. Keckstein, A. Wolf, and S. Wittek, "Status of the fallopian tube following pelviscopic surgery (conventional versus laser) of tubal pregnancy," *Archives of Gynecology and Obstetrics* 245 (Number 1–4, 1989): 416–18. (Published in German)

28. S. G. Krantz et al., "Time trends in risk factors and clinical outcome of ectopic pregnancy," *Fertility and Sterility* 54 (July 1990): 42–46.

29. A. Berenson et al., "Bacteriologic findings with ectopic pregnancy," *Journal of Reproductive Medicine* 36 (February 1991): 118–20.

30. A. H. DeCherney and M. P. Diamond, "Laparoscopic salpingostomy for ectopic pregnancy," *Obstetrics and Gynecology* 70 (December 1987): 948–50.

31. J. B. Dubuisson et al., "Should one operate on bifocal tubal lesions in 1984? Apropos of 54 cases," *Journal de Gynecologie, Obstetrique et Biologie de la Reproduction (Paris)* 13 (Number 8, 1984): 925–32. (Published in French)

32. D. M. Leiserowitz et al., "Fertility following adnexal surgery," *Acta Europaea Fertilitatis* 8 (September 1977): 239–43.

33. D. E. Mitchell, H. F. McSwain, and H. B. Peterson, "Fertility after ectopic pregnancy," *American Journal of Obstetrics and Gynecology* 161 (September 1989): 576–80.

34. T. C. Trimbos-Kemper, J. B. Trimbos, and E. V. van Hall, "Adhesion formation after tubal surgery: Results of the eighth-day laparoscopy in 188 patients," *Fertility and Sterility* 43 (March 1985): 395–400.

35. T. Speroff et al., "A risk-benefit analysis of elective bilateral oophorectomy: Effect of changes in compliance with estrogen therapy on outcome," *American Journal of Obstetrics and Gynecology* 164 (January 1991): 165–74.

36. G. W. Creasy and J. Morgan, "Hemolytic uremic syndrome after ectopic pregnancy: Postectopic nephrosclerosis," *Obstetrics and Gynecology* 69 (March 1987): 448–49.

37. G. Leiman and G. Naylor, "Mucinous metaplasia in scar endometriosis. Diagnosis by aspiration cytology," *Diagnostic Cytopathology* 1 (April–June 1985): 153–56.

38. F. D. Loffer and D. Pent, "Indications, contraindications and complications of laparoscopy," *Obstetrical and Gynecological Survey* 30 (July 1975): 407–27.

39. I. C. Chi, M. Potts, and L. Wilkens, "Rare events associated with tubal sterilizations: an international experience," *Obstetrical and Gynecological Survey* 41 (January 1986): 7–19.

40. L. M. Adler et al., "Bilateral compartment syndrome after a long gynecologic operation in the lithotomy position," *American Journal of Obstetrics and Gynecology* 162 (May 1990): 1271–72.

41. M. J. Webb, "Ovarian remnant syndrome," *Australian and New Zealand Journal of Obstetrics and Gynaecology* 29 (November 1989): 433–35.

42. J. P. Cederna et al., "Necrotizing fasciitis of the total abdominal wall after sterilization by partial salpingectomy," *American Journal of Obstetrics and Gynecology* 163 (July 1990): 138–39.

43. H. H. Sheikh, "Hysterosalpingographic follow-up of the partial salpingectomy type of sterilization," *American Journal of Obstetrics and Gynecology* 128 (15 August 1977): 858–61.

44. R. J. Paulson and M. V. Sauer, "Conservative surgical treatment of ectopic pregnancy. Avoiding partial salpingectomy," *Journal of Reproductive Medicine* 35 (January 1990): 22–24.

45. J. R. Zhao, R. Wing, and J. F. Hulka, "Ovarian function in monkeys after bilateral salpingectomy," *International Journal of Fertility* 29 (Number 2, 1984): 118–21.

46. H. Mecke, K. Semm, and E. Lehmann-Willenbrock, "Results of operative pelviscopy in 202 cases of ectopic pregnancy," *International Journal of Fertility* 34 (March–April 1989): 93–94, 97–100.

47. T. Tulandi and M. Guralnick, "Treatment of tubal ectopic pregnancy by salpingotomy with or without tubal suturing and salpingectomy," *Fertility and Sterility* 55 (January 1991): 53–55.

48. P. D. Silva, "A laparoscopic approach can be applied to most cases of ectopic pregnancy," *Obstetrics and Gynecology* 72 (December 1988): 944–47.

49. J. Keckstein et al., "The contact Nd:YAG laser: A new technique for conservation of the fallopian tube in unruptured ectopic pregnancy," *British Journal of Obstetrics and Gynaecology* 97 (April 1990): 352–56.

50. W. I. Onuigbo, "Elective appendectomy at salpingectomy for ectopic pregnancy: Is it desirable?" *Obstetrics and Gynecology* 49 (April 1977): 435–37.

51. G. Keckstein et al., "Tube-preserving endoscopic surgical procedures in unruptured tubal pregnancy. What significance does laser use have?" *Geburtshilfe und Frauenheilkunde* 50 (March 1990): 207–11. (Published in German)

Repair of Cystocele or Rectocele

1. J. H. Heslop, "Piles and rectoceles," *Australian and New Zealand Journal of Surgery* 57 (December 1987): 935–38.

2. J. H. Croushore and R. B. Black, "Scrotal cystocele," *Journal of Urology* 121 (April 1979): 541–42.

3. N. S. Curry, K. F. O'Connor, and C. O. Tubbs, "Scrotal cystocele diagnosed by computed tomography," *Urologic Radiology* 9 (Number 4, 1988): 247–48.

4. K. Delaere et al., "Hydronephrosis caused by cystocele. Treatment by colpopexy to sacral promontory," *Urology* 24 (October 1984): 364–65.

5. G. A. Macer, "Transabdominal repair of cystocele, a 20-year experience, compared with the traditional vaginal approach," *American Journal of Obstetrics and Gynecology* 131 (15 May 1978): 203–7.

6. M. W. Arnold, W. R. Stewart, and P. S. Aguilar, "Rectocele repair. Four years' experience," *Diseases of the Colon and Rectum* 33 (August 1990): 684–87.

7. I. T. Khubchandani et al., "Endorectal repair of rectocele," *Diseases of the Colon and Rectum* 26 (December 1983): 792–96.

8. I. R. Block, "Transrectal repair of rectocele using obliterative suture," *Diseases of the Colon and Rectum* 29 (November 1986): 707–11.

9. M. W. Arnold, W. R. Stewart, and P. S. Aguilar, "Rectocele repair. Four years' experience," *Diseases of the Colon and Rectum* 33 (August 1990): 684–87.

10. S. Sehapayak, "Transrectal repair of rectocele: An extended armamentarium of colorectal surgeons. A report of 355 cases," *Diseases of the Colon and Rectum* 28 (June 1985): 422–33.

11. S. Raz, C. G. Klutke, and J. Golomb, "Four-corner bladder and urethral suspension for moderate cystocele," *Journal of Urology* 142 (September 1989): 712–15.

Repair of Obstetric Laceration

1. L. Borgatta, S. L. Piening, and W. R. Cohen, "Association of episiotomy and delivery position with deep perineal laceration during spontaneous delivery in nulliparous women," *American Journal of Obstetrics and Gynecology* 160 (February 1989): 294–97.

2. L. S. Wilcox et al., "Episiotomy and its role in the incidence of perineal lacerations in a maternity center and a tertiary hospital obstetric service," *American Journal of Obstetrics and Gynecology* 160 (May 1989): 1047–52.

3. Ibid.

Repair of Obstetric Laceration of the Rectum and Anus

1. R. E. Perry et al., "Manometric diagnosis of anal sphincter injuries," *American Journal of Surgery* 159 (January 1990): 112–16; discussion 116–17.

2. G. G. Browning and R. W. Motson, "Anal sphincter injury. Management and results of Parks sphincter repair," *Annals of Surgery* 199 (March 1984): 351–57.

3. S. J. Snooks, M. M. Henry, and M. Swash, "Faecal incontinence due to external anal sphincter division in childbirth is associated with damage to the innervation of the pelvic floor musculature: A double pathology," *British Journal of Obstetrics and Gynaecology* 92 (August 1985): 824–28.

4. P. O. Jacobs et al., "Obstetric fecal incontinence. Role of pelvic floor denervation and results of delayed sphincter repair," *Diseases of the Colon and Rectum* 33 (June 1990): 494–97.

5. S. J. Snooks et al., "Injury to innervation of pelvic floor sphincter musculature in childbirth," *Lancet* 2 (8 September 1984): 546–50.

6. S. Mellerup Sorensen, "Perineal rupture following vaginal delivery. Long-term consequences," *ACTA Obstetricia et Gynecologica Scandinavica* 67 (Number 4, 1988): 315–18.

Repair of Vessel

1. R. R. Schenck and G. H. Derman, "An intraluminal silastic stent for small vessel repair," *Orthopedic Clinics of North America* 8 (April 1977): 265–71.

2. G. M. Williams et al., "Rejection and repair of endothelium in major vessel transplants," *Surgery* 78 (December 1975): 694–706.

3. S. J. Stricker, W. E. Burkhalter, and A. E. Ouellette, "Single-vessel forearm arterial repairs. Patency rates using nuclear angiography," *Orthopedics* 12 (July 1989): 963–65.

4. R. C. Wray and B. M. O'Brien, "The effects of suturing technique and vessel size on patency after microarterial repair," *Annals of Plastic Surgery* 2 (March 1979): 233–34.

Revision of Vascular Procedure

1. Y. Inoue et al., "Pathological considerations of reoperative vascular patients," *Bulletin of Tokyo Medical and Dental University* 34 (September 1987): 53–59.

2. R. K. Spence et al., "Exsanguinating upper extremity vascular injury: Is an initial approach by clavicular resection adequate?" *Journal of Cardiovascular Surgery (Torino)* 30 (May–June 1989): 450–53.

3. A. Nemes et al., "Development and treatment of false aneurysm following vascular intervention," *Journal of Cardiovascular Surgery (Torino)* 29 (January–February 1988): 1–7.

4. J. W. Dennis et al., "Anastomotic pseudoaneurysms. A continuing late complication of vascular reconstructive procedures," *Archives in Surgery* 121 (March 1986): 314–17.

5. D. Bergqvist and K. G. Ljungstrom, "Hemorrhagic complications resulting in reoperation after peripheral vascular surgery: A 14-year experience," *Journal of Vascular Surgery* 6 (August 1987): 134–38.

6. S. J. Stricker, W. E. Burkhalter, and A. E. Ouellette, "Single-vessel forearm arterial repairs. Patency rates using nuclear angiography," *Orthopedics* 12 (July 1989): 963–65.

7. R. C. Wray and B. M. O'Brien, "The effects of suturing technique and vessel size on patency after microarterial repair," *Annals of Plastic Surgery* 2 (March 1979): 233–34.

8. H. W. Kaebnick et al., "The microbiology of explanted vascular prostheses," *Surgery* 102 (October 1987): 756–62.

9. W. Hepp, N. Pallua, and J. Palenker, "Change in the therapeutic concept of deep wound infection following vascular surgery interventions," *Chirurg* 60 (May 1989): 340–45. (Published in German)

10. W. E. Evans, J. P. Hayes, and B. D. Vermilion, "Effect of a failed distal reconstruction on the level of amputation," *American Journal of Surgery* 160 (August 1990): 217–20.

11. K. S. Scher, "Sartorius transposition to protect vascular grafts in the groin," *American Surgeon* 55 (March 1989): 158–61.

12. R. A. Graor and P. L. Whitlow, "Transluminal atherectomy for occlusive peripheral vascular disease," *Journal of the American College of Cardiology* 15 (June 1990): 1551–58.

Right Hemicolectomy

1. R. S. Snell, *Clinical Anatomy for Medical Students,* 3rd ed. (Boston: Little, Brown, and Company, 1986), 281–83.

2. W. J. Hoskins et al., "Right hemicolectomy and ileal resection with primary reanastomosis for irradiation injury of the terminal ileum," *Gynecology and Oncology* 26 (February 1987): 215–24.

3. B. M. Smithers et al., "Emergency right hemicolectomy in colon carcinoma: A prospective study," *Australian and New Zealand Journal of Surgery* 56 (October 1986): 749–52.

4. W. P. Morgan et al., "Management of obstructing carcinoma of the left colon by extended right hemicolectomy," *American Journal of Surgery* 149 (March 1985): 327–29.

5. J. A. Riseman and K. Wichterman, "Evaluation of right hemicolectomy for unexpected cecal mass," *Archives of Surgery* 124 (September 1989): 1043–44.

6. Hoskins et al., "Right hemicolectomy and ileal resection with primary reanastomosis for irradiation injury of the terminal ileum," 215–24.

7. R. N. Garrison et al., "Evaluation of management of the emergency right hemicolectomy," *Journal of Trauma* 19 (October 1979): 734–39.

8. Hoskins et al., "Right hemicolectomy and ileal resection with primary reanastomosis for irradiation injury of the terminal ileum," 215–24.

9. B. A. Mizock, "Branched-chain amino acids in sepsis and hepatic failure," *Archives of Internal Medicine* 145 (July 1985): 1284–88.

Rotator Cuff Repair

1. R. S. Snell, *Clinical Anatomy for Medical Students,* 3rd ed. (Boston: Little, Brown, and Company, 1986), 444–45.

2. A. M. Wiley, "Arthroscopy for shoulder instability and a technique for arthroscopic repair," *Arthroscopy* 4 (Number 1, 1988): 25–30.

3. J. S. Neviaser, R. J. Neviaser, and T. J. Neviaser, "The repair of chronic massive ruptures of the rotator cuff of the shoulder by use of a freeze-dried rotator cuff," *Journal of Bone and Joint Surgery, American Volume* 60 (July 1978): 681–84.

4. S. C. Thomas and F. A. Matsen, III, "An approach to the repair of avulsion of the glenohumeral ligaments in the man-

agement of traumatic anterior glenohumeral instability," *Journal of Bone and Joint Surgery, American Volume* 71 (April 1989): 506–13.

5. J. M. Bjorkenheim et al., "Surgical repair of the rotator cuff and surrounding tissues. Factors influencing the results," *Clinical Orthopaedics and Related Research* (November 1988): 148–53.

6. R. W. Bassett and R. H. Cofield, "Acute tears of the rotator cuff. The timing of surgical repair," *Clinical Orthopaedics and Related Research* (May 1983): 18–24.

7. G. S. Kappakas and J. H. McMaster, "Repair of acromioclavicular separation using a Dacron prosthesis graft," *Clinical Orthopaedics and Related Research* (March–April 1978): 247–51.

8. D. J. Daluga and W. Dobozi, "The influence of distal clavicle resection and rotator cuff repair on the effectiveness of anterior acromioplasty," *Clinical Orthopaedics and Related Research* (October 1989): 117–23.

9. R. J. Hawkins and R. L. Angelo, "Glenohumeral osteoarthrosis. A late complication of the Putti-Platt repair," *Journal of Bone and Joint Surgery, American Volume* 72 (September 1990): 1193–97.

10. J. K. DeOrio and R. H. Cofield, "Results of a second attempt at surgical repair of a failed initial rotator cuff repair," *Journal of Bone and Joint Surgery, American Volume* 66 (April 1984): 563–67.

11. Ibid.

12. G. B. Ha'eri and A. M. Wiley, "Advancement of the supraspinatus muscle in the repair of ruptures of the rotator cuff," *Journal of Bone and Joint Surgery, American Volume* 63 (February 1981): 232–38.

13. L. Sedel and Y. Abols, "Iatrogenic lesions of the spinal accessory nerve. Microsurgical repair," *Presse Medicale* 12 (25 June 1983): 1711–13. (Published in French)

14. M. Post, "Rotator cuff repair with carbon filament. A preliminary report of five cases," *Clinical Orthopaedics and Related Research* (June 1985): 154–58.

Septoplasty

1. O. Fjermedal, C. Saunte, and S. Pedersen, "Septoplasty and/or submucous resection?" *Journal of Laryngology and Otology* 102 (September 1988): 796–98.

2. M. Jessen, A. Ivarsson, and L. Malm, "Nasal airway resistance and symptoms after functional septoplasty: Comparison of findings at nine months and nine years," *Clinical Otolaryngology* 14 (June 1989): 231–34.

3. K. Larsen and S. Kristensen, "Peak flow nasal patency indices and self-assessment in septoplasty," *Clinical Otolaryngology* 15 (August 1990): 327–34.

4. Jessen, Ivarsson, and Malm, "Nasal airway resistance and symptoms after functional septoplasty," 231–34.

5. M. Jessen and L. Malm, "The importance of nasal airway resistance and nasal symptoms in the selection of patients for septoplasty," *Rhinology* 22 (September 1984): 157–64.

6. K. Larsen and H. Oxhoj, "Spirometric forced volume measurements in the assessment of nasal patency after septoplasty. A prospective clinical study," *Rhinology* 26 (September 1988): 203–8.

7. P. O. Haraldsson, H. Nordemar, and A. Anggard, "Long-term results after septal surgery—submucous resection versus septoplasty," *ORL; Journal of Otorhinolaryngology and its Related Specialties* 49 (Number 4, 1987): 218–22.

8. G. H. Gottschalk, "An improved septoplasty: The microsurgical suture technique," *Annals of Plastic Surgery* 1 (January 1978): 30–33.

9. B. J. Cohen, J. D. Johnson, and M. J. Raff, "Septoplasty complicated by staphylococcal spinal osteomyelitis," *Archives of Internal Medicine* 145 (March 1985): 556–57.

10. K. L. Silk et al., "Absence of bacteremia during nasal septoplasty," *Archives of Otolaryngology—Head and Neck Surgery* 117 (January 1991): 54–55.

11. R. Wagner and J. M. Toback, "Toxic shock syndrome following septoplasty using plastic septal splints," *Laryngoscope* 96 (June 1986): 609–10.

12. I. T. Huang et al., "Toxic shock syndrome following septoplasty and partial turbinectomy," *Journal of Otolaryngology* 15 (October 1986): 310–12.

13. I. N. Lee and L. Vukovic, "Hemostatic suture for septoplasty: How we do it," *Journal of Otolaryngology* 17 (February 1988): 54–56.

14. S. R. Wullstein, "Septoplasty without postoperative nasal packing. Mucosal repair of the upper airway with human biologica glue," *HNO* 27 (September 1979): 322–24. (Published in German)

15. K. Paulsen, "How important are lower tunnels in the cottle septoplasty?" *HNO* 24 (March 1976): 106–7. (Published in German)

16. R. S. Snell, *Clinical Anatomy for Medical Students,* 3rd ed. (Boston: Little, Brown, and Company, 1986), 855.

17. J. H. Jensen and H. Dommerby, "Routine radiological examination of the sinuses before septoplasty," *Journal of Laryngology and Otology* 100 (August 1986): 893–96.

18. W. Pirsig, "Regeneration of septal cartilage in children after septoplasty. A histological study," *ACTA Oto-Laryngologica (Stockholm)* 79 (May–June 1975): 451–59. (Published in German)

19. L. F. Grymer et al., "Acoustic rhinometry: Evaluation of the nasal cavity with septal deviations, before and after septoplasty," *Laryngoscope* 99 (November 1989): 1180–87.

20. P. Broms, B. Jonson, and L. Malm, "Rhinomanometry. IV. A pre- and postoperative evaluation in functional septoplasty," *ACTA Oto-Laryngologica (Stockholm)* 94 (November–December 1982): 523–29.

21. B. Mayer and H. Henkes, "Mini-septoplasty—for function and form," *Laryngorhinootologie* 69 (June 1990): 303–7. (Published in German)

22. R. Haye and A. Freng, "Experimental septoplasty in the growing cat. A histological study," *ACTA Oto-Laryngologica (Stockholm)* 102 (July–August 1986): 113–17.

23. A. Freng and R. Haye, "Experimental nasal septoplasty; influence on nasomaxillary development. A roentgen cephalometric study in growing domestic cats," *ACTA Oto-Laryngologica (Stockholm)* 100 (September–October 1985): 309–15.

Shoulder Arthroplasty

1. A. P. Weiss et al., "Unconstrained shoulder arthroplasty. A five-year average follow-up study," *Clinical Orthopaedics and Related Research* (August 1990): 86–90.

2. S. R. McCoy et al., "Total shoulder arthroplasty in rheumatoid arthritis," *Journal of Arthroplasty* 4 (Number 2, 1989): 105–13.

3. D. Huten and J. Duparc, "Prosthetic arthroplasty in recent and old complex injuries of the shoulder," *Revue de Chirurgie Orthopedique et Reparatrice de L Appareil Moteur* 72 (Number 8, 1986): 517–29. (Published in French)

4. D. K. Paradis and D. C. Ferlic, "Shoulder arthroplasty in rheumatoid arthritis," *Physical Therapy* 55 (February 1975): 157–59.

5. W. A. Souter, "The surgical treatment of the rheumatoid shoulder," *Annals of the Academy of Medicine, Singapore* 12 (April 1983): 243–55.

6. H. C. Amstutz, A. L. Sew Hoy, and I. C. Clarke, "UCLA anatomic total shoulder arthroplasty," *Clinical Orthpaedics and Related Research* (March–April 1981): 7–20.

7. L. Marmor, "Hemiarthroplasty for the rheumatoid shoulder joint," *Clinical Orthopaedics and Related Research* (January–February 1977): 201–3.

8. B. J. Thomas, H. C. Amstutz, and A. Cracchiolo, "Shoulder arthroplasty for rheumatoid arthritis," *Clinical Orthopaedics and Related Research* (April 1991): 125–28.

9. Weiss et al., "Unconstrained shoulder arthroplasty," 86–90.

10. R. J. Hawkins, R. H. Bell, and B. Jallay, "Total shoulder arthroplasty," *Clinical Orthpaedics and Related Research* (May 1989): 188–94.

11. R. H. Cofield, "Total shoulder arthroplasty with the Neer prosthesis," *Journal of Bone and Joint Surgery, American Volume* 66 (July 1984): 899–906.

12. B. C. Brenner et al., "Survivorship of unconstrained total shoulder arthroplasty," *Journal of Bone and Joint Surgery, American Volume* 71 (October 1989): 1289–96.

13. R. H. Cofield and B. C. Edgerton, "Total shoulder arthroplasty: Complications and revision surgery," *Instructional Course Lectures* 39 (1990): 449–62.

14. C. S. Neer, II, "Unconstrained shoulder arthroplasty," *Instructional Course Lectures* 34 (1985): 278–86.

15. G. H. Johnston et al., "A complication of posterior glenoid osteotomy for recurrent posterior shoulder instability," *Clinical Orthopaedics and Related Research* (July–August 1984): 147–49.

16. P. Kjaersgaard-Andersen et al., "Heterotopic bone formation following total shoulder arthroplasty," *Journal of Arthroplasty* 4 (Number 2, 1989): 99–104.

17. H. E. Figgie, III, et al., "An analysis of factors affecting the long-term results of total shoulder arthroplasty in inflammatory arthritis," *Journal of Arthroplasty* 3 (Number 2, 1988): 123–30.

18. R. H. Cofield, "Shoulder arthrodesis and resection arthroplasty," *Instructional Course Lectures* 34 (1985): 268–77.

19. S. N. Bell and N. Gschwend, "Clinical experience with total arthroplasty and hemiarthroplasty of the shoulder using the Neer prosthesis," *International Orthopaedics* 10 (Number 4, 1986): 217–22.

20. A. D. Boyd, Jr., et al., "Total shoulder arthroplasty versus hemiarthroplasty. Indications for glenoid resurfacing," *Journal of Arthroplasty* 5 (December 1990): 329–36.

Sigmoidectomy

1. J. Sayfan et al., "Sutured posterior abdominal rectopexy with sigmoidectomy compared with Marlex rectopexy for rectal prolapse," *British Journal of Surgery* 77 (February 1990): 143–45.

2. G. D'Angelo, H. S. Stern, and E. Myers, "Rectal prolapse in scleroderma: Case report and review of the colonic complications of scleroderma," *Canadian Journal of Surgery* 28 (January 1985): 62–63.

3. T. Sugiyama and T. Kadowaki, "A case of vesicosigmoidal fistula," *Hinyokika Kiyo* 34 (April 1988): 692–95. (Published in Japanese)

4. M. L. Corman, "Rectal prolapse. Surgical techniques," *Surgical Clinics of North America* 68 (December 1988): 1255–65.

5. L. Pahlman et al., "Volvulus of the colon. A review of 93 cases and current aspects of treatment," *ACTA Chirurgica Scandinavica* 155 (Number 1, 1989): 53–56.

6. J. C. Le Neel et al., "Volvulus of the sigmoid colon," *Annales de Chirurgie de la Main* 43 (Number 5, 1989): 348–51. (Published in French)

7. J. A. Solla, D. A. Rothenberger, and S. M. Goldberg, "Colonic resection in the treatment of complete rectal prolapse," *Netherlands Journal of Surgery* 41 (December 1989): 132–35.

8. E. R. Letwin, "Diverticulitis of the colon. Clinical review of acute presentations and management," *American Journal of Surgery* 143 (May 1982): 579–81.

9. R. D. Fry, J. W. Fleshman, Jr., and I. J. Kodner, "Abdominal colectomy with ileorectal anastomosis," *Southern Medical Journal* 77 (June 1984): 711–14.

10. M. M. Henry, "Fecal incontinence and rectal prolapse," *Surgical Clinics of North America* 68 (December 1988): 1249–54.

11. R. H. Hunt, "The role of colonoscopy in complicated diverticular disease. A review," *ACTA Chirurgica Belgica* 78 (November–December 1979): 349–53.

12. F. T. Fork, C. Lindstrom, and G. R. Ekelund, "Reliability of routine double-contrast examination (DCE) of the large bowel in polyp detection: A prospective clinical study," *Gastrointestinal Radiology* 8 (Number 2, 1983): 163–72.

13. I. S. Grimm and L. S. Friedman, "Inflammatory bowel disease in the elderly," *Gastroenterology Clinics of North America* 19 (June 1990): 361–89.

14. T. Pohlman, "Diverticulitis," *Gastroenterology Clinics of North America* 17 (June 1988): 357–85.

15. Z. H. Krukowski and N. A. Matheson, "Emergency surgery for diverticular disease complicated by generalized and faecal peritonitis: A review," *British Journal of Surgery* 71 (December 1984): 921–27.

16. S. D. Smith et al., "Sigmoid volvulus in childhood," *Southern Medical Journal* 83 (July 1990): 778–81.

17. H. B. Kram et al., "Rectal prolapse caused by blunt abdominal trauma," *Surgery* 105 (June 1989): 790–92.

18. I. T. Jones and V. W. Fazio, "Colonic volvulus. Etiology and management," *Digestive Diseases and Sciences* 7 (Number 4, 1989): 203–9.

19. Le Neel et al., "Volvulus of the sigmoid colon," 348–51.

20. P. Vayre, "Surgical treatment of sigmoid diverticulitis," *Journal de Chirurgie (Paris)* 127 (November 1990): 547–51. (Published in French)

21. Jones and Fazio, "Colonic volvulus," 203–9.

22. J. F. Renier et al., "Surgical treatment of perforated diverticular sigmoiditis. A retrospective study apropos of 45 cases," *Journal de Chirurgie (Paris)* 126 (November 1989): 567–74. (Published in French)

23. J. M. Greif, G. Fried, and C. K. McSherry, "Surgical treatment of perforated diverticulitis of the sigmoid colon," *Diseases of the Colon and Rectum* 23 (October 1980): 483–87.

24. C. W. Chappuis and I. Cohn, Jr., "Acute colonic diverticulitis," *Surgical Clinics of North America* 68 (April 1988): 301–13.

Skin Suture

1. K. R. Brickman and R. W. Lambert, "Evaluation of skin stapling for wound closure in the emergency department," *Annals of Emergency Medicine* 18 (October 1989): 1122–25.

2. P. Lugani er al., "Skin suture with skin stapler in general surgery," *Minerva Chirurgica* 44 (15 May 1989): 1365–69. (Published in Italian)

3. R. G. Bennett, "Selection of wound closure materials," *Journal of the American Academy of Dermatology* 18 (April 1988): 619–37.

4. D. H. Bass et al., "Topical anaesthesia for repair of minor lacerations," *Archives of Disease in Childhood* 65 (November 1990): 1272–73.

5. M. S. Agren and L. Franzen, "Influence of zinc deficiency on breaking strength of three-week-old skin incisions in the rat," *ACTA Chirurgica Scandinavica* 156 (October 1990): 667–70.

Surgical Repair of Indirect Inguinal Hernia
Surgical Repair of Direct Inguinal Hernia
Surgical Repair of Unilateral Inguinal Hernia

1. M. Ganesaratnam, "Maydl's hernia: Report of a series of seven cases and review of the literature," *British Journal of Surgery* 72 (September 1985): 737–38.

2. V. S. Sidorin, S. M. Petrova, and A. Polotskaia, "Anaerobic clostridial infection of surgical wounds," *Arkhiv Patologii* 44 (Number 12, 1982): 69–72. (Published in Russian)

3. F. J. Rescorla and J. L. Grosfeld, "Inguinal hernia repair in the perinatal period and early infancy: Clinical considerations," *Journal of Pediatric Surgery* 19 (December 1984): 832–37.

4. G. R. Tingwald and M. Cooperman, "Inguinal and femoral hernia repair in geriatric patients," *Surgery, Gynecology, and Obstetrics* 154 (May 1982): 704–6.

5. M. Michelsen and F. Walter, "Comparison of outpatient and inpatient operations for inguinal hernia (1971 to 1978)," *Zentralblatt fur Chirurgie* 107 (Number 2, 1982): 94–102. (Published in German)

6. L. C. Chiedozi, I. O. Aboh, and N. E. Piserchia, "Mechanical bowel obstruction. Review of 316 cases in Benin City," *American Journal of Surgery* 139 (March 1980): 389–93.

7. N. J. Andrews, "Presentation and outcome of strangulated external hernia in a district general hospital," *British Journal of Surgery* 68 (May 1981): 329–32.

8. K. Singal et al., "Genital edema in patients on continuous ambulatory peritoneal dialysis. Report of three cases and review of the literature," *American Journal of Nephrology* 6 (Number 6, 1986): 471–75.

9. P. Pietri and F. Gabrielli, "Recurrent inguinal hernia," *International Surgery* 71 (July–September 1986): 164–68.

10. John L. Madden, *Atlas of Technics in Surgery*, 2nd ed. (Norwalk, Conn.: Appleton-Century-Crofts, 1964), 58–74.

11. E. Simchen, R. Rozin, and Y. Wax, "The Israeli study of surgical infection of drains and the risk of wound infection in operations for hernia," *Surgery, Gynecology, and Obstetrics* 170 (April 1990): 331–37.

12. J. Iles, "The management of elective hernia repair," *Annals of Plastic Surgery* 2 (June 1979): 538–41.

13. P. Cubertafond and A. Gainant, "Treatment of inguinal hernia by Shouldice type herniorrhaphy. Analysis of a series of 403 cases surgically treated," *Chirurgie* 115 (Number 2, 1989): 133–35. (Published in French)

14. J. W. Serpell, C. D. Johnson, and P. E. Jarrett, "A prospective study of bilateral inguinal hernia repair," *Annals of the Royal College of Surgeons of England* 72 (September 1990): 299–303.

15. A. R. Miller et al., "Simultaneous bilateral hernia repair. A case against conventional wisdom," *Annals of Surgery* 213 (March 1991): 272–76.

16. D. B. McGregor, K. Halverson, and C. B. McVay, "The unilateral pediatric inguinal hernia: Should the contralateral side be explored?" *Journal of Pediatric Surgery* 15 (June 1980): 313–17.

17. M. A. Stott, R. Sutton, and G. T. Royle, "Bilateral inguinal hernias: Simultaneous or sequential repair?" *Postgraduate Medical Journal* 64 (May 1988): 375–78.

18. F. C. Chang and G. J. Farha, "Inguinal herniorrhaphy under local anesthesia. A prospective study of 100 consecutive patients with emphasis of perioperative morbidity and patient acceptance," *Archives of Surgery* 112 (September 1977): 1069–71.

19. A. I. Gilbert, "Inguinal herniorrhaphy: Reduced morbidity, recurrences, and costs," *Southern Medical Journal* 72 (July 1979): 831–34.

20. M. Deysine, R. Grimson, and H. S. Soroff, "Herniorrhaphy in the elderly. Benefits of a clinic for the treatment of external abdominal wall hernias," *American Journal of Surgery* 153 (April 1987): 387–91.

21. P. Rabec and P. Sesboue, "Technic of surgical cure of inguinal hernia by interposition of a crinoplaque," *Annales de Chirurgie de la Main* 43 (Number 10, 1989): 804–10. (Published in French)

22. J. V. Blondiau, V. Verheyen, and M. Colard, "Cure of inguino-crural herniae through median preperitoneal route and teflon prosthesis. Personal series of 56 cases," *ACTA Chirurgica Belgica* 78 (September–October 1979): 317–23. (Published in French)

23. "The use of Mersilene mesh in repair of abdominal wall hernias: A clinical and experimental study," *Annals of Surgery* 181 (May 1975): 728–34.

24. Tingwald and Cooperman, "Inguinal and femoral hernia repair in geriatric patients," 704–6.

25. D. C. Lewis, C. G. Moran, and K. D. Vellacott, "Inguinal hernia repair in the elderly," *Journal of the Royal College of Surgeons, Edinburgh* 34 (April 1989): 101–3.

26. Madden, *Atlas of Technics in Surgery*, 58–74.

27. Deysine, Grimson, and Soroff, "Herniorrhaphy in the elderly," 387–91.

28. "Results of follow-up of operations in pediatric patients with indirect inguinal hernia," *Langenbecks Archiv fur Chirurgie* 371 (Number 2, 1987): 115–21. (Published in German)

29. Deysine, Grimson, and Soroff, "Herniorrhaphy in the elderly," 387–91.

30. Cubertafond and Gainant, "Treatment of inguinal hernia by Shouldice type herniorrhaphy," 133–5.

31. Tingwald and Cooperman, "Inguinal and femoral hernia repair in geriatric patients," 704–6.

32. E. Cahlin and L. Weiss, "Results of postoperative clinical examination of inguinal hernia after three years," *ACTA Chirurgica Scandinavica* 146 (Number 6, 1980): 421–26.

33. Miller et al., "Simultaneous bilateral hernia repair," 272–6.

34. Deysine, Grimson, and Sorof, "Herniorrhaphy in the elderly," 387–91.

35. Lewis, Moran, and Vellacott, "Inguinal hernia repair in the elderly," 101–3.

36. J. Beacon, R. W. Hoile, and H. Ellis, "A trial of suction drainage in inguinal hernia repair," *British Journal of Surgery* 67 (August 1980): 554–55.

37. J. A. Cox, "Inguinal hernia of childhood," *Surgical Clinics of North America* 65 (October 1985): 1331–42.

38. J. S. Azagra et al., "Ninety-four inguinal hernias treated by interposition of a prosthesis using medial and preperitoneal approach," *ACTA Chirurgica Belgica* 87 (January–February 1987): 15–18. (Published in French)

39. Blondiau, Verheyen, and Colard, "Cure of inguino-crural herniae through median preperitoneal route and teflon prosthesis," 317–23.

40. McGregor, Halverson, and McVay, "The unilateral pediatric inguinal hernia," 313–17.

41. Tingwald and Cooperman, "Inguinal and femoral hernia repair in geriatric patients," 704–6.

42. Cubertafond and Gainant, "Treatment of inguinal hernia by Shouldice type herniorrhaphy," 133–35.

43. Stott, Sutton, and Royle, "Bilateral inguinal hernias," 375–8.

44. Gilbert, "Inguinal herniorrhaphy," 831–4.

45. F. Glassow, "Inguinal hernia repair. A comparison of the Shouldice and Cooper ligament repair of the posterior inguinal wall," *American Journal of Surgery* 131 (March 1976): 306–11.

46. E. Cahlin and L. Weiss, "Results of postoperative clinical examination of inguinal hernia after three years," *ACTA Chirurgica Scandinavica* 146 (Number 6, 1980): 421–26.

47. L. M. Nyhus et al., "The preperitoneal approach and prosthetic buttress repair for recurrent hernia. The evolution of a technique," *Annals of Surgery* 208 (December 1988): 733–37.

48. F. Glassow, "Femoral hernia. Review of 2,105 repairs in a 17-year period," *American Journal of Surgery* 150 (September 1985): 353–56.

49. S. Mejdahl, H. J. Gyrtrup, and E. Kvist, "Outpatient operation of inguinal hernia in children," *British Journal of Surgery* 76 (April 1989): 406–7.

50. J. H. Solhaug, "Polyglycolic acid (Dexon) versus Mersilene in repair of inguinal hernia," *ACTA Chirurgica Scandinavica* 150 (Number 5, 1984): 385–87.

51. R. C. Read, "Recurrence after preperitoneal herniorrhaphy in the adult," *Archives of Surgery* 110 (May 1975): 666–71.

52. Miller et al., "Simultaneous bilateral hernia repair," 272–76.

53. Ibid.

54. I. L. Lichtenstein, "Herniorrhaphy. A personal experience with 6,321 cases," *American Journal of Surgery* 153 (June 1987): 553–59.

55. A. Sjogren and O. Elmer, "Outcome of inguinal hernia surgery," *Annales Chirurgiae et Gynaecologiae* 76 (Number 6, 1987): 314–17.

56. A. Shafik, "Invagination of the hernial sac stump. Technique for repair of inguinal hernia," *American Journal of Surgery* 140 (September 1980): 431–36.

57. M. H. Harvey, M. J. Johnstone, and D. P. Fossard, "In-

guinal herniotomy in children: A five-year survey," *British Journal of Surgery* 72 (June 1985): 485–87.

58. A. G. Greenburg, "Revisiting the recurrent groin hernia," *American Journal of Surgery* 154 (July 1987): 35–40.

59. R. C. Read, "Bilaterality and the prosthetic repair of large recurrent inguinal hernias," *American Journal of Surgery* 138 (December 1979): 788–93.

60. H. Lifschutz and G. L. Juler, "The inguinal darn," *Archives of Surgery* 121 (June 1986): 717–19.

61. Miller et al., "Simultaneous bilateral hernia repair," 272–76.

62. T. Dorflinger and J. Kiil, "Absorbable suture in hernia repair," *ACTA Chirurgica Scandinavica* 150 (Number 1, 1984): 41–43.

63. E. Kvist et al., "Outpatient orchiopexy and herniotomy in children," *ACTA Paediatrica Scandinavica* 78 (September 1989): 754–58.

64. J. R. Andersen et al., "Polyglycolic acid, silk, and topical ampicillin. Their use in hernia repair and cholecystectomy," *Archives of Surgery* 115 (March 1980): 293–95.

65. C. L. Slingluff, Jr., W. W. Burns, and C. Cooperberg, "Toxic shock syndrome after inguinal hernia repair. Report of a case with patient survival," *American Surgeon* 56 (October 1990): 610–12.

66. R. E. Stoppa, "The treatment of complicated groin and incisional hernias," *World Journal of Surgery* 13 (September–October 1989): 545–54.

67. A. G. Shulman, P. K. Amid, and I. L. Lichtenstein, "The 'plug' repair of 1402 recurrent inguinal hernias," *Archives of Surgery* 125 (February 1990): 265–67.

68. I. L. Lichtenstein, A. G. Shulman, and P. K. Amid, "Use of mesh to prevent recurrence of hernias," *Postgraduate Medicine* 87 (January 1990): 155–58, 160.

69. P. Platt et al., "Perioperative antibiotic prophylaxis for herniorrhaphy and breast surgery," *New England Journal of Medicine* 322 (18 January 1990): 153–60.

70. Simchen, Rozin, and Wax, "The Israeli Study of Surgical Infection of drains and the risk of wound infection in operations for hernia," 331–37.

71. H. W. Gilbert and W. G. Everett, "Clips or sutures for herniorrhaphy wounds?" *British Journal of Clinical Practice* 44 (August 1990): 306–8.

72. C. Tons et al., "Cremaster resection in Shouldice repair. A prospective controlled bi-center study," *Chirurg* 61 (February 1990): 109–11. (Published in German)

73. M. P. Elliott and G. L. Juler, "Comparison of Marlex mesh and microporous Teflon sheets when used for hernia repair in the experimental animal," *American Journal of Surgery* 137 (March 1979): 342–44.

Temporary Pacemaker System Insertion

1. J. E. Morin et al., "Temporary cardiac pacing following open-heart surgery," *Canadian Journal of Surgery* 25 (March 1982): 128–31.

2. V. Pekarsky et al., "Prevention of recurrent life-threatening ventricular arrhythmias by temporary cardiac pacing," *ACTA Medica Scandinavica* 217 (Number 1, 1985): 95–99.

3. C. E. Northcutt, J. D. Morgan, and R. E. Ligon, "Temporary transvenous pacemakers in the community hospital," *American Family Physician* 11 (May 1975): 115–18.

4. N. D. Berman, "Permanent pacemaker malfunction: diagnostic aspects of temporary pacing," *Canadian Medical Association Journal* 123 (August 1980): 190–93.

5. P. O. Littleford et al., "Clinical evaluation of a new temporary atrial pacing catheter: Results in 100 patients," *American Heart Journal* 107 (February 1984): 237–40.

6. E. G. Papasteriadis et al., "The use of the subclavian vein for temporary transvenous pacemaker therapy," *Angiology* 34 (July 1983): 480–83.

7. S. K. Krueger et al., "Temporary pacemaking by general internists," *Archives of Internal Medicine* 143 (August 1983): 1531–33.

8. W. Fairbanks et al., "Temporary transvenous cardiac pacemaking in rural family practice," *Journal of Family Practice* 4 (April 1977): 641–43.

9. D. L. Dunn and J. J. Gregory, "Noninvasive temporary pacing: experience in a community hospital," *Heart and Lung* 18 (January 1989): 23–28.

10. D. Inoue et al., "Devices external pulse generator: A reliable temporary pacemaker?" *Clinical Cardiology* 10 (December 1987): 815–17.

11. N. I. Jowett, D. R. Thompson, and J. E. Pohl, "Temporary transvenous cardiac pacing: Six years' experience in one coronary care unit," *Postgraduate Medical Journal* 65 (April 1989): 211–15.

12. J. L. Austin et al., "Analysis of pacemaker malfunction and complications of temporary pacing in the coronary care

unit," *American Journal of Cardiology* 49 (1 February 1982): 301–6.

13. K. D. Donovan and K. Y. Lee, "Indications for and complications of temporary transvenous cardiac pacing," *Anaesthesia and Intensive Care* 13 (February 1985): 63–70.

14. L. Hurtado Buen Abad et al., "Use of the temporary pacemaker in acute myocardial infarct," *Archivos del Instituto de Cardiologia de Mexico* 53 (July–August 1983): 303–12. (Published in Spanish)

15. N. G. Pandian, B. D. Kosowsky, and V. Gurewich, "Transfemoral temporary pacing and deep vein thrombosis," *American Heart Journal* 100 (December 1980): 847–51.

16. A. J. Nolewajka, M. D. Goddard, and T. C. Brown, "Temporary transvenous pacing and femoral vein thrombosis," *Circulation* 62 (September 1980): 646–50.

17. J. K. Hynes, D. D. Holmes, Jr., and C. E. Harrison, "Five-year experience with temporary pacemaker therapy in the coronary care unit," *Mayo Clinic Proceedings* 58 (February 1983): 122–26.

18. I. C. Gilchrist and A. Cameron, "Temporary pacemaker use during coronary arteriography," *American Journal of Cardiology* 60 (1 November 1987): 1051–54.

19. J. A. Smith and J. Tatoulis, "Right atrial perforation by a temporary epicardial pacing wire," *Annals of Thoracic Surgery* 50 (July 1990): 141–42.

20. C. Price and D. J. Keenan, "Injury to a saphenous vein graft during removal of a temporary epicardial pacing wire electrode," *British Heart Journal* 61 (June 1989): 546–47.

21. J. R. Harvey et al., "Use of balloon flotation pacing catheters for prophylactic temporary pacing during diagnostic and therapeutic catheterization procedures," *American Journal of Cardiology* 62 (1 November 1988): 941–44.

22. I. C. Gilchrist and A. Cameron, "Chronic bundle branch block and use of temporary transvenous pacemakers during coronary arteriography," *Catheterization and Cardiovascular Diagnosis* 15 (Number 4, 1988): 229–32.

23. L. W. Johnson, M. A. Bowser, and E. C. Lozner, "Use of temporary pacemakers during coronary angioplasty: An evolving experience with ventricular fibrillation in 400 cases," *Catheterization and Cardiovascular Diagnosis* 15 (Number 3, 1988): 150–54.

24. J. K. Madsen et al., "Transcutaneous pacing: Experience with the Zoll noninvasive temporary pacemaker," *American Heart Journal* 116 (July 1988): 7–10.

25. D. Berliner et al., "Transcutaneous temporary pacing in the operating room," *Journal of the American Medical Association* 254 (5 July 1985): 84–86.

Toe Amputation

1. J. Apelqvist et al., "Prognostic value of systolic ankle and toe blood pressure levels in outcome of diabetic foot ulcer," *Diabetes Care* 12 (June 1989): 373–78.

2. R. A. Mann, N. K. Poppen, and M. O'Konski, "Amputation of the great toe. A clinical and biomechanical study," *Clinical Orthopaedics and Related Research* (January 1988): 192–205.

3. N. K. Poppen et al., "Amputation of the great toe," *Foot and Ankle* 1 (May 1981): 333–37.

4. F. Hashimoto et al., "Free peroneal flap coverage of the great toe defect resulting from a wrap-around flap transfer," *Microsurgery* 7 (Number 4, 1986): 199–202.

5. B. O'Brien et al., "Microvascular second toe transfer for digital reconstruction," *Journal of Hand Surgery, American Volume* 3 (March 1978): 123–33.

6. R. Schiewe, E. Freund, and H. Schroder, "Toe transfer to a mid-hand stump covered with abdominal skin," *Handchirurgie, Mikrochirurgie, Plastische Chirurgie* 18 (January 1986): 30–34. (Published in German)

7. "Free toe transfer to the forearm stump following wrist amputation—a current alternative to the Krukenberg operation," *Handchirurgie, Mikrochirurgie, Plastische Chirurgie* 17 (March 1985): 92–97. (Published in German)

8. G. Foucher et al., "Toe-to-hand transfers in reconstructive surgery of the hand. Experience with 71 cases," *Annales de Chirurgie de la Main* 3 (Number 2, 1984): 124–38. (Published in English and French)

9. J. M. Mirra et al., "Primary osteosarcoma of toe phalanx: First documented case. Review of osteosarcoma of short tubular bones," *American Journal of Surgical Pathology* 12 (April 1988): 300–307.

10. B. A. Kraemer and M. Fremling, "Dermatofibrosarcoma protuberans of the toe," *Annals of Plastic Surgery* 25 (October 1990): 295–98.

11. I. F. Hitti et al., "Inverted variant of carcinoma cuniculatum of the toe," *Cutis* 39 (March 1987): 250–52.

12. L. M. Field, "An 'ultimate solution' for a painful toe," *Journal of Dermatologic Surgery and Oncology* 5 (May 1979): 402–3.

13. P. H. Julien et al., "Reconstruction of soft tissue defects about the great toe," *Journal of Foot Surgery* 27 (March–April 1988): 116–20.

14. Schiewe, Freund, and Schroder, "Toe transfer to a mid-hand stump covered with abdominal skin," 30–34.

15. T. M. Due and R. L. Jacobs, "Molded foot orthosis after great toe or medial ray amputations in diabetic feet," *Foot and Ankle* 6 (December 1985): 150–52.

16. N. K. Poppen et al., "Amputation of the great toe," *Foot and Ankle* 1 (May 1981): 333–37.

17. L. C. Chiedozi, "Gangrenous bowel. Benin experience," *American Journal of Surgery* 142 (November 1981): 622–24.

18. C. O. Castillo and S. C. Martinez, "Necrotizing perineal phlegmon (Fournier's gangrene)," *ACTAS Urologicas Espanolas* 13 (September–October 1989): 381–83. (Published in Spanish)

Tonsillectomy

1. R. M. Rosenfeld and R. P. Green, "Tonsillectomy and adenoidectomy: Changing trends," *Annals of Otology, Rhinology, and Laryngology* 99 (March 1990): 187–91.

2. I. Eliaschar et al., "Sleep apneic episodes as indications for adenotonsillectomy," *Archives of Otolaryngology* 106 (August 1980): 492–96.

3. G. Lugassy et al., "Clinical and pathological features of non-Hodgkin's lymphoma of the tonsil. Review of the literature and report of 10 cases," *Israel Journal of Medical Sciences* 25 (May 1989): 25–55.

4. "Unilateral tonsillectomy—indications and results," *Journal of Laryngology and Otology* 97 (December 1983): 1111–19.

5. D. J. Blum and H. B. Neel, III, "Current thinking on tonsillectomy and adenoidectomy," *Comprehensive Therapy* 9 (December 1983): 48–56.

6. M. D. Ying, "Immunological basis of indications for tonsillectomy and adenoidectomy," *ACTA Otolaryngologica, Supplement (Stockholm)* 454 (1988): 279–85.

7. Ibid.

8. H. B. Wong, "The problems of tonsils and adenoids," *Journal of the Singapore Paediatric Society* 31 (Number 3–4, 1989): 97–102.

9. H. Gastparm, "Indications for tonsillectomy in childhood from the current viewpoint," *Laryngologie, Rhinologie, Otologie* 63 (April 1984): 203–5. (Published in German)

10. HealthCare Knowledge Resources/Commission on Professional and Hospital Activities, *HealthWeek* (6 November 1989).

11. Ibid.

12. Blum and Neel, "Current thinking on tonsillectomy and adenoidectomy," 48–56.

13. J. B. Colclasure and S. S. Graham, "Complications of outpatient tonsillectomy and adenoidectomy: A review of 3,340 cases," *Ear, Nose, and Throat Journal* 69 (March 1990): 155–60.

14. B. C. Okafor, "Tonsillectomy: An appraisal of indications in developing countries," *ACTA Otolaryngologica (Stockholm)* 96 (November–December 1983): 517–22.

15. K. T. Kavanagh and N. S. Beckford, "Adenotonsillectomy in children: Indications and contraindications," *Southern Medical Journal* 81 (April 1988): 507–14.

16. J. P. LoGerfo et al., "Tonsillectomies, adenoidectomies, audits: Have surgical indications been met?" *Medical Care* 16 (November 1978): 950–55.

17. O. E. Brown, S. C. Manning, and B. Ridenour, "Cor pulmonale secondary to tonsillar and adenoidal hypertrophy: Management considerations," *International Journal of Pediatric Otorhinolaryngology* 16 (November 1988): 131–39.

18. K. E. Ellsbury, "Therapeutic alternatives and clinical outcomes in peritonsillitis," *Journal of Family Practice* 18 (January 1984): 69–73.

19. M. Echeverria and M. Olarieta, "Current surgical indications for tonsillar pathology," *ACTA Otorrinolaringologica Espanola* 40 (March–April 1989): 71–73. (Published in Spanish)

20. H. B. Neel, III, and T. J. McDonald, "Tonsillectomy and adenoidectomy. Are there any indications?" *Postgraduate Medicine* 70 (September 1981): 107–12.

21. J. H. Mandel, "Pharyngeal infections. Causes, findings, and management," *Postgraduate Medicine* 77 (15 February 1985): 187–93, 196–99.

22. Kavanagh and Beckford, "Adenotonsillectomy in children," 507–14.

23. B. E. Linden et al., "Morbidity in pediatric tonsillectomy," *Laryngoscope* 100 (February 1990): 120–24.

24. J. E. Wennberg et al., "Changes in tonsillectomy rates associated with feedback and review," *Pediatrics* 59 (June 1977): 821–26.

Tonsillectomy and Adenoidectomy

1. R. M. Rosenfeld and R. P. Green, "Tonsillectomy and adenoidectomy: Changing trends," *Annals of Otology, Rhinology, and Laryngology* 99 (March 1990): 187–91.

2. I. Eliaschar et al., "Sleep apneic episodes as indications for adenotonsillectomy," *Archives of Otolaryngology* 106 (August 1980): 492–96.

3. G. Lugassy et al., "Clinical and pathological features of non-Hodgkin's lymphoma of the tonsil. Review of the literature and report of 10 cases," *Israel Journal of Medical Sciences* 25 (May 1989): 251–55.

4. "Unilateral tonsillectomy—indications and results," *Journal of Laryngology and Otology* 97 (December 1983): 1111–19.

5. D. J. Blum and H. B. Neel, III, "Current thinking on tonsillectomy and adenoidectomy," *Comprehensive Therapy* 9 (December 1983): 48–56.

6. M. D. Ying, "Immunological basis of indications for tonsillectomy and adenoidectomy," *ACTA Otolaryngologica, Supplement (Stockholm)* 454 (1988): 279–85.

7. Ibid.

8. H. B. Wong, "The problems of tonsils and adenoids," *Journal of the Singapore Paediatric Society* 31 (Number 3–4, 1989): 97–102.

9. H. Gastparm, "Indications for tonsillectomy in childhood from the current viewpoint," *Laryngologie, Rhinologie, Otologie* 63 (April 1984): 203–5. (Published in German)

10. Blum and Neel, "Current thinking on tonsillectomy and adenoidectomy," 48–56.

11. Rosenfeld and Green, "Tonsillectomy and adenoidectomy," 187–91.

12. P. A. Shapiro, "Effects of nasal obstruction on facial development," *Journal of Allergy and Clinical Immunology* 81 (May 1988): 967–71.

13. Blum and Neel, "Current thinking on tonsillectomy and adenoidectomy," 48–56.

14. R. L. Doty and R. Frye, "Influence of nasal obstruction on smell function," *Otolaryngologic Clinics of North America* 22 (April 1989): 397–411.

15. M. Sagnelli et al., "Secretory otitis media: Current aspects and therapeutic role of adenoidectomy," *Medicina (Firenze)* 10 (January–March 1990): 16–22. (Published in Italian)

Total Abdominal Hysterectomy

1. D. A. Grimes and K. F. Schulz, "Morbidity and mortality from second-trimester abortions," *Journal of Reproductive Medicine* 30 (July 1985): 505–14.

2. W. Matuszewski, J. Rzempoluch, and G. Cieslar, "Hysterectomy within the scope of cesarean section," *Zentralblatt fur Gynakologie* 109 (Number 15, 1987): 956–61. (Published in German)

3. P. A. Wingo et al., "The mortality risk associated with hysterectomy," *American Journal of Obstetrics and Gynecology* 152 (1 August 1985): 803–8.

4. P. Hohlweg-Majert and R. Weidmann, "Hysterectomy in young women," *Fortschritte der Medizin* 101 (3 November 1983): 1851–54. (Published in German)

5. A. Chryssikopoulos and C. Loghis, "Indications and results of total hysterectomy," *International Surgery* 71 (July–September 1986): 188–94.

6. D. G. Gallup and R. T. Welham, "Vaginal hysterectomy by an anterior colpotomy technic," *Southern Medical Journal* 69 (June 1976): 752–54, 756.

7. P. Draca, "Complications following vaginal hysterectomy," *Jugoslavenska Ginekologija I Opstetricija* 16 (March–April 1976): 105–13. (Published in Serbo-Croatian, Roman)

8. K. Becker, E. Muller-Wuhr, and G. Stark, "Follow-up of 2,300 vaginal and abdominal hysterectomies," *Fortschritte der Medizin* 95 (9 June 1977): 1425–28. (Published in German)

9. R. Ranney and S. Abu-Ghazaleh, "The future function and fortune of ovarian tissue which is retained in vivo during hysterectomy," *American Journal of Obstetrics and Gynecology* 128 (15 July 1977): 626–34.

10. C. Schubring and E. Werner, "Urine drainage following vaginal gynecologic operations," *Geburtshilfe und Frauenheilkunde* 46 (July 1986): 459–61. (Published in German)

11. E. Harms, U. Christmann, and F. K. Klock, "Suprapubic urinary diversion following gynecologic operations," *Geburtshilfe und Frauenheilkunde* 45 (April 1985): 254–60. (Published in German)

12. A 1987 pamphlet, "Understanding Hysterectomy," from the American College of Obstetricians and Gynecologists, quoted in "Sexual Response After Hysterectomy," *HealthFacts* (New York: Center for Medical Consumers, 1990), Vol. XV, No. 139, p 1.

13. J. Dietl and K. Semm, "Conization and hysterectomy

from the viewpoint of the surgically treated woman," *Geburtshilfe und Frauenheilkunde* 43 (September 1983): 562–66. (Published in German)

14. G. Seidenschnur et al., "Attitude and sex behavior following hysterectomy," *Zentralblatt fur Gynakologie* 111 (Number 1, 1989): 53–59. (Published in German)

15. "The effects of 554 non-radical vaginal and abdominal hysterectomies on micturition symptoms and urinary incontinence," *ACTA Obstetricia et Gynecologica Scandinavica* 67 (Number 2, 1988): 141–46.

16. P. Kilkku, "Supravaginal uterine amputation versus hysterectomy with reference to subjective bladder symptoms and incontinence," *ACTA Obstetricia et Gynecologica Scandinavica* 64 (Number 5, 1985): 375–79.

17. R. C. Dicker et al., "Complications of abdominal and vaginal hysterectomy among women of reproductive age in the United States. The Collaborative Review of Sterilization," *American Journal of Obstetrics and Gynecology* 144 (1 December 1982): 841–48.

18. G. W. Morley and J. O. DeLancey, "Sacrospinous ligament fixation for eversion of the vagina," *American Journal of Obstetrics and Gynecology* 158 (April 1988): 872–81.

19. S. H. Cruikshank, "Preventing posthysterectomy vaginal vault prolapse and enterocele during vaginal hysterectomy," *American Journal of Obstetrics and Gynecology* 156 (June 1987): 1433–40.

20. C. F. Langmade and J. A. Oliver, Jr., "Partial colpocleisis," *American Journal of Obstetrics and Gynecology* 154 (June 1986): 1200–5.

21. P. M. Wisniewski et al., "Early diagnosis of a diverticular colovaginal fistula with colposcopy. A case report," *Journal of Reproductive Medicine* 33 (August 1988): 705–8.

22. M. Lev-Gur et al., "Pararenal hematoma as a complication of vaginal hysterectomy. A case report," *Journal of Reproductive Medicine* 32 (January 1987): 68–71.

23. D. Dargent and R. C. Rudigoz, "Vaginal hysterectomy. Our experience between the years 1970 to 1979," *Journal de Gynecologie, Obstetrique et Biologie de la Reproduction (Paris)* 9 (Number 8, 1980): 895–908. (Published in French)

24. S. C. Voss, H. C. Sharp, and J. R. Scott, "Abdominoplasty combined with gynecologic surgical procedures," *Obstetrics and Gynecology* 67 (February 1986): 181–85.

25. G. Ralph et al., "Functional disorders of the lower urinary tract following radical abdominal and vaginal surgery of cervix cancer," *Geburtshilfe und Frauenheilkunde* 47 (August 1987): 551–54. (Published in German)

26. O. E. Jaschevatzky et al., "Prostaglandin F2 alpha for prevention of urinary retention after vaginal hysterectomy," *Obstetrics and Gynecology* 66 (August 1985): 244–47.

27. P. Riss, R. Spernol, and W. Gruber, "Intravesical prostaglandin E2 and placebo in urinary retention after gynaecological surgery," *Geburtshilfe und Frauenheilkunde* (March 1982): 182–84. (Published in German)

28. R. Kudo et al., "Vaginal hysterectomy without ligation of the ligaments of the cervix uteri," *Surgery, Gynecology, and Obstetrics* 170 (April 1990): 299–305.

29. P. Cole and J. Berlin, "Elective hysterectomy," *American Journal of Obstetrics and Gynecology* 129 (15 September 1977): 117–23.

Total Cholecystectomy

1. J. C. Skillings, C. Kumai, and J. R. Hinshaw, "Cholecystostomy: A place in modern biliary surgery?" *American Journal of Surgery* 139 (June 1980): 865–69.

2. E. E. Vuori, "Treatment of cholecystitis: Cholecystostomy or cholecystectomy?" *American Journal of Surgery* 132 (July 1976): 75–80.

3. Ibid.

4. P. W. Houghton, L. R. Jenkinson, and L. A. Donaldson, "Cholecystectomy in the elderly: A prospective study," *British Journal of Surgery* 72 (March 1985): 220–22.

5. L. W. Ottinger, "Acute cholecystitis as a postoperative complication," *Annals of Surgery* 184 (August 1976): 162–65.

6. S. Nakamura et al., "Aggressive surgery for carcinoma of the gallbladder," *Surgery* 106 (September 1989): 467–73.

7. H. Winter Griffith, *Complete Guide to Symptoms, Illness, and Surgery* (Los Angeles: The Body Press, 1985), 707.

8. H. J. Burhenne and J. L. Stoller, "Minicholecystostomy and radiologic stone extraction in high-risk cholelithiasis patients," *American Journal of Surgery* 149 (May 1985): 632–35.

9. M. Tanaka et al., "The long-term fate of the gallbladder after endoscopic sphincterotomy. Complete follow-up study of 122 patients," *American Journal of Surgery* 154 (November 1987): 505–9.

10. *Physicians' Desk Reference* (Oradell, NJ: Medical Economics Co., 1991): 2180–82.

11. Based on a search of the National Library of Medicine

database, using PaperChase, and searching for the words "laparoscopic" and "cholecystectomy" through the July 1991 update.

12. E. J. Reddick et al., "Safe performance of difficult laparoscopic cholecystectomies," *American Journal of Surgery* 161 (March 1991): 377–81.

13. A. Cuschieri et al., "The European experience with laparoscopic cholecystectomy," *American Journal of Surgery* 161 (March 1991): 385–87.

14. J. Perissat et al., "Laparoscopic cholecystectomy using intracorporeal lithotripsy," *American Journal of Surgery* 161 (March 1991): 371–76.

15. S. K. Teplick et al., "Percutaneous interventional gallbladder procedures: Personal experience and literature review," *Gastrointestinal Radiology* 15 (Spring 1990): 133–36.

Total Hip Replacement

1. H. von Zippel, "Multi-morbidity and perioperative risk of total hip endoprosthesis," *Beitrage Zur Orthopadie und Traumatologie* 37 (April 1990): 193–203. (Published in German)

2. G. Assennato et al., "Hip prosthesis: Idea, indications, development," *Clinical Therapeutics* 134 (15 September 1990): 313–22. (Published in Italian)

3. R. M. Luba, G. L. Maistrelli, and T. W. Barrington, "The Madreporic cementless total hip arthroplasty: Short-term North American experience," *Canadian Journal of Surgery* 28 (November 1985): 515–17.

4. F. A. Sloan, J. M. Perrin, and J. Valvona, "In-hospital mortality of surgical patients: Is there an empiric basis for standard setting?" *Surgery* 99 (April 1986): 446–54.

5. B. M. Wroblewski, "Loosening of hip prostheses," *Orthopade* 18 (September 1989): 388–96. (Published in German)

6. B. Schoning, K. P. Schulitz, and T. Pfluger, "Statistical analysis of perioperative and postoperative mortality of patients with prosthetic replacement of the hip joint," *Archives of Orthopaedic and Traumatic Surgery* 97 (Number 1, 1980): 21–26.

7. von Zippel, "Multi-morbidity and perioperative risk of total hip endoprosthesis," 193–203.

8. D. Hernandez-Vaquero, "The risk of thromboembolism in prosthetic surgery of the hip, and its prevention by administration of individualized heparin dosages," *ACTA Ortho-

paedica Belgica* 56 (December 1990): 445–50. (Published in French)

9. R. Egbert et al., "Heart arrest in implantation of a cemented total hip joint endoprosthesis under spinal anesthesia—a case report," *Anasthesie, Intensivtherapie, Notfallmedizin* 24 (April 1989): 118–20. (Published in German)

10. C. Ulrich et al., "Intraoperative transesophageal two-dimensional echocardiography in total hip replacement," *Archives of Orthopaedic and Traumatic Surgery* 105 (Number 5, 1986): 274–78.

11. H. Maxeiner, "Fatal intraoperative lung fat embolism in endoprosthesis of the hip joint," *Beitrage Zur Gerichtlichen Medizin* 47 (1989): 415–27. (Published in German)

12. M. Hochmeister et al., "Intraoperative fatal fat and bone marrow embolism of the lung in implantation of a hip endoprosthesis with polymethylmethacrylate bone cement," *Zeitschrift fur Orthopadie und Ihre Grenzgebiete* 125 (May–June 1987): 337–39. (Published in German)

13. K. H. Andersen, "Air aspirated from the venous system during total hip replacement," *Anaesthesia* 38 (December 1983): 1175–78.

14. P. B. Harvey and J. A. Smith, "Prevention of air emboli in hip surgery. Femoral shaft insufflation with carbon dioxide," *Anaesthesia* 37 (July 1982): 714–17.

15. W. Seelig, U. Ludin, and E. Morscher, "Perioperative risks and problems in total hip joint replacement," *Schweizerische Rundschau fur Medizin Praxis* 78 (4 April 1989): 390–93. (Published in German)

16. S. Malingue et al., "Mortality after regular implantations of total hip prostheses," *Cahiers D'Anesthesiologie* 34 (May 1986): 227–30. (Published in French)

17. C. R. Covert and G. S. Fox, "Anaesthesia for hip surgery in the elderly," *Canadian Journal of Anaesthesia* 36 (May 1989): 311–19.

18. J. Raunest, A. Kaschner, and E. Derra, "Incidence of complications and early mortality in surgical management of coxal femoral fractures," *Langenbecks Archiv fur Chirurgie* 375 (Number 3, 1990): 156–60. (Published in German)

19. M. Katzner, S. Babin, and E. Schvingt, "Complications observed in a series of 2,018 total hip replacements," *Nouvelle Presse Medicale* 11 (23 January 1982): 181–83. (Published in French)

20. J. A. Duncan, "Intra-operative collapse or death related to the use of acrylic cement in hip surgery," *Anaesthesia* 44 (February 1989): 149–53.

21. Luba, Maistrelli, and Barrington, "The Madreporic cementless total hip arthroplasty," 515–17.

22. P. L. Broos et al., "Hip fractures in the elderly: mortality, functional results and probability of returning home," *Nederlands Tijdschrift Voor Geneeskunde* 134 (12 May 1990): 957–61. (Published in Dutch)

23. O. Soreide and J. Lillestol, "Mortality patterns following internal fixation for acute femoral neck fractures in the elderly with special emphasis on potential excess mortality following reoperations," *Age and Ageing* 9 (February 1980): 59–63.

24. H. Lindberg et al., "The overall mortality rate in patients with total hip arthroplasty, with special reference to coxarthrosis," *Clinical Orthopaedics and Related Research* (December 1984): 116–20.

25. G. D. Paiement and C. Desautels, "Deep vein thrombosis: Prophylaxis, diagnosis, and treatment—lessons from orthopedic studies," *Clinical Cardiology* 13 (April 1990, Supplement): VI19–22.

26. C. M. Kessler, "Modern treatment of pulmonary embolism," *Lung* 168 (1990, Supplement): 841–48.

27. R. W. Barnes et al., "Perioperative asymptomatic venous thrombosis: Role of duplex scanning versus venography," *Journal of Vascular Surgery* 9 (February 1989): 251–60.

28. H. Heinrich et al., "Transesophageal two-dimensional echocardiography in hip endoprostheses," *Anasthesist* 34 (March 1985): 118–23. (Published in German)

29. "Intraoperative detection of air embolism and corpuscular embolism using pulse oximetry and capnometry. Comparative studies with transesophageal echocardiography," *Anasthesie, Intensivtherapie, Notfallmedizin* 24 (February 1989): 20–26. (Published in German)

30. J. Thorburn, J. R. Louden, and R. Vallance, "Spinal and general anaesthesia in total hip replacement: Frequency of deep vein thrombosis," *British Journal of Anaesthesia* 52 (November 1980): 1117–21.

31. Y. Samra, Y. Shaked, and M. K. Maier, "Nontyphoid salmonellosis in patients with total hip replacement: Report of four cases and review of the literature," *Reviews of Infectious Diseases* 8 (November–December 1986): 978–83.

32. K. L. Garvin, E. A. Salvati, and B. D. Brause, "Role of gentamicin-impregnated cement in total joint arthroplasty," *Orthopedic Clinics of North America* 19 (July 1988): 605–10.

33. W. Oberthaler, R. Bauer, and K. Sattler, "Results of alloarthroplasty of the hip joint," *Archives of Orthopaedic and Traumatic Surgery* 96 (Number 4, 1980): 247–58.

34. E. Morscher, R. Babst, and H. Jenny, "Treatment of infected joint arthroplasty," *International Orthopaedics* 14 (Number 2, 1990): 161–65.

35. Wroblewski, "Loosening of hip prostheses," 388–96.

36. W. Plitz, "Biomechanical aspects of loosening of hip prostheses," *Orthopade* 18 (September 1989): 344–49. (Published in German)

37. G. Stringa et al., "Total hip prosthesis according to Charnley. Review of our cases," *Archivio Putti Di Chirurgia Degli Organi Di Movimento* 37 (Number 1, 1989): 9–35. (Published in Italian)

38. R. Schneider, "Total prosthesis of the hip: Procedure using cement," *Langenbecks Archiv fur Chirurgie* 372 (1987): 457–64. (Published in German)

39. D. C. Ayers et al., "Prevention of heterotopic ossification in high-risk patients by radiation therapy," *Clinical Orthopaedics and Related Research* (February 1991): 87–93.

40. B. Shaffer, "A critical review. Heterotopic ossification in total hip replacement," *Bulletin of the Hospital for Joint Diseases Orthopaedic Institute* 49 (Spring 1989): 55–74.

41. S. B. Warren, "Heterotopic ossification after total hip replacement," *Orthopaedic Review* 19 (July 1990): 603–11.

42. P. Kjaersgaard-Andersen and S. A. Schmidt, "Total hip arthroplasty. The role of anti-inflammatory medications in the prevention of heterotopic ossification," *Clinical Orthopaedics and Related Research* (February 1991): 78–86.

43. D. J. Callahan and C. K. Safley, "Cement dam. A simple device to prevent cement extrusion," *Orthopedics* 8 (June 1985): 752–55.

44. H. O. Dustmann and G. Godolias, "Experiences with cement-free implantation of the Zweymuller/Endler and Zweymuller total hip joint endoprosthesis," *Zeitschrift fur Orthopadie und Ihre Grenzgebiete* 126 (May–June 1988): 314–25. (Published in German)

45. P. Albrecht-Olsen et al., "Nine-year follow-up of the cementless Ring hip," *ACTA Orthopaedica Scandinavica* 60 (February 1989): 77–80.

46. T. A. Andrew et al., "The isoelastic, noncemented total hip arthroplasty. Preliminary experience with 400 cases," *Clinical Orthopaedics and Related Research* (May 1986): 127–38.

47. Ibid.

48. D. W. Mok and K. M. Bryant, "Ring uncemented plastic on metal hip replacements—results from an independent unit," *Journal of the Royal Society of Medicine* 82 (March 1989): 142–44.

49. H. U. Cameron and S. Bhimji, "Design rationale in early clinical trials with a hemispherical threaded acetabular com-

ponent," *Journal of Arthroplasty* 3 (Number 4, 1988): 299–304.

50. R. H. Turner, D. A. Mattingly, and A. Scheller, "Femoral revision total hip arthroplasty using a long-stem femoral component. Clinical and radiographic analysis," *Journal of Arthroplasty* 2 (Number 3, 1987): 247–58.

51. F. W. Wittmann and P. A. Ring, "Reduction in blood loss in total hip arthroplasty using topical Colgen," *Journal of Arthroplasty* 4 (September 1989): 253–56.

52. A. K. Vazeery and O. Lunde, "Controlled hypotension in hip joint surgery. An assessment of surgical haemorrhage during sodium nitroprusside infusion," *ACTA Orthopaedica Scandinavica* 50 (August 1979): 433–41.

53. G. Barbier-Bohm et al., "Comparative effects of induced hypotension and normovolaemic haemodilution on blood loss in total hip arthroplasty," *British Journal of Anaesthesia* 52 (October 1980): 1039–43.

54. "The review of 4,300 Charnley total hip replacements inserted between 1968 and 1979," *Revue de Chirurgie Orthopedique et Reparatrice de L Appareil Moteur* 66 (March 1980): 57–67. (Published in French)

55. A. Bullrich and E. Miltner, "Fatal hemorrhage in total endoprosthesis reimplantation. A case report and legal viewpoints," *Unfallchirurg* 92 (April 1989): 187–90. (Published in German)

56. S. A. Stuchin, "Femoral shaft fracture in porous and press-fit total hip arthroplasty," *Orthopaedic Review* 19 (February 1990): 153–59.

57. G. Mayer, H. W. Seide, and P. Patzak, "Femur shaft fractures in artificial hip joint replacement," *Zentralblatt fur Chirurgie* 110 (Number 12, 1985): 739–48. (Published in German)

58. C. M. Christensen, B. M. Seger, and R. B. Schultz, "Management of intraoperative femur fractures associated with revision hip arthroplasty," *Clinical Orthopaedics and Related Research* (November 1989): 177–80.

59. R. H. Fitzgerald, Jr., et al., "The uncemented total hip arthroplasty. Intraoperative femoral fractures," *Clinical Orthopaedics and Related Research* (October 1988): 61–66.

60. B. Nachbur, R. P. Meyer, and J. Baumgartner, "Vascular complications in surgery of the hip joint," *Orthopade* 18 (November 1989): 552–58. (Published in German)

61. J. Abrahamson and S. Eldar, "Acute cholecystitis after orthopaedic operations," *International Orthopaedics* 12 (Number 1, 1988): 93–95.

62. A. J. Timperley and D. J. Bracey, "Cardiac arrest follow-ing the use of hydrogen peroxide during arthroplasty," *Journal of Arthroplasty* 4 (December 1989): 369–70.

63. "Complications during implantation of 3,260 hip endoprostheses under spinal anesthesia," *Regional Anaesthesie* 12 (November 1989): 117–26. (Published in German)

64. "The review of 4,300 Charnley total hip replacements inserted between 1968 and 1979," 57–67.

65. H. P. Werner, "Complications and risks of suction drainage," *Zeitschrift fur Die Gesamte Hygiene und Ihre Grenzgebiete* 36 (February 1990): 94–99. (Published in German)

66. S. Jantsch et al., "Intra-operative shaft fissure—a possible cause of postoperative shaft pain following cement-free hip joint implantation," *Zeitschrift fur Orthopadie und Ihre Grenzgebiete* 128 (March–April 1990): 144–48. (Published in German)

67. R. D. Kaufman and L. F. Walts, "Tourniquet-induced hypertension," *British Journal of Anaesthesia* 54 (March 1982): 333–36.

68. B. J. Awbrey et al., "Late complications of total hip replacement from bone cement within the pelvis. A review of the literature and a case report involving dyspareunia," *Journal of Bone and Joint Surgery, British Volume* 66 (January 1984): 41–44.

69. I. Jakim, C. Barlin, and M. B. Sweet, "RM isoelastic total hip arthroplasty. A review of 34 cases," *Journal of Arthroplasty* 3 (Number 3, 1988): 191–99.

70. R. Rosso, "Five-year review of the isoelastic RM total hip endoprosthesis," *Archives of Orthopaedic and Traumatic Surgery* 107 (Number 2, 1988): 86–88.

71. G. L. Maistrelli et al., "A Valgus-extension osteotomy for osteoarthritis of the hip. Indications and long-term results," *Journal of Bone and Joint Surgery, British Volume* 72 (July 1990): 653–57.

72. Turner, Mattingly, and Scheller, "Femoral revision total hip arthroplasty using a long-stem femoral component," 247–58.

73. M. Slavik and V. Stedry, "Traumatic indications for total hip joint prosthesis," *ACTA Chirurgiae Orthopaedicae et Traumatologiae Cechoslovaca* 57 (July 1990): 328–38. (Published in Czech)

74. T. A. Andrew et al., "Long-term review of ring total hip arthroplasty," *Clinical Orthopaedics and Related Research* (December 1985): 111–22.

75. Mok and Bryant, "Ring uncemented plastic on metal hip replacements" 142–44.

76. C. Picault, C. R. Michel, and R. Vidil, "The review of

4,300 Charnley total hip replacements inserted between 1968 and 1979," *Revue de Chirurgie Orthopedique et Reparatrice de L Appareil Moteur* 66 (March 1980): 57–67. (Published in French)

77. P. Haentjens et al., "The Muller acetabular support ring. A preliminary review of indications and clinical results," *International Orthopaedics* 10 (Number 4, 1986): 223–30.

78. Luba, Maistrelli, and Barrington, "The Madreporic cementless total hip arthroplasty," 515–17.

79. Albrecht-Olsen et al., "Nine-year follow-up of the cementless Ring hip," 77–80.

80. Andrew et al., "The isoelastic, noncemented total hip arthroplasty," 127–38.

81. Dustmann and Godolias, "Experiences with cement-free implantation of the Zweymuller/Endler and Zweymuller total hip joint endoprosthesis," 314–25.

82. J. L. Stambough et al., "Conversion total hip replacement. Review of 140 hips with greater than six-year follow-up study," *Journal of Arthroplasty* 1 (February 1986): 261–69.

83. P. Vanclooster et al., "Treatment of unstable, intracapsular fractures of the femoral neck by the cementless self-locking cephalic endoprosthesis," *ACTA Chirurgica Belgica* 88 (January–February 1988): 21–25.

84. R. Turcotte et al., "Hip fractures and Parkinson's disease. A clinical review of 94 fractures treated surgically," *Clinical Orthopaedics and Related Research* (July 1990): 132–36.

85. C. E. Johnston et al., "Primary endoprosthetic replacement for acute femoral neck fractures. A review of 150 cases," *Clinical Orthopaedics and Related Research* (July 1982): 123–30.

Total Knee Replacement

1. I. Hvid, "Trabecular bone strength at the knee," *Clinical Orthopaedics and Related Research* (February 1988): 210–21.

2. R. D. Scott, "Total hip and knee arthroplasty in juvenile rheumatoid arthritis," *Clinical Orthopaedics and Related Research* (October 1990): 83–91.

3. K. M. Yaw and L. D. Wurtz, "Resection and reconstruction for bone tumors in the proximal tibia," *Orthopedic Clinics of North America* 22 (January 1991): 133–48.

4. M. R. Urist, "Acrylic cement stabilized joint replacements," *Current Problems in Surgery* (November 1975): 1–54.

5. HealthCare Knowledge Resources/Commission on Professional and Hospital Activities, *HealthWeek* (6 November 1989).

6. B. F. Morrey et al., "Complications and mortality associated with bilateral or unilateral total knee arthroplasty," *Journal of Bone and Joint Surgery, American Volume* 69 (April 1987): 484–88.

7. Richard S. Snell, *Clinical Anatomy for Medical Students* (Boston: Little, Brown and Company, 1986), 652 and 686.

8. D. L. Butler et al., "On the interpretation of our anterior cruciate ligament data," *Clinical Orthopaedics and Related Research* (June 1985): 26–34.

9. D. J. Zoltan, C. Reinecke, and P. A. Indelicato, "Synthetic and allograft anterior cruciate ligament reconstruction," *Clinics in Sports Medicine* 7 (October 1988): 773–84.

10. G. W. Brick and R. D. Scott, "The patellofemoral component of total knee arthroplasty," *Clinical Orthopaedics and Related Research* (June 1988): 163–78.

11. M. Alexiades et al., "Management of selected problems in revision knee arthroplasty," *Orthopedic Clinics of North America* 20 (April 1989): 211–19.

12. V. M. Goldberg, H. E. Figgie III, and M. P. Figgie, "Technical considerations in total knee surgery. Management of patella problems," *Orthopedic Clinics of North America* 20 (April 1989): 189–99.

13. R. Poss, "Current status of total joint arthroplasty: Observations and projections," *Journal of Rheumatology* (August 1987, Supplement): 40–45.

14. P. Cartier, M. Mammeri, and P. Villers, "Clinical and radiographic evaluation of modular knee replacement. A review of 95 cases," *International Orthopaedics* 6 (October 1982): 35–44.

15. F. F. Buechel and M. J. Pappas, "The New Jersey Low-Contact-Stress Knee Replacement System: Biomechanical rationale and review of the first 123 cemented cases," *Archives of Orthopaedic and Traumatic Surgery* 105 (Number 4, 1986): 197–204.

16. R. S. Laskin, "Total condylar knee replacement in rheumatoid arthritis. A review of 117 knees," *Journal of Bone and Joint Surgery, American Volume* 63 (January 1981): 29–35.

17. D. S. Barrett, S. P. Biswas, and R. P. MacKenney, "The Oxford knee replacement. A review from an independent centre," *Journal of Bone and Joint Surgery, British Volume* 72 (September 1990): 775–78.

18. J. A. Vanhegan, W. Dabrowski, and G. P. Arden, "A review of 100 Attenborough stabilised gliding knee prostheses," *Journal of Bone and Joint Surgery, British Volume* 61 (Number 4, 1979): 445–50.

19. A. E. Koch, "*Candida albicans* infection of a prosthetic knee replacement: A report and review of the literature," *Journal of Rheumatology* 15 (February 1988): 362–65.

20. J. A. Rand and R. S. Bryan, "Results of revision total knee arthroplasties using condylar prostheses. A review of 50 knees," *Journal of Bone and Joint Surgery* 70 (June 1988): 738–45.

21. E. M. Massarotti and H. Dinerman, "Septic arthritis due to *Listeria monocytogenes*," *Journal of Rheumatology* 17 (January 1990): 111–13.

22. C. J. Kershaw and A. E. Themen, "The Attenborough knee. A four- to 10-year review," *Journal of Bone and Joint Surgery, British Volume* 70 (January 1988): 89–93.

23. H. U. Cameron and D. M. Fedorkow, "Review of a failed knee replacement and some observations on the design of a knee resurfacing prosthesis," *Archives of Orthopaedic and Traumatic Surgery* 97 (Number 2, 1980): 87–89.

24. R. J. Minns, "The Minns meniscal knee prosthesis: Biomechanical aspects of the surgical procedure and a review of the first 165 cases," *Archives of Orthopaedic and Traumatic Surgery* 108 (Number 4, 1989): 231–35.

25. M. H. Huo and T. P. Sculco, "Complications in primary total knee arthroplasty," *Orthopaedic Review* 19 (September 1990): 781–88.

26. M. Levine, S. J. Rehm, and A. H. Wilde, "Infection with *Candida albicans* of a total knee arthroplasty," *Clinical Orthopaedics and Related Research* (January 1988): 235–39.

27. A. W. Heywood and I. D. Learmonth, "Total replacement of the rheumatoid knee: A review of currently available prostheses and a follow-up of 50 operations," *South African Medical Journal* 57 (23 February 1980): 272–77.

28. "Fungal prosthetic arthritis: Presentation of two cases and review of the literature," *Reviews of Infectious Diseases* 10 (September-October 1988): 1038–43.

29. E. Morscher, "Endoprosthetic surgery in 1988," *Annales Chirurgiae et Gynaecologiae* 78 (Number 3, 1989): 242–53.

30. J. G. Lee et al., "Review of the all-polyethylene tibial component in total knee arthroplasty. A minimum seven-year follow-up period," *Clinical Orthopaedics and Related Research* (November 1990): 87–92.

31. Y. H. Kim, "Knee arthroplasty using a cementless PCA prosthesis with a porous-coated central tibial stem. Clinical and radiographic review at five years," *Journal of Bone and Joint Surgery, British Volume* 72 (May 1990): 412–17.

32. T. M. Turner et al., "Bone ingrowth into the tibial component of a canine total condylar knee replacement prosthesis," *Journal of Orthopaedic Research* 7 (Number 6, 1989): 893–901.

33. C. O. Townley, "Total knee arthroplasty. A personal retrospective and prospective review," *Clinical Orthopaedics and Related Research* (November 1988): 8–22.

34. M. Porter and P. Hirst, "The Sheehan total knee arthroplasty. A retrospective review," *Clinical Orthopaedics and Related Research* (November 1988): 227–32.

35. G. G. Hallock, "Salvage of total knee arthroplasty with local fasciocutaneous flaps," *Journal of Bone and Joint Surgery, American Volume* 72 (September 1990): 1236–39.

36. H. A. Rose et al., "Peroneal-nerve palsy following total knee arthroplasty. A review of The Hospital for Special Surgery experience," *Journal of Bone and Joint Surgery, American Volume* 64 (March 1982): 347–51.

37. F. W. Sunderman, Jr., et al., "Cobalt, chromium, and nickel concentrations in body fluids of patients with porous-coated knee or hip prostheses," *Journal of Orthopaedic Research* 7 (Number 3, 1989): 307–15.

38. T. H. Shurley et al., "Unicompartmental arthroplasty of the knee: A review of three-five year follow-up," *Clinical Orthopaedics and Related Research* (April 1982): 236–40.

39. Porter and Hirst, "The Sheehan total knee arthroplasty," 227–32.

40. T. S. Thornhill and R. D. Scott, "Unicompartmental total knee arthroplasty," *Orthopedic Clinics of North America* 20 (April 1989): 245–56.

41. P. G. Wilcox and D. W. Jackson, "Unicompartmental knee arthroplasty," *Orthopaedic Review* 15 (August 1986): 490–95.

42. J. Black, "Requirements for successful total knee replacement. Material considerations," *Orthopedic Clinics of North America* 20 (January 1989): 1–13.

Transurethral Destruction of Bladder Lesion

1. F. Samdal and B. Brevik, "Laser combined with TURP in the treatment of localized prostatic cancer," *Scandinavian Journal of Urology and Nephrology* 24 (Number 3, 1990): 175–77.

2. M. Fall, "Conservative management of chronic interstitial cystitis: Transcutaneous electrical nerve stimulation and transurethral resection," *Journal of Urology* 133 (May 1985): 774–78.

3. H. J. Reuter, "Complications of cryosurgery in the treatment of prostatic tumors," *Archivos Espanoles de Urologia* 31 (May–June 1978): 213–24. (Published in Spanish)

4. W. G. Guerriero, "Operative injury to the lower urinary tract," *Urologic Clinics of North America* 12 (May 1985): 339–48.

5. Ibid.

6. A. Mosbah et al., "Iatrogenic urethral strictures of the male urethra," *Acta Urologica Belgica* 58 (Number 3, 1990): 87–93. (Published in French)

7. C. L. Strand et al., "Nosocomial *Pseudomonas aeruginosa* urinary tract infections," *Journal of the American Medical Association* 248 (1 October 1982): 1615–18.

8. R. A. Appell et al., "Occult bacterial colonization of bladder tumors," *Journal of Urology* 124 (September 1980): 345–46.

9. J. V. Ricos Torrent et al., "Incidence of vesico-ureteral reflux after endoscopic surgery of superficial tumors of the bladder," *Archivos Espanoles de Urologia* 43 (March 1990): 136–39. (Published in Spanish)

10. J. F. Gephart, "Endotoxin contamination of Foley catheters associated with fevers following transurethral resection of the prostate," *Infection Control* 5 (May 1984): 231–34.

11. C. Viville, R. de Petriconi, and L. Bietho, "Intravesical explosion during endoscopic resection," *Journal of Urology (Paris)* 90 (Number 5, 1984): 361–63. (Published in French)

12. M. Camey, "Bladder tumors. Diagnosis and therapeutic indications," *Rev Chirurgie* 111 (May–June 1976): 639–46. (Published in French)

13. W. Brannan et al., "Partial cystectomy in the treatment of transitional cell carcinoma of the bladder," *Transactions—American Association Genitourinary Surgeons* 69 (1977): 97–99.

14. G. D. Webster and N. Galloway, "Surgical treatment of interstitial cystitis," *Urology* 29 (April 1987, Supplement): 34–39.

15. A. Orandi and M. Orandi, "Urine cytology in the detection of bladder tumor recurrence," *Journal of Urology* 116 (November 1976): 568–69.

Transurethral Removal of Ureter Obstruction

1. A. J. LeRoy et al., "Percutaneous removal of small ureteral calculi," *American Journal of Roentgenology Medicine* 145 (July 1985): 109–12.

2. E. Q. Wiess, A. Leyva, and A. Hernandez, "Treatment of lithiasis by the forced injection of liquid and ureteral catheterization by the translumbar route," *International Surgery* 61 (August 1976): 419–22.

3. P. Recloux et al., "Ureteral obstruction in patients with breast cancer," *Cancer* 61 (May 1988): 1904–7.

4. C. D. Johnson et al., "Percutaneous balloon dilatation of ureteral strictures," *American Journal of Roentgenology* 148 (January 1987): 181–84.

5. M. D. Turner, R. Witherington, and J. J. Carswell, "Ureteral splints: Results of a survey," *Journal of Urology* 127 (April 1982): 654–56.

6. E. K. Lang, "Antegrade ureteral stenting for dehiscence, strictures, and fistulae," *American Journal of Roentgenology* 143 (October 1984): 795–801.

7. E. I. Leff et al., "Use of ureteral catheters in colonic and rectal surgery," *Diseases of the Colon and Rectum* 25 (July–August 1982): 457–60.

8. R. E. Symmonds, "Ureteral injuries associated with gynecologic surgery: Prevention and management," *Clinical Obstetrics and Gynecology* 19 (September 1976): 623–44.

9. M. P. Banner and H. M. Pollack, "Dilatation of ureteral stenoses: Techniques and experience in 44 patients," *American Journal of Roentgenology* 143 (October 1984): 789–93.

10. L. R. Bigongiari et al., "Percutaneous ureteral stent placement for stricture management and internal urinary drainage," *American Journal of Roentgenology Medicine* 133 (November 1979): 865–68.

11. Y. Hara et al., "Percutaneous dissolution of uric acid and cystine stones causing acute ureteral obstruction," *Hinyokika Kiyo* 36 (November 1990): 1271–76. (Published in Japanese)

12. R. I. Kahn, "Endourological treatment of ureteral calculi," *Journal of Urology* 135 (February 1986): 239–43.

13. W. S. Hare, "Ureteral calculi: Percutaneous removal using modified basket extractors and fluoroscopy," *Radiology* 160 (July 1986): 189–92.

14. J. M. Libby, R. B. Meacham, and D. P. Griffith, "The role of silicone ureteral stents in extracorporeal shock-wave

lithotripsy of large renal calculi," *Journal of Urology* 139 (January 1988): 15–17.

15. J. D. Barr, C. J. Tegtmeyer, and A. D. Jenkins, "In situ lithotripsy of ureteral calculi: Review of 261 cases," *Radiology* 174 (January 1990): 103–8.

16. A. D. Jenkins, "Dornier extracorporeal shock-wave lithotripsy for ureteral stones," *Urologic Clinics of North America* 15 (August 1988): 377–84.

17. G. Vallancien et al., "Ureteral flushing," *Annales D' Urologie (Paris)* 23 (Number 2, 1989): 137–39. (Published in French)

18. A. D. Smith et al., "Introduction of the Gibbons ureteral stent facilitated by antecedent percutaneous nephrostomy," *Journal of Urology* 120 (November 1978): 543–44.

19. S. P. Dretler, "An evaluation of ureteral laser lithotripsy: 225 consecutive patients," *Journal of Urology* 143 (February 1990): 267–72.

20. J. Nuzzarello, M. A. Rubenstein, and D. M. Norris, "Extracorporeal shock wave lithotripsy and the ureteral stone brush: Initial results," *Journal of Urology* 143 (February 1990): 261–62.

21. R. Chang, F. F. Marshall, and S. Mitchell, "Percutaneous management of benign ureteral strictures and fistulas," *Journal of Urology* 137 (June 1987): 1126–31.

22. J. E. Lingeman et al., "Management of upper ureteral calculi with extracorporeal shock-wave lithotripsy," *Journal of Urology* 138 (October 1987): 720–23.

23. H. H. Henry, II, and E. M. Tomlin, "Ureteral calculi: Review of 17 years of experience at a community hospital," *Journal of Urology* 113 (June 1975): 762–64.

24. G. W. Drach, "Transurethral ureteral stone manipulation," *Urologic Clinics of North America* 10 (November 1983): 709–17.

25. E. V. Macalalag, "Multiple ureteral tubation for stones," *Journal of Urology* 130 (July 1983): 35–36.

26. J. Franczyk and R. R. Gray, "Ureteral stenting in urosepsis: A cautionary note," *Cardiovascular Interventional Radiology* 12 (September–October 1989): 265–66.

27. L. V. Wagenknecht, "Indwelling ureteral splints. Retrospective study of applications and results of ureteral stents in Germany," *European Urology* 7 (Number 2, 1981): 61–64.

28. Lang, "Antegrade ureteral stenting for dehiscence, strictures, and fistulae," 795–801.

29. D. P. Finnerty et al., "Transluminal balloon dilation of ureteral strictures," *Journal of Urology* 131 (June 1984): 1056–60.

30. W. L. Gerber and A. S. Narayana, "Failure of the double-curved ureteral stent," *Journal of Urology* 127 (February 1982): 317–19.

31. Ibid.

32. A. Kar, F. F. Angwafo, and J. S. Jhunjhunwala, "Ureteroarterial and ureterosigmoid fistula associated with polyethylene indwelling ureteral stents," *Journal of Urology* 132 (October 1984): 755–57.

33. R. B. Smith, "Ureteral common iliac artery fistula: A complication of internal double-J ureteral stent," *Journal of Urology* 132 (July 1984): 113.

34. R. V. Kidd, III, D. J. Confer, and T. P. Ball, Jr., "Ureteral and renal vein perforation with placement into the renal vein as a complication of the pigtail ureteral stent," *Journal of Urology* 124 (September 1980): 424–26.

35. L. V. Wagenknecht, "Ureteral endosplints: A quiet revolution of urological treatment," *Scandinavian Journal of Urology and Nephrology, Supplement* 104 (1987): 133–39.

36. J. L. Pryor, M. J. Langley, and A. D. Jenkins, "Comparison of symptom characteristics of indwelling ureteral catheters," *Journal of Urology* 145 (April 1991): 719–22.

37. K. Bregg and R. A. Riehle, Jr., "Morbidity associated with indwelling internal ureteral stents after shock-wave lithotripsy," *Journal of Urology* 141 (March 1989): 510–12.

38. R. A. Riehle, Jr., "Selective use of ureteral stents before extracorporeal shock-wave lithotripsy," *Urologic Clinics of North America* 15 (August 1988): 499–506.

39. Y. Taki et al., "The ureteral stent: Is it useful?" *Hinyokika Kiyo* 31 (December 1985): 2203–7. (Published in Japanese)

40. R. de Petriconi et al., "Double-J ureteral catheter: A method without complications?" *Journal D'Urologie (Paris)* 93 (Number 5, 1987): 259–61. (Published in French)

41. K. Kohri et al., "Effects and side effects of ureteral stenting during extracorporeal shock-wave lithotripsy," *Nippon Hinyokika Gakkai Zasshi* 81 (October 1990): 1543–49. (Published in Japanese)

42. B. H. Branitz et al., "Effect of ureteral stent on urinary tract infections in renal transplantation," *Urology* 6 (December 1975): 687–928.

43. H. K. Mardis, T. W. Hepperlen, and H. Kammandel, "Double pigtail ureteral stent," *Urology* 14 (July 1979): 23–26.

44. M. D. Collier et al., "Proximal stent displacement as complication of pigtail ureteral stent," *Urology* 13 (April 1979): 372–75.

45. T. A. Flam et al., "Laser treatment of obstruction from

incrusted ureteral catheter," *Journal of Urology* 145 (February 1991): 337–38.

46. G. C. Oswalt, Jr., A. J. Bueschen, and I. K. Lloyd, "Upward migration of indwelling ureteral stents," *Journal of Urology* 122 (August 1979): 249–50.

47. A. Greenstein et al., "Potential pitfalls in the obstructive renal scan in patients with double-pigtail ureteral catheters," *Journal of Urology* 141 (February 1989): 283–84.

Transurethral Resection of the Prostate (TURP)

1. K. M. Jensen and J. T. Andersen, "Urodynamic implications of benign prostatic hyperplasia," *Urologe (Ausgabe A)* 29 (January 1990): 1–4.

2. M. J. Barry, "Epidemiology and natural history of benign prostatic hyperplasia," *Urologic Clinics of North America* 17 (August 1990): 495–507

3. L. Geder and F. Rapp, "Herpesviruses and prostate carcinogenesis," *Archives of Andrology* 4 (February 1980): 71–78.

4. H. K. Armenian et al., "Epidemiologic characteristics of patients with prostatic neoplasms," *American Journal of Epidemiology* 102 (July 1975): 47–54.

5. M. G. Mawhinney, "Etiological considerations for the growth of stroma in benign prostatic hyperplasia," *Federation Proceedings* 45 (October 1986): 2615–17.

6. S. Maehama et al., "Purification and partial characterization of prostate-derived growth factor," *Proceedings of the National Academy of Sciences of the U.S.* 83 (November 1986): 8162–66.

7. H. Araki et al., "High-risk group for benign prostatic hypertrophy," *Prostate* 4 (Number 3, 1983): 253–64.

8. H. Checkoway et al., "Medical, life-style, and occupational risk factors for prostate cancer," *Prostate* 10 (Number 1, 1987): 79–88.

9. Ibid.

10. HealthCare Knowledge Resources/Commission on Professional and Hospital Activities, *HealthWeek* (6 November 1989).

11. R. D. Leach, "Prostatectomy at a district general hospital," *Annals of the Royal College of Surgeons of England* 61 (November 1979): 459–62.

12. R. Sach and V. R. Marshall, "Prostatectomy: Its safety in an Australian teaching hospital," *British Journal of Surgery* 64 (March 1977): 210–14.

13. A. G. Graham, "Scottish prostates: A six-year review," *British Journal of Urology* 49 (Number 7, 1977): 679–82.

14. P. Perrin et al., "Forty years of transurethral prostatic resections," *Journal of Urology* 116 (December 1976): 757–58.

15. W. K. Mebust et al., "Transurethral prostatectomy: Immediate and postoperative complications. A cooperative study of 13 participating institutions evaluating 3,885 patients," *Journal of Urology* 141 (February 1989): 243–47.

16. T. Kolmert and H. Norlen, "Transurethral resection of the prostate. A review of 1,111 cases," *International Urology and Nephrology* 21 (Number 1, 1989): 47–55.

17. H. Tonnesen et al., "Influence of alcoholism on morbidity after transurethral prostatectomy," *Scandinavian Journal of Urology and Nephrology* 22 (Number 3, 1988): 175–77.

18. Mebust et al., "Transurethral prostatectomy," 243–47.

19. Kolmert and Norlen, "Transurethral resection of the prostate," 47–55.

20. P. Mangin, D. Beurton, and J. Cukier, "Transurethral resection of the prostate," *Journal D'Urologie (Paris)* 88 (Number 2, 1982): 117–23. (Published in French)

21. E. Hradec et al., "The obturator nerve block. Preventing damage of the bladder wall during transurethral surgery," *International Urology and Nephrology* 15 (Number 2, 1983): 149–53.

22. B. Kihl, A. E. Nilson, and S. Pettersson, "Thigh adductor contraction during transurethral resection of bladder tumours: Evaluation of inactive electrode placement and obturator nerve topography," *Scandinavian Journal of Urology and Nephrology* 15 (Number 2, 1981): 121–25.

23. R. C. Bruskewitz et al., "Three-year followup of urinary symptoms after transurethral resection of the prostate," *Journal of Urology* 136 (September 1986): 613–15.

24. C. Moller-Nielsen et al., "Sexual life following 'minimal' and 'total' transurethral prostatic resection," *Urologia Internationalis* 40 (Number 1, 1985): 3–4.

25. E. P. So et al., "Erectile impotence associated with transurethral prostatectomy," *Urology* 19 (March 1982): 259–62.

26. M. D. Wasserman et al., "Impaired nocturnal erections and impotence following transurethral prostatectomy," *Urology* 15 (July 1980): 552–55.

27. J. Bertrand et al., "Transurethral resection of the prostate (TURP syndrome), myth or reality? Analytic studies using a

radioactive isotope method," *Journal D'Urologie (Paris)* 87 (Number 1, 1981): 1–4. (Published in French)

28. Kolmert and Norlen, "Transurethral resection of the prostate," 47–55.

29. M. M. Kane, D. W. Fields, and E. D. Vaughan, Jr., "Medical management of benign prostatic hyperplasia," *Urology* 36 (November 1990, Supplement): 5–12.

30. D. J. Malenka et al., "Further study of the increased mortality following transurethral prostatectomy: A chart-based analysis," *Journal of Urology* 144 (August 1990): 224–27.

31. N. P. Roos and E. W. Ramsey, "A population-based study of prostatectomy: Outcomes associated with differing surgical approaches," *Journal of Urology* 137 (June 1987): 1184–88.

32. Malenka et al., "Further study of the increased mortality following transurethral prostatectomy," 224–27.

Unilateral External Simple Mastectomy

1. A. Nicolosi et al., "Carcinoma of the male breast. Review of the literature and case series contribution," *Minerva Chirurgica* 45 (Number 13–14, 1990): 947–52. (Published in Italian)

2. M. Stierer, H. Spoula, and H. R. Rosen, "Breast cancer in the male—a retrospective analysis of 15 cases," *Onkologie* 13 (April 1990): 128–31. (Published in German)

3. M. Molls et al., "Breast carcinoma in men: Radiotherapy and treatment results," *Strahlentherapie und Onkologie* 164 (October 1988): 574–80. (Published in German)

4. *Stedman's Medical Dictionary,* 25th ed. (Baltimore: Williams and Wilkins, 1990), 925.

5. See, for example, H. W. Griffith, *Complete Guide to Symptoms, Illness, and Surgery* (Los Angeles: The Body Press, 1985), 743–44.

6. S. Watt-Boolsen, K. Jacobsen, and M. Blichert-Toft, "Total mastectomy with special reference to surgical technique, extent of axillary dissection and complications," *Acta Oncologica* 27 (Number 6A, 1988): 663–65.

7. Ibid.

8. M. P. Osborne and P. I. Borgen, "Role of mastectomy in breast cancer," *Surgical Clinics of North America* 70 (October 1990): 1023–46.

9. A. Badr el Din et al., "Local postoperative morbidity following pre-operative irradiation in locally advanced breast cancer," *European Journal of Surgical Oncology* 15 (December 1989): 486–89.

10. Q. P. Zhuang, "Breast repair using a silicone gel-filled prosthesis. Report of 21 cases," *Chung Hua Wai Ko Tsa Chih* 27 (October 1989): 617–19, 639. (Published in Chinese)

11. H. P. Graversen et al., "Breast cancer: Risk of axillary recurrence in node-negative patients following partial dissection of the axilla," *European Journal of Surgical Oncology* 14 (October 1988): 407–12.

12. C. K. Axelsson and M. Blichert-Toft, "Low-risk breast cancer patients treated by mastectomy and lower axillary dissection. The present status of the Danish Breast Cancer Cooperative Group Trial 77-A," *Acta Oncologica* 27 (Number 6A, 1988): 605–9.

13. H. Johansen, S. Kaae, and T. Schiodt, "Simple mastectomy with postoperative irradiation versus extended radical mastectomy in breast cancer. A 25-year follow-up of a randomized trial," *Acta Oncologica* 29 (Number 6, 1990): 709–15.

14. T. Wobbes, J. G. Tinnemans, and R. F. van der Sluis, "Residual tumour after biopsy for non-palpable ductal carcinoma in situ of the breast," *British Journal of Surgery* 76 (February 1989): 185–86.

15. "Sector resection with or without postoperative radiotherapy for stage I breast cancer: A randomized trial. Uppsala-Orebro Breast Cancer Study Group," *Journal of the National Cancer Institute* 82 (21 February 1990): 277–82.

16. G. N. Hortobagyi et al., "Management of stage III primary breast cancer with primary chemotherapy, surgery, and radiation therapy," *Cancer* 62 (15 December 1988): 2507–16.

17. M. Baum et al., "The Cancer Research Campaign trials of adjuvant therapy for early breast cancer," *Acta Oncologica* 28 (Number 6, 1989): 907–12.

18. M. Overgaard et al., "Postmastectomy irradiation in high-risk breast cancer patients. Present status of the Danish Breast Cancer Cooperative Group trials," *Acta Oncologica* 27 (Number 6A, 1988): 707–14.

19. M. J. Lopez et al., "Multimodal therapy in locally advanced breast carcinoma," *American Journal of Surgery* 160 (December 1990): 669–74.

20. M. Castiglione, R. D. Gelber, and A. Goldhirsch, "Adjuvant systemic therapy for breast cancer in the elderly: Competing causes of mortality. International Breast Cancer Study

Group," *Journal of Clinical Oncology* 8 (March 1990): 519–26.

21. J. M. Morrison et al., "West Midlands Oncology Association trials of adjuvant chemotherapy in operable breast cancer: Results after a median follow-up of 7 years," *British Journal of Cancer* 60 (December 1989): 911–18.

22. Morrison et al., "West Midlands Oncology Association trials of adjuvant chemotherapy in operable breast cancer," 919–24.

23. F. W. Sellke, C. W. Loughry, and S. Kashkari, "Angiosarcoma of the breast: Report of two long-term survivals," *International Surgery* 73 (July–September 1988): 193–95.

24. S. Holt et al., "A randomised controlled trial of adjuvant hormono-chemotherapy in Stage II breast cancer," *European Journal of Surgical Oncology* 14 (December 1988): 663–67.

25. M. Overgaard et al., "Evaluation of radiotherapy in high-risk breast cancer patients: Report from the Danish Breast Cancer Cooperative Group (DBCG 82) Trial," *International Journal of Radiation Oncology, Biology, Physics* 19 (November 1990): 1121–24.

26. C. C. Bishop, S. Singh, and A. G. Nash, "Mastectomy and breast reconstruction preserving the nipple," *Annals of the Royal College of Surgeons of England* 72 (March 1990): 87–89.

27. R. G. Wilson, A. Hart, and P. J. Dawes, "Mastectomy or conservation: The patient's choice," *British Medical Journal* 297 (5 November 1988): 1167–69.

28. B. Fisher et al., "Eight-year results of a randomized clinical trial comparing total mastectomy and lumpectomy with or without irradiation in the treatment of breast cancer," *New England Journal of Medicine* 320 (30 March 1989): 822–28.

29. "Sector resection with or without postoperative radiotherapy for stage I breast cancer," 277–82.

30. M. H. Bailey et al., "Immediate breast reconstruction: Reducing the risks," *Plastic and Reconstructive Surgery* 83 (May 1989): 845–51.

31. Osborne and Borgen, "Role of mastectomy in breast cancer," 1023–46.

32. L. Barreau-Pouhaer et al., "Immediate breast reconstruction: Indications and techniques. Apropos of 120 cases treated at the Institut Gustave-Roussy," *Annales de Chirurgie Plastique et Esthetique* 34 (Number 2, 1989): 97–102. (Published in French)

33. P. Houpt et al., "The result of breast reconstruction after mastectomy for breast cancer in 109 patients," *Annals of Plastic Surgery* 21 (December 1988): 516–25.

34. S. Pompei, A. Varanese, and F. Fanini, "Immediate reconstructive approach in neoplastic pathology and 'high risk' of the breast," *Giornale Di Chirurgia* 11 (July–August 1990): 403–8. (Published in Italian)

35. M. Kaufmann et al., "Transposition and myocutaneous island flaps in primary or secondary locoregional surgical therapy of breast cancer," *Geburtshilfe und Frauenheilkunde* 48 (August 1988): 584–87. (Published in German)

36. B. A. Toth and M. C. Glafkides, "Immediate breast reconstruction with deepithelialized TRAM flaps: Techniques for improving breast reconstruction," *Plastic and Reconstructive Surgery* 85 (June 1990): 967–70.

37. E. Maunsell, J. Brisson, and L. Deschenes, "Psychological distress after initial treatment for breast cancer: A comparison of partial and total mastectomy," *Journal of Clinical Epidemiology* 42 (Number 8, 1989): 765–71.

38. A. V. Hughson et al., "Psychosocial consequences of mastectomy: Levels of morbidity and associated factors," *Journal of Psychosomatic Research* 32 (Number 4–5, 1988): 383–91.

39. J. M. McArdle, A. V. Hughson, and C. S. McArdle, "Reduced psychological morbidity after breast conservation," *British Journal of Surgery* 77 (November 1990): 1221–23.

Unilateral Salpingo-Oophorectomy

1. W. W. Liang, Y. N. Lin, and Y. N. Lee, "Malignant mixed mullerian tumor of fallopian tube. Report of a case and review of literature," *Chung-Hua Fu Chan Ko Tsa Chih* 45 (April 1990): 272–75.

2. H. G. Muntz et al., "Primary adenocarcinoma of the fallopian tube," *European Journal of Gynaecological Oncology* 10 (Number 4, 1989): 239–49.

3. W. H. Wolberg, "Adjunctive chemotherapy as an alternative to ovarian ablation in premenopausal women with carcinoma of the breast," *Surgery, Gynecology and Obstetrics* 165 (December 1987): 563–66.

4. M. Izuo, "Breast cancer and hormone therapy," *Gan To Kagaku Ryoho* 14 (October 1987): 2830–36. (Published in Japanese)

5. K. I. Pritchard and D. J. Sutherland, "The use of endocrine therapy," *Hematology/Oncology Clinics of North America* 3 (December 1989): 765–805.

6. W. R. Miller, "Fundamental research leading to improved

endocrine therapy for breast cancer," *Journal of Steroid Biochemistry* 27 (Number 1–3, 1987): 477–85.

7. I. Jacobs and D. Oram, "Prophylactic oophorectomy," *British Journal of Hospital Medicine* 38 (November 1987): 440–44, 448–49.

8. M. Hernandez Avila, A. M. Walker, and H. Jick, "Use of replacement estrogens and the risk of myocardial infarction," *Epidemiology* 1 (March 1990): 128–33.

9. L. Weinstein, "Hormonal therapy in the patient with surgical menopause," *Obstetrics and Gynecology* 75 (April 1990, Supplement): 47S–50S.

10. F. V. Price, R. Edwards, and H. J. Buchsbaum, "Ovarian remnant syndrome: Difficulties in diagnosis and management," *Obstetrical and Gynecological Survey* 45 (March 1990): 151–56.

11. M. M. Zaitoon, "Ureteral obstruction secondary to retained ovarian remnants: A case report and review of the literature," *Journal of Urology* 137 (May 1987): 973–74.

12. P. Loizzi et al., "Removal or preservation of ovaries during hysterectomy: A six-year review," *International Journal of Gynaecology and Obstetrics* 31 (March 1990): 257–61.

13. A. Birnkrant, J. Sampson, and P. H. Sugarbaker, "Ovarian metastasis from colorectal cancer," *Diseases of the Colon and Rectum* 29 (November 1986): 767–71.

Unilateral Thyroid Lobectomy

1. A. al Muhanna et al., "Thyroid lobectomy for removal of a fish bone," *Journal of Laryngology and Otology* 104 (June 1990): 511–12.

2. J. M. Lore, Jr., D. J. Kim, and S. Elias, "Preservation of the laryngeal nerves during total thyroid lobectomy," *Annals of Otology, Rhinology, and Laryngology* 86 (November–December 1977): 777–88.

3. I. D. Hay et al., "Ipsilateral lobectomy versus bilateral lobar resection in papillary thyroid carcinoma: A retrospective analysis of surgical outcome using a novel prognostic scoring system," *Surgery* 102 (December 1987): 1088–95.

4. P. Blondeau, A. Legros, and L. Rene, "Is unilateral total lobectomy adequate treatment for a single malignant thyroid nodule?" *Nouvelle Presse Medicale* 6 (10 September 1977): 2583–87. (Published in French)

Ureteral Catheterization

1. M. K. Elyaderani et al., "Facilitation of difficult percutaneous ureteral stent insertion," *Journal of Urology* 128 (December 1982): 1173–76.

2. A. J. LeRoy et al., "Percutaneous removal of small ureteral calculi," *American Journal of Roentgenology* 145 (July 1985): 109–12.

3. E. Q. Wiess, A. Leyva, and A. Hernandez, "Treatment of lithiasis by the forced injection of liquid and ureteral catheterization by the translumbar route," *International Surgery* 61 (August 1976): 419–22.

4. P. Recloux et al., "Ureteral obstruction in patients with breast cancer," *Cancer* 61 (May 1988): 1904–7.

5. C. D. Johnson et al., "Percutaneous balloon dilatation of ureteral strictures," *American Journal of Roentgenology* 148 (January 1987): 181–84.

6. M. D. Turner, R. Witherington, and J. J. Carswell, "Ureteral splints: Results of a survey," *Journal of Urology* 127 (April 1982): 654–56.

7. E. K. Lang, "Antegrade ureteral stenting for dehiscence, strictures, and fistulae," *American Journal of Roentgenology* 143 (October 1984): 795–801.

8. E. I. Leff et al., "Use of ureteral catheters in colonic and rectal surgery," *Diseases of the Colon and Rectum* 25 (July–August 1982): 457–60.

9. R. E. Symmonds, "Ureteral injuries associated with gynecologic surgery: Prevention and management," *Clinical Obstetrics and Gynecology* 19 (September 1976): 623–44.

10. M. P. Banner and H. M. Pollack, "Dilatation of ureteral stenoses: Techniques and experience in 44 patients," *American Journal of Roentgenology* 143 (October 1984): 789–93.

11. L. R. Bigongiari et al., "Percutaneous ureteral stent placement for stricture management and internal urinary drainage," *American Journal of Roentgenology* 133 (November 1979): 865–68.

12. Y. Hara et al., "Percutaneous dissolution of uric acid and cystine stones causing acute ureteral obstruction," *Hinyokika Kiyo* 36 (November 1990): 1271–76. (Published in Japanese)

13. R. I. Kahn, "Endourological treatment of ureteral calculi," *Journal of Urology* 135 (February 1986): 239–43.

14. W. S. Hare, "Ureteral calculi: Percutaneous removal us-

ing modified basket extractors and fluoroscopy," *Radiology* 160 (July 1986): 189–92.

15. J. M. Libby, R. B. Meacham, and D. P. Griffith, "The role of silicone ureteral stents in extracorporeal shock-wave lithotripsy of large renal calculi," *Journal of Urology* 139 (January 1988): 15–17.

16. J. D. Barr, C. J. Tegtmeyer, and A. D. Jenkins, "In situ lithotripsy of ureteral calculi: Review of 261 cases," *Radiology* 174 (January 1990): 103–8.

17. A. D. Jenkins, "Dornier extracorporeal shock-wave lithotripsy for ureteral stones," *Urologic Clinics of North America* 15 (August 1988): 377–84.

18. G. Vallancien et al., "Ureteral flushing," *Annales D' Urologie (Paris)* 23 (Number 2, 1989): 137–39. (Published in French)

19. A. D. Smith et al., "Introduction of the Gibbons ureteral stent facilitated by antecedent percutaneous nephrostomy," *Journal of Urology* 120 (November 1978): 543–44.

20. S. P. Dretler, "An evaluation of ureteral laser lithotripsy," *Journal of Urology* 143 (February 1990): 267–72.

21. J. Nuzzarello, M. A. Rubenstein, and D. M. Norris, "Extracorporeal shock wave lithotripsy and the ureteral stone brush: Initial results," *Journal of Urology* 143 (February 1990): 261–62.

22. R. Chang, F. F. Marshall, and S. Mitchell, "Percutaneous management of benign ureteral strictures and fistulas," *Journal of Urology* 137 (June 1987): 1126–31.

23. J. E. Lingeman et al., "Management of upper ureteral calculi with extracorporeal shock wave lithotripsy," *Journal of Urology* 138 (October 1987): 720–23.

24. J. D. Daughtry et al., "Balloon dilation of the ureter: A means to facilitate passage of ureteral and renal calculi," *Journal of Urology* 136 (November 1986): 1063–65.

25. H. H. Henry II and E. M. Tomlin, "Ureteral calculi: Review of 17 years of experience at a community hospital," *Journal of Urology* 113 (June 1975): 762–64.

26. G. W. Drach, "Transurethral ureteral stone manipulation," *Urologic Clinics of North America* 10 (November 1983): 709–17.

27. E. V. Macalalag, "Multiple ureteral tubation for stones," *Journal of Urology* 130 (July 1983): 35–36.

28. J. Franczyk and R. R. Gray, "Ureteral stenting in urosepsis: A cautionary note," *Cardiovascular Interventional Radiology* 12 (September–October 1989): 265–66.

29. L. V. Wagenknecht, "Indwelling ureteral splints. Ret-rospective study of applications and results of ureteral stents in Germany," *European Urology* 7 (Number 2, 1981): 61–64.

30. Lang, "Antegrade ureteral stenting for dehiscence, strictures, and fistulae," 795–801.

31. D. P. Finnerty et al., "Transluminal balloon dilation of ureteral strictures," *Journal of Urology* 131 (June 1984): 1056–60.

32. W. L. Gerber and A. S. Narayana, "Failure of the double-curved ureteral stent," *Journal of Urology* 127 (February 1982): 317–19.

33. Ibid.

34. A. Kar, F. F. Angwafo, and J. S. Jhunjhunwala, "Ureteroarterial and ureterosigmoid fistula associated with polyethylene indwelling ureteral stents," *Journal of Urology* 132 (October 1984): 755–57.

35. R. B. Smith, "Ureteral common iliac artery fistula: A complication of internal double-J ureteral stent," *Journal of Urology* 132 (July 1984): 113.

36. R. V. Kidd III, D. J. Confer, and T. P. Ball, Jr., "Ureteral and renal vein perforation with placement into the renal vein as a complication of the pigtail ureteral stent," *Journal of Urology* 124 (September 1980): 424–26.

37. L. V. Wagenknecht, "Ureteral endosplints: A quiet revolution of urological treatment," *Scandinavian Journal of Urology and Nephrology, Supplement* 104 (1987): 133–39.

38. J. L. Pryor, M. J. Langley, and A. D. Jenkins, "Comparison of symptom characteristics of indwelling ureteral catheters," *Journal of Urology* 145 (April 1991): 719–22.

39. K. Bregg and R. A. Riehle, Jr., "Morbidity associated with indwelling internal ureteral stents after shock wave lithotripsy," *Journal of Urology* 141 (March 1989): 510–12.

40. R. A. Riehle, Jr., "Selective use of ureteral stents before extracorporeal shock-wave lithotripsy," *Urologic Clinics of North America* 15 (August 1988): 499–506.

41. Y. Taki et al., "The ureteral stent: Is it useful?" *Hinyokika Kiyo* 31 (December 1985): 2203–7. (Published in Japanese)

42. R. de Petriconi et al., "Double-J ureteral catheter: A method without complications?" *Journal D'Urologie (Paris)* 93 (Number 5, 1987): 259–61. (Published in French)

43. K. Kohri et al., "Effects and side effects of ureteral stenting during extracorporeal shock-wave lithotripsy," *Nippon Hinyokika Gakkai Zasshi* 81 (October 1990): 1543–49. (Published in Japanese)

44. B. H. Branitz et al., "Effect of ureteral stent on urinary

tract infections in renal transplantation," *Urology* 6 (December 1975): 687–928.

45. H. K. Mardis, T. W. Hepperlen, and H. Kammandel, "Double pigtail ureteral stent," *Urology* 14 (July 1979): 23–26.

46. M. D. Collier et al., "Proximal stent displacement as complication of pigtail ureteral stent," *Urology* 13 (April 1979): 372–75.

47. T. A. Flam et al., "Laser treatment of obstruction from incrusted ureteral catheter," *Journal of Urology* 145 (February 1991): 337–38.

48. G. C. Oswalt, Jr., A. J. Bueschen, and I. K. Lloyd, "Upward migration of indwelling ureteral stents," *Journal of Urology* 122 (August 1979): 249–50.

49. A. Greenstein et al., "Potential pitfalls in the obstructive renal scan in patients with double-pigtail ureteral catheters," *Journal of Urology* 141 (February 1989): 283–84.

Uterine Lesion Destruction

1. Y. Sakaguchi, "Determination of residual lesion in remaining uterus after conization," *Nippon Sanka Fujinka Gakkai Zasshi* 38 (June 1986): 924–32. (Published in Japanese)

2. C. P. West and M. A. Lumsden, "Fibroids and menorrhagia," *Baillieres Clinical Obstetrics and Gynaecology* 3 (June 1989): 357–74.

3. B. McLucas, "Intrauterine applications of the resectoscope," *Surgery, Gynecology and Obstetrics* 172 (June 1991): 425–31.

Vacuum Extraction Delivery with Episiotomy

1. D. L. Healy, M. A. Quinn, and R. J. Pepperell, "Rotational delivery of the fetus: Kielland's forceps and two other methods compared," *British Journal of Obstetrics and Gynaecology* 89 (July 1982): 501–6.

2. HealthCare Knowledge Resources/Commission on Professional and Hospital Activities, *HealthWeek* (6 November 1989).

3. L. Meyer et al., "Maternal and neonatal morbidity in instrumental deliveries with the Kobayashi vacuum extractor

and low forceps," *ACTA Obstetricia et Gynecologica Scandinavica* 66 (Number 7, 1987): 643–47.

4. *Stedman's Medical Dictionary,* 25th ed. (Baltimore: Williams and Wilkins, 1990), 409.

5. D. L. Dell, S. E. Sightler, and W. C. Plauche, "Soft cup vacuum extraction: A comparison of outlet delivery," *Obstetrics and Gynecology* 66 (Number 5, 1985): 624–28.

6. J. B. Greis, J. Bieniarz, and A. Scommegna, "Comparison of maternal and fetal effects of vacuum extraction with forceps or cesarean deliveries," *Obstetrics and Gynecology* 57 (May 1981): 571–77.

7. P. Altmann et al., "About the choice of extraction instrument for vaginal operative termination in vertex presentation," *Geburtshilfe und Frauenheilkunde* 35 (December 1975): 949–55. (Published in German)

8. S. T. Nilsen, "Boys born by forceps and vacuum extraction examined at 18 years of age," *ACTA Obstetricia et Gynecologica Scandinavica* 63 (Number 6, 1984): 549–54.

9. J. Endl, G. Wolf, and A. Schaller, "Problems and results of skull x-ray following vacuum extraction," *Geburtshilfe und Frauenheilkunde* 35 (December 1975): 943–48. (Published in German)

10. Meyer et al., "Maternal and neonatal morbidity in instrumental deliveries with the Kobayashi vacuum extractor and low forceps," 643–47.

11. K. E. Thacker, T. Lim, and J. H. Drew, "Cephalhaematoma: a 10-year review," *Australian and New Zealand Journal of Obstetrics and Gynaecology* 27 (August 1987): 210–12.

12. G. M. Maryniak and J. B. Frank, "Clinical assessment of the Kobayashi vacuum extractor." *Obstetrics and Gynecology* 64 (September 1984): 431–35.

13. W. C. Plauche, "Fetal cranial injuries related to delivery with the Malmstrom vacuum extractor," *Obstetrics and Gynecology* 53 (June 1979): 750–57.

14. F. F. Broekhuizen et al., "Vacuum extraction versus forceps delivery: Indications and complications, 1979 to 1984," *Obstetrics and Gynecology* 69 (March 1987): 338–42.

15. W. C. Plauche, "Subgaleal hematoma. A complication of instrumental delivery," *Journal of the American Medical Association* 244 (3 October 1980): 1597–98.

16. R. Besio et al., "Neonatal retinal hemorrhages and influence of perinatal factors," *American Journal of Ophthalmology* 87 (January 1979): 74–76.

17. F. A. Chervenak et al., "Is routine cesarean section necessary for vertex-breech and vertex-transverse twin gesta-

tions?" *American Journal of Obstetrics and Gynecology* 148 (1 January 1984): 1–5.

18. H. Schrocksnadel, K. Heim, and O. Dapunt, "The clavicular fracture—a questionable achievement in modern obstetrics," *Geburtshilfe und Frauenheilkunde* 49 (May 1989): 481–84. (Published in German)

19. H. Y. Ngan, G. W. Tang, and H. K. Ma, "Vacuum extractor: A safe instrument?" *Australian and New Zealand Journal of Obstetrics and Gynaecology* 26 (August 1986): 177–81.

20. Maryniak and Frank, "Clinical assessment of the Kobayashi vacuum extractor," 431–35.

21. H. A. Krone and H. Heidegger, "Maternal mortality, its definition and assessment. Report of maternal mortality at the Bamberg Gynecologic Clinic 1963–1988," *Geburtshilfe und Frauenheilkunde* 49 (July 1989): 666–72. (Published in German)

22. D. B. Schwartz, M. Miodovnik, and J. P. Lavin, Jr., "Neonatal outcome among low birth weight infants delivered spontaneously or by low forceps," *Obstetrics and Gynecology* 62 (September 1983): 283–86.

23. S. Scherjon, "A comparison between the organization of obstetrics in Denmark and The Netherlands," *British Journal of Obstetrics and Gynaecology* 93 (July 1986): 684–89.

24. M. Tew, "Do obstetric intranatal interventions make birth safer?" *British Journal of Obstetrics and Gynaecology* 93 (July 1986): 659–74.

25. P. Bergsjo, E. Schmidt, and D. Pusch, "Differences in the reported frequencies of some obstetrical interventions in Europe," *British Journal of Obstetrics and Gynaecology* 90 (July 1983): 628–32.

Vaginal Hysterectomy

1. R. K. Laros and B. A. Work, "Female sterilization," *Obstetrics and Gynecology* 46 (August 1975): 215–20.

2. A. C. Naylor, "Hysterectomy—analysis of 2,901 personally performed procedures," *South African Medical Journal* 65 (18 February 1984): 242–45.

3. R. Schwarz and H. H. Buttner, "Vaginal radical surgery using the Schauta-Amreich method. Results from the years 1959 to 1970 and consequences for determining indications," *Zentralblatt fur Gynakologie* 98 (Number 19, 1976): 1162–67. (Published in German)

4. W. Lotze and P. Richter, "Recurrence following staged treatment of cervical cancer in stage Ia," *Zentralblatt fur Gynakologie* (Number 7, 1985): 411–17. (Published in German)

5. R. Kudo et al., "Vaginal semiradical hysterectomy: A new operative procedure for microinvasive carcinoma of the cervix," *Obstetrics and Gynecology* 64 (December 1984): 810–15.

6. S. E. Jaszczak and T. N. Evans, "Intrafascial abdominal and vaginal hysterectomy: A reappraisal," *Obstetrics and Gynecology* 59 (April 1982): 435–44.

7. R. Kudo et al., "Vaginal hysterectomy without ligation of the ligaments of the cervix uteri," *Surgery, Gynecology, and Obstetrics* 170 (April 1990): 299–305.

8. J. J. Mikuta et al., "The 'problem' radical hysterectomy," *American Journal of Obstetrics and Gynecology* 128 (15 May 1977): 119–27.

9. P. Hohlweg-Majert et al., "Clinical aspects of vaginal hysterectomy," *Geburtshilfe und Frauenheilkunde* 47 (December 1987): 864–67. (Published in German)

10. P. A. Wingo et al., "The mortality risk associated with hysterectomy," *American Journal of Obstetrics and Gynecology* 152 (1 August 1985): 803–8.

11. A. Ellenbogen, A. Agranat, and S. Grunstein, "The role of vaginal hysterectomy in the aged woman," *Journal of the American Geriatrics Society* 29 (September 1981): 426–28.

12. A. Chryssikopoulos and C. Loghis, "Indications and results of total hysterectomy," *International Surgery* 71 (July–September 1986): 188–94.

13. D. G. Gallup and R. T. Welham, "Vaginal hysterectomy by an anterior colpotomy technique," *Southern Medical Journal* 69 (June 1976): 752–54, 756.

14. P. Draca, "Complications following vaginal hysterectomy," *Jugoslavenska Ginekologija I Opstetricija* 16 (March–April 1976): 105–13. (Published in Serbo-Croatian, Roman)

15. K. Becker, E. Muller-Wuhr, and G. Stark, "Follow-up of 2,300 vaginal and abdominal hysterectomies," *Fortschritte der Medizin* 95 (9 June 1977): 1425–28. (Published in German)

16. N. G. Osborne, R. C. Wright, and M. Dubay, "Preoperative hot conization of the cervix: A possible method to reduce postoperative febrile morbidity following vaginal hysterectomy," *American Journal of Obstetrics and Gynecology* 133 (15 February 1979): 374–78.

17. J. H. Grossman, III, et al., "Endometrial and vaginal cuff bacteria recovered at elective hysterectomy during a trial of antibiotic prophylaxis," *American Journal of Obstetrics and Gynecology* 130 (1 February 1978): 312–16.

18. J. P. Forney et al., "Impact of cephalosporin prophylaxis

on conization-vaginal hysterectomy morbidity," *American Journal of Obstetrics and Gynecology* 125 (1 May 1976): 100.

19. J. W. Orr, Jr., et al., "Single-center study results of cefotetan and cefoxitin prophylaxis for abdominal or vaginal hysterectomy," *American Journal of Obstetrics and Gynecology* 158 (March 1988): 714–16.

20. S. F. Gordon, "Results of a single-center study of cefotetan prophylaxis in abdominal or vaginal hysterectomy," *American Journal of Obstetrics and Gynecology* 158 (March 1988): 710–14.

21. A. S. Berkeley et al., "Comparison of cefotetan and cefoxitin prophylaxis for abdominal and vaginal hysterectomy," *American Journal of Obstetrics and Gynecology* 158 (March 1988): 706–9.

22. M. J. Ohm and R. P. Galask, "The effect of antibiotic prophylaxis on patients undergoing vaginal operations," *American Journal of Obstetrics and Gynecology* 123 (15 November 1975): 590–96.

23. D. L. Hemsell, M. O. Menon, and A. J. Friedman, "Ceftriaxone or cefazolin prophylaxis for the prevention of infection after vaginal hysterectomy," *American Journal of Surgery* 148 (19 October 1984): 22–26.

24. D. D. Mathews et al., "A double-blind trial of single-dose chemoprophylaxis with co-trimoxazole during vaginal hysterectomy and repair," *British Journal of Obstetrics and Gynaecology* 86 (September 1979): 737–40.

25. C. Petersen and H. H. Brautigam, "Short-term perioperative prophylaxis with cefotaxime in obstetric and gynecological surgery," *Deutsche Medizinische Wochenschrift* 110 (6 September 1985): 1369–74. (Published in German)

26. C. R. Wheeless, Jr., J. H. Dorsey, and L. R. Wharton, Jr., "An evaluation of prophylactic doxycycline in hysterectomy patients," *Journal of Reproductive Medicine* 21 (September 1978): 146–50.

27. S. Roy et al., "Efficacy and safety of single-dose ceftizoxime vs. multiple-dose cefoxitin in preventing infection after vaginal hysterectomy," *Journal of Reproductive Medicine* 33 (January 1988, Supplement): 149–53.

28. S. Faro, "Prevention of infections after obstetric and gynecologic surgery," *Journal of Reproductive Medicine* 33 (January 1988, Supplement): 154–58.

29. J. T. DiPiro et al., "Prophylactic parenteral cephalosporins in surgery. Are the newer agents better?" *Journal of the American Medical Association* 252 (21 December 1984): 3277–79.

30. C. Jackson and M. S. Amstey, "Prophylactic ampicillin therapy for vaginal hysterectomy," *Surgery, Gynecology, and Obstetrics* 141 (November 1975): 755–57.

31. P. Jackson and W. J. Ridley, "Simplified antibiotic prophylaxis for vaginal hysterectomy," *Australian and New Zealand Journal of Obstetrics and Gynaecology* 19 (November 1979): 225–27.

32. R. H. Jennings, "Prophylactic antibiotics in vaginal and abdominal hysterectomy," *Southern Medical Journal* 71 (March 1978): 251–54.

33. W. H. Swartz, "Prophylaxis of minor febrile and major infectious morbidity following hysterectomy," *Obstetrics and Gynecology* 54 (September 1979): 284–88.

34. R. M. Pitkin, "Vaginal hysterectomy in obese women," *Obstetrics and Gynecology* 49 (May 1977): 567–69.

35. J. F. Holman, J. E. McGowan, and J. D. Thompson, "Perioperative antibiotics in major elective gynecologic surgery," *Southern Medical Journal* 71 (April 1978): 417–20.

36. D. L. Hemsell et al., "Cefoxitin for prophylaxis in premenopausal women undergoing vaginal hysterectomy," *Obstetrics and Gynecology* 56 (November 1980): 629–34.

37. A. Mickal, D. Curole, and C. Lewis, "Cefoxitin sodium: Double-blind vaginal hysterectomy prophylaxis in premenopausal patients," *Obstetrics and Gynecology* 56 (August 1980): 222–25.

38. P. Duff and R. C. Park, "Antibiotic prophylaxis in vaginal hysterectomy: A review," *Obstetrics and Gynecology* 55 (May 1980, Supplement): 193S–202S.

39. J. H. Grossman, III, et al., "Prophylactic antibiotics in gynecologic surgery," *Obstetrics and Gynecology* 53 (May 1979): 537–44.

40. J. Mendelson et al., "Effect of single and multidose cephradine prophylaxis on infectious morbidity of vaginal hysterectomy," *Obstetrics and Gynecology* 53 (January 1979): 31–35.

41. J. M. Roberts and H. D. Homesley, "Low-dose carbenicillin prophylaxis for vaginal and abdominal hysterectomy," *Obstetrics and Gynecology* 52 (July 1978): 83–87.

42. J. V. Hirschmann and T. S. Inui, "Antimicrobial prophylaxis: A critique of recent trials," *Reviews of Infectious Diseases* 2 (January–February 1980): 1–23.

43. D. L. Hemsell, P. G. Hemsell, and B. J. Nobles, "Doxycycline and cefamandole prophylaxis for premenopausal women undergoing vaginal hysterectomy," *Surgery, Gynecology, and Obstetrics* 161 (November 1985): 462–64.

44. T. Tabei, "Effects of antibiotics in the prevention of infections following vaginal and abdominal hysterectomy: An

evaluation by febrile morbidity and fever index," *Japanese Journal of Antibiotics* 36 (July 1983): 1569–80. (Published in Japanese)

45. D. L. Hemsell et al., "Single-dose piperacillin versus triple-dose cefoxitin prophylaxis at vaginal and abdominal hysterectomy," *Southern Medical Journal* 82 (April 1989): 438–42.

46. R. Ranney and S. Abu-Ghazaleh, "The future function and fortune of ovarian tissue which is retained in vivo during hysterectomy," *American Journal of Obstetrics and Gynecology* 128 (15 July 1977): 626–34.

47. C. Schubring and E. Werner, "Urine drainage following vaginal gynecologic operations," *Geburtshilfe und Frauenheilkunde* 46 (July 1986): 459–61. (Published in German)

48. E. Harms, U. Christmann, and F. K. Klock, "Suprapubic urinary diversion following gynecologic operations," *Geburtshilfe und Frauenheilkunde* 45 (April 1985): 254–60. (Published in German)

49. A 1987 pamphlet, "Understanding Hysterectomy," from the American College of Obstetricians and Gynecologists, quoted in "Sexual Response After Hysterectomy," *HealthFacts* (New York: Center for Medical Consumers, 1990), Vol. XV, No. 139., p. 1.

50. J. Dietl and K. Semm, "Conization and hysterectomy from the viewpoint of the surgically treated woman," *Geburtshilfe und Frauenheilkunde* 43 (September 1983): 562–66. (Published in German)

51. G. Seidenschnur et al., "Attitude and sex behavior following hysterectomy," *Zentralblatt für Gynakologie* 111 (Number 1, 1989): 53–59. (Published in German)

52. "The effects of 554 nonradical vaginal and abdominal hysterectomies on micturition symptoms and urinary incontinence," *ACTA Obstetricia et Gynecologica Scandinavica* 67 (Number 2, 1988): 141–46.

53. P. Kilkku, "Supravaginal uterine amputation versus hysterectomy with reference to subjective bladder symptoms and incontinence," *ACTA Obstetricia et Gynecologica Scandinavica* 64 (Number 5, 1985): 375–79.

54. R. C. Dicker et al., "Complications of abdominal and vaginal hysterectomy among women of reproductive age in the United States. The Collaborative Review of Sterilization," *American Journal of Obstetrics and Gynecology* 144 (1 December 1982): 841–48.

55. S. K. Samra, B. A. Friedman, and P. J. Beitler, "A study of blood utilization in association with hysterectomy," *Transfusion* 23 (November–December 1983): 490–95.

56. G. W. Morley and J. O. DeLancey, "Sacrospinous ligament fixation for eversion of the vagina," *American Journal of Obstetrics and Gynecology* 158 (April 1988): 872–81.

57. S. H. Cruikshank, "Preventing posthysterectomy vaginal vault prolapse and enterocele during vaginal hysterectomy," *American Journal of Obstetrics and Gynecology* 156 (June 1987): 1433–40.

58. C. F. Langmade and J. A. Oliver, Jr., "Partial colpocleisis," *American Journal of Obstetrics and Gynecology* 154 (June 1986): 1200–1205.

59. G. H. Barker and D. W. Roberts, "Spontaneous extrusion of Hulka-Clemens spring-loaded clips after vaginal hysterectomy: Two case reports," *British Journal of Obstetrics and Gynaecology* 84 (December 1977): 954–55.

60. P. M. Wisniewski et al., "Early diagnosis of a diverticular colovaginal fistula with colposcopy. A case report," *Journal of Reproductive Medicine* 33 (August 1988): 705–8.

61. M. Lev-Gur et al., "Pararenal hematoma as a complication of vaginal hysterectomy. A case report," *Journal of Reproductive Medicine* 32 (January 1987): 68–71.

62. J. E. Oesterling, S. M. Goldman, and F. C. Lowe, "Intravesical herniation of small bowel after bladder perforation," *Journal of Urology* 138 (November 1987): 1236–38.

63. D. Dargent and R. C. Rudigoz, "Vaginal hysterectomy. Our experience between the years 1970 to 1979," *Journal de Gynecologie, Obstetrique et Biologie de la Reproduction (Paris)* 9 (Number 8, 1980): 895–908. (Published in French)

64. S. C. Voss, H. C. Sharp, and J. R. Scott, "Abdominoplasty combined with gynecologic surgical procedures," *Obstetrics and Gynecology* 67 (February 1986): 181–85.

65. G. Ralph et al., "Functional disorders of the lower urinary tract following radical abdominal and vaginal surgery of cervix cancer," *Geburtshilfe und Frauenheilkunde* 47 (August 1987): 551–54. (Published in German)

66. O. E. Jaschevatzky et al., "Prostaglandin F2 alpha for prevention of urinary retention after vaginal hysterectomy," *Obstetrics and Gynecology* 66 (August 1985): 244–47.

67. P. Riss, R. Spernol, and W. Gruber, "Intravesical prostaglandin E2 and placebo in urinary retention after gynaecological surgery," *Geburtshilfe und Frauenheilkunde* (March 1982): 182–84. (Published in German)

68. Kudo et al., "Vaginal hysterectomy without ligation of the ligaments of the cervix uteri," 299–305.

69. A. S. Tondare et al., "Femoral neuropathy: A complication of lithotomy position under spinal anaesthesia," *Ca-*

nadian Anaesthetists Society Journal 30 (January 1983): 84–86.

70. P. Draca, "Vaginal hysterectomy by means of morcellation," European Journal of Obstetrics, Gynecology, and Reproductive Biology 22 (August 1986): 237–42.

71. "Tumour of the ovary after hysterectomy," Geburtshilfe und Frauenheilkunde 40 (December 1980): 1087–92. (Published in German)

72. W. Heidenreich and B. Mlasowsky, "Spontaneous splenic rupture as a cause of postoperative hemorrhage," Geburtshilfe und Frauenheilkunde 46 (December 1986): 910–11. (Published in German)

73. P. Cole and J. Berlin, "Elective hysterectomy," American Journal of Obstetrics and Gynecology 129 (15 September 1977): 117–23.

74. S. N. Hajj, "A simplified surgical technique for the treatment of the vault in vaginal hysterectomy," American Journal of Obstetrics and Gynecology 133 (15 April 1979): 851–54.

75. A. Yilmazturk et al., "Complete closure or open healing of the skin of the vaginal stump in vaginal hysterectomy," Zentralblatt fur Gynakologie 112 (Number 13, 1990): 827–33. (Published in German)

76. B. McNulty and W. S. Roberts, "Elective cesarean hysterectomy versus vaginal hysterectomy for the treatment of cervical intraepithelial neoplasia," Southern Medical Journal 80 (August 1987): 984–86.

Vascular Shunt and Bypass

1. J. S. Dorsey and J. A. Cogordan, "Pleuroperitoneal shunt for intractable pleural effusion," Canadian Journal of Surgery 27 (November 1984): 598–99.

2. J. K. Kim, R. Maynulet, and A. Goldfarb, "Use of Denver shunt in recurrent hepatic hydrothorax," Postgraduate Medicine 71 (May 1982): 236–37, 240–41.

3. R. S. Foster et al., "Use of a caval-atrial shunt for resection of a caval tumor thrombus in renal cell carcinoma," Journal of Urology 140 (December 1988): 1370–71.

4. T. Tsubokawa, S. Nakamura, and K. Satoh, "Effect of temporary subdural-peritoneal shunt on subdural effusion with subarachnoid effusion," Childs Brain 11 (Number 1, 1984): 47–59.

5. D. A. Bettenay et al., "The anaesthetic and perioperative management of the patient undergoing insertion of a peritoneovenous shunt," Anaesthesia and Intensive Care 10 (May 1982): 108–12.

6. J. H. Raaf and J. R. Stroehlein, "Palliation of malignant ascites by the LeVeen peritoneo-venous shunt," Cancer 45 (1 March 1980): 1019–24.

7. H. Van Damme, W. Vaneerdeweg, and E. Schoofs, "The Denver shunt in malignant ascites," ACTA Chirurgica Belgica 85 (January–February 1985): 43–52. (Published in Dutch)

8. C. Smadja and D. Franco, "The LeVeen shunt in the elective treatment of intractable ascites in cirrhosis. A prospective study on 140 patients," Annals of Surgery 201 (April 1985): 488–93.

9. H. H. LeVeen, "The LeVeen shunt," Annual Review of Medicine 36 (1985): 453–69.

10. H. E. Nervino and F. C. Gebhardt, "Peritoneovenous shunt for intractable malignant ascites. A single case report of metastatic peritoneal mesothelioma implanted via LeVeen shunt," Cancer 54 (15 November 1984): 2231–33.

11. R. C. Prokesch and D. Rimland, "Infectious complications of the peritoneovenous shunt," American Journal of Gastroenterology 78 (April 1983): 235–40.

12. A. E. Hirst and F. C. Saunders, "Fatal air embolism following perforation of the cecum in a patient with peritoneovenous shunt for ascites," American Journal of Gastroenterology 76 (November 1981): 453–55.

13. W. K. Jacobsen et al., "Air embolism in association with LeVeen shunt," Critical Care Medicine 8 (November 1980): 659–60.

14. L. F. Fenster, R. F. Wheelis, and J. A. Ryan, Jr., "Acute respiratory distress syndrome after peritoneovenous shunt," American Review of Respiratory Diseases 125 (February 1982): 244–45.

15. P. E. Donahue, D. Spigos, and S. C. Kukreja, "Malposition of venous end of LeVeen shunt: A preventable complication," American Surgeon 47 (June 1981): 259–61.

16. R. Downing, J. Black, and C. W. Windsor, "Palliation of malignant ascites by the Denver peritoneovenous shunt," Annals of the Royal College of Surgeons of England 66 (September 1984): 340–43.

17. H. H. LeVeen et al., "Peritoneovenous shunt occlusion. Etiology, diagnosis, therapy," Annals of Surgery 200 (August 1984): 212–23.

18. M. O'Connor, J. I. Allen, and M. L. Schwartz, "Peritoneovenous shunt therapy for leaking ascites in the cirrhotic patient," Annals of Surgery 200 (July 1984): 66–69.

19. M. V. Ragni, J. H. Lewis, and J. A. Spero, "Ascites-

induced LeVeen shunt coagulopathy," *Annals of Surgery* 198 (July 1983): 91–95.

20. J. R. Darsee et al., "Hemodynamics of LeVeen shunt pulmonary edema," *Annals of Surgery* 194 (August 1981): 189–92.

21. J. E. Rosenman, D. C. Allison, and D. E. Smith, "Colonic perforation as a complication of peritoneovenous shunt: A case report," *Surgery* 95 (May 1984): 619–21.

22. A. W. Silberman, "The 'bedside' peritoneovenous shunt," *Surgery* 91 (June 1982): 669–70.

Wound Debridement and Excision

1. B. Haury et al., "Debridement: An essential component of traumatic wound care," *American Journal of Surgery* 135 (February 1978): 238–42.

2. M. L. Hamer et al., "Quantitative bacterial analysis of comparative wound irrigations," *Annals of Surgery* 181 (June 1975): 819–22.

3. A. Trelstad and D. Osmundson, "Water Piks: Wound cleansing alternative," *Plastic Surgical Nursing* 9 (Fall 1989): 117–19.

4. H. R. Mancusi-Ungaro, Jr., and N. H. Rappaport, "Preventing wound infections," *American Family Physician* 33 (April 1986): 147–53.

5. L. S. Nichter and J. Williams, "Ultrasonic wound debridement," *Journal of Hand Surgery, American Volume* 13 (January 1988): 142–46.

6. W. H. Hartl and H. L. Klammer, "Gunshot and blast injuries to the extremities. Management of soft tissue wounds by a modified technique of delayed wound closure," *ACTA Chirurgica Scandinavica* 154 (September 1988): 495–99.

7. H. M. Tian et al., "Quantitative bacteriological study of the wound track," *Journal of Trauma* 28 (January 1988, Supplement): S215–S216.

8. S. J. Mathes, L. J. Feng, and T. K. Hunt, "Coverage of the infected wound," *Annals of Surgery* 198 (October 1983): 420–29.

9. W. Terranova and F. A. Crawford, Jr., "Treatment of median sternotomy wound infection and sternal necrosis in an infant," *Annals of Thoracic Surgery* 48 (July 1989): 122–23.

10. J. A. Majure et al., "Reconstruction of the infected median sternotomy wound," *Annals of Thoracic Surgery* 42 (July 1986): 9–12.

11. J. Mahoney, "Treatment of the chronically infected median sternotomy wound with muscle flaps," *Canadian Journal of Surgery* 28 (September 1985): 453–55.

12. J. B. Eckman, Jr., et al., "Wound and serum levels of tobramycin with the prophylactic use of tobramycin-impregnated polymethylmethacrylate beads in compound fractures," *Clinical Orthopaedics and Related Research* (December 1988): 213–15.

13. M. J. Spebar and R. B. Lindberg, "Fungal infection of the burn wound," *American Journal of Surgery* 138 (December 1979): 879–82.

14. J. H. Kendrick et al., "The complicated septic abdominal wound," *Archives of Surgery* 117 (April 1982): 464–68.

15. S. J. Mathes, L. J. Feng, and T. K. Hunt, "Coverage of the infected wound," *Annals of Surgery* 198 (October 1983): 420–29.

16. E. Levy et al., "Septic necrosis of the midline wound in postoperative peritonitis. Successful management by debridement, myocutaneous advancement, and primary skin closure," *Annals of Surgery* 207 (April 1988): 470–79.

17. J. P. Anthony and S. J. Mathes, "The recalcitrant perineal wound after rectal extirpation. Applications of muscle flap closure," *Archives of Surgery* 125 (October 1990): 1371–76.

18. L. G. Prevosti et al., "A comparison of the open and closed methods in the initial treatment of sternal wound infections," *Journal of Cardiovascular Surgery (Torino)* 30 (September–October 1989): 757–63.

19. D. H. Parks, H. A. Linares, and P. D. Thomson, "Surgical management of burn wound sepsis," *Surgery, Gynecology, and Obstetrics* 153 (September 1981): 374–76.

20. R. J. Leicester et al., "Sexual function and perineal wound healing after intersphincteric excision of the rectum for inflammatory bowel disease," *Diseases of the Colon and Rectum* 27 (April 1984): 244–48.

21. R. McLeod et al., "Primary perineal wound closure following excision of the rectum," *Canadian Journal of Surgery* 26 (March 1983): 122–24.

22. T. T. Irvin and J. C. Goligher, "A controlled clinical trial of three different methods of perineal wound management following excision of the rectum," *British Journal of Surgery* 62 (April 1975): 287–91.

23. O. Terranova et al., "Management of the perineal wound after rectal excision for neoplastic disease: A controlled clinical trial," *Diseases of the Colon and Rectum* 22 (May–June 1979): 228–33.

24. J. R. Oakley et al., "Management of the perineal wound

after rectal excision for ulcerative colitis," *Diseases of the Colon and Rectum* 28 (December 1985): 885–88.

25. J. D'Auria, S. Lipson, and J. M. Garfield, "Fatal iodine toxicity following surgical debridement of a hip wound," *Journal of Trauma* 30 (March 1990): 353–55.

26. W. B. Riley, Jr., "Wound healing," *American Family Physician* 24 (November 1981): 107–13.

27. B. G. MacMillan, "Closing the burn wound," *Surgical Clinics of North America* 58 (December 1978): 1205–31.

28. Z. G. Wang et al., "Early pathomorphologic characteristics of the wound track caused by fragments," *Journal of Trauma* 28 (January 1988, Supplement): S89–S95.

29. R. G. Brunner and W. F. Fallon, Jr., "A prospective, randomized clinical trial of wound debridement versus conservative wound care in soft-tissue injury from civilian gunshot wounds," *American Surgeon* 56 (February 1990): 104–7.

30. M. L. Fackler et al., "Open wound drainage versus wound excision in treating the modern assault rifle wound," *Surgery* 105 (May 1989): 576–84.

31. J. M. Ryan et al., "Field surgery on a future conventional battlefield: Strategy and wound management," *Annals of the Royal College of Surgeons of England* 73 (January 1991): 13–20.

32. R. M. Coupland, "Technical aspects of war wound excision," *British Journal of Surgery* 76 (July 1989): 663–67.

33. K. Hell, "Characteristics of the ideal antibiotic for prevention of wound sepsis among military forces in the field," *Reviews of Infectious Diseases* 13 (January–February 1991, Supplement): S164–S169.

34. M. K. Reames, C. Christensen, and E. A. Luce, "The use of maggots in wound debridement," *Annals of Plastic Surgery* 21 (October 1988): 388–91.

35. M. H. Desai et al., "Early burn wound excision significantly reduces blood loss," *Annals of Surgery* 211 (June 1990): 753–59.

36. P. J. Carley and S. F. Wainapel, "Electrotherapy for acceleration of wound healing: Low intensity direct current," *Archives of Physical Medicine and Rehabilitation* 66 (July 1985): 443–46.

37. B. A. Levine, K. R. Sirinek, and B. A. Pruitt, Jr., "Wound excision to fascia in burn patients," *Archives of Surgery* 113 (April 1978): 403–7.

38. W. F. McManus, A. D. Mason, Jr., and B. A. Pruitt, Jr., "Excision of the burn wound in patients with large burns," *Archives of Surgery* 124 (June 1989): 718–20.

39. S. E. Efem, "Clinical observations on the wound healing properties of honey," *British Journal of Surgery* 75 (July 1988): 679–81.

Index

controversies surrounding operations, 21
information available on, xiii–xiv
interviewing with, 9, 25
partnership between patients and, xv, 3
questions to ask, 9–10
reputations of, 7–8
resources available on, 10
selection of, 5–10, 24–25
specialists and, xiii, 11–13
surgical training of, 6, 25
where to get names of, 8
surgery and surgeries:
alternatives to, 39
appropriateness of, 39
assessing chances of surviving, 37
checklist, 24–27
complications associated with, 9
conditions treated by, 36
controversial issues associated with, 35, 39–40
definition of, xiii
descriptions and discussions of, 35–36
determining most frequently performed, 31–32
fear of, xiii–xiv, 24
Good Operations—Bad Operations Quick Rating Guide for, 35
how they are performed, 36
inpatient, 14–15, 22–23, 31
long-term side effects of, 21
looking them up, 35–40
mortality statistics on, 20–21, 35–38
nosocomial infection rates associated with, 9
in past, xiii–xiv
prevalence of, xiii, 19, 23
recovery time after, 32
risks of, 16–18
settings for, 14–18, 22–23
sources for information on, 33–35
success rates of, 9–10
therapy after, 32
time needed for, 32
unnecessary, 19–23
where they are performed, 36
who they are performed by, 36
surgery centers, 14–16, 23
surgical residencies, 5–6
sutures and suturing:
and appendectomies, 111
and arterial catheterizations, 43, 45
and cataract surgery, 123–24
and hemorrhoidectomies, 153

and local destruction of ovarian lesions, 174
and open reduction and internal fixation of fractures of femurs, 186
and partial small bowel resections, 191, 193
and peritoneal adhesiolysis, 198
and placement of central venous catheters, 200
and removals of tubes and ectopic pregnancies, 203
and repairs of cystoceles or rectoceles, 207
and repairs of incisional hernias, 155–156
and repairs of inguinal hernias, 230, 232–34
and repairs of vessels, 213
and revisions of vascular procedures, 215
and rotator cuff repairs, 219
and septoplasties, 221
and shoulder arthroplasties, 224–25
and sigmoidectomies, 227
of skin, 229–30
and toe amputations, 237
and total abdominal hysterectomies, 244
and unilateral external simple mastectomies, 272
and wound debridement and excision, 298
Swan-Ganz catheters, 43–46, 201
systemic problems, 101–2
systemic therapy, 46

tamoxifen, 274
teaching hospitals, 14–15
telangiectasias, 176
temporary pacemaker system insertions, 234–36
tendons:
cruciate ligament repairs and, 136–37
rotator cuff repairs and, 218–20
shoulder arthroplasties and, 224–25
total knee replacements and, 258–59
vaginal hysterectomies and, 289
terminal ileum, 165
testicles, 63–64, 158, 231
Theirry forceps, 181
thighs, 138–40, 270
thoracic aorta, 100–101
thoracic surgeons, 12–13
thoracotomies, 69, 79
throat, 12, 238–39, 241

thromboembolectomies, 103
thromboembolisms, 53, 132, 190, 247, 255, 260
thrombosed hemorrhoids, 154
thrombosis, 54
arterial catheterizations and, 45
and closed fracture reductions of tibiae and fibulae, 132
and combined right and left cardiac catheterizations, 53
and contrast phlebograms of legs, 60
dialysis arteriovenostomies and, 140
hemorrhoidectomies and, 153
joint replacement revisions and, 163
and ligation and stripping of varicose veins of legs, 169
and open reduction and internal fixation of fractures of tibiae and fibulae, 190
temporary pacemaker system insertions and, 235
total hip replacements and, 254–55
through-the-knee amputations, 104
thyroid gland, 12, 278–79
thyroid storms, 278
tibiae:
closed fracture reductions of, 132–33
cruciate ligament repairs and, 135–36
open reduction and internal fixation of fractures of, 189–91
single-component replacements and, 261–62
total knee replacements and, 258–59
toe amputations, 236–38
tongue cancer, 45
tonsillectomies, xiii, 14, 21, 238–41
total abdominal hysterectomies, xiii, 14, 243–47, 265, 280, 288–94
cone biopsies and, 48
as elective, 32
ovary removal in, 118
prophylactic, 21
and unilateral salpingo-oophorectomies or salpingo-ovariectomies, 277
unnecessary, 20–21
uterine lesion destruction and, 283–84
vaginal hysterectomies vs., 294
total cholecystectomies, 14, 39, 248–52
total hip replacements, 252–57
total knee replacements, 257–62
total mastectomies, 272–73, 275
total parenteral nutrition (TPN), 192–93
toxemia, 112
toxic megacolon, 71, 228
toxic shock syndrome, 222, 233